Jekel's Epidemiology, Biostatistics, Preventive Medicine, and Public Health

Jekel's Epidemiology, Biostatistics, Preventive Medicine, and Public Health

Fourth Edition

David L. Katz, MD, MPH, FACPM, FACP

Director, Prevention Research Center
Yale University School of Medicine
Director, Integrative Medicine Center
Griffin Hospital
Derby, Connecticut

Joann G. Elmore, MD, MPH

Professor of Medicine, Department of Internal Medicine
University of Washington School of Medicine
Attending Physician
Harborview Medical Center
Adjunct Professor of Epidemiology, School of Public Health
Seattle, Washington

Dorothea M.G. Wild, MD, MPH

Lecturer, School of Epidemiology
Yale University School of Medicine
New Haven, Connecticut
President, Griffin Faculty Practice Plan
Associate Program Director, Combined Internal Medicine/Preventive
*   Medicine Residency Program, Griffin Hospital*
Derby, Connecticut

Sean C. Lucan, MD, MPH, MS

Assistant Professor, Family and Social Medicine
Albert Einstein College of Medicine
Attending Physician, Family and Social Medicine
Montefiore Medical Center
Bronx, New York

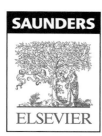

SAUNDERS

ELSEVIER

SAUNDERS

1600 John F. Kennedy Blvd.
Ste 1800
Philadelphia, PA 19103-2899

JEKEL'S EPIDEMIOLOGY, BIOSTATISTICS, PREVENTIVE MEDICINE
AND PUBLIC HEALTH

ISBN: 978-1-4557-0658-7

Notices

Knowledge and best practice in this field are constantly changing. As new research and experience broaden
our understanding, changes in research methods, professional practices, or medical treatment may become
necessary.

Practitioners and researchers must always rely on their own experience and knowledge in evaluating
and using any information, methods, compounds, or experiments described herein. In using such
information or methods they should be mindful of their own safety and the safety of others, including
parties for whom they have a professional responsibility.

With respect to any drug or pharmaceutical products identified, readers are advised to check the most
current information provided (i) on procedures featured or (ii) by the manufacturer of each product to be
administered, to verify the recommended dose or formula, the method and duration of administration,
and contraindications. It is the responsibility of practitioners, relying on their own experience and
knowledge of their patients, to make diagnoses, to determine dosages and the best treatment for each
individual patient, and to take all appropriate safety precautions.

To the fullest extent of the law, neither the Publisher nor the authors, contributors, or editors, assume
any liability for any injury and/or damage to persons or property as a matter of products liability,
negligence or otherwise, or from any use or operation of any methods, products, instructions, or ideas
contained in the material herein.

International Standard Book Number
978-1-4557-0658-7

Senior Content Strategist: James Merritt
Content Development Managers: Barbara Cicalese, Marybeth Thiel
Publishing Services Manager: Patricia Tannian
Senior Project Manager: Sarah Wunderly
Design Direction: Louis Forgione

Working together to grow
libraries in developing countries

www.elsevier.com | www.bookaid.org | www.sabre.org

ELSEVIER   BOOK AID International   Sabre Foundation

Printed in the United States of America

Last digit is the print number: 9 8 7 6 5 4 3 2

About the Authors

David L. Katz, MD, MPH, FACPM, FACP, is the founding director of Yale University's Prevention Research Center. He is a two-time diplomate of the American Board of Internal Medicine and a board-certified specialist in Preventive Medicine/Public Health. Dr. Katz is known internationally for expertise in nutrition, weight management, and chronic disease prevention. He has published roughly 150 scientific articles, innumerable blogs and columns, nearly 1,000 newspaper articles, and 14 books to date. He is the Editor-in-Chief of the journal *Childhood Obesity*, President-Elect of the American College of Lifestyle Medicine, and founder and President of the non-profit Turn the Tide Foundation. Dr. Katz is the principal inventor of the Overall Nutritional Quality Index (patents pending) that is used in the NuVal® nutrition guidance program (www.nuval.com). He has been recognized three times by the Consumers Research Council of America as one of the nation's top physicians in preventive medicine and was nominated for the position of United States Surgeon General to the Obama Administration by the American College of Physicians, the American College of Preventive Medicine, and the Center for Science in the Public Interest, among others. www.davidkatzmd.com

Joann G. Elmore, MD, MPH, is Professor of Medicine at the University of Washington (UW) School of Medicine and Adjunct Professor of Epidemiology at the UW School of Public Health, Seattle, Washington. Dr. Elmore's clinical and scientific interests include variability in cancer screening, diagnostic testing, and the evaluation of new technologies. She is an expert on breast cancer–related issues, including variability in mammographic interpretation. She was Associate Director of the Robert Wood Johnson Clinical Scholars program at Yale and the University of Washington and recipient of the Robert Wood Johnson Generalist Faculty Award. For the past two decades, her research has been continuously well funded by the National Institutes of Health (NIH) and non-profit foundations, and she has to her credit more than 150 peer-reviewed publications in such journals as the *New England Journal of Medicine* and the *Journal of the American Medical Association.* Dr. Elmore has served on national advisory committees for the Institute of Medicine, NIH, American Cancer Society, Foundation for Informed Medical Decision Making, and the Robert Wood Johnson Foundation.

Dorothea M.G. Wild, MD, MPH, Dr.med., is a Research Affiliate in Public Health at the Yale University Schools of Medicine and Public Health and Associate Program Director of the combined Internal Medicine/Preventive Medicine residency program at Griffin Hospital. Dr. Wild is President of the Griffin Faculty Practice Plan at Griffin Hospital, where she also works as a hospitalist. She has a special interest in health policy, patient-centered care, cost-effectiveness analysis in medicine, and in development of systems to reduce medical errors.

Sean C. Lucan, MD, MPH, MS, is a practicing family physician in the Bronx and a former Robert Wood Johnson Clinical Scholar. His research focuses on how different aspects of urban food environments may influence what people eat, and what the implications are for obesity and chronic diseases, particularly in low-income and minority communities. Dr. Lucan has published over 30 papers in peer-reviewed journals, given at least as many presentations at national and international scientific meetings, delivered invited talks around the United States on his research, and been honored with national awards for his scholarship. Notably, Dr. Lucan is a three-time recipient of NIH support for his work on health disparities. He belongs to several professional societies and reviews for a number of journals that address health promotion, public health, family medicine, and nutrition.

Guest Authors

Meredith A. Barrett, PhD
Robert Wood Johnson Foundation Health & Society
    Scholar
Center for Health & Community at the University of
    California, San Francisco
School of Public Health at the University of California,
    Berkeley
San Francisco, California

Hannah Blencowe, MBChB, MRCPCH, Msc
London School of Tropical Medicine
London, England

Joshua S. Camins, BA, BS
Graduate Student, Department of Psychology
Towson University
Towson, Maryland

Linda Degutis, DrPH, MSN, FRSPH (Hon.)
Director, National Center for Injury Prevention and
    Control
Centers for Disease Control and Prevention
Atlanta, Georgia

Eugene M. Dunne, MA
Department of Psychology
Towson University
Towson, Maryland

Elizabeth C. Katz, PhD
Director, MA Program in Clinical Psychology
Assistant Professor, Department of Psychology
Towson University
Towson, Maryland

Joy E. Lawn, MB, BS, MRCP (Paeds), MPH, PhD
Director, Global Evidence and Policy
Saving Newborn Lives
Save the Children
Cape Town, South Africa

Samantha Lookatch, MA
Clinical Psychology
University of Tennessee
Knoxville, Tennessee

Elizabeth M. McClure, PhD-c
Epidemiologist, Department of Epidemiology
University of North Carolina
Chapel Hill, North Carolina

Thiruvengadam Muniraj, MD, PhD, MRCP(UK)
Clinical Instructor of Medicine
Yale University
New Haven, Connecticut
Hospitalist, Medicine
Griffin Hospital
Derby, Connecticut

Steven A. Osofsky, DVM
Director, Wildlife Health Policy
Wildlife Conservation Society
Bronx, New York

Mark Russi, MD, MPH
Professor of Medicine and Public Health
Yale University
Director, Occupational Health
Yale-New Haven Hospital
New Haven, Connecticut

Patricia E. Wetherill, MD
Clinical Assistant Professor of Medicine
New York Medical College
Valhalla, New York
Attending, Department of Medicine
Norwalk Hospital
Norwalk, Connecticut
Former Senior Consultant, Division of Infectious Diseases
National University Health System, Singapore

Acknowledgments

My co-authors and I are enormously grateful to Jim Jekel, both for initiating this journey with the first edition of the text and for entrusting the current edition to us. We are thankful to our senior editor at Elsevier, Jim Merritt, for able and experienced guidance throughout the process and crucial insights at crucial moments. We are most grateful to our production editor, Barbara Cicalese, in whose capable hands a great deal of material was turned into a book. Personally, I acknowledge and thank my wife, Catherine, and my children for graciously accommodating the many hours of undisturbed solitude that book writing requires, and for waiting with eager expectation for the day the job is done and we get to rediscover the exotic concept of a weekend together! —DLK

I acknowledge the important influence students have had in shaping our text and the meticulous and valuable editorial assistance that Raymond Harris, PhD, provided on the epidemiology chapters for this fourth edition. I personally thank my son, Nicholas R. Ransom, for his support and patience during the preparation of each new edition of this text. —JE

I gratefully acknowledge the helpful reviews and thoughtful comments from Drs. Earl Baker, Doug Shenson, Majid Sadigh, and Lionel Lim, and those of Patrick Charmel, Todd Liu, and Stephan and Gerlind Wild. —DW

I gratefully acknowledge several contributors who assisted with generating content for online supplemental material: Dr. Himabindu Ekanadham, Dr. Ruth A. Christoforetti, Alice Beckman, Dr. Manisha Sharma, Dr. Joel Bumol, Nandini Nair, Dr. Jessica Marrero, Luis Torrens, Ben Levy, and Jackie Rodriguez. I also gratefully acknowledge the chair of my department, Dr. Peter A. Selwyn, for encouraging me to take on this work, and my wife, Danielle, and my son, Max, for putting up with me when I did. —SL

Preface

We are very pleased and proud to bring you this fourth edition of what proved to be in earlier editions a best-selling title in its content area of epidemiology, biostatistics, and preventive medicine. We are, as well, a bit nervous about our efforts to honor that pedigree because this is the first edition not directly overseen by Dr. James Jekel, who set this whole enterprise in motion almost 20 years ago. We hasten to note that Dr. Jekel is perfectly well and was available to help us out as the need occasionally arose. But after some years of a declared retirement that looked like more than a full-time job for any reasonable person, Jim has finally applied his legendary good sense to himself and is spending well-earned time in true retirement with his large extended family. A mentor to several of us, Jim remains an important presence in this edition, both by virtue of the content that is preserved from earlier editions, and by virtue of the education he provided us. When the book is at its best, we gratefully acknowledge Dr. Jekel's influence. If ever the new edition falls short of that standard, we blame ourselves. We have done our best, but the bar was set high!

To maximize our chances of clearing the bar, we have done the prudent thing and brought in reinforcements. Most notable among them is Dr. Sean Lucan, who joined us as the fourth member of the main author team. Sean brought to the project an excellent fund of knowledge, honed in particular by the Robert Wood Johnson Clinical Scholars program at the University of Pennsylvania, as well as a keen editorial eye and a sharp wit. The book is certainly the better for his involvement, and we are thankful he joined us.

Also of note are five new chapters we did not feel qualified to write, and for which we relied on guest authors who most certainly were. Their particular contributions are noted in the contents list and on the title page of the chapters in question. We are grateful to this group of experts for bringing to our readers authoritative treatment of important topics we could not have addressed half so well on our own.

Readers of prior editions, and we thank you for that brand loyalty, will note a substantial expansion from 21 chapters to 30. This was partly the result of unbundling the treatment of preventive medicine and public health into separate sections, which the depth and breadth of content seemed to require. These domains overlap substantially, but are distinct and are now handled accordingly in the book. The expansion also allowed the inclusion of important topics that were formerly neglected: from the epidemiology of mental health disorders, to disaster planning, to health care reform, to the One Health concept that highlights the indelible links among the health of people, other species, and the planet itself.

Return readers will note that some content is simply preserved. We applied the "if it ain't broke, don't fix it!" principle to our efforts. Many citations and illustrations have stood the test of time and are as informative now as they ever were. We resisted the inclination to "update" such elements simply for the sake of saying we had done so. There was plenty of content that did require updating, and readers will also note a large infusion of new figures, tables, passages, definitions, illustrations, and citations. Our hopes in this regard will be validated if the book feels entirely fresh and current and clear to new and return readers alike, yet comfortably familiar to the latter group.

Any book is subject to constraints on length and scope, and ours is no exception. There were, therefore, predictable challenges regarding inclusions and exclusions, depth versus breadth. We winced at some of the harder trade-offs and did the best we could to strike the optimal balance.

Such, then, are the intentions, motivations, and aspirations that shaped this new edition of *Epidemiology, Biostatistics, Preventive Medicine, and Public Health*. They are all now part of a process consigned to our personal histories, and the product must be judged on its merits. The verdict, of course, resides with you.

David L. Katz
for the authors

Preface to the Third Edition

As the authors of the second edition of this textbook, we were pleased to be asked to write the third edition. The second edition has continued to be used for both courses and preventive medicine board review. Writing a revision every five years forces the authors to consider what the major developments have been since the last edition that need to be incorporated or emphasized. In the past five years, in addition to incremental developments in all health fields, some issues have become more urgent.

In the area of **medical care organization** and **financing**, after a period of relatively modest inflationary pressures following the introduction of the prospective payment system, we are now approaching a new crisis in the payment for medical care. In an attempt to remain globally competitive, employers either are not providing any medical insurance at all or are shifting an increasing proportion of the costs directly to the employees, many of whom cannot afford it. The costs are thus passed on to the providers, especially hospitals. In addition, the pressure for hospitals to demonstrate quality of care and avoid medical errors has become more intense.

Second, there have been major changes in **infectious diseases** since the last edition. Bovine spongiform encephalopathy has come to North America, and the world has experienced an epidemic of a new disease, severe acute respiratory syndrome (SARS). Even more significant, as this is being written the world is deeply concerned about the possibility of a true pandemic of the severe avian form of H5N1 influenza.

It has also become clear since the second edition that the United States and, to a lesser extent, much of the world are entering a time of **epidemic overweight** and **obesity**. This has already increased the incidence of many chronic diseases such as type II diabetes in adults and even in children.

In the past five years, questions about **screening for disease** have become more acute, because of both financial concerns and a better understanding of the use and limitations of screening in the prevention of symptomatic disease. The screening methods that have been subjected to the most study and debate have been mammography for breast cancer and determination of prostate-specific antigen and other techniques for prostate cancer.

Thus, major changes have occurred in the fields of health care policy and financing, infectious disease, chronic disease, and disease prevention technology. In this edition, we have sought to provide up-to-date guidance for these issues especially, and for preventive medicine generally. We wish to give special thanks to our developmental editor, Nicole DiCicco, for her helpful guidance throughout this process.

For this edition, we are pleased that Dr. Dorothea M.G. Wild, a specialist in health policy and management with a special interest in medical care quality, has joined us as a coauthor.

James F. Jekel
David L. Katz
Joann G. Elmore
Dorothea M.G. Wild

Contents

Epidemiology

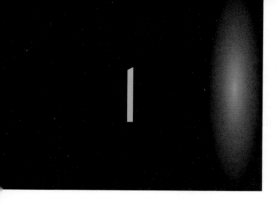

Basic Epidemiologic Concepts and Principles

I. WHAT IS EPIDEMIOLOGY?

Epidemiology is usually defined as the study of factors that determine the occurrence and distribution of disease in a population. As a scientific term, epidemiology was introduced in the 19th century, derived from three Greek roots: *epi,* meaning "upon"; *demos,* "people" or "population"; and *logos,* "discussion" or "study." Epidemiology deals with much more than the study of **epidemics,** in which a disease spreads quickly or extensively, leading to more cases than normally seen.

Epidemiology can best be understood as the basic science of public health. It provides methods to study disease, injury, and clinical practice. Whereas health care practitioners collect data on a single patient, **epidemiologists** collect data on an entire population. The scientific methods used to collect such data are described in the Epidemiology section of this text, Chapters 1 to 7, and the methods used to analyze the data are reviewed in the Biostatistics section, Chapters 8 to 13.

The scientific study of disease can be approached at the following four levels:

1. Submolecular or molecular level (e.g., cell biology, genetics, biochemistry, and immunology)
2. Tissue or organ level (e.g., anatomic pathology)
3. Level of individual patients (e.g., clinical medicine)
4. Level of populations (e.g., epidemiology).

Perspectives gained from these four levels are related, so the scientific understanding of disease can be maximized by coordinating research among the various disciplines.

Some people distinguish between classical epidemiology and clinical epidemiology. **Classical epidemiology,** which is population oriented, studies the community origins of health problems, particularly those related to infectious agents; nutrition; the environment; human behavior; and the psychological, social, economic, and spiritual state of a population. Classical epidemiologists are interested in discovering risk factors that might be altered in a population to prevent or delay disease, injury, and death.

Investigators involved in **clinical epidemiology** often use research designs and statistical tools similar to those used by classical epidemiologists. However, clinical epidemiologists study patients in health care settings rather than in the community at large. Their goal is to improve the prevention, early detection, diagnosis, treatment, prognosis, and care of illness in individual patients who are at risk for, or already affected by, specific diseases.[1]

Many illustrations from classical epidemiology concern infectious diseases, because these were the original impetus for the development of epidemiology and have often been its focus. Nevertheless, classical methods of surveillance and outbreak investigation remain relevant even for such contemporary concerns as **bioterrorism,** undergoing modification as they are marshaled against new challenges. One example of such an adapted approach is **syndromic epidemiology,** in which epidemiologists look for patterns of signs and symptoms that might indicate an origin in bioterrorism.

Epidemiology can also be divided into **infectious disease epidemiology** and **chronic disease epidemiology.** Historically, infectious disease epidemiology has depended more heavily on laboratory support (especially microbiology and serology), whereas chronic disease epidemiology has depended on complex sampling and statistical methods. However, this distinction is becoming less significant with the increasing use of molecular laboratory markers (genetic and other) in chronic disease epidemiology and complex statistical analyses in infectious disease epidemiology. Many illnesses, including tuberculosis and acquired immunodeficiency syndrome (AIDS), may be regarded as both infectious and chronic.

The name of a given medical discipline indicates both a method of research into health and disease and the body of knowledge acquired by using that method. *Pathology* is a field of medical research with its own goals and methods, but investigators and clinicians also speak of the "pathology of lung cancer." Similarly, *epidemiology* refers to a field of research that uses particular methods, but it can also be used to denote the resulting body of knowledge about the distribution and natural history of diseases—that is, the nutritional, behavioral, environmental, and genetic sources of disease as identified through epidemiologic studies.

II. ETIOLOGY AND NATURAL HISTORY OF DISEASE

The term **etiology** is defined as the cause or origin of a disease or abnormal condition. The way a disease progresses in the absence of medical or public health intervention is often called the **natural history** of the disease. Public health and medical personnel take advantage of available knowledge about the stages, mechanisms, and causes of disease to determine how and when to intervene. The goal of intervention, whether preventive or therapeutic, is to alter the natural history of a disease in a favorable way.

A. Stages of Disease

The development and expression of a disease occur over time and can be divided into three stages: predisease, latent, and symptomatic. During the **predisease stage,** before the disease process begins, early intervention may avert exposure to the agent of disease (e.g., lead, *trans*-fatty acids, microbes), preventing the disease process from starting; this is called **primary prevention.** During the **latent stage,** when the disease process has already begun but is still asymptomatic, screening for the disease and providing appropriate treatment may prevent progression to symptomatic disease; this is called **secondary prevention.** During the **symptomatic stage,** when disease manifestations are evident, intervention may slow, arrest, or reverse the progression of disease; this is called **tertiary prevention.** These concepts are discussed in more detail in Chapters 15 to 17.

B. Mechanisms and Causes of Disease

When discussing the etiology of disease, epidemiologists distinguish between the **biologic mechanisms** and the **social, behavioral, and environmental causes** of disease. For example, *osteomalacia* is a bone disease that may have both social and biologic causes. Osteomalacia is a weakening of the bone, often through a deficiency of vitamin D. According to the custom of purdah, which is observed by many Muslims, women who have reached puberty avoid public observation by spending most of their time indoors, or by wearing clothing that covers virtually all of the body when they go outdoors. Because these practices block the action of the sun on bare skin, they prevent the irradiation of ergosterol in the skin. However, irradiated ergosterol is an important source of D vitamins, which are necessary for growth. If a woman's diet is also deficient in vitamin D during the rapid growth period of puberty, she may develop osteomalacia as a result of insufficient calcium absorption. Osteomalacia can adversely affect future pregnancies by causing the pelvis to become distorted (more pear shaped), making the pelvic opening too small for the fetus to pass through. In this example, the social, nutritional, and environmental *causes* set in motion the biochemical and other biologic *mechanisms* of osteomalacia, which may ultimately lead to maternal and infant mortality.

Likewise, excessive fat intake, smoking, and lack of exercise are behavioral factors that contribute to the biologic mechanisms of *atherogenesis,* such as elevated blood levels of low-density lipoprotein (LDL) cholesterol or reduced blood levels of high-density lipoprotein (HDL) cholesterol. These behavioral risk factors may have different effects, depending on the genetic pattern of each individual and the interaction of genes with the environment and other risk factors.

Epidemiologists attempt to go as far back as possible to discover the social and behavioral causes of disease, which offer clues to methods of prevention. Hypotheses introduced by epidemiologists frequently guide laboratory scientists as they seek biologic mechanisms of disease, which may suggest methods of treatment.

C. Host, Agent, Environment, and Vector

The causes of a disease are often considered in terms of a triad of factors: the host, the agent, and the environment. For many diseases, it is also useful to add a fourth factor, the vector (Fig. 1-1). In measles, the *host* is a human who is susceptible to measles infection, the *agent* is a highly infectious virus that can produce serious disease in humans, and the *environment* is a population of unvaccinated individuals, which enables unvaccinated susceptible individuals to be exposed to others who are infectious. The *vector* in this case is relatively unimportant. In malaria, however, the host, agent, and environment are all significant, but the vector, the *Anopheles* mosquito, assumes paramount importance in the spread of disease.

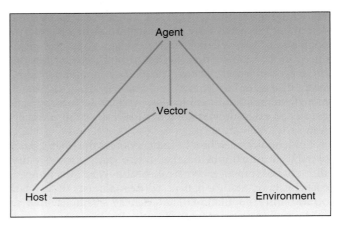

Figure I-I **Factors involved in natural history of disease.**

Host factors are responsible for the degree to which the individual is able to adapt to the stressors produced by the agent. Host resistance is influenced by a person's genotype (e.g., dark skin reduces sunburn), nutritional status and body mass index (e.g., obesity increases susceptibility to many diseases), immune system (e.g., compromised immunity reduces resistance to cancer as well as microbial disease), and social behavior (e.g., physical exercise enhances resistance to many diseases, including depression). Several factors can work synergistically, such as nutrition and immune status. Measles is seldom fatal in well-nourished children, even in the absence of measles immunization and modern medical care. By contrast, 25% of children with marasmus (starvation) or kwashiorkor (protein-calorie malnutrition related to weaning) may die from complications of measles.

Agents of disease or illness can be divided into several categories. **Biologic agents** include allergens, infectious organisms (e.g., bacteria, viruses), biologic toxins (e.g., botulinum toxin), and foods (e.g., high-fat diet). **Chemical agents** include chemical toxins (e.g., lead) and dusts, which can cause acute or chronic illness. **Physical agents** include kinetic energy (e.g., involving bullet wounds, blunt trauma, and crash injuries), radiation, heat, cold, and noise. Epidemiologists now are studying the extent to which **social and psychological stressors** can be considered agents in the development of health problems.

The **environment** influences the probability and circumstances of contact between the host and the agent. Poor restaurant sanitation increases the probability that patrons will be exposed to *Salmonella* infections. Poor roads and adverse weather conditions increase the number of automobile collisions and airplane crashes. The environment also includes social, political, and economic factors. Crowded homes and schools make exposure to infectious diseases more likely, and the political structure and economic health of a society influence the nutritional and vaccine status of its members.

Vectors of disease include insects (e.g., mosquitoes associated with spread of malaria), arachnids (e.g., ticks associated with Lyme disease), and mammals (e.g., raccoons associated with rabies in eastern U.S.). The concept of the *vector* can be applied more widely, however, to include human groups (e.g., vendors of heroin, cocaine, and methamphetamine) and even inanimate objects that serve as vehicles to transmit disease (e.g., contaminated needles associated with hepatitis and AIDS). A vector may be considered part of the environment, or it may be treated separately (see Fig. 1-1). To be an effective transmitter of disease, the vector must have a specific relationship to the agent, the environment, and the host.

In the case of human malaria, the vector is a mosquito of the genus *Anopheles*, the agent is a parasitic organism of the genus *Plasmodium*, the host is a human, and the environment includes standing water that enables the mosquito to breed and to come into contact with the host. Specifically, the plasmodium must complete part of its life cycle within the mosquito; the climate must be relatively warm and provide a wet environment in which the mosquito can breed; the mosquito must have the opportunity to bite humans (usually at night, in houses where sleeping people lack screens and mosquito nets) and thereby spread the disease; the host must be bitten by an infected mosquito; and the host must be susceptible to the disease.

D. Risk Factors and Preventable Causes

Risk factors for disease and preventable causes of disease, particularly life-threatening diseases such as cancer, have been the subject of much epidemiologic research. In 1964 a World Health Organization (WHO) expert committee estimated that the *majority* of cancer cases were potentially preventable and were caused by "extrinsic factors." Also that year, the U.S. Surgeon General released a report indicating that the risk of death from lung cancer in smokers was almost 11 times that in nonsmokers.[2]

Advances in knowledge have consolidated the WHO findings to the point where few, if any, researchers now question its main conclusion.[3] Indeed, some have gone further, substituting figures of 80% or even 90% as the proportion of potentially preventable cancers, in place of WHO's more cautious estimate of the "majority." Unfortunately, the phrase "extrinsic factors" (or its near-synonym, "environmental factors") has often been misinterpreted to mean only manmade chemicals, which was certainly not the intent of the WHO committee. In addition to man-made or naturally occurring carcinogens, the 1964 report included viral infections, nutritional deficiencies or excesses, reproductive activities, and a variety of other factors determined "wholly or partly by personal behavior."

The WHO conclusions are based on research using a variety of epidemiologic methods. Given the many different types of cancer cells, and the large number of causal factors to be considered, how do epidemiologists estimate the percentage of deaths caused by preventable risk factors in a country such as the United States?

One method looks at each type of cancer and determines (from epidemiologic studies) the percentage of individuals in the country who have identifiable, preventable causes of that cancer. These percentages are added up in a weighted manner to determine the total percentage of all cancers having identifiable causes.

A second method examines annual age-specific and gender-specific cancer incidence rates in countries that have the lowest rates of a given type of cancer and maintain an effective infrastructure for disease detection. For a particular cancer type, the low rate in such a country presumably results from a low prevalence of the risk factors for that cancer. Researchers calculate the number of cases of each type of cancer that would be expected to occur annually in each age and gender group in the United States, if the lowest observed rates had been true for the U.S. population. Next, they add up the expected numbers for the various cancer types in the U.S. They then compare the total number of expected cases with the total number of cases actually diagnosed in the U.S. population. Using these methods, epidemiologists have estimated that the U.S. has about five times as many total cancer cases as would be expected, based on the lowest rates in the world. Presumably, the excess cancer cases in the U.S. are caused by the prevalence of risk factors for cancer, such as smoking.

1. BEINGS Model

The acronym **BEINGS** can serve as a mnemonic device for the major categories of risk factors for disease, some of which are easier to change or eliminate than others (Box 1-1). Currently, genetic factors are among the most difficult

Box 1-1	BEINGS Acronym for Categories of Preventable Cause of Disease

Biologic factors and Behavioral factors
Environmental factors
Immunologic factors
Nutritional factors
Genetic factors
Services, Social factors, and Spiritual factors

to change, although this field is rapidly developing and becoming more important to epidemiology and prevention. Immunologic factors are usually the easiest to change, if effective vaccines are available.

"B"—BIOLOGIC AND BEHAVIORAL FACTORS

The risk for particular diseases may be influenced by gender, age, weight, bone density, and other biologic factors. In addition, human behavior is a central factor in health and disease. *Cigarette smoking* is an obvious example of a behavioral risk factor. It contributes to a variety of health problems, including myocardial infarction (MI); lung, esophageal, and nasopharyngeal cancer; and chronic obstructive pulmonary disease. Cigarettes seem to be responsible for about 50% of MI cases among smokers and about 90% of lung cancer cases. Because there is a much higher probability of MI than lung cancer, cigarettes actually cause more cases of MI than lung cancer.

Increasing attention has focused on the rapid increase in *overweight* and *obesity* in the U.S. population over the past two decades. The number of deaths per year that can be attributed to these factors is controversial. In 2004 the U.S. Centers for Disease Control and Prevention (CDC) estimated that 400,000 deaths annually were caused by obesity and its major risk factors, *inactivity* and an *unhealthy diet*.[4] In 2005, using newer survey data and controlling for more potential confounders, other CDC investigators estimated that the number of deaths attributable to obesity and its risk factors was only 112,000.[5] Regardless, increasing rates of obesity are found worldwide as part of a cultural transition related to the increased availability of calorie-dense foods and a simultaneous decline in physical activity, resulting in part from mechanized transportation and sedentary lifestyles.[6-11]

Obesity and overweight have negative health effects, particularly by reducing the age at onset of, and increasing the prevalence of, *type 2 diabetes.* Obesity is established as a major contributor to premature death in the United States,[12,13] although the exact magnitude of the association remains controversial, resulting in part from the complexities of the causal pathway involved (i.e., obesity leads to death indirectly, by contributing to the development of chronic disease).

Multiple behavioral factors are associated with the spread of some diseases. In the case of AIDS, the spread of human immunodeficiency virus (HIV) can result from unprotected sexual intercourse between men and from shared syringes among intravenous drug users, which are the two predominant routes of transmission in the United States.

HIV infection can also result from unprotected vaginal intercourse, which is the predominant transmission route in Africa and other parts of the world. Other behaviors that can lead to disease, injury, or premature death (before age 65) are excessive intake of alcohol, abuse of both legal and illegal drugs, driving while intoxicated, and homicide and suicide attempts. In each of these cases, as in cigarette smoking and HIV infection, changes in behavior could prevent the untoward outcomes. Many efforts in health promotion depend heavily on modifying human behavior, as discussed in Chapter 15.

"E"—ENVIRONMENTAL FACTORS

Epidemiologists are frequently the first professionals to respond to an apparent outbreak of new health problems, such as *legionnaires' disease* and *Lyme disease,* which involve important environmental factors. In their investigations, epidemiologists describe the patterns of the disease in the affected population, develop and test hypotheses about causal factors, and introduce methods to prevent further cases of disease. Chapter 3 describes the standard approach to investigating an epidemic.

During an outbreak of severe pneumonia among individuals attending a 1976 American Legion conference in Philadelphia, epidemiologists conducted studies suggesting that the epidemic was caused by an infectious agent distributed through the air-conditioning and ventilation systems of the primary conference hotels. Only later, after the identification of *Legionella pneumophila*, was it discovered that this small bacterium thrives in air-conditioning cooling towers and warm-water systems. It was also shown that respiratory therapy equipment that is merely rinsed with water can become a reservoir for *Legionella*, causing hospital-acquired legionnaires' disease.

An illness first reported in 1975 in Old Lyme, Connecticut, was the subject of epidemiologic research suggesting that the arthritis, rash, and other symptoms of the illness were caused by infection with an organism transmitted by a tick. This was enough information to enable preventive measures to begin. By 1977 it was clear that the disease, then known as Lyme disease, was spread by *Ixodes* ticks, opening the way for more specific prevention and research. Not until 1982, however, was the causative agent, *Borrelia burgdorferi*, discovered and shown to be spread by the *Ixodes* tick.

"I"—IMMUNOLOGIC FACTORS

Smallpox is the first infectious disease known to have been eradicated from the globe (although samples of the causative virus remain stored in U.S. and Russian laboratories). Smallpox eradication was possible because vaccination against the disease conferred individual immunity and produced herd immunity. **Herd immunity** results when a vaccine diminishes an immunized person's ability to spread a disease, leading to reduced disease transmission.

Most people now think of AIDS when they hear of a deficiency of the immune system, but **immunodeficiency** also may be caused by genetic abnormalities and other factors. Transient immune deficiency has been noted after some infections (e.g., measles) and after the administration of certain vaccines (e.g., live measles vaccine). This result is potentially serious in malnourished children. The use of cancer chemotherapy and the long-term use of corticosteroids also produce immunodeficiency, which may often be severe.

"N"—NUTRITIONAL FACTORS

In the 1950s it was shown that Japanese Americans living in Hawaii had a much higher rate of MI than people of the same age and gender in Japan, while Japanese Americans in California had a still higher rate of MI than similar individuals in Japan.[14-16] The investigators believed that dietary variations were the most important factors producing these differences in disease rates, as generally supported by subsequent research. The Japanese eat more fish, vegetables, and fruit in smaller portions.

Denis Burkitt, the physician after whom Burkitt's lymphoma was named, spent many years doing epidemiologic research on the critical role played by dietary fiber in good health. From his cross-cultural studies, he made some stunning statements, including the following[17]:

"By world standards, the entire United States is constipated."
"Don't diagnose appendicitis in Africa unless the patient speaks English."
"African medical students go through five years of training without seeing coronary heart disease or appendicitis."
"Populations with large stools have small hospitals. Those with small stools have large hospitals."

Based on cross-cultural studies, Burkitt observed that many of the diseases commonly seen in the United States, such as diabetes and hypertension, were rarely encountered in indigenous populations of tropical Africa (Box 1-2). This observation was true even of areas with good medical care, such as Kampala, Uganda, when Burkitt was there, indicating that such diseases were not being missed because of lack of diagnosis. These differences could not be primarily genetic in origin because African Americans in the United States experience these diseases at about the same rate as other U.S. groups. Cross-cultural differences suggest that the current heavy burden of these diseases in the United States is *not* inevitable. Burkitt suggested mechanisms by which a high intake of dietary fiber might prevent these diseases or greatly reduce their incidence.

"G"—GENETIC FACTORS

It is well established that the genetic inheritance of individuals interacts with diet and environment in complex ways to promote or protect against a variety of illnesses, including heart disease and cancer. As a result, **genetic epidemiology** is a growing field of research that addresses, among other things, the distribution of normal and abnormal genes in a population, and whether or not these are in equilibrium. Considerable research examines the possible interaction of various genotypes with environmental, nutritional, and behavioral factors, as well as with pharmaceutical treatments. Ongoing research concerns the extent to which environmental adaptations can reduce the burden of diseases with a heavy genetic component.

Genetic disease now accounts for a higher proportion of illness than in the past, not because the incidence of genetic disease is increasing, but because the incidence of noninherited disease is decreasing and our ability to identify genetic diseases has improved. Scriver[18] illustrates this point as follows:

> Heritability refers to the contribution of genes relative to all determinants of disease. Rickets, a genetic disease, recently showed an abrupt fall in incidence and an increase in heritability in Quebec. The fall in incidence followed universal supplementation of dairy milk with calciferol. The rise in heritability reflected the disappearance of a major environmental cause of rickets (vitamin D deficiency) and the persistence of Mendelian disorders of calcium and phosphate homeostasis, without any change in their incidence.

Genetic screening is important for identifying problems in newborns, such as phenylketonuria and congenital hypothyroidism, for which therapy can be extremely beneficial if instituted early enough. Screening is also important for identifying other genetic disorders for which counseling can be beneficial. In the future, the most important health benefits from genetics may come from identifying individuals who are at high risk for specific problems, or who would respond particularly well (or poorly) to specific drugs. Examples might include individuals at high risk for MI; breast or ovarian cancer (e.g., carriers of *BRCA1* and *BRCA2* genetic mutations); environmental asthma; or reactions to certain foods, medicines, or behaviors. Screening for *susceptibility genes* undoubtedly will increase in the future, but there are ethical concerns about potential problems, such as medical insurance carriers hesitating to insure individuals with known genetic risks. For more on the prevention of genetic disease, see Section 3, particularly Chapter 20.

"S"—SERVICES, SOCIAL FACTORS, AND SPIRITUAL FACTORS

Medical care services may be beneficial to health but also can be dangerous. One of the important tasks of epidemiologists is to determine the benefits and hazards of medical care in different settings. **Iatrogenic disease** occurs when a disease is induced inadvertently by treatment or during a diagnostic procedure. A U.S. Institute of Medicine report estimated that 2.9% to 3.7% of hospitalized patients experience "adverse events" during their hospitalization. Of these events, about 19% are caused by medication errors and 14% by wound infections.[19] Based on 3.6 million hospital admissions cited in a 1997 study, this report estimated that about 44,000 deaths each year are associated with medical errors in hospital. Other medical care–related causes of illness include unnecessary or inappropriate diagnostic or surgical

Box 1-2	Diseases that Have Been Rare in Indigenous Populations of Tropical Africa
Appendicitis	Diverticulitis
Breast cancer	Gallstones
Colon cancer	Hemorrhoids
Coronary heart disease	Hiatal hernia
Diabetes mellitus	Varicose veins

Data from Burkitt D: Lecture, Yale University School of Medicine, 1989.

procedures. For example, more than 50% of healthy women who undergo annual screening mammography over a 10-year period will have at least one mammogram interpreted as suspicious for breast cancer and will therefore be advised to undergo additional testing, even though they do not have cancer.[20]

The effects of **social and spiritual factors** on disease and health have been less intensively studied than have other causal factors. Evidence is accumulating, however, that personal beliefs concerning the meaning and purpose of life, perspectives on access to forgiveness, and support received from members of a social network are powerful influences on health. Studies have shown that experimental animals and humans are better able to resist noxious stressors when they are receiving social support from other members of the same species. Social support may be achieved through the family, friendship networks, and membership in various groups, such as clubs and churches. One study reviewed the literature concerning the association of religious faith with generally better health and found that strong religious faith was associated with better health and quality of life.[21] The effects of meditation and massage on quality of life in patients with advanced disease (e.g., AIDS) have also been studied.[22]

Many investigators have explored factors related to health and disease in Mormons and Seventh-Day Adventists. Both these religious groups have lower-than-average age-adjusted death rates from many common types of disease and specifically from heart disease, cancer, and respiratory disorders. Part of their protection undoubtedly arises from the behaviors proscribed or prescribed by these groups. Mormons prohibit the use of alcohol and tobacco. Seventh-Day Adventists likewise tend to avoid alcohol and tobacco, and they strongly encourage (but do not require) a vegetarian diet. It is unclear, however, that these behaviors are solely responsible for the health differences. As one study noted, "It is difficult … to separate the effects of health practices from other aspects of lifestyle common among those belonging to such religions, for example, differing social stresses and network systems."[23] Another study showed that for all age cohorts, the greater one's participation in churches or other groups and the stronger one's social networks, the lower the observed mortality.[24]

The work of the psychiatrist Victor Frankl also documented the importance of having a meaning and purpose in life, which can alleviate stress and improve coping.[25] Such factors are increasingly being studied as important in understanding the web of causation for disease.

III. ECOLOGICAL ISSUES IN EPIDEMIOLOGY

Classical epidemiologists have long regarded their field as "human ecology," "medical ecology," or "geographic medicine," because an important characteristic of epidemiology is its **ecological perspective.**[26] People are seen not only as individual organisms, but also as members of communities, in a social context. The world is understood as a complex ecosystem in which disease patterns vary greatly from one country to another. The types and rates of diseases in a country are a form of "fingerprint" that indicates the standard of living, the lifestyle, the predominant occupations, and the climate, among other factors. Because of the

tremendous growth in world population, now more than 7 billion, and rapid technologic developments, humans have had a profound impact on the global environment, often with deleterious effects. The existence of wide biodiversity, which helps to provide the planet with greater adaptive capacity, has become increasingly threatened. Every action that affects the ecosystem, even an action intended to promote human health and well-being, produces a reaction in the system, and the result is not always positive. (See http://www.cdc.gov and http://www.census.gov/main/www/popclock.html.)

A. Solution of Public Health Problems and Unintended Creation of New Problems

One of the most important insights of ecological thinking is that as people change one part of a system, they inevitably change other parts. An epidemiologist is constantly alert for possible negative side effects that a medical or health intervention might produce. In the United States the reduced mortality in infancy and childhood has increased the prevalence of chronic degenerative diseases because now most people live past retirement age. Although nobody would want to go back to the public health and medical care of 100 years ago, the control of infectious diseases has nevertheless produced new sets of medical problems, many of them chronic. Table 1-1 summarizes some of the new health and societal problems introduced by the solution of earlier health problems.

I. Vaccination and Patterns of Immunity

Understanding **herd immunity** is essential to any discussion of current ecological problems in immunization. A vaccine provides herd immunity if it not only protects the immunized individual, but also prevents that person from

Table I-I Examples of Unintended Consequences from Solution of Earlier Health Problems

Initial Health Problem	Solution	Unintended Consequences
Childhood infections	Vaccination	Decrease in the level of immunity during adulthood, caused by a lack of repeated exposure to infection
High infant mortality rate	Improved sanitation	Increase in the population growth rate; appearance of epidemic paralytic poliomyelitis
Sleeping sickness in cattle	Control of tsetse fly (the disease vector)	Increase in the area of land subject to overgrazing and drought, caused by an increase in the cattle population
Malnutrition and need for larger areas of tillable land	Erection of large river dams (e.g., Aswan High Dam, Senegal River dams)	Increase in rates of some infectious diseases, caused by water system changes that favor the vectors of disease

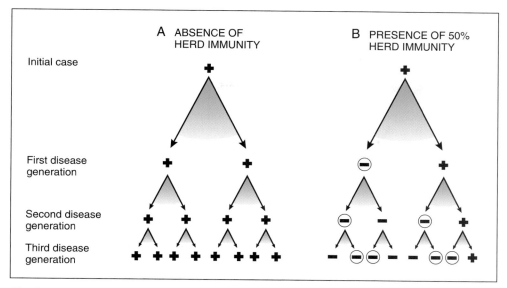

Figure I-2 Effect of herd immunity on spread of infection. Diagrams illustrate how an infectious disease, such as measles, could spread in a susceptible population if each infected person were exposed to two other persons. **A,** In the absence of herd immunity, the number of cases doubles each disease generation. **B,** In the presence of 50% herd immunity, the number of cases remains constant. The *plus sign* represents an infected person; the *minus sign* represents an uninfected person; and the *circled minus sign* represents an immune person who will not pass the infection to others. The *arrows* represent significant exposure with transmission of infection (if the first person is infectious) or equivalent close contact without transmission of infection (if the first person is not infectious).

transmitting the disease to others. This causes the prevalence of the disease organism in the population to decline. Herd immunity is illustrated in Figure 1-2, where it is assumed that each infected person comes into sufficient contact with two other persons to expose both of them to the disease if they are susceptible. Under this assumption, if there is no herd immunity against the disease and everyone is susceptible, the number of cases doubles every *disease generation* (Fig. 1-2, *A*). However, if there is 50% herd immunity against the disease, the number of cases is small and remains approximately constant (Fig. 1-2, *B*). In this model, if there is greater than 50% herd immunity, as would be true in a well-immunized population, the infection should die out eventually. The degree of immunity necessary to eliminate a disease from a population varies depending on the type of infectious organism, the time of year, and the density and social patterns of the population.

Immunization may seem simple: immunize everybody in childhood, and there will be no problems from the targeted diseases. Although there is some truth to this, in reality the control of diseases by immunization is more complex. The examples of diphtheria, smallpox, and poliomyelitis are used here to illustrate issues concerning vaccination programs and population immunity, and syphilis is used to illustrate natural herd immunity to infection.

DIPHTHERIA

Vaccine-produced immunity in humans tends to decrease over time. This phenomenon has a different impact at present, when infectious diseases such as diphtheria are less common, than it did in the past. When diphtheria was a more common disease, people who had been vaccinated against it were exposed more frequently to the causative

agent, and this exposure could result in a mild reinfection. The reinfection would produce a **natural booster effect** and maintain a high level of immunity. As diphtheria became less common because of immunization programs, fewer people were exposed, resulting in fewer subclinical *booster* infections.

In Russia, despite the wide availability of diphtheria vaccine, many adults who had not recently been in the military were found to be susceptible to *Corynebacterium diphtheriae*. Beginning in 1990, a major epidemic of diphtheria appeared in Russia. By 1992, about 72% of the reported cases were found among individuals older than 14 years. This was not caused by lack of initial immunization, because more than 90% of Russian adults had been fully immunized against diphtheria when they were children. The disease in older people was apparently caused by a decline in adult immunity levels. Before the epidemic was brought under control, it produced more than 125,000 cases of diphtheria and caused 4000 deaths.[27] An additional single vaccination is now recommended for adults to provide a booster.

SMALLPOX

As mentioned earlier, the goal of worldwide eradication of smallpox has now been met by immunizing people against the disease. Early attempts at preventing smallpox included actions reportedly by a Buddhist nun who would grind scabs from patients with the mild form and blow into the nose of nonimmune individuals; this was called *variolation*. The term *vaccination* comes from *vaca*, or "cow"; epidemiologists noted that milkmaids developed the less severe form of smallpox.

Attempts at eradication included some potential risks. The dominant form of smallpox in the 1970s was *variola minor* (alastrim). This was a relatively mild form of smallpox that, although often disfiguring, had a low mortality rate. However, alastrim provided individual and herd immunity against the much more disfiguring and often fatal *variola major* form of the disease (classical smallpox). To eliminate alastrim while increasing rates of variola major would have been a poor exchange. Fortunately, the smallpox vaccine was effective against both forms of smallpox, and the immunization program was successful in eradicating both variola minor and variola major.

POLIOMYELITIS

The need for herd immunity was also shown by poliomyelitis. The inactivated or *killed* polio vaccine (IPV), which became available in 1955, provided protection to the immunized individual, but did not produce much herd immunity. Although it stimulated the production of blood antibodies against the three types of poliovirus, it did not produce cell-mediated immunity in the intestine, where the polioviruses multiplied. For this reason, IPV did little to interrupt viral replication in the intestine. Declining rates of paralytic poliomyelitis lulled many people into lack of concern, and immunization rates for newborns decreased, leading to periodic small epidemics of poliomyelitis in the late 1950s and early 1960s because poliovirus was still present.

The live, attenuated Sabin oral polio vaccine (OPV) was approved in the early 1960s. OPV produced cell-mediated immunity, preventing the poliovirus from replicating in the intestine, and it also provided herd immunity. After the widespread use of OPV in the United States, the prevalence of all three types of the wild poliovirus declined rapidly, as monitored in waste sewage. Poliovirus now seems to have been eradicated from the Western Hemisphere, where the last known case of paralytic poliomyelitis caused by a wild poliovirus was confirmed in Peru in 1991.[28]

It might seem from this information that OPV is always superior, but this is not true. When the health department for the Gaza Strip used only OPV in its polio immunization efforts, many cases of paralytic poliomyelitis occurred among Arab children. Because of inadequate sanitation, the children often had other intestinal infections when they were given OPV, and these infections interfered with the OPV infection in the gut. As a result, the oral vaccine often did not "take," and many children remained unprotected.[29] The health department subsequently switched to an immunization program in which children were injected first with the inactivated vaccine to produce adequate blood immunity. Later, they were given OPV as a booster vaccine to achieve herd immunity.

Now that OPV has succeeded in eradicating wild poliovirus from the Western Hemisphere, the only indigenous cases of paralytic poliomyelitis occurring in the United States since 1979 have been iatrogenic (vaccine-induced) polio caused by the oral (live, attenuated) vaccine itself. Since 1999, to eliminate vaccine-caused cases, the CDC has recommended that infants be given the IPV instead of the OPV.[30] Some OPV is still held in reserve for outbreaks.

Polio was officially eradicated in 36 Western Pacific countries, including China and Australia in 2000. Europe was declared polio free in 2002. Polio remains endemic in only a few countries.

SYPHILIS

Syphilis is caused by infection with bacteria known as spirochetes and progresses in several stages. In the primary stage, syphilis produces a highly infectious skin lesion known as a chancre, which is filled with spirochete organisms. This lesion subsides spontaneously. In the secondary stage, a rash or other lesions may appear; these also subside spontaneously. A latent period follows, after which a tertiary stage may occur. Untreated infection typically results in immunity to future infection by the disease agent, but this immunity is not absolute. It does not protect individuals from progressive damage to their own body. It does provide some herd immunity, however, by making the infected individual unlikely to develop a new infection if he or she is exposed to syphilis again.[31] Ironically, when penicillin came into general use, syphilis infections were killed so quickly that *chancre immunity* did not develop, and high-risk individuals continued to repeatedly reacquire and spread the disease.

2. Effects of Sanitation

In the 19th century, diarrheal diseases were the primary killer of children, and tuberculosis was the leading cause of adult mortality. The sanitary revolution, which began in England about the middle of the century, was the most important factor in reducing infant mortality. However, the reduction of infant mortality contributed in a major way to increasing the effective birth rate and the overall rate of population growth. The sanitary revolution was therefore one of the causes of today's worldwide population problem. The current world population (>7 billion) has a profound and often unappreciated impact on the production of pollutants, the global fish supply, the amount of land available for cultivation, worldwide forest cover, and climate.

Care must be taken to avoid oversimplifying the factors that produce population growth, which continues even as the global rate of growth seems to be slowing down. On the one hand, a reduction in infant mortality temporarily helps to produce a significant difference between the birth and death rates in a population, resulting in rapid population growth, the **demographic gap.** On the other hand, the control of infant mortality seems to be necessary before specific populations are willing to accept population control. When the infant mortality rate is high, a family needs to have a large number of children to have reasonable confidence that one or two will survive to adulthood. This is not true when the infant mortality rate is low. Although it may seem paradoxical, reduced infant mortality seems to be both a cause of the population problem and a requirement for population control.

In addition to affecting population growth, the sanitary revolution of the 19th century affected disease patterns in unanticipated ways. In fact, improvements in sanitation were a fundamental cause of the appearance of epidemic paralytic poliomyelitis late in the 19th century. This may seem counterintuitive, but it illustrates the importance of an ecological perspective and offers an example of the so-called iceberg phenomenon, discussed later. The three polioviruses are enteric viruses transmitted by the fecal-oral route. People who have developed antibodies to all three types of poliovirus are immune to their potentially paralytic effects and show no symptoms or signs of clinical disease if they are exposed. Newborns receive passive antibodies from their mothers, and these maternal antibodies normally prevent polioviruses from invading the central nervous system early in an infant's first year of life. As a result, exposure of a young infant to polioviruses rarely leads to paralytic disease, but instead produces a subclinical (largely asymptomatic) infection, which causes infants to produce their own active antibodies and cell-mediated immunity.

Although improved sanitation reduced the proportion of people who were infected with polioviruses, it also delayed the time when most infants and children were exposed to the polioviruses. Most were exposed after they were no longer protected by maternal immunity, with the result that a higher percentage developed the paralytic form of the disease. Epidemic paralytic poliomyelitis can therefore be seen as an unwanted side effect of the sanitary revolution. Further, because members of the upper socioeconomic groups had the best sanitation, they were hit first and most severely, until the polio vaccine became available.

3. Vector Control and Land Use Patterns

Sub-Saharan Africa provides a disturbing example of how negative side effects from vectors of disease can result from positive intentions of land use. A successful effort was made to control the tsetse fly, which is the vector of African sleeping sickness in cattle and sometimes in humans. Control of the vector enabled herders to keep larger numbers of cattle, and this led to overgrazing. Overgrazed areas were subject to frequent droughts, and some became dust bowls with little vegetation.[32] The results were often famine and starvation for cattle and humans.

4. River Dam Construction and Patterns of Disease

For a time, it was common for Western nations to build large river dams in developing countries to produce electricity and increase the amount of available farmland by irrigation. During this period, the warnings of epidemiologists about potential negative effects of such dams went unheeded. The Aswan High Dam in Egypt provides a case in point. Directly after the dam was erected, the incidence of schistosomiasis increased in the areas supplied by the dam, just as epidemiologists predicted. Similar results followed the construction of the main dam and tributary dams for the Senegal River Project in West Africa. Before the dams were erected, the sea would move far inland during the dry season and mix with fresh river water, making the river water too salty to support the larvae of the blood flukes responsible for schistosomiasis or the mosquitoes that transmit malaria, Rift Valley fever, and dengue fever.[33] Once the dams were built, the incidence of these diseases increased until clean water, sanitation, and other health interventions were provided.

B. Synergism of Factors Predisposing to Disease

There may be a synergism between diseases or between factors predisposing to disease, such that each makes the other worse or more easily acquired. Sexually transmitted diseases, especially those that produce open sores, facilitate the spread of HIV. This is thought to be a major factor in countries where HIV is usually spread through heterosexual activity. In addition, the compromised immunity caused by AIDS permits the reactivation of previously latent infections, such as tuberculosis, which is now resurging in many areas of the globe.

The relationship between malnutrition and infection is similarly complex. Not only does malnutrition make infections worse, but infections make malnutrition worse as well. A malnourished child has more difficulty making antibodies and repairing tissue damage, which makes the child less resistant to infectious diseases and their complications. This scenario is observed in the case of measles. In isolated societies without medical care or measles vaccine, less than 1% of well-nourished children may die from measles or its complications, whereas 25% of malnourished children may die. Infection can worsen malnutrition for several reasons. First, infection puts greater demands on the body, so the relative deficiency of nutrients becomes greater. Second, infection tends to reduce the appetite, so intake is reduced. Third, in the presence of infection, the diet frequently is changed to emphasize bland foods, which often are deficient in proteins and vitamins. Fourth, in patients with gastrointestinal infection, food rushes through the irritated bowel at a faster pace, causing diarrhea, and fewer nutrients are absorbed.

Ecological and genetic factors can also interact to produce new strains of influenza virus. Many of the new, epidemic strains of influenza virus have names that refer to China (e.g., Hong Kong flu, Beijing flu) because of agricultural practices. In rural China, domesticated pigs are in close contact with ducks and people. The duck and the human strains of influenza infect pigs, and the genetic material of the two influenza strains may mix in the pigs, producing a new variant of influenza. These new variants can then infect humans. If the genetic changes in the influenza virus are major, the result is called an **antigenic shift,** and the new virus may produce a **pandemic,** or widespread, outbreak of influenza that could involve multiple continents. If the genetic changes in the influenza virus are minor, the phenomenon is called an **antigenic drift,** but this still can produce major regional outbreaks of influenza. The avian influenza (H5N1) virus from Southeast Asia differs greatly from human strains, and it has caused mortality in most people who contract the infection from birds. Should this strain of influenza acquire the capacity to spread from one human to another, the world is likely to see a **global pandemic** (worldwide epidemic).

The same principles apply to chronic diseases. Overnutrition and sedentary living interact so that each one worsens the impact of the other. As another example, the coexistence of cigarette smoking and pneumoconiosis (especially in coal workers) makes lung cancer more likely than a simple sum of the individual risks.

IV. CONTRIBUTIONS OF EPIDEMIOLOGISTS

A. Investigating Epidemics and New Diseases

Using the surveillance and investigative methods discussed in detail in Chapter 3, epidemiologists often have provided the initial hypotheses about disease causation for other scientists to test in the laboratory. Over the past 40 years,

Table I-2 **Early Hypotheses by Epidemiologists on Natural History and Prevention Methods for More Recent Diseases**

Disease	Date of Appearance	Epidemiologic Hypotheses	
		Agent and Route of Spread	Methods of Prevention
Lyme disease	1975	Infectious agent, spread by ticks	Avoid ticks
Legionnaires' disease	1976	Small infectious agent, spread via air-conditioning systems	Treat water in air-conditioning systems
Toxic shock syndrome	1980	Staphylococcal toxin, associated with use of tampons (especially Rely brand)	Avoid using long-lasting tampons
Acquired immunodeficiency syndrome (AIDS)	1981	Viral agent, spread via sexual activity, especially male homosexual activity, and via sharing of needles and exchange of blood and blood products during intravenous drug use and transfusions	Use condoms Avoid sharing needles Institute programs to exchange needles and screen blood
Eosinophilia-myalgia syndrome	1989	Toxic contaminant, associated with use of dietary supplements of L-tryptophan	Change methods of product manufacturing
Hantavirus pulmonary syndrome	1993	Hantavirus, spread via contact with contaminated droppings of deer mice	Avoid contact with excreta of deer mice
New-variant Creutzfeldt-Jakob disease	1996	Prions, spread via ingestion of beef infected with bovine spongiform encephalopathy	Avoid eating infected beef Avoid feeding animal remains to cattle
Severe acute respiratory syndrome (SARS)	2003	Animal coronavirus transferred to humans by handling and eating unusual food animals	Avoid handling, killing, and eating nonstandard food animals

epidemiologic methods have suggested the probable type of agent and modes of transmission for the diseases listed in Table 1-2 and others, usually within months of their recognition as new or emergent diseases. Knowledge of the modes of transmission led epidemiologists to suggest ways to prevent each of these diseases before the causative agents were determined or extensive laboratory results were available. Laboratory work to identify the causal agents, clarify the pathogenesis, and develop vaccines or treatments for most of these diseases still continues many years after this basic epidemiologic work was done.

Concern about the many, more recently discovered and resurgent diseases[34] is currently at a peak, both because of a variety of newly emerging disease problems and because of the threat of bioterrorism.[35] The rapid growth in world population; increased travel and contact with new ecosystems, such as rain forests; declining effectiveness of antibiotics and insecticides; and many other factors encourage the development of new diseases or the resurgence of previous disorders. In addition, global climate change may extend the range of some diseases or help to create others.

B. Studying the Biologic Spectrum of Disease

The first identified cases of a new disease are often fatal or severe, leading observers to conclude that the disease is always severe. As more becomes known about the disease, however, less severe (and even asymptomatic) cases usually are discovered. With infectious diseases, asymptomatic infection may be uncovered either by finding elevated antibody titers to the organism in clinically well people or by culturing the organism from such people.

This variation in the severity of a disease process is known as the **biologic spectrum of disease,** or the **iceberg phenomenon.**[36] The latter term is appropriate because most of an iceberg remains unseen, below the surface, analogous to

asymptomatic and mild cases of disease. An outbreak of diphtheria illustrates this point. When James F. Jekel worked with the CDC early in his career, he was assigned to investigate an epidemic of diphtheria in an Alabama county. The diphtheria outbreak caused two deaths; symptoms of clinical illness in 12 children who recovered; and asymptomatic infection in 32 children, some of whom had even been immunized against diphtheria. The 32 cases of asymptomatic infection were discovered by extensive culturing of the throats of the school-age children in the outbreak area. In this iceberg (Fig. 1-3), 14 infections were visible, but the 32 asymptomatic carriers would have remained invisible without extensive epidemiologic surveillance.[37] The iceberg phenomenon is paramount to epidemiology, because studying only symptomatic individuals may produce a misleading picture of the disease pattern and severity.[38] The biologic spectrum also applies to viral disease.[39]

C. Surveillance of Community Health Interventions

Randomized trials of preventive measures in the field (**field trials**) are an important phase of evaluating a new vaccine before it is given to the community at large. Field trials, however, are only one phase in the evaluation of immunization programs. After a vaccine is introduced, ongoing surveillance of the disease and vaccine side effects is essential to ensure the vaccine's continued safety and effectiveness.

The importance of continued surveillance can be illustrated in the case of immunization against poliomyelitis. In 1954, large-scale field trials of the Salk inactivated polio vaccine were done, confirming the value and safety of the vaccine.[40] In 1955, however, the polio surveillance program of the CDC discovered an outbreak of vaccine-associated poliomyelitis, which was linked to vaccine from one specific

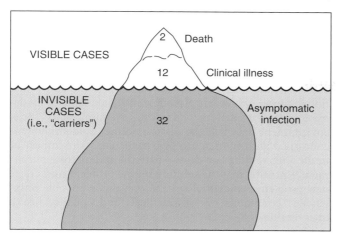

Figure 1-3 Iceberg phenomenon, as illustrated by a diphtheria epidemic in Alabama. In epidemics, the number of people with severe forms of the disease (part of iceberg above water) may be much smaller than the number of people with mild or asymptomatic clinical disease (part of iceberg below water). (Data from Jekel JF et al: *Public Health Rep* 85:310, 1970.)

laboratory.[41] Ultimately, 79 vaccinated individuals and 105 of their family members were found to have developed poliomyelitis. Apparently, a slight change from the recommended procedure for producing the vaccine had allowed clumping of the poliovirus to occur, which shielded some of the virus particles in the center of the clumps so that they were not killed by formaldehyde during vaccine production. As a result, some people received a vaccine containing live virus. It was only through the vaccine surveillance program that the problem was detected quickly and the dangerous vaccine removed from use.

Likewise, ongoing surveillance programs were responsible for detecting outbreaks of measles that occurred in 1971, 1977, and 1990, after impressive initial progress in vaccination against the disease. Epidemiologists were able to show that much of the unexpected disease occurred in college students and others who had received measles vaccine before 12 months of age without a later booster dose. The timing of the vaccine was important, because if given while maternal antibodies against measles persisted in the infants, the antigenicity of the vaccine was reduced.[42] Such findings have led to the current recommendations to provide measles vaccine initially at 15 months of age and to give a booster dose at 4 to 6 years of age.[30]

Routine smallpox vaccination among the entire American population stopped in 1972 after the eradication of the disease was announced. However, after the terrorist attacks on September 11, 2001, the United States developed a smallpox response plan in case of future bioterrorism events. Surveillance of the small number of persons vaccinated against smallpox since 2000 then revealed cases of vaccine-associated cardiomyopathy, and this outcome encouraged the CDC to curtail a large-scale vaccination program. As part of its response plan, the U.S. now has a stockpile of smallpox vaccines sufficient to vaccinate everyone in the country in the event of a smallpox emergency. Epidemiologists are thus contributing to national security by helping to establish new approaches to surveillance (**syndromic surveillance**) that

identify not only changes in disease occurrence, but also increases in potentially suspicious symptom patterns.

D. Setting Disease Control Priorities

Disease control priorities should be based not only on the currently existing size of the problem, but also on the potential of a disease to spread to others; its likelihood of causing death and disability; and its cost to individuals, families, and the community. U.S. legislatures often fund disease control efforts inappropriately, by considering only the number of cases reported. In the 1950s, a sharp drop in reported syphilis rates quickly led to declining support for syphilis control in the United States, which contributed to its subsequent rebound.[24] Sometimes health funding is influenced when powerful individuals lobby for more money for research or control efforts for a particular disease or injury.

Although relatively few people in the United States were infected with HIV in the early 1980s, epidemiologists recognized that the potential threat to society posed by AIDS was far greater than the absolute numbers of infected individuals and associated costs suggested at that time. Accordingly, a much larger proportion of national resources was allocated to the study and control of AIDS than to efforts focused on other diseases affecting similar numbers of people. Special concerns with AIDS included the rapid increase in incidence over a very brief period, the high case fatality ratio during the initial outbreak and before therapy was developed and available, the substantial medical and social costs, the ready transmissibility of the disease, and known methods of prevention not being well applied.

In the 21st century, a degree of control has been achieved over AIDS through antiretroviral drugs. However, new trends in other diseases have emerged. Most importantly, increased caloric intake and sedentary living have produced a rapid increase in overweight and obesity, leading to an increase in type 2 diabetes. In addition, new respiratory diseases have appeared in Asia. The first, *severe acute respiratory syndrome* (SARS), appeared in China in 2003 and was caused by an animal coronavirus traced to unusual food animals. If the new form of avian influenza (H5N1) spreads worldwide, it likely would move to the top of the priority list until it was controlled.

E. Improving Diagnosis, Treatment, and Prognosis of Clinical Disease

The application of epidemiologic methods to clinical questions helps us to improve clinical medicine, particularly in the diagnosis, therapy, and prognosis of disease. This is the domain of clinical epidemiology.

Diagnosis is the process of identifying the nature and cause of a disease through evaluation of the clinical history, review of symptoms, examination or testing. Epidemiologic methods are used to improve disease diagnosis through the selection of the best diagnostic tests, the determination of the best cutoff points for such tests, and the development of strategies to use in screening for disease. These issues are discussed in Chapters 7 and 8, as well as in the preventive medicine section of this book.

The methods of clinical epidemiology frequently are used to determine the most effective **treatment** in a given situation. One study used a randomized controlled clinical trial in many U.S. centers to test the hypothesis that pharmaceutical therapy with methylprednisolone reduced spinal cord damage and improved residual motor function after acute spinal cord injury. The hypothesis was confirmed.[43]

Epidemiologic methods also help improve our understanding of a patient's **prognosis,** or probable course and outcome of a disease.[44] Patients and families want to know the likely course of their illness, and investigators need accurate prognoses to stratify patients into groups with similar disease severity in research to evaluate treatments.

Epidemiologic methods permit **risk estimation.** These are perhaps best developed in various cardiac risk estimators using data from the Framingham Heart Study (see www.framinghamheartstudy.org/risk/index.html) and in the Gail model for breast cancer risk (see http://www.cancer.gov/search/results).

F. Improving Health Services Research

The principles and methods of epidemiology are used in planning and evaluating medical care. In health planning, epidemiologic measures are employed to determine present and future community health needs. Demographic projection techniques can estimate the future size of different age groups. Analyses of patterns of disease frequency and use of services can estimate future service needs.[45] Additional epidemiologic methods can be used to determine the effects of medical care in health program evaluation as well as in the broader field of cost-benefit analysis (see Chapter 29).

G. Providing Expert Testimony in Courts of Law

Increasingly, epidemiologists are being called on to testify regarding the state of knowledge about such topics as product hazards and the probable risks and effects of various environmental exposures or medications. The many types of lawsuits that may rely on epidemiologic data include those involving claims of damage from general environmental exposures (e.g., possible association of magnetic fields or cellular phone use and brain cancer), occupational illness claims (e.g., occupational lung damage from workplace asbestos), medical liability (e.g., adverse effects of vaccines or medications), and product liability (e.g., association of lung cancer with tobacco use, of toxic shock syndrome with tampon use, and of cyclooxygenase-1 inhibitor medications with cardiovascular disease). Frequently, the answers to these questions are unknown or can only be estimated by epidemiologic methods. Therefore, expert medical testimony often requires a high level of epidemiologic expertise.[46]

V. SUMMARY

Epidemiology is the study of the occurrence, distribution, and determinants of diseases, injuries, and other health-related issues in specific populations. As such, it is concerned with all the biologic, social, behavioral, spiritual, economic, and psychological factors that may increase the frequency of disease or offer opportunities for prevention. Epidemiologic methods are often the first scientific methods applied to a new health problem to define its pattern in the population and to develop hypotheses about its causes, methods of transmission, and prevention.

Epidemiologists generally describe the causes of a disease in terms of the host, agent, and environment, sometimes adding the vector as a fourth factor for consideration. In exploring the means to prevent a given disease, they look for possible behavioral, genetic, and immunologic causes in the host. They also look for biologic and nutritional causes, which are usually considered agents. Epidemiologists consider the physical, chemical, and social environment in which the disease occurs. Epidemiology is concerned with human ecology, particularly the impact of health interventions on disease patterns and on the environment. Knowing that the solution of one problem may create new problems, epidemiologists also evaluate possible unintended consequences of medical and public health interventions.

Contributions of epidemiologists to medical science include the following:

- Investigating epidemics and new diseases
- Studying the biologic spectrum of disease
- Instituting surveillance of community health interventions
- Suggesting disease control priorities
- Improving the diagnosis, treatment, and prognosis of clinical disease
- Improving health services research
- Providing expert testimony in courts of law

References

1. Haynes RB, Sackett DL, Guyatt GH, et al: *Clinical epidemiology,* ed 3, Boston, 2006, Little, Brown.
2. US Surgeon General: *Smoking and health,* Public Health Service Pub No 1103, Washington, DC, 1964, US Government Printing Office.
3. Doll R, Peto R: *The causes of cancer,* Oxford, 1981, Oxford University Press.
4. Mokdad AH, Marks JS, Stroup DF, et al: Actual causes of death in the United States, 2000. *JAMA* 291:1238–1245, 2004.
5. Flegal KM, Graubard BI, Williamson DF, et al: Excess deaths associated with underweight, overweight, and obesity. *JAMA* 293:1861–1867, 2005.
6. Kimm SY, Glynn NW, Kriska AM, et al: Decline in physical activity in black girls and white girls during adolescence. *N Engl J Med* 347:709–715, 2002.
7. Swinburn BA, Sacks G, Hall KD, et al: The global obesity pandemic: shaped by global drivers and local environments. *Lancet* 378(9793):804–814, 2011. PubMed PMID: 21872749.
8. Lakdawalla D, Philipson T: The growth of obesity and technological change. *Econ Hum Biol* 7:283–293, 2009. PubMed PMID: 19748839; PubMed Central PMCID: PMC2767437.
9. Kumanyika SK: Global calorie counting: a fitting exercise for obese societies (review). *Annu Rev Public Health* 29:297–302, 2008. PubMed PMID: 18173383.
10. Popkin BM: Global nutrition dynamics: the world is shifting rapidly toward a diet linked with noncommunicable diseases. *Am J Clin Nutr* 84:289–298, 2006. PubMed PMID: 16895874.
11. Anderson PM, Butcher KE: Childhood obesity: trends and potential causes (review). *Future Child* 16:19–45, 2006. PubMed PMID: 16532657.
12. Berenson GS: Health consequences of obesity. Bogalusa Heart Study group. *Pediatr Blood Cancer* 58:117–121, 2012. doi: 10.1002/pbc.23373. PubMed PMID: 22076834.
13. Mehta NK, Chang VW: Mortality attributable to obesity among middle-aged adults in the United States. *Demography* 46:851–872, 2009. PubMed PMID: 20084832; PubMed Central PMCID: PMC2831354.

14. Gordon T: Mortality experience among the Japanese in the United States, Hawaii, and Japan. *Public Health Rep* 72:543–553, 1957.

15. Keys A: The peripatetic nutritionist. *Nutr Today* 13:19–24, 1966.

16. Keys A: Summary: coronary heart disease in seven countries. *Circulation* 42(suppl 1):186–198, 1970.

17. Burkitt D: Lecture, New Haven, Conn, 1989, Yale University School of Medicine.

18. Scriver CR: Human genes: determinants of sick populations and sick patients. *Can J Public Health* 79:222–224, 1988.

19. US Institute of Medicine: *To err is human.* Washington, DC, 2000, National Academy Press.

20. Elmore JG, Barton MB, Moceri VM, et al: Ten-year risk of false positive screening mammograms and clinical breast examinations. *N Engl J Med* 338:1089–1096, 1998.

21. Larson DB: *Scientific research on spirituality and health: a consensus report,* Rockville, Md, 1998, National Institute for Healthcare Research.

22. Williams A, Selwyn PA, Liberti L, et al: Randomized controlled trial of meditation and massage effects on quality of life in people with advanced AIDS: a pilot study. *J Palliat Med* 8:939–952, 2005.

23. Berkman LF, Breslow L: *Health and ways of living: the Alameda County Study,* New York, 1983, Oxford University Press.

24. Berkman LF, Syme LS: Social networks, host resistance, and mortality: a nine-year follow-up of Alameda County residents. *Am J Epidemiol* 109:186–204, 1979.

25. Frankl VE: *Man's search for meaning: an introduction to logotherapy,* New York, 1963, Washington Square Press.

26. Kilbourne ED, Smillie WG: *Human ecology and public health,* ed 4, London, 1969, Macmillan.

27. US Centers for Disease Control and Prevention: Update: diphtheria epidemic in the newly independent states of the former Soviet Union, January 1995–March 1996. *MMWR* 45:693–697, 1996.

28. US Centers for Disease Control and Prevention: Progress toward global eradication of poliomyelitis, 1988–1993. *MMWR* 43:499–503, 1994.

29. Lasch E: Personal communication, 1979.

30. US Centers for Disease Control and Prevention: Recommended childhood and adolescent immunization schedule—United States, 2006. *MMWR* 53, 2006.

31. Jekel JF: Role of acquired immunity to *Treponema pallidum* in the control of syphilis. *Public Health Rep* 83:627–632, 1968.

32. Ormerod WE: Ecological effect of control of African trypanosomiasis. *Science* 191:815–821, 1976.

33. Jones K: The silent scourge of development. *Yale Med* 18–23, 2006.

34. Jekel JF: Communicable disease control and public policy in the 1970s: hot war, cold war, or peaceful coexistence? *Am J Public Health* 62:1578–1585, 1972.

35. US Institute of Medicine: *Emerging infections,* Washington, DC, 1992, National Academy Press.

36. Morris JN: *The uses of epidemiology,* Edinburgh, 1967, E & S Livingstone.

37. Jekel JF, et al: *Corynebacterium diphtheriae* survives in a partly immunized group. *Public Health Rep* 85:310, 1970.

38. Evans AS: Subclinical epidemiology. *Am J Epidemiol* 125:545–555, 1987.

39. Zerr DM, Meier AS, Selke SS, et al: A population-based study of primary human herpesvirus 6 infection. *N Engl J Med* 352:768–776, 2005.

40. Francis T, Jr, Korns RF, Voight RB, et al: An evaluation of the 1954 poliomyelitis vaccine trials. *Am J Public Health* 45(pt 2):1–63, 1955.

41. Langmuir AD: The surveillance of communicable diseases of national importance. *N Engl J Med* 268:182–192, 1963.

42. Marks JS, Halpin TJ, Orenstein WA, et al: Measles vaccine efficacy in children previously vaccinated at 12 months of age. *Pediatrics* 62:955–960, 1978.

43. Bracken MB, Shepard MJ, Collins WF, et al: A randomized controlled trial of methylprednisolone or naloxone in the treatment of acute spinal cord injury. *N Engl J Med* 322:1405–1411, 1990.

44. Horwitz RI, Cicchetti DV, Horwitz SM: A comparison of the Norris and Killip coronary prognostic indices. *J Chronic Dis* 37:369–375, 1984.

45. Connecticut Hospital Association: Impact of an aging population on utilization and bed needs of Connecticut hospitals. *Conn Med* 42:775–781, 1978.

46. Greenland S: Relation of probability of causation to relative risk and doubling dose: a methodologic error that has become a social problem. *Am J Public Health* 89:1166–1169, 1999.

Select Readings

Elmore JG, Barton MB, Moceri VM, et al: Ten-year risk of false positive screening mammograms and clinical breast examinations. *N Engl J Med* 338:1089–1096, 1998.

Gordis L: *Epidemiology,* ed 3, Philadelphia, 2004, Saunders. [An excellent text.]

Kelsey JL, Whittemore AS, Evans AS, et al: *Methods in observational epidemiology,* ed 2, New York, 1996, Oxford University Press. [Classical epidemiology.]

US Centers for Disease Control and Prevention: *Principles of epidemiology,* ed 2. [Available from the Public Health Foundation, Washington, DC.]

US Institute of Medicine: *Emerging infections,* Washington, DC, 1992, National Academy Press. [Medical ecology.]

US Institute of Medicine: *To err is human,* Washington, DC, 2000, National Academy Press.

Websites

Centers for Disease Control and Prevention: http://www.cdc.gov/
Global population: http://www.census.gov/main/www/popclock.html
Morbidity and Mortality Weekly Report: http://www.cdc.gov/mmwr/

Epidemiologic Data Measurements

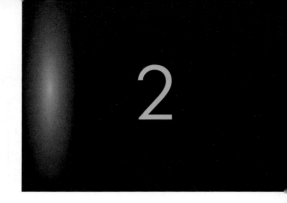

2

Clinical phenomena must be measured accurately to develop and test hypotheses. Because epidemiologists study phenomena in populations, they need measures that summarize what happens at the population level. The fundamental epidemiologic measure is the frequency with which an event of interest (e.g., disease, injury, or death) occurs in the population of interest.

I. FREQUENCY

The frequency of a disease, injury, or death can be measured in different ways, and it can be related to different denominators, depending on the purpose of the research and the availability of data. The concepts of incidence and prevalence are of fundamental importance to epidemiology.

A. Incidence (Incident Cases)

Incidence is the frequency of occurrences of disease, injury, or death—that is, the number of transitions from well to ill, from uninjured to injured, or from alive to dead—in the study population *during the time period of the study*. The term *incidence* is sometimes used incorrectly to mean incidence rate (defined in a later section). Therefore, to avoid confusion, it may be better to use the term *incident cases*, rather than *incidence*. Figure 2-1 shows the annual number of incident cases of acquired immunodeficiency syndrome (AIDS) by year of report for the United States from 1981 to 1992, using the definition of AIDS in use at that time.

B. Prevalence (Prevalent Cases)

Prevalence (sometimes called point prevalence) is the number of persons in a defined population who have a specified disease or condition *at a given point in time*, usually the time when a survey is conducted. The term *prevalence* is sometimes used incorrectly to mean prevalence rate (defined in a later section). Therefore, to avoid confusion, the awkward term *prevalent cases* is usually preferable to *prevalence*.

1. Difference between Point Prevalence and Period Prevalence

This text uses the term *prevalence* to mean **point prevalence**—i.e., prevalence at a specific point in time. Some articles in the literature discuss **period prevalence,** which refers to the number of persons who had a given disease at any time during the specified time interval. Period prevalence is the sum of the point prevalence at the beginning of the interval plus the incidence during the interval. Because period prevalence is a mixed measure, composed of point prevalence and incidence, it is not recommended for scientific work.

C. Illustration of Morbidity Concepts

The concepts of incidence (incident cases), point prevalence (prevalent cases), and period prevalence are illustrated

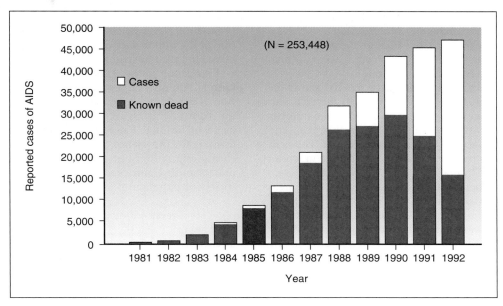

Figure 2-1 Incident cases of acquired immunodeficiency syndrome in United States, by year of report, 1981-1992. The full height of a bar represents the number of incident cases of AIDS in a given year. The darkened portion of a bar represents the number of patients in whom AIDS was diagnosed in a given year, but who were known to be dead by the end of 1992. The clear portion represents the number of patients who had AIDS diagnosed in a given year and were still living at the end of 1992. Statistics include cases from Guam, Puerto Rico, the U.S. Pacific Islands, and the U.S. Virgin Islands. (From Centers for Disease Control and Prevention: Summary of notifiable diseases—United States, 1992. *MMWR* 41:55, 1993.)

in Figure 2-2, based on a method devised in 1957.[1] Figure 2-2 provides data concerning eight persons who have a given disease in a defined population in which there is no emigration or immigration. Each person is assigned a case number (case no. 1 through case no. 8). A line begins when a person becomes ill and ends when that person either recovers or dies. The symbol t_1 signifies the beginning of the study period (e.g., a calendar year) and t_2 signifies the end.

In case no. 1, the patient was already ill when the year began and was still alive and ill when it ended. In case nos. 2, 6, and 8, the patients were already ill when the year began, but recovered or died during the year. In case nos. 3 and 5, the patients became ill during the year and were still alive and ill when the year ended. In case nos. 4 and 7, the patients became ill during the year and either recovered or died during the year. On the basis of Figure 2-2, the following calculations can be made. There were four incident cases during the year (case nos. 3, 4, 5, and 7). The point prevalence at t_1 was four (the prevalent cases were nos. 1, 2, 6, and 8). The point prevalence at t_2 was three (case nos. 1, 3, and 5). The period prevalence is equal to the point prevalence at t_1 plus the incidence between t_1 and t_2, or in this example, $4 + 4 = 8$. Although a person can be an incident case only once, he or she could be considered a prevalent case at many points in time, including the beginning and end of the study period (as with case no. 1).

D. Relationship between Incidence and Prevalence

Figure 2-1 provides data from the U.S. Centers for Disease Control and Prevention (CDC) to illustrate the complex relationship between incidence and prevalence. It uses the example of AIDS in the United States from 1981, when it was

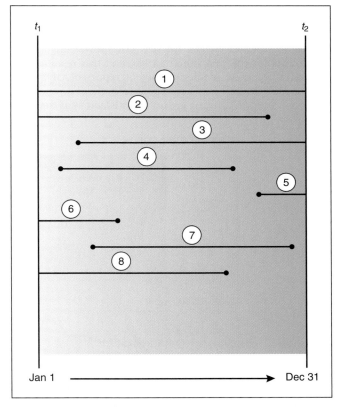

Figure 2-2 Illustration of several concepts in morbidity. Lines indicate when eight persons became ill (start of a line) and when they recovered or died (end of a line) between the beginning of a year (t_1) and the end of the same year ($\pm t_2$). Each person is assigned a case number, which is circled in this figure. Point prevalence: $t_1 = 4$ and $t_2 = 3$; period prevalence = 8. (Based on Dorn HF: A classification system for morbidity concepts. *Public Health Rep* 72:1043–1048, 1957.)

first recognized, through 1992, after which the definition of AIDS underwent a major change. Because AIDS is a clinical syndrome, the present discussion addresses the prevalence of AIDS, rather than the prevalence of its causal agent, human immunodeficiency virus (HIV) infection.

In Figure 2-1, the full height of each year's bar shows the total number of new AIDS cases reported to the CDC for that year. The darkened part of each bar shows the number of people in whom AIDS was diagnosed in that year, and who were known to be dead by December 31, 1992. The clear space in each bar represents the number of people in whom AIDS was diagnosed in that year, and who presumably were still alive on December 31, 1992. The sum of the clear areas represents the **prevalent cases** of AIDS as of the last day of 1992. Of the people in whom AIDS was diagnosed between 1990 and 1992 and who had had the condition for a relatively short time, a fairly high proportion were still alive at the cutoff date. Their survival resulted from the recency of their infection and from improved treatment. However, almost all people in whom AIDS was diagnosed during the first 6 years of the epidemic had died by that date.

The total number of cases of an epidemic disease reported over time is its **cumulative incidence.** According to the CDC, the cumulative incidence of AIDS in the United States through December 31, 1991, was 206,392, and the number known to have died was 133,232.[2] At the close of 1991, there were 73,160 prevalent cases of AIDS (206,392 − 133,232). If these people with AIDS died in subsequent years, they would be removed from the category of prevalent cases.

On January 1, 1993, the CDC made a major change in the criteria for defining AIDS. A backlog of patients whose disease manifestations met the new criteria was included in the counts for the first time in 1993, and this resulted in a sudden, huge spike in the number of reported AIDS cases (Fig. 2-3). Because of this change in criteria and reporting, the more recent AIDS data are not as satisfactory as the older

data for illustrating the relationship between incidence and prevalence. Nevertheless, Figure 2-3 provides a vivid illustration of the importance of a consistent definition of a disease in making accurate comparisons of trends in rates over time.

Prevalence is the result of many factors: the periodic (annual) number of new cases; the immigration and emigration of persons with the disease; and the average duration of the disease, which is defined as the time from its onset until death or healing. The following is an approximate general formula for prevalence that cannot be used for detailed scientific estimation, but that is conceptually important for understanding and predicting the **burden of disease** on a society or population:

$$\text{Prevalence} = \text{Incidence} \times (\text{average}) \text{ Duration}$$

This conceptual formula works only if the incidence of the disease and its duration in individuals are stable for an extended time. The formula implies that the prevalence of a disease can increase as a result of an increase in the following:

- Yearly numbers of new cases
  or
- Length of time that symptomatic patients survive before dying (or recovering, if that is possible)

In the specific case of AIDS, its incidence in the United States is declining, whereas the duration of life for people with AIDS is increasing as a result of antiviral agents and other methods of treatment and prophylaxis. These methods have increased the length of survival proportionately more than the decline in incidence, so that prevalent cases of AIDS continue to increase in the United States. This increase in prevalence has led to an increase in the burden of patient care in terms of demand on the health care system and dollar cost to society.

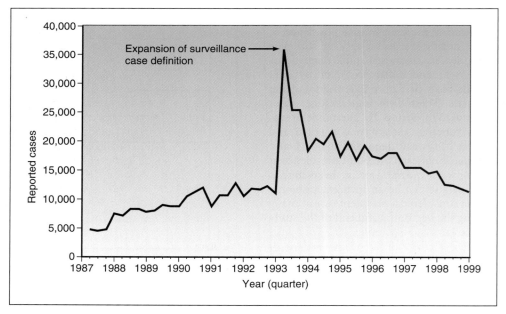

Figure 2-3 **Incident cases of AIDS in United States, by quarter of report, 1987-1999.** Statistics include cases from Guam, Puerto Rico, the U.S. Pacific Islands, and the U.S. Virgin Islands. On January 1, 1993, the CDC changed the criteria for defining AIDS. The expansion of the surveillance case definition resulted in a huge spike in the number of reported cases. (From Centers for Disease Control and Prevention: Summary of notifiable diseases—United States, 1998. MMWR 47:20, 1999.)

A similar situation exists with regard to cardiovascular disease. Its age-specific incidence has been declining in the United States in recent decades, but its prevalence has not. As advances in technology and pharmacotherapy forestall death, people live longer with disease.

II. RISK

A. Definition

In epidemiology, **risk** is defined as the proportion of persons who are unaffected at the beginning of a study period, but who experience a **risk event** during the study period. The risk event may be death, disease, or injury, and the people at risk for the event at the beginning of the study period constitute a **cohort.** If an investigator follows everyone in a cohort for several years, the denominator for the risk of an event does not change (unless people are lost to follow-up). In a cohort, the denominator for a 5-year risk of death or disease is the same as for a 1-year risk, because in both situations the denominator is the number of persons counted at the beginning of the study.

Care is needed when applying actual risk estimates (which are derived from populations) to individuals. If death, disease, or injury occurs in an individual, the person's risk is 100%. As an example, the best way to approach patients' questions regarding the risk related to surgery is probably *not* to give them a number (e.g., "Your chances of survival are 99%"). They might then worry whether they would be in the 1% group or the 99% group. Rather, it is better to put the risk of surgery in the context of the many other risks they may take frequently, such as the risks involved in a long automobile trip.

B. Limitations of the Concept of Risk

Often it is difficult to be sure of the correct denominator for a measure of risk. Who is truly at risk? Only women are at risk for becoming pregnant, but even this statement must be modified, because for practical purposes, only women aged 15 to 44 years are likely to become pregnant. Even in this group, some proportion is not at risk because they use birth control, do not engage in heterosexual relations, have had a hysterectomy, or are sterile for other reasons.

Ideally, for risk related to infectious disease, only the **susceptible population**—that is, people without antibody protection—would be counted in the denominator. However, antibody levels are usually unknown. As a practical compromise, the denominator usually consists of either the total population of an area or the people in an age group who probably lack antibodies.

Expressing the risk of death from an infectious disease, although seemingly simple, is quite complex. This is because such a risk is the product of many different proportions, as can be seen in Figure 2-4. Numerous **subsets of the population** must be considered. People who **die** of an infectious disease are a subset of people who are **ill** from the disease, who are a subset of the people who are **infected** by the disease agent, who are a subset of the people who are **exposed** to the infection, who are a subset of the people who are **susceptible** to the infection, who are a subset of the **total population.**

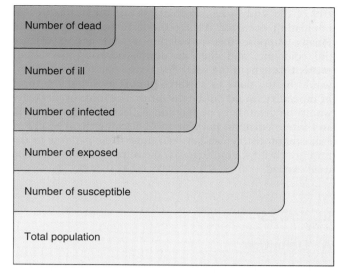

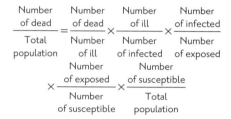

Figure 2-4 **Graphic representation of why the death rate from an infectious disease is the product of many proportions.** The formula may be viewed as follows:

$$\frac{\text{Number of dead}}{\text{Total population}} = \frac{\text{Number of dead}}{\text{Number of ill}} \times \frac{\text{Number of ill}}{\text{Number of infected}} \times \frac{\text{Number of infected}}{\text{Number of exposed}}$$
$$\times \frac{\text{Number of exposed}}{\text{Number of susceptible}} \times \frac{\text{Number of susceptible}}{\text{Total population}}$$

If each of the five fractions to the right of the equal sign were 0.5, the persons who were dead would represent 50% of those who were ill, 25% of those who were infected, 12.5% of those who were exposed, 6.25% of those who were susceptible, and 3.125% of the total population.

The proportion of clinically ill persons who die is the **case fatality ratio;** the higher this ratio, the more **virulent** the infection. The proportion of infected persons who are clinically ill is often called the **pathogenicity** of the organism. The proportion of exposed persons who become infected is sometimes called the **infectiousness** of the organism, but infectiousness is also influenced by the conditions of exposure. A full understanding of the epidemiology of an infectious disease would require knowledge of all the ratios shown in Figure 2-4. Analogous characterizations may be applied to noninfectious disease.

The concept of risk has other limitations, which can be understood through the following thought experiment. Assume that three different populations of the same size and age distribution (e.g., three nursing homes with no new patients during the study period) have the same overall risk of death (e.g., 10%) in the same year (e.g., from January 1 to December 31 in year X). Despite their similarity in risk, the deaths in the three populations may occur in very different patterns over time. Suppose that population A suffered a serious influenza epidemic in January (the beginning of the study year), and that most of those who died that year did so in the first month of the year. Suppose that the influenza epidemic did not hit population B until December (the end of the study year), so that most of the deaths in that population occurred during the last month of the year. Finally, suppose that population C did not experience the epidemic, and that its deaths occurred (as usual) evenly throughout the year. The 1-year risk of death (10%) would be the *same* in all three populations, but the **force of mortality** would not be the same. The force of mortality would be greatest in population A, least in population B, and intermediate in population C. Because the measure of risk cannot distinguish between these three patterns in the timing of deaths, a more precise measure—the rate—may be used instead.

III. RATES

A. Definition

A *rate* is the number of events that occur in a defined time period, divided by the *average* number of people at risk for the event during the period under study. Because the population at the middle of the period can usually be considered a good estimate of the average number of people at risk during that period, the midperiod population is often used as the denominator of a rate. The formal structure of a rate is described in the following equation:

$$Rate = \frac{Numerator}{Denominator} \times Constant\ multiplier$$

Risks and rates usually have values less than 1 unless the event of interest can occur repeatedly, as with colds or asthma attacks. However, decimal fractions are awkward to think about and discuss, especially if we try to imagine fractions of a death (e.g., "one one-thousandth of a death per year"). Rates are usually multiplied by a **constant multiplier**—100, 1000, 10,000, or 100,000—to make the numerator larger than 1 and thus easier to discuss (e.g., "one death per thousand people per year"). When a constant multiplier is used, the numerator and the denominator are multiplied by the same number, so the value of the ratio is not changed.

The **crude death rate** illustrates why a constant multiplier is used. In 2011, this rate for the United States was estimated as 0.00838 per year. However, most people find it easier to multiply this fraction by 1000 and express it as 8.38 deaths per 1000 individuals in the population per year. The general form for calculating the rate in this case is as follows:

Crude death rate =

$$\frac{No.\ deaths\,(same\ place\ and\ time\ period)}{Midperiod\ population\,(same\ place\ and\ time\ period)} \times 1000$$

Rates can be thought of in the same way as the velocity of a car. It is possible to talk about **average rates** or average velocity for a period of time. The average velocity is obtained by dividing the miles traveled (e.g., 55) by the time required (e.g., 1 hour), in which case the car averaged 55 miles per hour. This does not mean that the car was traveling at exactly 55 miles per hour for every instant during that hour. In a similar manner, the average rate of an event (e.g., death) is equal to the total number of events for a defined time (e.g., 1 year) divided by the average population exposed to that event (e.g., 12 deaths per 1000 persons per year).

A rate, as with a velocity, also can be understood as describing reality at an instant in time, in which case the death rate can be expressed as an **instantaneous death rate** or **hazard rate**. Because death is a discrete event rather than a continuous function, however, instantaneous rates cannot actually be measured; they can only be estimated. (Note that the rates discussed in this book are average rates unless otherwise stated.)

B. Relationship between Risk and Rate

In an example presented in section II.B, populations A, B, and C were similar in size, and each had a 10% overall risk of death in the same year, but their patterns of death differed greatly. Figure 2-5 shows the three different patterns and illustrates how, in this example, the concept of rate is superior to the concept of risk in showing differences in the force of mortality.

Because most of the deaths in population A occurred before July 1, the midyear population of this cohort would be the smallest of the three, and the resulting death rate would be the highest (because the denominator is the smallest and the numerator is the same size for all three populations). In contrast, because most of the deaths in population B occurred at the end of the year, the midyear population of this cohort would be the largest of the three, and the death rate would be the lowest. For population C, both the number of deaths before July 1 and the death rate would be intermediate between those of A and B. Although the 1-year risk for these three populations did not show differences in the force of mortality, cohort-specific rates did so by reflecting more accurately the timing of the deaths in the three populations. This quantitative result agrees with the graph and with intuition, because if we assume that the quality of life was reasonably good, most people would prefer to be in population B. More days of life are lived by those in population B during the year, because of the lower force of mortality.

Rates are often used to estimate risk. A rate is a good approximation of risk if the:

- Event in the numerator occurs only once per individual during the study interval.
- Proportion of the population affected by the event is small (e.g., <5%).
- Time interval is relatively short.

If the time interval is long or the percentage of people who are affected is large, the rate is noticeably larger than the risk. If the event in the numerator occurs more than once during the study—as can happen with colds, ear infections, or asthma attacks—a related statistic called **incidence density** (discussed later) should be used instead of rate.

In a cohort study, the denominator for a 5-year risk is the same as the denominator for a 1-year risk. However, the denominator for a rate is constantly changing. It decreases as some people die and others emigrate from the population, and it increases as some immigrate and others are born. In most real populations, all four of these changes—birth, death, immigration, and emigration—are occurring at the same time. The rate reflects these changes by using the midperiod population as an estimate of the average population at risk.

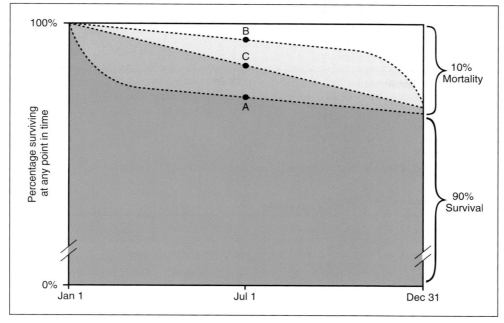

Figure 2-5 Circumstances under which the concept of rate is superior to the concept of risk. Assume that populations *A*, *B*, and *C* are three different populations of the same size; that 10% of each population died in a given year; and that most of the deaths in population *A* occurred early in the year, most of the deaths in population *B* occurred late in the year, and the deaths in population *C* were evenly distributed throughout the year. In all three populations, the risk of death would be the same—10%—even though the patterns of death differed greatly. The rate of death, which is calculated using the midyear population as the denominator, would be the highest in population *A*, the lowest in population *B*, and intermediate in population *C*, reflecting the relative magnitude of the force of mortality in the three populations.

C. Quantitative Relationship between Risk and Rate

As noted earlier, a rate may be a good approximation of a risk if the time interval under study is short. If the time interval is long, the rate is higher than the risk because the rate's denominator is progressively reduced by the number of risk events (e.g., deaths) that occur up to the midperiod. When the rate and risk are both small, the difference between the rate and the corresponding risk is also small. These principles can be shown by examining the relationship between the **mortality rate** and the **mortality risk** in population C in Figure 2-5. Population C had an even mortality risk throughout the year and a total yearly mortality risk of 10%. By the middle of the year, death had occurred in 5%. The mortality rate would be 0.10/(1 − 0.05) = 0.10/0.95 = 0.1053 = 105.3 per 1000 persons per year. In this example, the denominator is 0.95 because 95% of population C was still living at midyear to form the denominator. The yearly rate is higher than the yearly risk because the **average population at risk** is smaller than the **initial population at risk**.

What would be the **cumulative mortality risk** for population C at the end of 2 years, assuming a **constant yearly mortality rate** of 0.1053? It cannot be calculated by simply multiplying 2 years times the yearly risk of 10%, because the number still living and subject to the force of mortality by the beginning of the second year would be smaller (i.e., it would be 90% of the original population). Likewise, the cumulative risk of death over 10 years cannot be calculated by simply multiplying 10 years times 10%. This would mean that 100% of population C would be dead after one decade, yet intuition suggests that at least some of the population would live more than 10 years. In fact, if the mortality rate

remained constant, the cumulative risks at 2 years, 5 years, 10 years, and 15 years would be 19%, 41%, 65%, and 79%. Box 2-1 describes a straightforward way to determine the cumulative risk for any number of years, and the calculations can be done easily on most handheld calculators.

D. Criteria for Valid Use of the Term *Rate*

To be valid, a rate must meet certain criteria with respect to the correspondence between numerator and denominator. First, all the events counted in the numerator must have happened to persons in the denominator. Second, all the persons counted in the denominator must have been at risk for the events in the numerator. For example, the denominator of a cervical cancer rate should contain no men.

Before comparisons of rates can be made, the following must also be true: The numerators for all groups being compared must be defined or diagnosed in the same way; the constant multipliers being used must be the same; and the time intervals must be the same. These criteria may seem obvious, but it is easy to overlook them when making comparisons over time or between populations. For example, numerators may not be easy to compare if the quality of medical diagnosis differs over time. In the late 1800s, there was no diagnostic category called *myocardial infarction*, but many persons were dying of *acute indigestion*. By 1930, the situation was reversed: Almost nobody died of acute indigestion, but many died of myocardial infarction. It might be tempting to say that the acute indigestion of the late 1800s was really myocardial infarction, but there is no certainty that this is true. Another example of the problems implicit in studying causes of disease over time relates to changes in commonly used classification systems. In 1948, there was a

| Box 2-1 | Calculation of Cumulative Mortality Risk in a Population with a Constant Yearly Mortality Rate |

PART 1 Beginning Data (see Fig. 2-5)

Population C in Figure 2-5 had an even mortality risk throughout the year and a total yearly **mortality risk** of 10%. By the middle of the year, death had occurred in 5%. The **mortality rate** would be $0.10/(1 - 0.05) = 0.10/0.95 = 0.1053 = 105.3$ per 1000 persons per year. If this rate of 0.1053 remained constant, what would be the cumulative mortality risk at the end of 2 years, 5 years, 10 years, and 15 years?

PART 2 Formula

$$R(t) = 1 - e^{-\mu t},$$

where R = risk; t = number of years of interest; e = the base for natural logarithms; and μ = the mortality rate.

PART 3 Calculation of the Cumulative 2-Year Risk

$$R(2) = 1 - e^{-(0.1053)(2)}$$
$$= 1 - e^{-0.2106}$$

Exponentiate the second term (i.e., take the anti–natural logarithm, or anti-ln, of the second term)

$$= 1 - 0.8101$$
$$= 0.1899$$
$$= \textbf{19\% risk} \text{ of death in 2 years}$$

PART 4 Calculation of Cumulative Risks on a Handheld Calculator

To calculate cumulative risks on a handheld calculator, the calculator must have a key for natural logarithms (i.e., a key for logarithms to the base $e = 2.7183$). The logarithm key is labeled "ln" (not "log," which is a key for logarithms to the base 10).

Begin by entering the number of years (t), which in the above example is 2. Multiply the number by the mortality rate (μ), which is 0.1053. The product is 0.2106. Hit the "+/−" button to change the sign to negative. Then hit the "INV" (inverse) button and the "ln" (natural log) button. The result at this point is 0.810098. Hit the "M in" (memory) button to put this result in memory. Clear the register. Then enter 1 − "MR" (memory recall) and hit the "=" button. The result should be 0.189902. Rounded off, this is the same 2-year risk shown above (19%).

Calculations for 5-year, 10-year, and 15-year risks can be made in the same way, yielding the following results:

No. Years	Cumulative Risk of Death
1	0.100 (10%)
2	0.190 (19%)
5	0.409 (41%)
10	0.651 (65%)
15	0.794 (79%)

As these results show, the cumulative risk cannot be calculated or accurately estimated by merely multiplying the number of the years by the 1-year risk. If it could, at 10 years, the risk would be 100%, rather than 65%. The results shown here are based on a constant mortality rate. Because in reality the mortality rate increases with time (particularly for an older population), the longer-term calculations are not as useful as the shorter-term calculations. The techniques described here are most useful for calculating a population's cumulative risks for intervals of up to 5 years.

major revision in the *International Classification of Diseases* (ICD), the international coding manual for classifying diagnoses. This revision of the ICD was followed by sudden, major changes in the reported numbers and rates of many diseases.

It is difficult not only to track changes in causes of death over time, but also to make accurate comparisons of cause-specific rates of disease between populations, especially populations in different countries. Residents of different countries have different degrees of access to medical care, different levels in the quality of medical care available to them, and different styles of diagnosis. It is not easy to determine how much of any apparent difference is real, and how much is caused by variation in medical care and diagnostic styles.

E. Specific Types of Rates

The concepts of incidence (incident cases) and prevalence (prevalent cases) were discussed earlier. With the concept of a rate now reviewed, it is appropriate to define different types of rates, which are usually developed for large populations and used for public health purposes.

1. Incidence Rate

The incidence rate is calculated as the number of incident cases over a defined study period, divided by the population at risk at the midpoint of that study period. An incidence rate is usually expressed per 1000, per 10,000, or per 100,000 population.

2. Prevalence Rate

The so-called prevalence rate is actually a proportion and not a rate. The term is in common use, however, and is used here to indicate the proportion (usually expressed as a percentage) of persons with a defined disease or condition at the time they are studied. The 2009 Behavioral Risk Factor Survey reported that the prevalence rate for self-report of physician-diagnosed arthritis varied from a low of 20.3% in California to a high of 35.6% in Kentucky.[3]

Prevalence rates can be applied to risk factors, to knowledge, and to diseases or other conditions. In selected states, the prevalence rate of rarely or never using seat belts among high school students varied from 4% in Utah to 17.2% in North Dakota.[2] Likewise, the percentage of people recognizing stroke signs and symptoms in a 17-state study varied from 63.3% for some signs to 94.1% for others.[3]

3. Incidence Density

Incidence density refers to the number of new events per *person-time* (e.g., per person-months or person-years). Suppose that three patients were followed after tonsillectomy and adenoidectomy for recurrent ear infections. If one patient was followed for 13 months, one for 20 months, and one for 17 months, and if 5 ear infections occurred in these 3 patients during this time, the incidence density would be 5 infections per 50 person-months of follow-up or 10 infections per 100 person-months.

Incidence density is especially useful when the event of interest (e.g., colds, otitis media, myocardial infarction) can occur in a person more than once during the study period. For methods of statistical comparison of two incidence densities, see Chapter 11.

IV. SPECIAL ISSUES ON USE OF RATES

Rates or risks are typically used to make one of three types of comparison. The first type is a comparison of an observed rate (or risk) with a target rate (or risk). For example, the United States set national health goals for 2020, including the expected rates of various types of death, such as the infant mortality rate. When the final 2020 statistics are published, the observed rates for the nation and for subgroups will be compared with the target objectives set by the government.

The second type is a comparison of two different populations *at the same time*. This is probably the most common type. One example involves comparing the rates of death or disease in two different countries, states, or ethnic groups for the same year. Another example involves comparing the results in treatment groups to the results in control groups participating in randomized clinical trials. A major research concern is to ensure that the two populations are not only similar but also measured in exactly the same way.

The third type is a comparison involving the same population *at different times*. This approach is used to study time trends. Because there also are trends over time in the composition of a population (e.g., increasing proportion of elderly people in U.S. population), adjustments must be made for such changes before concluding that there are real differences over time in the rates under study. Changes over

time (usually improvement) in diagnostic capabilities must also be taken into account.

A. Crude Rates versus Specific Rates

There are three broad categories of rates: crude, specific, and standardized. Rates that apply to an entire population, without reference to any characteristics of the individuals in it, are **crude rates.** The term *crude* simply means that the data are presented without any processing or adjustment. When a population is divided into more homogeneous subgroups based on a particular characteristic of interest (e.g., age, sex/gender, race, risk factors, or comorbidity), and rates are calculated within these groups, the result is **specific rates** (e.g., age-specific rates, gender-specific rates). Standardized rates are discussed in the next section.

Crude rates are valid, but they are often misleading. Here is a quick challenge: Try to guess which of the following three countries—Sweden, Ecuador, or the United States—has the highest and lowest crude death rate. Those who guessed that Ecuador has the highest and Sweden the lowest have the sequence exactly reversed. Table 2-1 lists the estimated crude death rates and the corresponding life expectancy at birth. For 2011, Ecuador had the lowest crude death rate and Sweden the highest, even though Ecuador had the highest age-specific mortality rates and the shortest life expectancy, and Sweden had just the reverse.

Table 2-1 Crude Death Rate and Life Expectancy for Three Countries (2011 estimate)

Country	Crude Death Rate	Life Expectancy at Birth
Ecuador	5.0 per 1000	75.73 years
United States	8.4 per 1000	78.37 years
Sweden	10.2 per 1000	81.07 years

Data from CIA Factbook, under the name of the country. http://www.cia.gov/library/publications/the-world-factbook/

This apparent anomaly occurs primarily because the crude death rates do not take age into account. For a population with a young age distribution, such as Ecuador (median age 26 years), the birth rate is likely to be relatively high, and the crude death rate is likely to be relatively low, although the **age-specific death rates** (ASDRs) for each age group may be high. In contrast, for an older population, such as Sweden, a low crude birth rate and a high crude death rate would be expected. This is because age has such a profound influence on the force of mortality that an old population, even if it is relatively healthy, inevitably has a high overall death rate, and vice versa. The huge impact of age on death rates can be seen in Figure 2-6, which shows data on probability of death at different ages in the United States in 2001. As a general principle, investigators should never make comparisons of the risk of death or disease between populations without controlling for age (and sometimes for other characteristics as well).

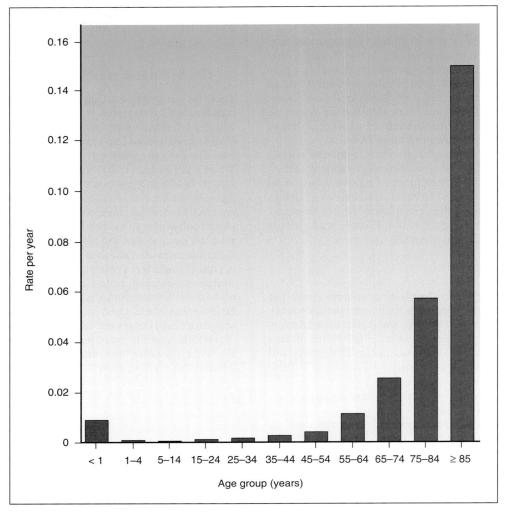

Figure 2-6 **Age-specific death rates (ASDRs) for deaths from all causes—United States, 2001.** Graph illustrates the profound impact of age on death rates. (Data from National Center for Health Statistics: *Natl Vital Stat Rep* 52(3), 2003. Recent data can be found at www.cdc.gov/nchs/data/nvsr/.)

Why not avoid crude rates altogether and use specific rates? There are many circumstances when it is not possible to use specific rates if the:

- Frequency of the event of interest (i.e., the numerator) is unknown for the subgroups of a population.
- Size of the subgroups (i.e., the denominator) is unknown.
- Numbers of people at risk for the event are too small to provide stable estimates of the specific rates.

If the number of people at risk is large in each of the subgroups of interest, however, specific rates provide the most information, and these should be sought whenever possible.

Although the biasing effect of age can be controlled for in several ways, the simplest (and usually the best) method is to calculate the ASDRs, so that the rates can be compared in similar age groups. The formula is as follows:

Age-specific death rate =

$$\frac{\text{No. deaths to people in a particular}}{\substack{\text{age group (defined place and time period)}\\ \text{Midperiod population}\\ \text{(same age group, place, and time period)}}} \times 1000$$

Crude death rates are the sum of the ASDRs in each of the age groups, weighted by the relative size of each age group. The underlying formula for any summary rate is as follows:

$$\text{Summary rate} = \Sigma w_i r_i$$

where w_i = the individual weights (proportions) of each age-specific group, and r_i = the rates for the corresponding age group. This formula is useful for understanding why crude rates can be misleading. In studies involving two age-specific populations, a difference in the relative weights (sizes) of the old and young populations will result in different weights for the high and low ASDRs, and no fair comparison can be made. This general principle applies not only to demography and population epidemiology, where investigators are interested in comparing the rates of large groups, but also to clinical epidemiology, where investigators may want to compare the risks or rates of two patient groups who have different proportions of severely ill, moderately ill, and mildly ill patients.[4]

A similar problem occurs when investigators want to compare death rates in different hospitals to measure the quality of care. To make fair comparisons among hospitals, investigators must make some adjustment for differences in the types and severity of illness and surgery in the patients who are treated. Otherwise, the hospitals that care for the sickest patients would be at an unfair disadvantage in such a comparison.

B. Standardization of Death Rates

Standardized rates, also known as **adjusted rates,** are crude rates that have been modified (adjusted) to control for the effects of age or other characteristics and allow valid comparisons of rates. To obtain a summary death rate that is free from age bias, investigators can age-standardize (age-adjust) the crude rates by a direct or indirect method. Standardization is usually applied to death rates, but it may be used to adjust any type of rate.

I. Direct Standardization

Direct standardization is the most common method to remove the biasing effect of differing age structures in different populations. In direct standardization, the ASDRs of the populations to be compared are applied to a single, standard population. This is done by multiplying each ASDR from each population under comparison by the number of persons in the corresponding age group in the standard population. Because the age structure of the standard population is the same for all the death rates applied to it, the distorting effect of different age distributions in the real

populations is eliminated. Overall death rates can then be compared without age bias.

The standard population may be any real (or realistic) population. In practice, it is often a larger population that contains the subpopulations to be compared. For example, the death rates of two cities in the same state can be compared by using the state's population as the standard population. Likewise, the death rates of states may be compared by using the U.S. population as the standard.

The direct method shows the total number of deaths that *would have occurred* in the standard population *if* the ASDRs of the individual populations were applied. The total expected number of deaths from each of the comparison populations is divided by the standard population to give a standardized *crude* death rate, which may be compared with any other death rate that has been standardized in the same way. The direct method may also be applied to compare incidence rates of disease or injury as well as death.

Standardized rates are *fictitious.* They are "what if" rates only, but they do allow investigators to make fairer comparisons of death rates than would be possible with crude rates. Box 2-2 shows a simplified example in which two populations, A and B, are divided into "young," "middle-aged," and "older" subgroups, and the ASDR for each age group in population B is twice as high as that for the corresponding age group in population A. In this example, the standard population is simply the sum of the two populations being compared. Population A has a higher overall crude death rate

---

Box 2-2 | **Direct Standardization of Crude Death Rates of Two Populations, Using the Combined Weights as the Standard Population (Fictitious Data)**

PART I Calculation of Crude Death Rates

| | Population A | | | | | Population B | | | | |
Age Group	Population Size		Age-Specific Death Rate		Expected No. Deaths	Population Size		Age-Specific Death Rate		Expected No. Deaths
Young	1000	×	0.001	=	1	4000	×	0.002	=	8
Middle-aged	5000	×	0.010	=	50	5000	×	0.020	=	100
Older	4000	×	0.100	=	400	1000	×	0.200	=	200
Total	10,000				451	10,000				308
Crude death rate					$\frac{451}{10,000} = 4.51\%$					$\frac{308}{10,000} = 3.08\%$

PART 2 Direct Standardization Rates of the Above Crude Death Rates, with the Two Populations Combined to Form the Standard Weights

| | Population A | | | | | Population B | | | | |
Age Group	Population Size		Age-Specific Death Rate		Expected No. Deaths	Population Size		Age-Specific Death Rate		Expected No. Deaths
Young	5000	×	0.001	=	5	5000	×	0.002	=	10
Middle-aged	10,000	×	0.010	=	100	10,000	×	0.020	=	200
Older	5000	×	0.100	=	500	5000	×	0.200	=	1000
Total	20,000				605	20,000				1210
Standardized death rate					$\frac{605}{20,000} = 3.03\%$					$\frac{1210}{20,000} = 6.05\%$

(4.51%) than population B (3.08%), despite the ASDRs in B being twice the ASDRs in A. After the death rates are standardized, the adjusted death rate for population B correctly reflects the fact that its ASDRs are twice as high as those of population A.

2. Indirect Standardization

Indirect standardization is used if ASDRs are unavailable in the population whose crude death rate needs to be adjusted. It is also used if the population to be standardized is small, such that ASDRs become statistically unstable. The indirect method uses **standard rates** and applies them to the known age groups (or other specified groups) in the population to be standardized.

Suppose that an investigator wanted to see whether the death rates in a given year for male employees of a particular company, such as workers in an offshore oil rig, were similar to or greater than the death rates for all men in the U.S. population. To start, the investigator would need the observed crude death rate and the ASDRs for all U.S. men for a similar year. These would serve as the **standard death rates.** Next, the investigator would determine the number of male workers in each of the age categories used for the U.S. male

population. The investigator would then determine the observed total deaths for 1 year for all the male workers in the company.

The first step for indirect standardization is to multiply the standard death rate for each age group in the standard population by the number of workers in the corresponding age group in the company. This gives the number of deaths that would be *expected* in each age group of workers if they had the same death rates as the standard population. The expected numbers of worker deaths for the various age groups are then summed to obtain the total number of deaths that would be expected in the entire worker group, if the ASDRs for company workers were the same as the ASDRs for the standard population. Next, the total number of *observed* deaths among the workers is divided by the total number of *expected* deaths among the workers to obtain a value known as the **standardized mortality ratio** (SMR). Lastly, the SMR is multiplied by 100 to eliminate fractions, so that the expected mortality rate in the standard population equals 100. If the employees in this example had an SMR of 140, it would mean that their mortality was 40% greater than would be expected on the basis of the ASDRs of the standard population. Box 2-3 presents an example of indirect standardization.

| Box 2-3 | Indirect Standardization of Crude Death Rate for Men in a Company, Using the Age-Specific Death Rates for Men in a Standard Population (Fictitious Data) |

PART 1 Beginning Data

	Men in Standard Population				Men in Company		
Age Group	Proportion of Standard Population		Age-Specific Death Rate	Observed Death Rate	No. Workers	Age-Specific Death Rate	Observed No. Deaths
Young	0.40	×	0.001 =	0.00004	2000	× ? =	?
Middle-aged	0.30	×	0.010 =	0.00030	3000	× ? =	?
Older	0.30	×	0.100 =	0.00300	5000	× ? =	?
Total	1.00			0.00334	10,000		
Observed death rate	0.00334, or 334/100,000				48/10,000, or 480/100,000		

PART 2 Calculation of Expected Death Rate, Using Indirect Standardization of Above Rates and Applying Age-Specific Death Rates from the Standard Population to the Numbers of Workers in the Company

	Men in Standard Population				Men in Company		
Age Group	Proportion of Standard Population		Age-Specific Death Rate	Observed Death Rate	No. Workers	Age-Specific Death Rate	Observed No. Deaths
Young	0.40	×	0.001 =	0.00004	2000	× 0.0001 =	0.2
Middle-aged	0.30	×	0.010 =	0.00030	3000	× 0.0010 =	3.0
Older	0.30	×	0.100 =	0.00300	5000	× 0.0100 =	50.0
Total	1.00			0.00334	10,000		53.2
Expected death rate						53.2/10,000, or 532/100,000	

PART 3 Calculation of Standardized Mortality Ratio (SMR)

SMR = Observed death rate for men in the company/Expected death rate for men in the company × 100

= 0.00480/0.00532 × 100

= (0.90)(100) = 90

= Men in the company actually had a death rate that was only 90% of the standard population.

C. Cause-Specific Rates

Remember that rates refer to events in the numerator, occurring to a population in the denominator. To compare the rates of events among comparable populations, the denominators must be made comparable. For example, making rates gender or age specific would allow a comparison of events among groups of men or women or among people in a certain age bracket. Because the numerator describes the specific events that are occurring, the numerators are comparable when rates are cause specific. A particular event (e.g., gunshot wound, myocardial infarction) could be compared among differing populations. Comparing cause-specific death rates over time or between countries is often risky, however, because of possible differences in diagnostic style or efficiency. In countries with inadequate medical care, 10% to 20% of deaths may be diagnosed as "symptoms, signs, and ill-defined conditions." Similar uncertainties may also apply to people who die without adequate medical care in more developed countries.[5]

Cause-specific death rates have the following general form:

Cause-specific death rate =

$$\frac{\begin{array}{c}\text{No. deaths due to a particular cause} \\ \text{(defined place and time period)}\end{array}}{\begin{array}{c}\text{Midperiod population} \\ \text{(same place and time period)}\end{array}} \times 100,000$$

Table 2-2 provides data on the leading causes of death in the United States for 1950 and 2000, as reported by the National Center for Health Statistics (NCHS) and based on the underlying cause of death indicated on death certificates. These data are rarely accurate enough for epidemiologic studies of causal factors,[6] but are useful for understanding the relative importance of different disease groups and for studying trends in causes of death over time. For example, the table shows that age-specific rates for deaths caused by

cardiac disease and cerebrovascular disease are less than half of what they were in 1950, whereas rates for deaths caused by malignant neoplasms have remained almost steady.

V. COMMONLY USED RATES THAT REFLECT MATERNAL AND INFANT HEALTH

Many of the rates used in public health, especially the infant mortality rate, reflect the health of mothers and infants. The terms relating to the reproductive process are especially important to understand.

A. Definitions of Terms

The international definition of a **live birth** is the delivery of a product of conception that shows any sign of life after complete removal from the mother. A **sign of life** may consist of a breath or a cry, any spontaneous movement, a pulse or a heartbeat, or pulsation of the umbilical cord.

Fetal deaths are categorized as early, intermediate, or late. An **early fetal death,** commonly known as a **miscarriage,** occurs when a dead fetus is delivered within the first 20 weeks of gestation. According to international agreements, an **intermediate fetal death** is one in which a dead fetus is delivered between 20 and 28 weeks of gestation. A fetus born dead at 28 weeks of gestation or later is a **late fetal death,** commonly known as a **stillbirth.** An **infant death** is the death of a live-born infant before the infant's first birthday. A **neonatal death** is the death of a live-born infant before the completion of the infant's 28th day of life. A **postneonatal death** is the death of an infant after the 28th day of life but before the first birthday.

B. Definitions of Specific Types of Rates

1. Crude Birth Rate

The crude birth rate is the number of live births divided by the midperiod population, as follows:

$$\text{Crude birth rate} = \frac{\begin{array}{c}\text{No. live births} \\ \text{(defined place and time period)}\end{array}}{\begin{array}{c}\text{Midperiod population} \\ \text{(same place and time period)}\end{array}} \times 1000$$

2. Infant Mortality Rate

Because the health of infants is unusually sensitive to maternal health practices (especially maternal nutrition and use of tobacco, alcohol, and drugs), environmental factors, and the quality of health services, the infant mortality rate (IMR) is often used as an overall index of the health status of a nation. This rate has the added advantage of being both age specific and available for most countries. The numerator and the denominator of the IMR are obtained from the same type of data collection system (i.e., vital statistics reporting), so in areas where infant deaths are reported, births are also likely to be reported, and in areas where reporting is poor, births and deaths are equally likely to be affected. The formula for the IMR is as follows:

Table 2-2 **Age-Adjusted (Age-Standardized) Death Rates for Select Causes of Death in the United States, 1950 and 2000**

Cause of Death	Age-Adjusted Death Rate per 100,000 per Year*	
	1950	2000
Cardiac diseases	586.8	257.6
Malignant neoplasms	193.9	199.6
Cerebrovascular disease	180.7	60.9
Unintentional injuries	78.0	34.9
Influenza and pneumonia	48.1	23.7
Diabetes	23.1	25.0
Suicide	13.2	10.4
Chronic liver disease and cirrhosis	11.3	9.5
Homicide	5.1	5.9
HIV disease	—	5.2
All causes	*1446*	*869*

From National Center for Health Statistics: *Health, United States, 2003,* Hyattsville, Md, 2003, NCHS.

HIV, Human immunodeficiency virus.

*The age-adjusted death rates for 1950 reflect the National Center for Health Statistics switch to the U.S. population as shown by the year 2000 Census (NCHS previously used the 1940 U.S. Census). This emphasizes that adjusted (standardized) rates are not actual rates, but rather *relative* rates based on the standard population chosen.

$$IMR = \frac{\begin{array}{c}\text{No. deaths to infants} <1 \text{ year of age} \\ \text{(defined place and time period)}\end{array}}{\begin{array}{c}\text{No. live births} \\ \text{(same place and time period)}\end{array}} \times 1000$$

Most infant deaths occur in the first week of life and are caused by prematurity or intrauterine growth retardation. Both conditions often lead to respiratory failure. Some infant deaths in the first month are caused by congenital anomalies.

A subtle point, which is seldom of concern in large populations, is that for any given year, there is not an exact correspondence between the numerator and denominator of the IMR. This is because some of the infants born in a given calendar year will not die until the following year, whereas some of the infants who die in a given year were born in the previous year. Although this lack of exact correspondence does not usually influence the IMR of a large population, it might do so in a small population. To study infant mortality in small populations, it is best to accumulate data over 3 to 5 years. For detailed epidemiologic studies of the causes of infant mortality, it is best to link each infant death with the corresponding birth.

3. Neonatal and Postneonatal Mortality Rates

Epidemiologists distinguish between neonatal and postneonatal mortality. The formulas for the rates are as follows:

$$\text{Neonatal mortality rate} = \frac{\begin{array}{c}\text{No. deaths to infants} <28 \text{ days old} \\ \text{(defined place and time period)}\end{array}}{\begin{array}{c}\text{No. live births} \\ \text{(same place and time period)}\end{array}} \times 1000$$

$$\text{Postneonatal mortality rate} = \frac{\begin{array}{c}\text{No. deaths to infants} \\ 28\text{-}365 \text{ days old} \\ \text{(defined place and time period)}\end{array}}{\begin{array}{cc}\text{No. live births} & \text{No. neonatal deaths} \\ \text{(same place and} - & \text{(same place and} \\ \text{time period)} & \text{time period)}\end{array}} \times 1000$$

The formula for the neonatal mortality rate is obvious, because it closely resembles the formula for the IMR. For the postneonatal mortality rate, however, investigators must keep in mind the criteria for a valid rate, especially the condition that all those counted in the denominator must be at risk for the numerator. Infants born alive are not at risk for dying in the postneonatal period if they die during the neonatal period. The correct denominator for the postneonatal mortality rate is the number of live births *minus* the number of neonatal deaths. When the number of neonatal deaths is small, however, as in the United States, with less than 5 per 1000 live births, the following approximate formula is adequate for most purposes:

$$\text{Approximate postneonatal mortality rate} = \\ \text{Infant mortality rate} - \text{Neonatal mortality rate}$$

As a general rule, the neonatal mortality rate reflects the quality of medical services and of maternal prenatal behavior (e.g., nutrition, smoking, alcohol, drugs), whereas the postneonatal mortality rate reflects the quality of the home environment.

4. Perinatal Mortality Rate and Ratio

The use of the IMR has its limitations, not only because the probable causes of death change rapidly as the time since birth increases, but also because the number of infants born alive is influenced by the effectiveness of prenatal care. It is conceivable that an improvement in medical care could actually increase the IMR. This would occur, for example, if the improvement in care kept very sick fetuses viable long enough to be born alive, so that they die after birth and are counted as infant deaths rather than as stillbirths. To avoid this problem, the **perinatal mortality rate** was developed. The term *perinatal* means "around the time of birth." This rate is defined slightly differently from country to country. In the United States, it is defined as follows:

$$\text{Perinatal mortality rate} = \frac{\begin{array}{cc}\text{No. stillbirths} & \text{No. deaths to} \\ \text{(defined place and} + & \text{infants} <7 \text{ days old} \\ \text{time period)} & \text{(same place and time period)}\end{array}}{\begin{array}{cc}\text{No. stillbirths} & \text{No. live births} \\ \text{(same place and} + & \text{(same place and} \\ \text{time period)} & \text{time period)}\end{array}} \times 1000$$

In the formula shown here, stillbirths are included in the numerator to capture deaths that occur around the time of birth. Stillbirths are also included in the denominator because of the criteria for a valid rate. Specifically, all fetuses that reach the 28th week of gestation are at risk for late fetal death or live birth.

An approximation of the perinatal mortality rate is the **perinatal mortality ratio**, in which the denominator does not include stillbirths. In another variation, the numerator uses neonatal deaths instead of deaths at less than 7 days of life (also called *hebdomadal* deaths). The primary use of the perinatal mortality rate is to evaluate the care of pregnant women before and during delivery, as well as the care of mothers and their infants in the immediate postpartum period.

A recent development in the study of perinatal mortality involves the concept of **perinatal periods of risk.** This approach focuses on perinatal deaths and their excess over the deaths expected in low-risk populations. Fetuses born dead with a birth weight of 500 to 1499 g constitute one group, for which *maternal health* would be investigated. Such cases are followed up to examine community and environmental factors that predispose to immaturity. Fetuses born dead with a birth weight of 1500 g or more constitute another group, for which *maternal care* is examined. For neonatal deaths involving birth weights of 1500 g or more, *care during labor and delivery* is studied. For postneonatal deaths of 1500 g or more, *infant care* is studied. Although this is a promising approach to community analysis, its ultimate value has yet to be fully established.

5. Maternal Mortality Rate

Although generally considered a *normal* biologic process, pregnancy unquestionably puts considerable strain on women and places them at risk for numerous hazards they would not usually face otherwise, such as hemorrhage, infection, and toxemia of pregnancy. Pregnancy also complicates the course of other conditions, such as heart disease, diabetes, and tuberculosis. A useful measure of the progress of a nation in providing adequate nutrition and medical care for pregnant women is the **maternal mortality rate,** calculated as follows:

$$\text{Maternal mortality rate} = \frac{\substack{\text{No. pregnancy-related deaths} \\ \text{(defined place and time period)}}}{\substack{\text{No. live births} \\ \text{(same place and time period)}}} \times 100,000$$

The equation is based on the number of **pregnancy-related** (puerperal) deaths. In cases of accidental injury or homicide, however, the death of a woman who is pregnant or has recently delivered is not usually considered "pregnancy related." Technically, the denominator of the equation should be the number of pregnancies rather than live births, but for simplicity, the number of live births is used to estimate the number of pregnancies. The constant multiplier used is typically 100,000 because in recent decades the maternal mortality rate in many developed countries has declined to less than 1 per 10,000 live births. Nevertheless, the U.S. maternal mortality rate in 2006 was 13.3 per 100,000 live births, slightly higher than 1 per 10,000. Of note, the 2006 rate was lower for white Americans (9.5) than for all other races, with African American women experiencing a much higher maternal mortality rate of 32.7 per 100,000 live births.[7]

VI. SUMMARY

Much of the data for epidemiologic studies of public health are collected routinely by various levels of government and

---

Box 2-4	Definitions of Basic Epidemiologic Concepts and Measurements

Incidence (incident cases): The frequency (number) of new occurrences of disease, injury, or death—that is, the number of transitions from well to ill, from uninjured to injured, or from alive to dead—in the study population during the time period being examined.

Point prevalence (prevalent cases): The number of persons in a defined population who had a specified disease or condition at a particular point in time, usually the time a survey was done.

Period prevalence: The number of persons who had a specified disease at any time during a specified time interval. Period prevalence is the sum of the point prevalence at the beginning of the interval plus the incidence during the interval. Because period prevalence combines incidence and prevalence, it must be used with extreme care.

Incidence density: The frequency (density) of new events per person-time (e.g., person-months or person-years). Incidence density is especially useful when the event of interest (e.g., colds, otitis media, myocardial infarction) can occur in a person more than once during the period of study.

Cohort: A clearly defined group of persons who are studied over a period of time to determine the incidence of death, disease, or injury.

Risk: The proportion of persons who are unaffected at the beginning of a study period, but who undergo the risk event (death, disease, or injury) during the study period.

Rate: The frequency (number) of new events that occur in a defined time period, divided by the average population at risk. Often, the midperiod population is used as the average number of persons at risk (see *Incidence rate*). Because a rate is almost always less than 1.0 (unless everybody dies or has the risk event), a constant multiplier is used to increase the numerator and the denominator to make the rate easier to think about and discuss.

Incidence rate: A rate calculated as the number of incident cases (see above) over a defined study period, divided by the population at risk at the midpoint of that study period. Rates of the occurrence of births, deaths, and new diseases all are forms of an incidence rate.

Prevalence rate: The proportion (usually expressed as a percentage) of a population that has a defined disease or condition at a particular point in time. Although usually called a rate, it is actually a *proportion.*

Crude rates: Rates that apply to an entire population, with no reference to characteristics of the individuals in the population. Crude rates are generally not useful for comparisons because populations may differ greatly in composition, particularly with respect to age.

Specific rates: Rates that are calculated after a population has been categorized into groups with a particular characteristic. Examples include age-specific rates and gender-specific rates. Specific rates generally are needed for valid comparisons.

Standardized (adjusted) rates: Crude rates that have been modified (adjusted) to control for the effects of age or other characteristics and allow for valid comparisons of rates.

Direct standardization: The preferred method of standardization if the specific rates come from large populations and the needed data are available. The direct method of standardizing death rates, for example, applies the age distribution of some population—the standard population—to the actual age-specific death rates of the different populations to be compared. This removes the bias that occurs if an old population is compared with a young population.

Indirect standardization: The method of standardization used when the populations to be compared are small (so that age-specific death rates are unstable) or when age-specific death rates are unavailable from one or more populations but data concerning the age distribution and the crude death rate are available. Here standard death rates (from the standard population) are applied to the corresponding age groups in the different population or populations to be studied. The result is an "expected" (standardized crude) death rate for each population under study. These "expected" values are those that would have been expected if the standard death rates had been true for the populations under study. Then the standardized mortality ratio is calculated.

Standardized mortality ratio (SMR): The observed crude death rate divided by the expected crude death rate. The SMR generally is multiplied by 100, with the standard population having a value of 100. If the SMR is greater than 100, the **force of mortality** is higher in the study population than in the standard population. If the SMR is less than 100, the force of mortality is lower in the study population than in the standard population.

Box 2-5	Equations for the Most Commonly Used Rates from Population Data

(1) Crude birth rate $= \dfrac{\text{No. live births (defined place and time period)}}{\text{Midperiod population (same place and time period)}} \times 1000$

(2) Crude death rate $= \dfrac{\text{No. deaths (defined place and time period)}}{\text{Midperiod population (same place and time period)}} \times 1000$

(3) Age-specific death rate $= \dfrac{\substack{\text{No. deaths to people in a particular age group} \\ \text{(defined place and time period)}}}{\substack{\text{Midperiod population} \\ \text{(same age group, place, and time period)}}} \times 1000$

(4) Cause-specific death rate $= \dfrac{\text{No. deaths due to a particular cause (defined place and time period)}}{\text{Midperiod population (same place and time period)}} \times 100,000$

(5) Infant mortality rate $= \dfrac{\text{No. deaths to infants <1 year old (defined place and time period)}}{\text{No. live births (same place and time period)}} \times 1000$

(6) Neonatal mortality rate $= \dfrac{\text{No. deaths to infants <28 days old (defined place and time period)}}{\text{No. live births (same place and time period)}} \times 1000$

(7) Postneonatal mortality rate $= \dfrac{\text{No. deaths to infants 28-365 days old (defined place and time period)}}{\substack{\text{No. live births} \\ \text{(same place and time period)}} - \substack{\text{No. neonatal deaths} \\ \text{(same place and time period)}}} \times 1000$

(8) Approximate postneonatal mortality rate $=$ Infant mortality rate $-$ Neonatal mortality rate

(9) Perinatal mortality rate* $= \dfrac{\substack{\text{No. stillbirths} \\ \text{(defined place and time period)}} + \substack{\text{No. deaths to infants <7 days old} \\ \text{(same place and time period)}}}{\substack{\text{No. stillbirths} \\ \text{(same place and time period)}} + \substack{\text{No. live births} \\ \text{(same place and time period)}}} \times 1000$

(10) Maternal mortality rate $= \dfrac{\text{No. pregnancy-related deaths (defined place and time period)}}{\text{No. live births (same place and time period)}} \times 100,000$

*Several similar formulas are in use around the world.

made available to local, state, federal, and international groups. The United States and most other countries undertake a complete population census on a periodic basis, with the U.S. census occurring every 10 years. Community-wide epidemiologic measurement depends on accurate determination and reporting of the following:

- Numerator data, especially events such as births, deaths, becoming ill (incident cases), and recovering from illness
- Denominator data, especially the population census

Prevalence data are determined by surveys. These types of data are used to create community rates and ratios for planning and evaluating health progress. The collection of such data is the responsibility of individual countries. Most countries report their data to the United Nations, which publishes large compendia on the World Wide Web.[8,9]

To be valid, a rate must meet certain criteria with respect to the denominator and numerator. First, all the people counted in the denominator must have been at risk for the events counted in the numerator. Second, all the events counted in the numerator must have happened to people included in the denominator. Before rates can be compared, the numerators for all groups in the comparison must be defined or diagnosed in the same way; the constant multipliers in use must be the same; and the time intervals under study must be the same.

Box 2-4 provides definitions of the basic epidemiologic concepts and measurements discussed in this chapter. Box 2-5 lists the equations for the most commonly used population rates.

References

1. US Centers for Disease Control and Prevention: Prevalence of doctor-diagnosed arthritis and possible arthritis—30 states, 2002. *MMWR* 52:383–386, 2004.
2. Youth risk behavior surveillance—United States, 2003. *MMWR* 53(SS-2)1–96, 2004.
3. US Centers for Disease Control and Prevention. Awareness of stroke warning signs—17 states and the U.S. Virgin Islands, 2001. *MMWR* 52:359–362, 2004.

4. Chan CK, Feinstein AR, Jekel JF, et al: The value and hazards of standardization in clinical epidemiologic research. *J Clin Epidemiol* 41:1125–1134, 1988.

5. Becker TM, Wiggins CL, Key CR, et al: Symptoms, signs, and ill-defined conditions: a leading cause of death among minorities. *Am J Epidemiol* 131:664–668, 1990.

6. Burnand B, Feinstein AR: The role of diagnostic inconsistency in changing rates of occurrence for coronary heart disease. *J Clin Epidemiol* 45:929–940, 1992.

7. Heron M, Doyert DL, Murphy SL, et al: Deaths: Final data for 2006. *National Vital Statistics Report* 57(14), Hyattsville, Maryland, 2009, National Center for Health Statistics.

8. Dorn HF: A classification system for morbidity concepts. *Public Health Reports* 72:1043–1048, 1957.

9. US Centers for Disease Control and Prevention: The second 100,000 cases of acquired immunodeficiency syndrome: United States, June 1981 to December 1991. *MMWR* 41:28–29, 1992.

Select Readings

Brookmeyer R, Stroup DF: *Monitoring the health of populations: statistical principles and methods for public health surveillance,* New York, 2004, Oxford University Press.

Chan CK, Feinstein AR, Jekel JF, et al: The value and hazards of standardization in clinical epidemiologic research. *J Clin Epidemiol* 41:1125–1134, 1988. [Standardization of rates.]

Elandt-Johnson RC: Definition of rates: some remarks on their use and misuse. *Am J Epidemiol* 102:267–271, 1975. [Risks, rates, and ratios.]

Epidemiologic Surveillance and Epidemic Outbreak Investigation

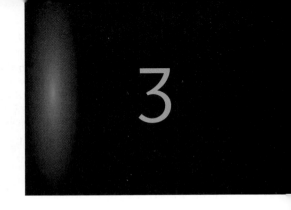

3

This chapter describes the importance of disease surveillance and early identification of epidemics. **Epidemics,** or disease outbreaks, are defined as the occurrence of disease at an unusual or unexpected, elevated frequency. Reliable surveillance to define the usual rates of disease in an area is necessary before rates that are considerably elevated can be identified.

I. SURVEILLANCE OF DISEASE

A. Responsibility for Surveillance

Surveillance is the entire process of collecting, analyzing, interpreting, and reporting data on the incidence of death, diseases, and injuries and the prevalence of certain conditions, knowledge of which is considered important for promoting and safeguarding public health. Surveillance is generally considered the foundation of disease control efforts. In the United States the Centers for Disease Control and Prevention (CDC) is the federal agency responsible for the surveillance of most types of acute diseases and the investigation of outbreaks. The CDC conducts surveillance if requested by a state or if an outbreak has the potential to affect more than one state. Data for disease surveillance are passed from local and state governments to the CDC, which evaluates the data and works with the state and local agencies regarding further investigation and control of any problems discovered.

According to the U.S. Constitution, the federal government has jurisdiction over matters concerning interstate commerce, including disease outbreaks with **interstate implications** (outbreaks that originated in one state and have spread to other states or have the potential to do so). Each state government has jurisdiction over disease outbreaks with **intrastate implications** (outbreaks confined within one state's borders). If a disease outbreak has interstate implications, the CDC is a first responder and takes immediate action, rather than waiting for a request for assistance from a state government.

B. Creating a Surveillance System

The development of a surveillance system requires clear objectives regarding the diseases or conditions to be covered (e.g., infectious diseases, side effects of vaccines, elevated lead levels, pneumonia-related deaths in patients with influenza). Also, the objectives for each surveillance item should be clear, including surveillance of an infectious disease to determine whether a vaccine program is effective, the search for possible side effects of new vaccines or vaccine programs, and the determination of progress toward meeting U.S. health objectives for 2020 for a particular disease.

The criteria for defining a case of a reportable disease or condition must be known to develop standardized reporting procedures and reporting forms. As discussed later, the case definition usually is based on clinical findings; laboratory results; and epidemiologic data on the time, place, and characteristics of affected persons. The intensity of the planned surveillance (active vs. passive) and duration of the surveillance (ongoing vs. time-limited) must be known in advance.

The types of analysis needed (e.g., incidence, prevalence, case fatality ratio, years of potential life lost, quality-adjusted life years, costs) should be stated in advance. In addition, plans should be made for disseminating the findings on the Internet and in other publication venues.

These objectives and methods should be developed with the aid of the investigators charged with collecting, reporting, and using the data. A pilot test should be performed and evaluated in the field, perhaps in one or more demonstration areas, before the full system is attempted. When it is operational, the full system also should be continually evaluated. The CDC has extensive information on surveillance at its website, www.cdc.gov.

C. Methods and Functions of Disease Surveillance

Surveillance may be either passive or active. Most surveillance conducted on a routine basis is passive surveillance. In **passive surveillance,** physicians, clinics, laboratories, and hospitals that are required to report disease are given the appropriate forms and instructions, with the expectation that they will record all cases of reportable disease that come to their attention. **Active surveillance,** on the other hand, requires periodic (usually weekly) telephone calls, electronic contact or personal visits to the reporting individuals and institutions to obtain the required data. Active surveillance is more labor intensive and costly, so it is seldom done on a routine basis.

The percentage of patients with reportable diseases that are actually reported to public health authorities varies considerably.[1] One group estimated that the percentage reported to state-based passive reporting systems in the United States varied from 30% to 62% of cases.

Sometimes a change in medical care practice uncovers a previously invisible disease surveillance issue. For example, a hospital in Connecticut began reporting many cases of pharyngeal gonorrhea in young children. This apparently localized outbreak in one hospital was investigated by a rapid response team, who discovered that the cases began to appear only after the hospital started examining all throat cultures in children for gonococci and for beta-hemolytic streptococci.[2]

In contrast to infectious diseases, the reporting of most other diseases, injuries, and conditions is less likely to be rapid or nationwide, and the associated surveillance systems tend to develop on a problem-by-problem basis. Without significant support and funding from governments, surveillance systems are difficult to establish. Even with such support, most systems tend to begin as demonstration projects in which a few areas participate. Later the systems expand to include participation by all areas or states.

As discussed in Chapter 24, several states and regions have cancer registries, but the United States has no national cancer registry. Fatal diseases can be monitored to some extent by death certificates, but such diagnoses are often inaccurate, and reporting is seldom rapid enough for the detection of disease outbreaks. (The reporting systems for occupational and environmental diseases and injuries are discussed in Section 3 of this book.)

I. Establishment of Baseline Data

Usual (baseline) rates and patterns of diseases can be known only if there is a regular reporting and surveillance system.

Epidemiologists study the patterns of diseases by the time and geographic location of cases and the characteristics of the persons involved. Continued surveillance allows epidemiologists to detect deviations from the usual pattern of data, which prompt them to explore whether an epidemic (i.e., an unusual incidence of disease) is occurring or whether other factors (e.g., alterations in reporting practices) are responsible for the observed changes.

2. Evaluation of Time Trends

SECULAR (LONG-TERM) TRENDS

The implications of secular (or long-term) trends in disease are usually different from those of outbreaks or epidemics and often carry greater significance. The graph in Figure 3-1 from a CDC surveillance report on salmonellosis shows that the number of reported cases of salmonellosis in the United Sates has increased over time. The first question to ask is whether the trend can be explained by changes in disease detection, disease reporting, or both, as is frequently the case when an apparent outbreak of a disease is reported. The announcement of a real or suspected outbreak may increase suspicion among physicians practicing in the community and thus lead to increased diagnosis and increased reporting of diagnosed cases. Nevertheless, epidemiologists concluded that most of the observed increase in salmonellosis from 1955 to 1985 was real, because they noted increasing numbers of outbreaks and a continuation of the trend over an extended time. This was especially true for the East Coast, where a sharp increase in outbreaks caused by *Salmonella enteritidis* was noted beginning about 1977. A long-term increase in a disease in one U.S. region, particularly when it is related to a single serotype, is usually of greater public health significance than a localized outbreak because it suggests the existence of a more widespread problem.

Figure 3-2 shows the decline in the reported incidence and mortality from diphtheria in the United States. The data in this figure are presented in the form of a **semilogarithmic graph,** with a **logarithmic scale** used for the vertical y-axis and an **arithmetic scale** for the horizontal x-axis. The figure illustrates one advantage of using a logarithmic scale: The lines showing incidence and mortality trace an approximately parallel decline. On a logarithmic scale, this means that the decline in rates was **proportional,** so that the percentage of cases that resulted in death—the **case fatality ratio**—remained relatively constant at about 10% over the years shown. This relative constancy suggests that prevention of disease, rather than treatment of people who were ill, was responsible for the overall reduction in diphtheria mortality in the United States.

SEASONAL VARIATION

Many infectious diseases show a strong seasonal variation, with periods of highest incidence usually depending on the **route of spread.** To determine the usual number of cases or rates of disease, epidemiologists must therefore incorporate any expected seasonal variation into their calculations.

Infectious diseases that are spread by the **respiratory route,** such as influenza, colds, measles, and varicella (chickenpox), have a much higher incidence in the winter and early spring in the Northern Hemisphere. Figure 3-3 shows the

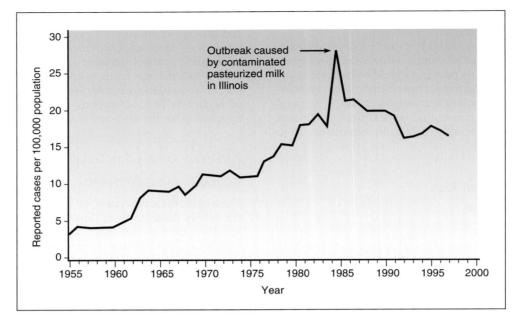

Figure 3-1 Incidence rates of salmonellosis (excluding typhoid fever) in the United States, by year of report, 1955-1997. (Data from Centers for Disease Control and Prevention: Summary of notifiable diseases, United States, 1992. *MMWR* 41:41, 1992; and Summary of notifiable diseases, United States, 1997. *MMWR* 46:18, 1998.)

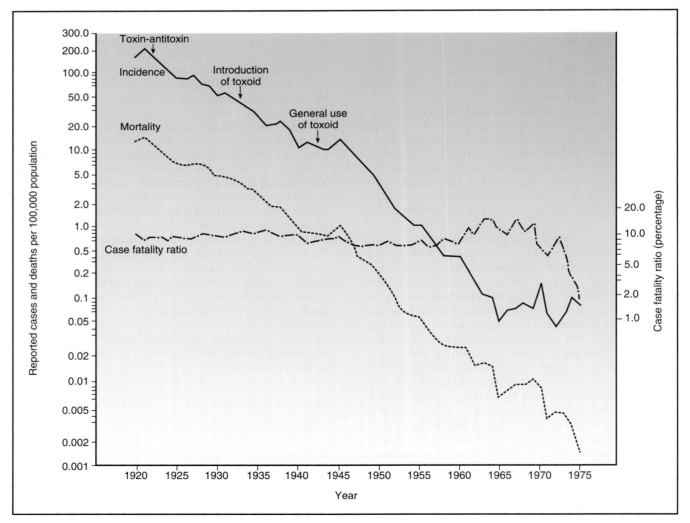

Figure 3-2 Incidence rates, mortality rates, and case fatality ratios for diphtheria in the United States, by year of report, 1920-1975. (Data from Centers for Disease Control and Prevention: Diphtheria surveillance summary. Pub No (CDC) 78-8087, Atlanta, 1978, CDC.)

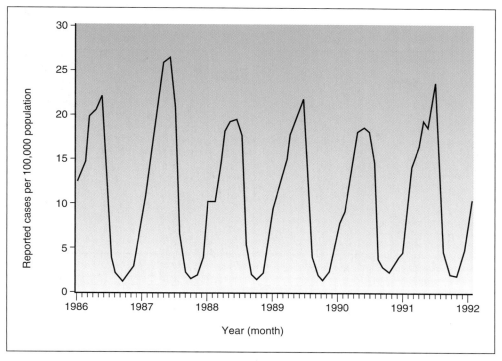

Figure 3-3 Incidence rates of varicella (chickenpox) in the United States, by month of report, 1986-1992. (Data from Centers for Disease Control and Prevention: Summary of notifiable diseases, United States, 1992. *MMWR* 41:53, 1992.)

seasonal variation for varicella in the United States, by month, over a 6-year period. Notice the peaks after January and before summer of each year. Such a pattern is thought to occur during these months because people spend most of their time close together indoors, where the air changes slowly. The drying of mucous membranes, which occurs in winter because of low humidity and indoor heating, may also play a role in promoting respiratory infections. Since the introduction of varicella vaccine, this seasonal pattern has been largely eliminated.

Diseases that are spread by **insect or arthropod vectors** (e.g., viral encephalitis from mosquitoes) have a strong predilection for the summer or early autumn. Lyme disease, spread by *Ixodes* ticks, is usually acquired in the late spring or summer, a pattern explained by the seasonally related life cycle of the ticks and the outdoor activity of people wearing less protective clothing during warmer months.

Infectious diseases that are spread by the **fecal-oral route** are most common in the summer, partly because of the ability of the organisms to multiply more rapidly in food and water during warm weather. Figure 3-4 shows the summer seasonal pattern of waterborne outbreaks of gastrointestinal disease. The peak frequency of outbreaks attributable to drinking water occurs from May to August, whereas the peak for outbreaks attributable to recreational water (e.g., lakes, rivers, swimming pools) occurs from June to October.

Figure 3-5 shows a late-summer peak for aseptic meningitis, which is usually caused by viral infection spread by the fecal-oral route or by insects. Figure 3-6 shows a pattern that is similar but has sharper and narrower peaks in late summer

and early autumn. It describes a known arthropod-borne viral infection caused by California-serogroup viruses of the central nervous system.

Because the peaks of different disease patterns occur at different times, the CDC sometimes illustrates the incidence of diseases by using an "epidemiologic year." In contrast to the **calendar year,** which runs from January 1 of one year to December 31 of the same year, the **epidemiologic year** for a given disease runs from the month of lowest incidence in one year to the same month in the next year. The advantage of using the epidemiologic year when plotting the incidence of a disease is that it puts the high-incidence months near the center of a graph and avoids having the high-incidence peak split between the two ends of the graph, as would occur with many respiratory diseases if they were graphed for a calendar year.

OTHER TYPES OF VARIATION

Health problems can vary by the day of the week; Figure 3-7 shows that recreational drowning occurs more frequently on weekends than on weekdays, presumably because more people engage in water recreation on weekends.

3. Identification and Documentation of Outbreaks

An **epidemic,** or **disease outbreak,** is the occurrence of disease at an unusual (or unexpected) frequency. Because the word "epidemic" tends to create fear in a population, that term usually is reserved for a problem of wider-than-local implications, and the term "outbreak" typically is used for a

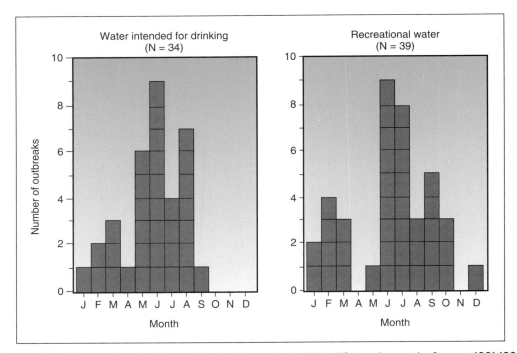

Figure 3-4 **Incidence of waterborne outbreaks of gastrointestinal disease in the United States, by month of report, 1991-1992.** (Data from Centers for Disease Control and Prevention: Surveillance for waterborne disease outbreaks, United States, 1991-1992. *MMWR* 42(SS-5):1, 1993.)

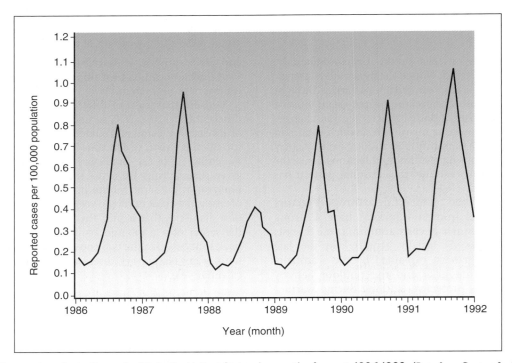

Figure 3-5 **Incidence rates of aseptic meningitis in the United States, by month of report, 1986-1992.** (Data from Centers for Disease Control and Prevention: Summary of notifiable diseases, United States, 1992. *MMWR* 41:20, 1992.)

localized epidemic. Nevertheless, the two terms often are used interchangeably.

It is possible to determine that the level of a disease is unusual only if the usual rates of the disease are known and reliable surveillance shows that current rates are considerably elevated. To determine when and where influenza and pneumonia outbreaks occur, the CDC uses a seasonally adjusted *expected* percentage of influenza and pneumonia deaths in the United States and a number called the **epidemic threshold** to compare with the reported percentage. (Pneumonias are included because influenza-induced pneumonias may be signed out on the death certificate as "pneumonia," with no mention of influenza.)

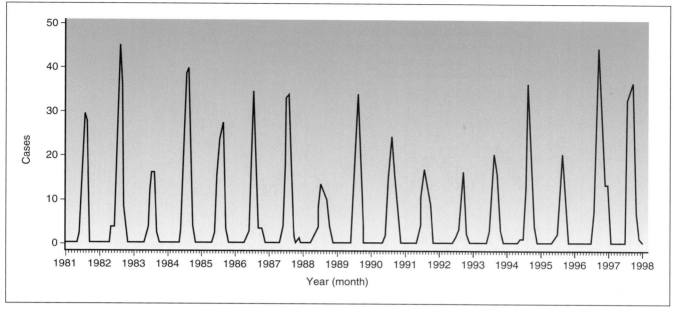

Figure 3-6 Incidence of central nervous system infections caused by California-serogroup viruses in the United States, by month of report, **1981-1997.** (Data from Centers for Disease Control and Prevention: Summary of notifiable diseases, United States, 1992. *MMWR* 41:18, 1992; and Summary of notifiable diseases, United States, 1997. *MMWR* 46:20, 1998.)

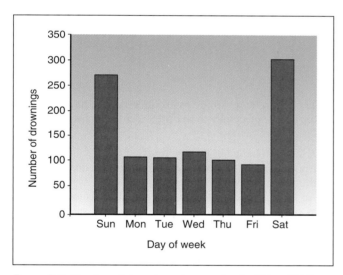

Figure 3-7 Number of drownings at recreation facilities of U.S. Army Corps of Engineers, by day of week of report, 1986-1990. (Data from Centers for Disease Control and Prevention: Drownings at U.S. Army Corps of Engineers recreation facilities, 1986-1990. *MMWR* 41:331, 1992.)

Figure 3-8 provides data concerning the expected percentage of deaths caused by pneumonia and influenza in 122 U.S. cities for 1994 through 2000. The lower *(solid)* sine wave is the seasonal baseline, which is the expected percentage of pneumonia and influenza deaths per week in these cities. The upper *(dashed)* sine wave is the epidemic threshold, with essentially no influenza outbreak in winter 1994-1995, a moderate influenza outbreak in winter 1995-1996, and major outbreaks in the winters of 1996-1997, 1997-1998, and 1998-1999, as well as in autumn 1999. No other disease has

Box 3-1	Diseases Considered Major Threats for Bioterrorism
Anthrax	Smallpox
Botulism	Tularemia (inhalational)
Plague	Viral hemorrhagic fevers

such a sophisticated prediction model, but the basic principles apply to any determination of the occurrence of an outbreak.

SURVEILLANCE FOR BIOTERRORISM

For at least a century, epidemiologists have worried about the use of biologic agents for military or terrorist purposes. The basic principles of disease surveillance are still valid in these domains, but there are special concerns worth mentioning. The most important need is for rapid detection of a problem. With regard to bioterrorism, special surveillance techniques are being developed to enable rapid detection of major increases in the most likely biologic agents[3] (Box 3-1). Detection is made more difficult if the disease is scattered over a wide geographic area, as with the anthrax outbreak in the United States after terrorist attacks in late 2001.

A technique developed for more rapid detection of epidemics and possible bioterrorism is **syndromic surveillance.**[3] The goal of this surveillance is to characterize "syndromes" that would be consistent with agents of particular concern and to prime the system to report any such syndromes quickly. Rather than trying to establish a specific diagnosis before sounding an alert, this approach might provide an early warning of a bioterrorism problem.

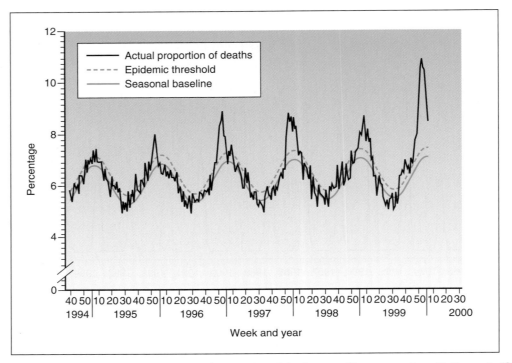

Figure 3-8 Epidemic threshold, seasonal baseline, and actual proportion of deaths caused by pneumonia and influenza in 122 U.S. cities, 1994-2000. The epidemic threshold is 1.645 standard deviations above the seasonal baseline. The expected seasonal baseline is projected using a robust regression procedure in which a periodic regression model is applied to observed percentages of deaths from pneumonia and influenza since 1983. (Data from Centers for Disease Control and Prevention: Update: influenza activity—United States and worldwide, 1999-2000. *MMWR* 49:174, 2000.)

4. Evaluation of Public Health and Disease Interventions

The introduction of major interventions intended to change patterns of disease in a population, especially the introduction of new vaccines, should be followed by surveillance to determine if the intended changes were achieved. Figure 3-9 shows the impact of the two types of polio vaccine—the inactivated (Salk) vaccine and the oral (Sabin) vaccine—on the reported incident cases of poliomyelitis. The large graph in this figure has a logarithmic scale on the *y*-axis. It is used here because the decline in the poliomyelitis incidence rate was so steep that on an arithmetic scale, no detail would be visible at the bottom after the early 1960s. A logarithmic scale compresses the high rates on a graph compared with the lower rates, so that the detail of the latter can be seen.

Figure 3-9 shows that after the inactivated vaccine was introduced in 1955, the rates of paralytic disease declined quickly. The public tended to think the problem had gone away, and many parents became less concerned about immunizing newborns. Because the inactivated vaccine did not provide herd immunity, however, the unimmunized infants were at great risk. A recurrent poliomyelitis spike occurred in 1958 and 1959, when most of the new cases of paralytic poliomyelitis were in young children who had not been immunized. The rates declined again in 1960 and thereafter because the public was shaken out of its complacency to obtain vaccine and because a newer oral vaccine was introduced. This live, attenuated oral vaccine provided both herd immunity and individual immunity (see Figure 1-2).

The failure of a vaccine to produce satisfactory immunity or the failure of people to use the vaccine can be detected by one of the following:

- A lack of change in disease rates
- An increase in disease rates after an initial decrease, as in the previous example of the polio vaccine
- An increase in disease rates in a recently vaccinated group, as occurred after the use of defective lots of inactivated polio vaccine in the 1950s.

The importance of postmarketing surveillance was underscored through continued evaluation and close surveillance of measles rates in the United States. Investigators were able to detect the failure of the initial measles vaccines and vaccination schedules to provide long-lasting protection (see Chapter 1). Research into this problem led to a new set of recommendations for immunization against measles. According to the 2006 recommendations, two doses of measles vaccine should be administered to young children. The first dose should be given when the child is 12 to 15 months old (to avoid a higher failure rate if given earlier) and the second dose when the child is 4 to 6 years old, before school entry.[4] A third dose at about age 18 is also recommended.

With regard to medications, the importance of postmarketing surveillance was affirmed by the discovery of an increased incidence of cardiovascular events in people who took newly introduced cyclooxygenase-2 (COX-2) inhibitors. The discovery resulted in some COX-2 inhibitors being removed from the market.

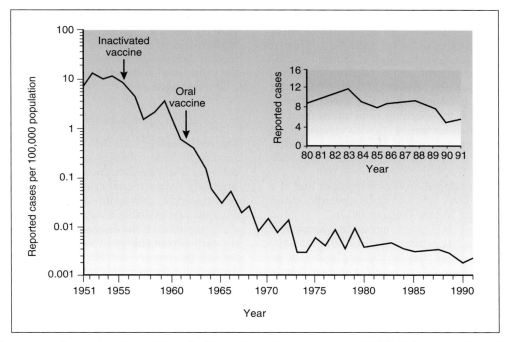

Figure 3-9 Incidence rates of paralytic poliomyelitis in the United States, by year of report, 1951-1991. (Data from Centers for Disease Control and Prevention: Summary of notifiable diseases, United States, 1991. *MMWR* 40:37, 1991.)

5. Setting of Disease Control Priorities

Data on the patterns of diseases for the current time and recent past can help governmental and voluntary agencies establish priorities for disease control efforts. This is not a simple counting procedure. A disease is of more concern if its rates increase rapidly, as with acquired immunodeficiency syndrome (AIDS) in the 1980s, than if its rates are steady or declining. The *severity* of the disease is a critical feature, which usually can be established by good surveillance. AIDS received high priority because surveillance demonstrated its severity and its potential for epidemic spread.

6. Study of Changing Patterns of Disease

By studying the patterns of occurrence of a particular disease over time in populations and subpopulations, epidemiologists can better understand the changing patterns of the disease. Data derived from the surveillance of syphilis cases in New York City during the 1980s, when crack cocaine came into common use, proved valuable in suggesting the source of changing patterns of acquired and congenital syphilis. As shown in Figure 3-10, the reported number of cases of primary and secondary syphilis among women increased substantially beginning in 1987. Both this trend and the concurrent increase in congenital syphilis were strongly associated with the women's use of crack (trading sex for drugs) and with their lack of prenatal care (a situation that allowed their syphilis to go undetected and untreated).

A new **pattern** of occurrence may be more ominous than a mere increase in the incidence of a disease. In the case of tuberculosis in the United States, yearly incidence decreased steadily from 1953 (when reporting began) until 1985, when 22,201 cases were reported. Thereafter, yearly incidence began to rise again. Of special concern was the association of this rise with the increasing impact of the AIDS epidemic

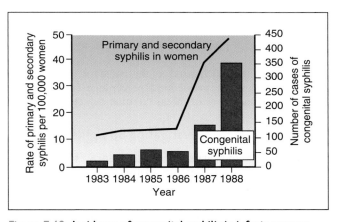

Figure 3-10 Incidence of congenital syphilis in infants younger than 1 year *(bars)* and incidence of primary and secondary syphilis in women *(line)* in New York City, by year of report, 1983-1988. (Data from Centers for Disease Control and Prevention: Congenital syphilis, New York City, 1983-1988. *MMWR* 38:825, 1989.)

and the increasing resistance of *Mycobacterium tuberculosis* to antimicrobial agents. This concern led to greater efforts to detect tuberculosis in people with AIDS and to use directly observed therapy to prevent antimicrobial resistance. Tuberculosis rates peaked in 1992, when 26,673 cases were reported, and then began declining again.

II. INVESTIGATION OF EPIDEMICS

A. Nature of Epidemics

The common definition of an **epidemic** is the unusual occurrence of a disease; the term is derived from Greek roots meaning "upon the population." Although people usually think of an epidemic as something that involves large numbers of people, it is possible to name circumstances under which just one case of a disease could be considered an epidemic. Because smallpox has been eliminated worldwide, a single case would represent a smallpox epidemic. Similarly, if a disease has been eradicated from a particular region (e.g., paralytic poliomyelitis in the Western Hemisphere) or if a disease is approaching elimination from an area and has the potential for spread (as with measles in the U.S.), the report of even one case in the geographic region might be considered unexpected and become a cause for concern.

When a disease in a population occurs regularly and at a more or less constant level, it is said to be **endemic,** based on Greek roots meaning "within the population."

Epidemiologists use analogous terms to distinguish between usual and unusual patterns of diseases in animals. A disease outbreak in an animal population is said to be **epizootic** ("upon the animals"), whereas a disease deeply entrenched in an animal population but not changing much is said to be **enzootic** ("within the animals").

Investigators of acute disease outbreaks ordinarily use a measure of disease frequency called the **attack rate,** particularly when the period of exposure is short (i.e., considerably less than 1 year). Rather than being a true rate, the attack rate is really the proportion of exposed persons that becomes ill. It is calculated as follows:

Attack rate = Number of new cases of a disease/
        Number of persons exposed in a particular outbreak × 100

In this equation, 100 is used as the constant multiplier so that the rate can be expressed as a percentage. (For a discussion of other measures of disease frequency, see Chapter 2.)

B. Procedures for Investigating an Epidemic

The forces for and against the occurrence of disease are usually in equilibrium. If an epidemic occurs, this equilibrium has been disrupted. The goal of investigation is to discover and correct recent changes so that the balance can be restored and the epidemic controlled. The physician who is alert to possible epidemics not only would be concerned to give the correct treatment to individual patients, but also would ask, "Why did this patient become sick with this disease at this time and place?"

Outbreak investigation is similar to crime investigation; both require "a lot of shoe leather."[5] Although there is no simple way to teach imagination and creativity in the investigation of disease outbreaks, there is an organized way of approaching and interpreting the data that assist in solving problems. This section outlines the series of steps to follow in investigating a disease outbreak.[6]

I. Establish the Diagnosis

Establishing the diagnosis may seem obvious, but it is surprising how many people start investigating an outbreak without taking this first step. Many cases are solved just by making the correct diagnosis and showing that the disease occurrence was not unusual after all. A health department in North Carolina received panic calls from several people who were concerned about the occurrence of smallpox in their community. A physician assigned to investigate quickly discovered that the reported case of smallpox was actually a typical case of chickenpox in a young child. The child's mother did not speak English well, and the neighbors heard the word "pox" and panicked. The outbreak was stopped by a correct diagnosis.

2. Establish Epidemiologic Case Definition

The epidemiologic case definition is the list of specific criteria used to decide whether or not a person has the disease of concern. The case definition is not the same as a clinical diagnosis. Rather, it establishes consistent criteria that enable epidemiologic investigations to proceed before definitive diagnoses are available. Establishing a case definition is especially important if the disease is unknown, as was the case in the early investigations of legionnaires' disease, AIDS, hantavirus pulmonary syndrome, eosinophilia-myalgia syndrome, and severe acute respiratory syndrome. The CDC case definition for eosinophilia-myalgia syndrome included the following:

- A total eosinophil count greater than 1000 cells/µL
- Generalized myalgia (muscle pain) at some point during the course of the illness, of sufficient severity to limit the ability to pursue normal activities
- Exclusion of other neoplastic or infectious conditions that could account for the syndrome

The use of these epidemiologic and clinical criteria assisted in the outbreak investigation.

No case definition is perfect because there are always some **false positives** (i.e., individuals without the disease who are wrongly included in the group considered to have the disease) and **false negatives** (i.e., diseased individuals wrongly considered to be disease free). Nevertheless, the case definition should be developed carefully and adhered to in the collection and analysis of data. The case definition also permits epidemiologists to make comparisons among the findings from different outbreak investigations.

3. Is an Epidemic Occurring?

Even if proven, cases must occur in sufficient numbers to constitute an epidemic. As emphasized previously, it is difficult to assess whether the number of cases is high unless the *usual* number is known by ongoing surveillance. It may be assumed, however, that a completely new disease or syndrome meets the criteria for an epidemic.

4. Characterize Epidemic by Time, Place, and Person

The epidemic should be characterized by time, place, and person, using the criteria in the case definition. It is unwise to start data collection until the case definition has been established, because it determines the data needed to classify persons as affected or unaffected.

TIME

The time dimension of the outbreak is best described by an **epidemic time curve.** This is a graph with time on the *x*-axis and the number of new cases on the *y*-axis. The epidemic time curve should be created so that the units of time on the *x*-axis are considerably smaller than the probable incubation period, and the *y*-axis is simply the number of cases that became symptomatic during each time unit. Rates usually are not used in creating the curve.

The epidemic time curve provides several important clues about what is happening in an outbreak and helps the epidemiologist answer the following questions:

- What was the **type of exposure** (single source or spread from person to person)?
- What was the probable **route of spread** (respiratory, fecal-oral, skin-to-skin contact, exchange of blood or body fluids, or via insect or animal vectors)?
- When were the affected persons exposed? What was the incubation period?
- In addition to **primary cases** (persons infected initially by a common source), were there **secondary cases?** (Secondary cases represent person-to-person transmission of disease from primary cases to other persons, often members of the same household.)

In a **common source exposure**, many people come into contact with the same source, such as contaminated water or food, usually over a short time. If an outbreak is caused by this type of exposure, the epidemic curve usually has a sudden onset, a peak, and a rapid decline. If the outbreak is caused by **person-to-person spread,** however, the epidemic curve usually has a prolonged, irregular pattern, often known as a **propagated** outbreak.

Figure 3-11 shows the epidemic time curve from an outbreak of gastrointestinal disease caused by a common source exposure to *Shigella boydii* at Fort Bliss, Texas. In this outbreak, spaghetti was contaminated by a food handler. The time scale in this figure is shown in 12-hour periods. Note the rapid increase and rapid disappearance of the outbreak.

Figure 3-12 shows the epidemic time curve from a propagated outbreak of bacillary dysentery caused by *Shigella sonnei*, which was transmitted from person to person at a training school for mentally retarded individuals in Vermont. In this outbreak, the disease spread when persons, clothing, bedding, and other elements of the school environment were contaminated with feces. The time scale is shown in 5-day periods. Note the prolonged appearance of the outbreak.

Under certain conditions, a respiratory disease spread by the person-to-person route may produce an epidemic time curve that closely resembles that of a common-source epidemic. Figure 3-13 shows the spread of measles in an elementary school. A widespread exposure apparently occurred at a school assembly, so the air in the school auditorium can almost be regarded as a common source. The first person infected in this situation is called the **index case**—the case that introduced the organism into the population. Sequential individual cases, however, can be seen every 12 days or so during the prior 2 months. The first of these measles cases should have warned school and public health officials to immunize all students immediately. If that had happened, the outbreak probably would have been avoided.

Sometimes an epidemic has more than one peak, either because of multiple common source exposures or because of secondary cases. Figure 3-14 shows the epidemic time curve for an outbreak of shigellosis among students who attended

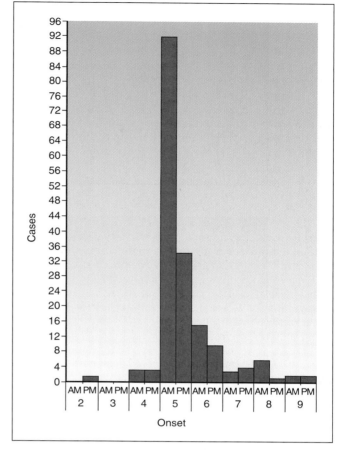

Figure 3-11 Epidemic time curve showing onset of cases of gastrointestinal disease caused by *Shigella boydii* in Fort Bliss, Texas, in November 1976. The onset is shown in 12-hour periods for dates in November. (Data from Centers for Disease Control and Prevention: Food and waterborne disease outbreaks: annual summary, 1976, Atlanta, 1977, CDC.)

a summer camp in the eastern United States. The campers who drank contaminated water on the trip were infected with *Shigella* organisms. After they returned home, they infected others with shigellosis.

Epidemiologists occasionally encounter situations in which two different common-source outbreaks have the same time and place of exposure, but different incubation periods. Suppose that a group of people is exposed to contaminated shellfish in a restaurant. The exposure might cause an outbreak of shigellosis in 24 to 72 hours and an outbreak of hepatitis A about 2 to 4 weeks later in the same population.

The epidemic time curve is useful to ascertain the type of exposure and the time when the affected persons were exposed. If the causative organism is known, and the exposure seems to be a common source, epidemiologists can use knowledge about that organism's usual incubation period to determine the probable time of exposure. Two methods typically are used for this purpose. The data in Figure 3-14, which pertain to *Shigella* infection among campers, assist in illustrating each method.

Method 1 involves taking the shortest and longest known incubation period for the causative organism and calculating

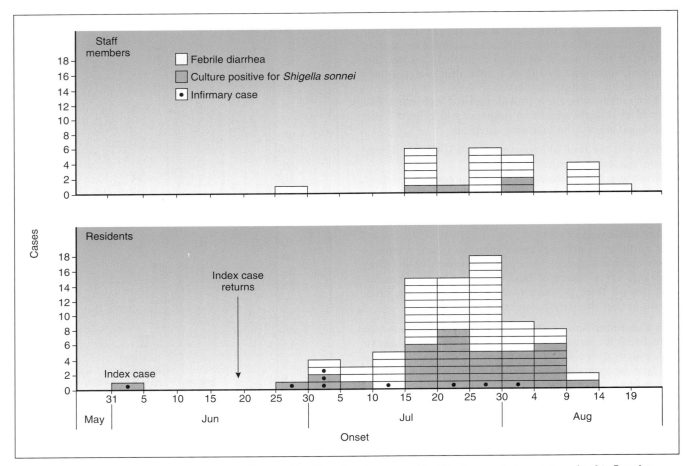

Figure 3-12 **Epidemic time curve showing onset of cases of bacillary dysentery caused by** *Shigella sonnei* **at a training school in Brandon, Vermont, from May to August 1974.** The onset is shown in 5-day periods for dates in May, June, July, and August. (Data from Centers for Disease Control and Prevention: *Shigella* surveillance. Report No 37, Atlanta, 1976, CDC.)

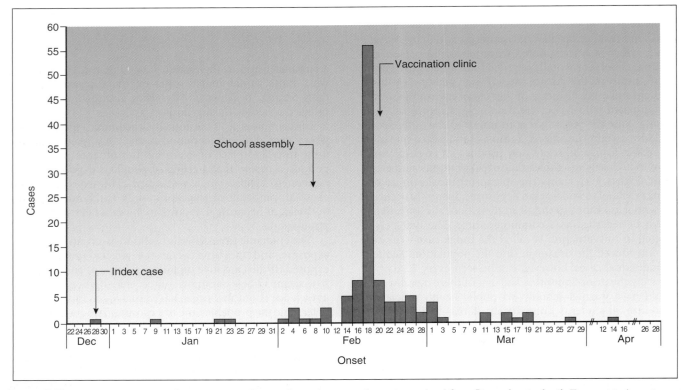

Figure 3-13 **Epidemic time curve showing onset of cases of measles at an elementary school from December to April.** The onset is shown in 2-day periods for dates in December 1975 and in January, February, March, and April 1976. (Data from Centers for Disease Control and Prevention: Measles surveillance, 1973-1976. Report No 10, Atlanta, 1977, CDC.)

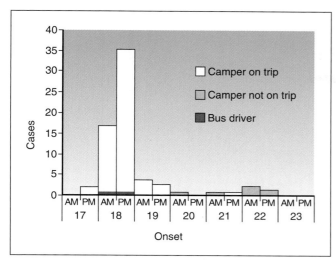

Figure 3-14 **Epidemic time curve showing onset of cases of shigellosis in campers from New Jersey and New York in August.** The onset is shown in 12-hour periods for dates in August 1971. (Data from Centers for Disease Control and Prevention: *Shigella* surveillance: annual summary, 1971, Atlanta, 1972, CDC.)

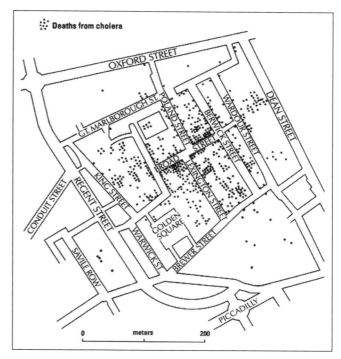

Figure 3-15 **Spot map of cholera deaths in the Soho district of London, 1854, based on a map prepared by John Snow in 1855.** The deaths centered on the intersection of Broad and Lexington streets, where there was a popular community well (near the "L" of Lexington Street in the map). This well apparently was the source of the contamination. The present name of Broad Street is "Broadwick Street," and the John Snow pub is on the southwest corner of Broadwick and Lexington streets. (Modified from http://www.doe.k12.de.us/infosuites/staff/ci/content_areas/files/ss/Cholera_in_19thc_London.pdf.)

backward in time from the first and last cases. If reasonably close together, these estimates bracket the probable time of exposure. For example, the incubation period for *Shigella* organisms is usually 1 to 3 days (24-72 hours), but it may range from 12 to 96 hours.[7] Figure 3-14 shows that the first two cases of shigellosis occurred after noon on August 17. If these cases had a 12-hour incubation period, the exposure was sometime before noon on August 17 (without knowing the exact hours, it is not possible to be more specific). The longest known incubation period for *Shigella* is 96 hours, and the last camper case was August 21 after noon; 96 hours before that would be August 17 after noon. The most probable exposure time was either before noon or after noon on August 17. If the same procedure is used but applied to the *most common* incubation period (24-72 hours), the result is an estimate of after noon on August 16 (from the earliest cases) and an estimate of after noon on August 18 (from the last case). These two estimates still center on August 17, so it is reasonable to assume that the campers were exposed sometime on that date.

Method 2 is closely related to the previous method, but it involves taking the average incubation period and measuring backward from the epidemic peak, if that is clear. In Figure 3-14, the peak is after noon on August 18. An average of 48 hours (2 days) earlier would be after noon on August 16, slightly earlier than the previous estimates. The most probable time of exposure was either after noon on August 16 or at any time on August 17.

PLACE

The accurate characterization of an epidemic involves defining the location of all cases, because a geographic clustering of cases may provide important clues. Usually, however, the geographic picture is not sufficient by itself, and other data are needed to complete the interpretation.

Sometimes a *spot map* that shows where each affected person lives, works, or attends school is helpful in solving an

epidemic puzzle. The most famous of all public health spot maps was prepared in 1855 in London by John Snow. By mapping the location of cholera deaths in the epidemic of 1854, Snow found that they centered on the Broad Street water pump in London's Soho district (Fig. 3-15). His map showed that most of the persons killed by the outbreak lived in the blocks immediately surrounding the Broad Street pump. Based on this information, Snow had the pump handle removed to prevent anyone from drinking the water (although by the time he did this, the epidemic was already waning).

The use of spot maps currently is limited in outbreak investigations because these maps show only the numerator (number of cases) and do not provide information on the denominator (number of persons in the area). Epidemiologists usually prefer to show incidence rates by *location,* such as by hospital ward (in a hospital infection outbreak), by work area or classroom (in an occupational or school outbreak), or by block or section of a city (in a community outbreak). An outbreak of respiratory fungal infection in an Arkansas school shows how incidence rates by classroom can provide a major clue to the cause of such outbreaks.[5] All except one of the classrooms in the school had three or fewer cases each. The exception, the Liberace Room, had 14 cases. This room was located directly over a coal chute, and coal had been dumped on the ground and shoveled into the chute during several windy days. As a result, the Liberace Room

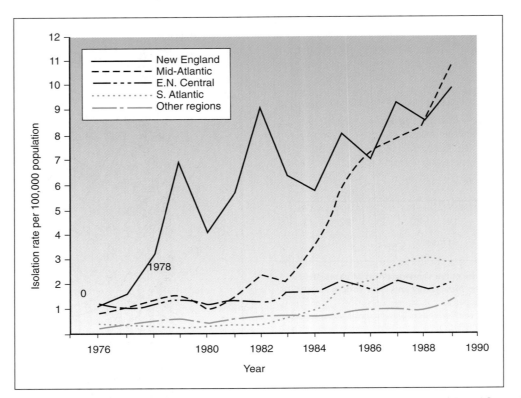

Figure 3-16 **Isolation rate of *Salmonella enteritidis* infections per 100,000 population in various regions of the United States, by year of report, 1976-1989.** (Data from Centers for Disease Control and Prevention: Update: *Salmonella enteritidis* infections and shell eggs, United States, 1990. *MMWR* 39:909, 1990.)

became dusty from the coal, which had come from a strip mine and had been contaminated with *Histoplasma capsulatum* from the soil before delivery to the school. The children had inhaled the coal dust and become ill with histoplasmosis.

When epidemiologists want to determine the general location of a disease and how it is spreading, they may compare trends in incidence rates in different regions. Figure 3-16 shows the rates of reported *Salmonella enteritidis* infections by region in the United States for 1976 through 1989. There was an unusually high rate for the New England region from 1978 to 1989. Beginning in about 1984, the Mid-Atlantic States also began to show an excessive rate of salmonellosis from the same serotype, suggesting that the problem was spreading down the East Coast.

Figure 3-17 uses a map to show the spread of epidemic cholera in South and Central America from January 1991 through July 1992.

A special problem in recent years has involved reports of clusters of cancer or other types of disease in neighborhoods or other small areas. From the theory of random sampling, epidemiologists would expect clusters of disease to happen by chance alone, but that does not comfort the people involved.

Distinguishing "chance" clusters from "real" clusters is often difficult, but identifying the types of cancer in a cluster may help epidemiologists decide fairly quickly whether the cluster represents an environmental problem. If the types of cancer in the cluster vary considerably and belong to the more common cell types (e.g., lung, breast, colon, prostate),

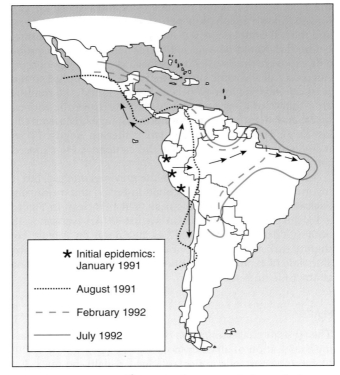

Figure 3-17 **Map showing spread of epidemic cholera in Latin America from January 1991 to July 1992.** (Data from Centers for Disease Control and Prevention: Update: Cholera, Western Hemisphere. *MMWR* 41:667, 1992.)

the cluster probably is not caused by a hazardous local exposure.[8-10] However, if most of the cases represent only one type or a small number of related types of cancer (especially leukemia or thyroid or brain cancer), a more intensive investigation may be indicated.

The next step is to begin at the time the cluster is reported and observe the situation prospectively. The **null hypothesis** is that the unusual number of cases will not continue. Because this is a **prospective hypothesis** (see Chapter 10), an appropriate statistical test can be used to decide whether the number of cases continues to be excessive. If the answer is "yes," there may be a true environmental problem in the area.

PERSON

Knowing the characteristics of persons affected by an outbreak may help clarify the problem and its cause. Important characteristics include age; gender; race; ethnicity; religion; source of water, milk, and food; immunization status; type of work or schooling; and contacts with other affected persons.

Figures 3-18 and 3-19 illustrate the value of analyzing the personal characteristics of affected individuals for clues regarding the cause of the outbreak. Figure 3-18 shows the age distribution of measles cases among children in the Navajo Nation, and Figure 3-19 shows the age distribution of measles cases among residents of Cuyahoga County, Ohio. The fact that measles in the Navajo Nation tended to occur in very young children is consistent with the hypothesis that the outbreak was caused by lack of immunization of preschool-age children. In contrast, the fact that very young children in Cuyahoga County were almost exempt from measles, while school-age children tended to be infected, suggests that the younger children had been immunized, and that the outbreak in this situation resulted from the failure of measles vaccine to produce long-lasting immunity. If they were not immunized early, the children of Cuyahoga County probably would have had measles earlier in life and would have been immune by the time they entered school. Fortunately, this type of outbreak has been almost eliminated by the requirement that children receive a second dose of measles vaccine before entering school.

5. Develop Hypotheses Regarding Source, Patterns of Spread, and Mode of Transmission

The **source of infection** is the person (the index case) or vehicle (e.g., food, water) that initially brought the infection into the affected community. The source of infection in the outbreak of gastrointestinal illness at Fort Bliss was an infected food handler, who contaminated spaghetti that was eaten by many people more or less simultaneously (see Fig. 3-11).

The **pattern of spread** is the pattern by which infection can be carried from the source to the individuals infected. The primary distinction is between a **common-source pattern,** such as occurs when contaminated water is drunk by many people in the same time period, and a **propagated pattern,** in which the infection propagates itself by spreading directly from person to person over an extended period. There is also a **mixed pattern,** in which persons acquire a disease through a common source and spread it to family

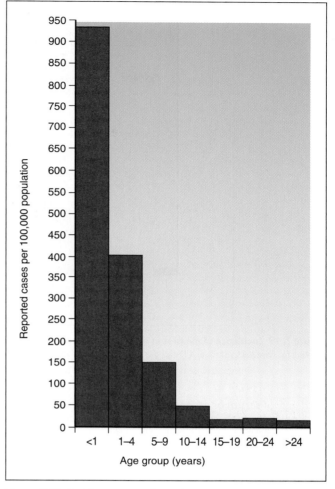

Figure 3-18 **Incidence rates of measles in members of the Navajo Nation, by age group, 1972-1975.** (Data from Centers for Disease Control. Measles surveillance, 1973-1976. Report No 10, Atlanta, CDC, 1977.)

members or others (secondary cases) by personal contact (see Fig. 3-14).

Affected persons in common-source outbreaks may only have one brief **point-source exposure,** or they may have a **continuous common-source exposure.** In the Fort Bliss outbreak, the infected spaghetti was the point source. In Milwaukee in 1993, an epidemic of *Cryptosporidium* infection was caused by contamination of the public water supply for the southern part of the city over a several-day period; this was a continuous common-source exposure.[11]

Many types of infections have more than one pattern of spread. *Shigella* infection can be spread through contaminated water (continuous common source) or through person-to-person contact (propagated spread). Human immunodeficiency virus (HIV) can be spread to several intravenous drug users through the sharing of a single infected syringe (continuous common source), and HIV can be passed from one person to another through sexual contact (propagated spread).

The **mode of transmission** of epidemic disease may be respiratory, fecal-oral, vector-borne, skin-to-skin, or through

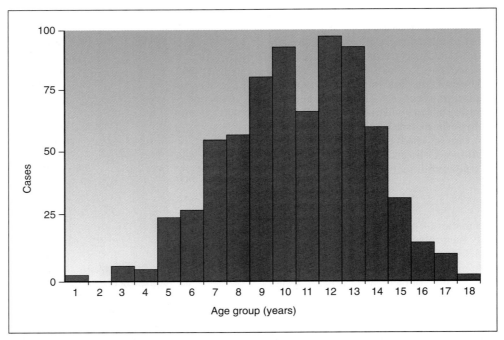

Figure 3-19 **Incidence of measles in residents of Cuyahoga County, Ohio, by age group, from October 1973 to February 1974.** (Data from Centers for Disease Control and Prevention: Measles surveillance, 1973-1976. Report No 10, Atlanta, 1977, CDC.)

exchange of serum or other body fluids. In some cases, transmission is through contact with **fomites**—objects that can passively carry organisms from one person to another, such as soiled sheets or doorknobs.

6. Test Hypotheses

Laboratory studies are important in testing epidemiologic hypotheses and may include one or more of the following:

- Cultures from patients and, if appropriate, from possible vehicles, such as food or water
- Stool examinations for ova and parasites
- Serum tests for antibodies to the organism suspected of causing the disease (e.g., tests of *acute* and *convalescent* serum samples to determine if there has been an increase in antibodies to the organism over time)
- Tests for nonmicrobiologic agents, such as toxins or drugs

A common, efficient way of testing hypotheses is to conduct **case-control studies** (see Chapter 5). For a foodborne outbreak of disease, the investigator assembles the persons who have the disease (cases) and a sample of the persons who ate at the same place at the suspected time of exposure but do not have the disease (controls). The investigator looks for possible risk factors (e.g., food items eaten) that were considerably more common in the cases than in the controls. Both groups are questioned regarding the specific foods they did or did not eat before the outbreak. For each item of food and drink, the percentage of controls who consumed it is subtracted from the percentage of cases who consumed it. The food item showing the greatest difference in consumption percentage between cases and controls is the most likely risk factor.

The case-control method also can be used in an epidemic of noninfectious disease. In 1971 it was noted that eight young women with adenocarcinoma of the vagina were treated at one hospital between 1966 and 1969.[12] Because of the rarity of this type of cancer, the number of cases would qualify as an outbreak. When the investigators performed a case-control study, they used 32 controls (4 matched controls for every case). They were able to show that the only significant difference between the 8 cases and 32 controls was that 7 of the 8 cancer patients had been exposed to diethylstilbestrol (DES) in utero. Their mothers had been given DES, a synthetic estrogen, during the first semester of pregnancy in an effort to prevent miscarriage or premature labor. In contrast, none of the 32 controls was the offspring of mothers given DES during pregnancy. The probability of finding this distribution by chance alone was infinitesimal. DES is no longer used for any purpose during pregnancy.

7. Initiate Control Measures

When an outbreak is noted, it is usually accompanied by a general outcry that something must be done immediately. Therefore, it may be necessary to start taking control measures before the source of the outbreak and the route of spread are known for certain. If possible, control measures should be initiated in such a way so as not to interfere with the investigation of the outbreak. Four common types of intervention are used to control an outbreak, as follows:

1. **Sanitation** often involves modification of the environment. Sanitation efforts may consist of removing the pathogenic agent from the sources of infection (e.g., water, food); removing the human source of infection from environments where he or she can spread it to others (quarantine); or preventing contact with the source, perhaps by cleaning the environment or removing susceptible people from the environment (evacuation).

2. **Prophylaxis** implies putting a barrier to the infection, such as a vaccine, within the susceptible hosts. Although a variety of immunizations are recommended for the entire population and usually are initiated during infancy, other measures that offer short-term protection are also available for people who plan to travel to countries with endemic diseases. Examples include antimalarial drugs and hyperimmune globulin against hepatitis A.

3. **Diagnosis and treatment** are performed for the persons who are infected (e.g., in outbreaks of tuberculosis, syphilis, and meningococcal meningitis) so that they do not spread the disease to others.

4. **Control of disease vectors** includes mosquitoes (involved in malaria, dengue, and yellow fever) and *Ixodes* ticks (involved in Lyme disease).

Although a disease outbreak may require one or more of these interventions, some outbreaks simply fade away when the number of infected people is so high that few susceptible individuals remain.

One important aspect of the control effort is the written and oral communication of findings to the appropriate authorities, the appropriate health professionals, and the public. This communication (1) enables other agencies to assist in disease control, (2) contributes to the professional fund of knowledge about the causes and control of outbreaks, and (3) adds to the available information on prevention.

8. Initiate Specific Follow-up Surveillance to Evaluate Control Measures

No medical or public health intervention is adequate without follow-up surveillance of the disease or problem that initially caused the outbreak. The importance of a sound surveillance program not only involves detecting subsequent outbreaks but also evaluating the effect of the control measures. If possible, the surveillance after an outbreak should be *active* because this is more reliable than passive surveillance (see section I.C).

C. Example of Investigation of an Outbreak

In January 1991 a liberal arts college in New England with a population of about 400 students reported 82 cases of acute gastrointestinal illness, mostly among students, over 102 hours. The college president sought help from local and state health authorities to determine whether the college cafeteria should be closed or the entire college should be closed and the students sent home—an option that would have disrupted the entire academic year.

Initial investigation focused on making a diagnosis. Clinical data suggested that the illness was of short duration, with most students found to be essentially well in 24 hours. The data also suggested that the illness was relatively mild. Only one student was hospitalized, and the need for hospitalization in this case was uncertain. In most cases the symptoms consisted of nausea and vomiting, with minimal or no diarrhea and only mild systemic symptoms, such as headache and malaise. Examination revealed only a low-grade fever. Initial food and stool cultures for pathogenic bacteria yielded negative results.

Based on this information, the investigating team developed a case definition. A case was defined as any person in the college who complained of diarrhea or vomiting between Monday, January 28, and Thursday, January 31. The large percentage of cases over this short time made it clear that the situation was unusual, and that the problem could be considered a disease outbreak.

The people who met the criteria of the case definition included resident students, commuter students, and employees. When the investigating team interviewed some of the affected people, they found that most, but not all, of the resident students had eaten only at the campus cafeteria. The epidemic time curve suggested that if cafeteria food were the source, one or more meals on 2 days in January could have been responsible, although a few cases had occurred before and after the peak of the outbreak (Fig. 3-20). Near the beginning of the outbreak, two food handlers had worked while feeling ill with gastrointestinal symptoms. Health department records revealed, however, that the school cafeteria had always received high scores for sanitation, and officials who conducted an emergency reinspection of the facilities and equipment during the outbreak found no change. They detected no problem with sanitary procedures, except that the food handlers had worked while not feeling well.

Most of the commuter students with symptoms had brought food from home during the time in question. Almost none of them had eaten at the college cafeteria, although a few had eaten at an independently run snack bar on campus. Further questioning revealed that the family members of several of the affected commuter students also reported a similar illness, either during the weeks preceding the outbreak or concurrent with it. One public school in a nearby town had closed briefly because of a similar illness in most of the students and staff members.

Although a college-wide questionnaire was distributed and analyzed, this process took several days, and the president wanted answers as soon as possible. Within 2 days of being summoned, the investigating team was able to make the following recommendations: the college, including the cafeteria, should remain open; college-wide assemblies and indoor sports events should be canceled for 2 weeks; and no person should be allowed to work as a food handler while ill. To show their confidence in the cafeteria, the members of the investigating team ate lunch there while sitting in a prominent place. The outbreak quickly faded away, and the college schedule was able to proceed more or less normally.

How was the investigating team able to make these recommendations so quickly? Although the epidemic time curve and information gathered from interviews offered numerous clues, past knowledge gained from similar outbreaks, from disease surveillance, and from research on the natural history of diseases all helped the investigators make their recommendations with confidence. In particular, the following observations made the diagnosis of bacterial infection unlikely: the self-limiting, mild course of disease; the lack of reported diarrhea, even though it was in the original case definition; and the fact that no bacterial pathogens could be cultured from the food and stool samples that had been collected. A staphylococcal toxin was considered initially, but the consistent story of a low-grade fever made a toxin unlikely; fever is a sign of infection, but not of an external (ingested) toxin.

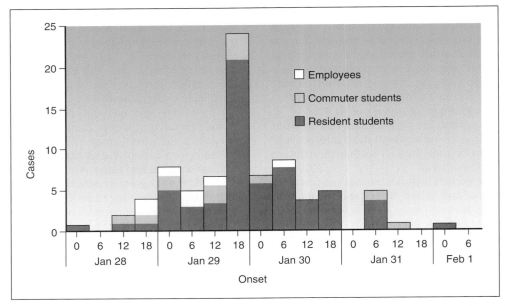

Figure 3-20 Epidemic time curve showing onset of cases of gastroenteritis at a small college in New England from January 28 to February 1, 1991. The onset is shown in 6-hour periods for dates in January and February.

The clinical and epidemiologic pattern was most consistent with an outbreak caused by a norovirus (the laboratory demonstration of a norovirus at that time was exceedingly difficult and costly, but we can now use real-time polymerase chain reaction testing). For noroviruses, the fecal-oral route of spread had been demonstrated for food and water, but many outbreaks revealed a pattern that also suggested a respiratory (propagated) route of spread, even though that possibility had not been confirmed. The latter possibility was the reason for suggesting the cancellation of assemblies and indoor sports events.

The outbreak investigation team was comfortable in recommending that the cafeteria remain open, because the commuters who had become ill had not eaten at the cafeteria, and because a similar illness was reported in the surrounding community. These factors made it unlikely that the cafeteria was the only source of infection, although there was a chance that infected food handlers had spread their illness to some people. The short duration and mild nature of the illness meant that there was no need to close the college, although a certain amount of disruption and class absenteeism would likely continue for a few more days.

Continued surveillance was established at the college, and this confirmed that the outbreak was waning. Cultures continued to yield negative results for bacterial pathogens, and analysis of the college-wide questionnaire did not change any conclusions. This outbreak illustrates that even without a definitive diagnosis, epidemiologic analysis enabled the investigators to rule out bacterial food contamination with a high degree of probability. This case also illustrates a principle discussed in Chapter 1: the ability of epidemiologic methods, even in the early phase of an outbreak, to guide control methods. In this outbreak, negative evidence (i.e., evidence that showed what the problem was not) permitted epidemiologists to calm a nervous population.

D. Example of Preparedness and Response to a Global Health Threat

In addition to severe illness, pandemic diseases cause numerous adverse effects, including fear, economic instability, and premature deaths.[13] Over time, epidemiologists have improved their ability to detect and respond to new pandemic threats. These improvements are attributable to increased communication among countries through the Internet, media, and organized public health systems and to advances in laboratory and diagnostic testing. Also, innovative surveillance systems monitor indirect signals of disease activity, such as influenza surveillance based on tracking call volume to telephone triage advice lines, over-the-counter drug sales, and health information–seeking behavior in the form of queries to online search engines.[14-17] In collaboration with multiple countries and using the International Health Regulations (in force since 2007) as a framework, the World Health Organization (WHO) and the CDC Global Disease Detection Operations Center have implemented epidemic alert and rapid response systems to help control international outbreaks and strengthen international public health security.

A representative example of improved preparedness for global health threats is the rapid, effective global response to the 2009 influenza A (H1N1) pandemic that affected more than 200 countries and territories. Ongoing disease surveillance detected the increased number of cases of patients with influenza-like signs and symptoms, allowing epidemiologists to identify and characterize the pandemic virus quickly. Epidemiologic investigations and surveillance characterized the severity, risk groups, and burden of disease; within 20 weeks of virus detection, diagnostic testing was made available to 146 countries, and through an international donation program, a vaccine was developed and made available to 86 countries. This collaborative effort was one of the great public health achievements of the first decade of the 21st century.

III. SUMMARY

Surveillance of disease activity is the foundation of public health control of disease. It may be active or passive. Its functions include determining the baseline rates of disease, detecting outbreaks, and evaluating control measures. Surveillance data are used for setting disease control policy. The investigation of disease outbreaks is a primary function of public health agencies, but the practicing physician makes important contributions in detecting and reporting acute outbreaks. A standard approach to the investigation of disease outbreaks was developed in the 20th century. This procedure involves making a diagnosis, establishing a case definition, and determining whether or not there is a definite outbreak.

If an outbreak is occurring, the cases of disease are characterized by time (especially using an epidemic time curve), place (usually determining rates in people who live and work in different locations), and person (determining the personal characteristics and patterns of the people involved in the outbreak and ascertaining how they differ from those of people not involved). This characterization is followed by the development and testing of hypotheses regarding the source of the infection, the pattern of spread, and the mode of transmission. These hypotheses are then tested using laboratory data (e.g., cultures, paired sera, analysis for toxins) or research methods (e.g., case-control studies), depending on the hypotheses. Control measures and follow-up surveillance are initiated as soon as is practical.

References

1. Harkess JF, Gildon BA, Archer PW, et al: Is passive surveillance always insensitive? *Am J Epidemiol* 128:878–881, 1988.
2. Helgerson SD, Jekel JF, Hadler JL: Training public health students to investigate disease outbreaks: examples of community service. *Public Health Rep* 103:72–76, 1988.
3. Emergency preparedness and response. www.bt.cdc.gov.
4. US Centers for Disease Control and Prevention: Recommended childhood and adolescent immunization schedule, United States, 2006. *MMWR* 53, 2006.
5. Roueché B: *The medical detectives,* New York, 1981, Truman Talley Books.
6. Information on CDC epidemiology training courses. www.cdc.gov or at wonder.cdc.gov.
7. Heymann DL, editor: *Control of communicable diseases manual,* ed 18, Washington, DC, 2004, American Public Health Association.
8. Brooks-Robinson S, et al: An epidemiologic investigation of putative cancer clusters in two Connecticut towns. *J Environ Health* 50:161–164, 1987.
9. Jacquez GM, editor: Workshop on statistics and computing in disease clustering. *Stat Med* 12:1751–1968, 1993.
10. National Conference on Clustering of Health Events. *Am J Epidemiol* 132:S1–202, 1990.
11. MacKenzie WR, Hoxie NJ, Proctor ME, et al: A massive outbreak in Milwaukee of *Cryptosporidium* infection transmitted through the public water supply. *N Engl J Med* 331:161–167, 1994.
12. Herbst AL, Ulfelder H, Poskanzer DC: Adenocarcinoma of the vagina: association of maternal stilbestrol therapy with tumor appearance in young women. *N Engl J Med* 284:878–881, 1971.
13. Ten great public health achievements—worldwide, 2001–2010. *JAMA* 306(5):484–487, 2011.
14. Espino JU, Hogan WR, Wagner MM: Telephone triage: a timely data source for surveillance of influenza-like diseases. *AMIA Annu Symp Proc* 215–219, 2003.
15. Magruder S: Evaluation of over-the-counter pharmaceutical sales as a possible early warning indicator of human disease. *Johns Hopkins University Applied Physics Laboratory Technical Digest* 24:349–353, 2003.
16. Eysenbach G: Infodemiology: tracking flu-related searches on the Web for syndromic surveillance. *AMIA Annu Symp Proc* 244–248, 2006.
17. Ginsberg J, Mohebbi MH, Patel RS, et al: Detecting influenza epidemics using search engine query data. *Nature* 457(7232):1012–1014, 2009.

Select Readings

Brookmeyer R, Stroup DF: *Monitoring the health of populations: statistical principles and methods for public health surveillance,* New York, 2004, Oxford University Press.
Goodman RA, Buehler JW, Koplan JP: The epidemiologic field investigation: science and judgment in public health practice. *Am J Epidemiol* 132:9–16, 1990. [Outbreak investigation.]
Kelsey JL, Whittemore AS, Evans AS, et al: *Methods in observational epidemiology,* ed 2, New York, 1996, Oxford University Press. [Outbreak investigation; see especially Chapter 11, Epidemic Investigation.]

Websites

Updated guidelines for evaluating public health surveillance systems: recommendations from the Guidelines Working Group: http://www.cdc.gov/mmwr/preview/mmwrhtml/rr5013a1.htm
CDC case definitions for infectious conditions under public health surveillance: http://www.cdc.gov/osels/ph_surveillance/nndss/casedef/index.htm

The Study of Risk Factors and Causation

4

Epidemiologists are frequently involved in studies to determine causation—that is, to find the specific cause or causes of a disease. This is a more difficult and elusive task than might be supposed, and it leaves considerable room for obfuscation, as shown in a newspaper article on cigarette smoking.[1] The article quoted a spokesman for the Tobacco Institute (a trade association for cigarette manufacturers) as saying that "smoking was a risk factor, though not a cause, of a variety of diseases."

Is a risk factor a cause, or is it not? To answer this question, we begin with a review of the basic concepts concerning causation. Studies can yield statistical associations between a disease and an exposure; epidemiologists need to interpret the meaning of these relationships and decide if the associations are artifactual, noncausal, or causal.

I. TYPES OF CAUSAL RELATIONSHIPS

Most scientific research seeks to identify causal relationships. The three fundamental types of causes, as discussed next

in order of decreasing strength, are (A) sufficient cause, (B) necessary cause, and (C) risk factor (Box 4-1).

A. Sufficient Cause

A sufficient cause precedes a disease and has the following relationship with the disease: if the cause is present, the disease will always occur. However, examples in which this proposition holds true are surprisingly rare, apart from certain genetic abnormalities that, if homozygous, inevitably lead to a fatal disease (e.g., Tay-Sachs disease).

Smoking is not a sufficient cause of bronchogenic lung cancer, because many people who smoke do not acquire lung cancer before they die of something else. It is unknown whether all smokers would eventually develop lung cancer if they continued smoking and lived long enough, but within the human life span, smoking cannot be considered a sufficient cause of lung cancer.

B. Necessary Cause

A necessary cause precedes a disease and has the following relationship with the disease: the cause must be present for the disease to occur, although it does not always result in disease. In the absence of the organism *Mycobacterium tuberculosis*, tuberculosis cannot occur. *M. tuberculosis* can thus be called a necessary cause, or prerequisite, of tuberculosis. It cannot be called a sufficient cause of tuberculosis, however, because it is possible for people to harbor the *M. tuberculosis* organisms all their lives and yet have no symptoms of the disease.

Cigarette smoking is not a necessary cause of bronchogenic lung cancer because lung cancer can and does occur in the absence of cigarette smoke. Exposure to other agents, such as radioactive materials (e.g., radon gas), arsenic, asbestos, chromium, nickel, coal tar, and some organic chemicals, has been shown to be associated with lung cancer, even in the absence of active or passive cigarette smoking.[2]

C. Risk Factor

A risk factor is an exposure, behavior, or attribute that, if present and active, clearly increases the probability of a particular disease occurring in a group of people compared with an otherwise similar group of people who lack the risk factor. A risk factor, however, is neither a necessary nor a sufficient cause of disease. Although smoking is the most important risk factor for bronchogenic carcinoma, producing 20 times as high a risk of lung cancer in men who are heavy smokers

Sufficient cause: If the factor (cause) is present, the effect (disease) will always occur.

Necessary cause: The factor (cause) must be present for the effect (disease) to occur; however, a necessary cause may be present without the disease occurring.

Risk factor: If the factor is present, the probability that the effect will occur is increased.

Directly causal association: The factor exerts its effect in the absence of intermediary factors (intervening variables).

Indirectly causal association: The factor exerts its effect through intermediary factors.

Noncausal association: The relationship between two variables is statistically significant, but no causal relationship exists because the temporal relationship is incorrect (the presumed cause comes after, rather than before, the effect of interest) or because another factor is responsible for the presumed cause and the presumed effect.

---

as in men who are nonsmokers, smoking is neither a sufficient nor a necessary cause of lung cancer.

What about the previously cited quotation, in which the spokesman from the Tobacco Institute suggested that "smoking was a risk factor, though not a cause, of a variety of diseases"? If by "cause" the speaker included only necessary and sufficient causes, he was correct. However, if he included situations in which the presence of the risk factor clearly increased the probability of the disease, he was wrong. An overwhelming proportion of scientists who have studied the question of smoking and lung cancer believe the evidence shows not only that cigarette smoking is a cause of lung cancer, but also that it is the most important cause, even though it is neither a necessary nor a sufficient cause of the disease.

D. Causal and Noncausal Associations

The first and most basic requirement for a causal relationship to exist is an **association** between the outcome of interest (e.g., a disease or death) and the presumed cause. The outcome must occur either significantly more often or significantly less often in individuals who are exposed to the presumed cause than in individuals who are not exposed. In other words, exposure to the presumed cause must make a difference, or it is not a cause. Because some differences would probably occur as a result of random variation, an association must be **statistically significant,** meaning that the difference must be large enough to be unlikely if the exposure really had no effect. As discussed in Chapter 10, "unlikely" is usually defined as likely to occur no more than 1 time in 20 opportunities (i.e., 5% of the time, or 0.05) by chance alone.

If an association is causal, the causal pathway may be direct or indirect. The classification depends on the absence or presence of **intermediary factors,** which are often called **intervening variables, mediating variables,** or **mediators.**

A **directly causal association** occurs when the factor under consideration exerts its effect without intermediary factors. A severe blow to the head would cause brain damage and death without other external causes being required.

An **indirectly causal association** occurs when one factor influences one or more other factors through intermediary variables. Poverty itself may not cause disease and death, but by preventing adequate nutrition, housing, and medical care, poverty may lead to poor health and premature death. In this case, the nutrition, housing, and medical care would be called intervening variables. Education seems to lead to better health indirectly, presumably because it increases the amount of knowledge about health, the level of motivation to maintain health, and the ability to earn an adequate income.

A statistical association may be strong but may not be causal. In such a case, it would be a **noncausal association.** An important principle of data analysis is that association does not prove causation. If a statistically significant association is found between two variables, but the presumed cause occurs **after** the effect (rather than before it), the association is not causal. For example, studies indicated that estrogen treatments for postmenopausal women were associated with endometrial cancer, so that these treatments were widely considered to be a cause of the cancer. Then it was realized that estrogens often were given to control early symptoms of undiagnosed endometrial cancer, such as bleeding. In cases where estrogens were prescribed after the cancer had started, the presumed cause (estrogens) was actually caused by the cancer. Nevertheless, estrogens are sometimes prescribed long before symptoms of endometrial cancer appear, and some evidence indicates that estrogens may contribute to endometrial cancer. As another example, quitting smoking is associated with an increased incidence of lung cancer. However, it is unlikely that quitting causes lung cancer or that continuing to smoke would be protective. What is much more likely is that smokers having early, undetectable or undiagnosed lung cancer start to feel sick because of their growing malignant disease. This sick feeling prompts them to stop smoking and thus, temporarily, they feel a little better. When cancer is diagnosed shortly thereafter, it appears that there is a causal association, but this is false. The cancer started before the quitting was even considered. The temporality of the association precludes causation.

Likewise, if a statistically significant association is found between two variables, but some other factor is responsible for both the presumed cause and the presumed effect, the association is not causal. For example, baldness may be associated with the risk of coronary artery disease (CAD), but baldness itself probably does not cause CAD. Both baldness and CAD are probably functions of age, gender, and dihydrotestosterone level.

Finally, there is always the possibility of **bidirectional causation.** In other words, each of two variables may reciprocally influence the other. For example, there is an association between the density of fast-food outlets in neighborhoods and people's purchase and consumption of fast foods. It is possible that people living in neighborhoods dense with sources of fast food consume more of it because fast food is so accessible and available. It is also possible that fast-food outlets choose to locate in neighborhoods where people's purchasing and consumption patterns reflect high demand. In fact, the association is probably true to some extent in both directions. This bidirectionality creates somewhat of a feedback loop, reinforcing the placement of new outlets (and potentially the movement of new consumers) into neighborhoods already dense with fast food.

II. STEPS IN DETERMINATION OF CAUSE AND EFFECT

Investigators must have a model of causation to guide their thinking. The scientific method for determining causation can be summarized as having three steps, which should be considered in the following order[3]:

- Investigation of the statistical association
- Investigation of the temporal relationship
- Elimination of all known alternative explanations

These steps in epidemiologic investigation are similar in many ways to the steps followed in an investigation of murder, as discussed next.

A. Investigation of Statistical Association

Investigations may test hypotheses about risk factors or protective factors. For causation to be identified, the presumed **risk factor** must be present significantly more often in persons with the disease of interest than in persons without the disease. To eliminate chance associations, this difference must be large enough to be considered statistically significant. Conversely, the presumed **protective factor** (e.g., a vaccine) must be present significantly less often in persons with the disease than in persons without it. When the presumed factor (either a risk factor or a protective factor) is not associated with a statistically different frequency of disease, the factor cannot be considered causal. It might be argued that an additional, unidentified factor, a **"negative" confounder** (see later), could be obscuring a real association between the factor and the disease. Even in that case, however, the principle is not violated, because proper research design and statistical analysis would show the real association.

The first step in an epidemiologic study is to show a statistical association between the presumed risk or protective factor and the disease. The equivalent early step in a murder investigation is to show a geographic and temporal association between the murderer and the victim—that is, to show that both were in the same place at the same time, or that the murderer was in a place from which he or she could have caused the murder.

The relationship between smoking and lung cancer provides an example of how an association can lead to an understanding of causation. The earliest epidemiologic studies showed that smokers had an average overall death rate approximately two times that of nonsmokers; the same studies also indicated that the death rate for lung cancer among all smokers was approximately 10 times that of nonsmokers.[4] These studies led to further research efforts, which clarified the role of cigarette smoking as a risk factor for lung cancer and for many other diseases as well.

In epidemiologic studies the research design must allow a statistical association to be shown, if it exists. This usually means comparing the rate of disease before and after exposure to an intervention that is designed to reduce the disease of interest, or comparing groups with and without exposure to risk factors for the disease, or comparing groups with and without treatment for the disease of interest. Statistical analysis is needed to show that the difference associated with the intervention or exposure is greater than would be expected by chance alone, and to estimate how large this difference is. Research design and statistical analysis work closely together (see Chapter 5).

If a statistically significant difference in risk of disease is observed, the investigator must first consider the direction and extent of the difference. Did therapy make patients better or worse, on average? Was the difference large enough to be etiologically or clinically important? Even if the observed difference is real and large, statistical association does not prove causation. It may seem initially that an association is causal, when in fact it is not. For example, in the era before antibiotics were developed, syphilis was treated with arsenical compounds (e.g., salvarsan), despite their toxicity. An outbreak of fever and jaundice occurred in many of the patients treated with arsenicals.[5] At the time, it seemed obvious that the outbreak was caused by the arsenic. Many years later, however, medical experts realized that such outbreaks were most likely caused by an infectious agent, probably hepatitis B or C virus, spread by inadequately sterilized needles during administration of the arsenical compounds. Any statistically significant association can only be caused by one of four possibilities: true causal association, chance (see Chapter 12), random error, or systematic error (bias or its special case, confounding, as addressed later).

Several criteria, if met, increase the probability that a statistical association is true and causal[6] (Box 4-2). (These criteria often can be attributed to the 19th-century philosopher John Stuart Mill.) In general, a statistical association is more likely to be **causal** if the criteria in Box 4-2 are true:

Figure 4-1 shows an example of a dose-response relationship based on an early investigation of cigarette smoking and lung cancer.[7] The investigators found the following rates of lung cancer deaths, expressed as the number of deaths per 100,000 population per year: 7 deaths in men who did not smoke, 47 deaths in men who smoked about one-half pack of cigarettes a day, 86 deaths in men who smoked about one pack a day, and 166 deaths in men who smoked two or more packs a day.

Box 4-2	**Statistical Association and Causality: Factors that Increase Likelihood of Statistical Association Being Causal**

- The association shows **strength;** the difference in rates of disease between those with the risk factor and those without the risk factor is large.
- The association shows **consistency;** the difference is always observed if the risk factor is present.
- The association shows **specificity;** the difference does not appear if the risk factor is absent.
- The association has **biologic plausibility;** the association makes sense, based on what is known about the natural history of the disease.
- The association exhibits **dose-response relationship;** the risk of disease is greater with stronger exposure to the risk factor.

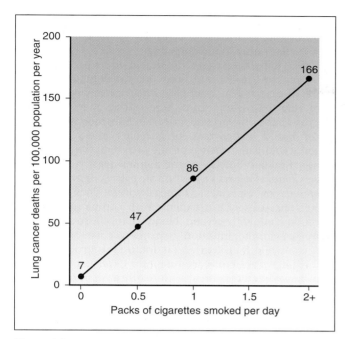

Figure 4-1 Example of dose-response relationship in epidemiology. The x-axis is the approximate *dose* of cigarettes per day, and the y-axis is the rate of deaths from lung cancer. (Data from Doll R, Hill AB: *BMJ* 2:1071, 1956.)

Even if all the previously cited criteria for a statistically significant association hold true, the proof of a causal relationship also depends on the demonstration of the necessary temporal relationship and the elimination of alternative explanations, which are the next two steps discussed.

B. Investigation of Temporal Relationship

Although some philosophical traditions consider time as circular, Western science assumes that time runs only one way. To show causation, the suspected causal factor must have occurred or been present before the effect (e.g., the disease) developed. Proving the time relationship is more complex than it might seem unless **experimental control** is possible—randomization followed by measurement of the risk factor and disease in both groups before and after the experimental intervention.

With chronic diseases, the timing of the exposure to the risk factor and onset of the effect on the chronic disease is often unclear. When did atherosclerosis begin? When did the first bronchial cell become cancerous? Likewise, the onset of the risk factor may be unclear. When did the blood pressure begin to increase? When did the diet first become unhealthy? Because of long but varying **latent periods** between the onset of risk factors and the onset of the resulting diseases, the temporal relationships may be obscured. These associations can be complex and can form vicious cycles. A chronic disease such as obesity can cause osteoarthritis, which can lead to inactivity that makes the obesity worse. Research design has an important role in determining the temporal sequence of cause and effect (see Chapter 5). If information on the cause and the effect is obtained simultaneously, it is

difficult to decide whether the presumed cause or the presumed effect began first. On the one hand, basic demographic variables such as gender and race—internal factors that are present from birth—presumably would have begun to have an effect before diseases caused by any external factors began. On the other hand, it is often impossible in a survey or in a single medical visit to determine which variables occurred first.

With respect to temporal relationships, parallels can be drawn between epidemiologic investigations and murder investigations, as noted earlier. In the case of a murder, the guilty party must have been in the presence of the victim immediately before the victim's death (unless some remote technique was used). In fictional murder mysteries, an innocent but suspect individual often stumbles onto the crime scene immediately after the murder has taken place and is discovered bending over the body. The task of a defense attorney in such a case would be to show that the accused individual actually appeared *after* the murder, and that someone *else* was there at the time of the murder.

C. Elimination of All Known Alternative Explanations

In a murder case, the verdict of "not guilty" (i.e., "not proved beyond a reasonable doubt") usually can be obtained for the defendant if his or her attorney can show that there are other possible scenarios to explain what happened, and that one of them is at least as likely as the scenario that implicates the defendant. Evidence that another person was at the scene of the crime, and had a motive for murder as strong as or stronger than the motive of the accused person, would cast sufficient doubt on the guilt of the accused to result in an acquittal.

In the case of an epidemiologic investigation concerning the causation of disease, even if the presumed causal factor is associated statistically with the disease and occurs before the disease appears, it is necessary to show that there are no other likely explanations for the association.

On the one hand, proper research design can reduce the likelihood of competing causal explanations. *Randomization,* if done correctly, ensures that neither self-selection nor investigator bias influences the allocation of participants into treatment (or experimental) group and control group. Randomization also means that the treatment and control groups should be reasonably comparable with regard to disease susceptibility and severity. The investigator can work to reduce measurement bias (discussed later) and other potential problems, such as a difference between the number of participants lost to follow-up.

On the other hand, the criterion that all alternative explanations be eliminated can *never* be met fully for all time because it is violated as soon as someone proposes a new explanation that fits the data and cannot be ruled out. The classic theory of the origin of peptic ulcers (stress and hypersecretion) was challenged by the theory that *Helicobacter pylori* infection is an important cause of these ulcers.[8] The fact that scientific explanations are always tentative—even when they seem perfectly satisfactory and meet the criteria for statistical association, timing, and elimination of known alternatives—is shown in the following examples on the causation of cholera and coronary heart disease.

1. Alternative Explanation for Cholera in 1849

In 1849, there was an almost exact correspondence between the predicted and observed cholera rates in London at various levels of elevation above the Thames River (Fig. 4-2). At the time, the accuracy of this prediction was hailed as an impressive confirmation of "miasma theory," on which the rates had been based.[9] According to this theory, cholera was caused by *miasmas* (noxious vapors), which have their highest and most dangerous concentrations at low elevations. The true reason for the association between cholera infection and elevation was that the higher the elevation, the less likely that wells would be infected by water from the Thames (which was polluted by pathogens that cause cholera) and the less likely that people would use river water for drinking. In later decades the *germ theory* of cholera became popular, and this theory has held to the present. Although nobody accepts miasma theory now, it would be difficult to improve on the 1849 prediction of cholera rates that were based on that theory.

2. Alternative Explanations for Coronary Heart Disease

Several studies of atherosclerosis and myocardial infarction have questioned the adequacy of the reigning paradigm, according to which hyperlipidemia, hypertension, and smoking are causes of coronary heart disease. Some years ago, the primary challenge to the hyperlipidemia hypothesis was the argument that coronary heart disease is caused by excess levels of iron in the body, which in turn result from oxidation of cholesterol.[10,11] Subsequently, the fact that treatment of hyperlipidemia with so-called statin drugs reduced the number of negative cardiac events convinced most investigators that iron is not a major factor in coronary heart

disease. In all probability, many factors contribute to the end result of atherosclerosis, so that many hypotheses are complementary, rather than competing.

Other hypotheses have implicated the role of chronic inflammation from infections in developing coronary heart disease.[12] For example, when germ-free chickens were infected with a bird herpesvirus, they developed atherosclerosis-like arterial disease.[13] Subsequently, investigators found higher rates of coronary artery disease in patients who had evidence of one of several types of infection, particularly infection with a gram-negative bacterium (e.g., *Chlamydia pneumoniae* or *H. pylori*) or with certain herpesviruses (especially cytomegalovirus). They also found higher rates of CAD in patients with chronic periodontal infection and with certain blood factors associated with acute or chronic infection (e.g., C-reactive protein and serum amyloid A protein). A randomized controlled clinical trial (RCT) of antibiotic treatment for *C. pneumoniae* infection showed that treatment with roxithromycin reduced the number of cardiac events (e.g., heart attacks) in patients with CAD.[14] However, not all studies have found that antibiotic treatment reduces the number of cardiac events.

Reigning hypotheses are always open to challenge. Whether or not the chronic inflammation hypothesis is supported by further research, the cholesterol hypothesis for coronary heart disease can be expected to face challenges by other hypotheses in the 21st century.

III. COMMON PITFALLS IN CAUSAL RESEARCH

Among the most frequently encountered pitfalls in causal research are bias, random error, confounding, synergism, and effect modification (Box 4-3).

A. Bias

Bias, also known as **differential error,** is a dangerous source of inaccuracy in epidemiologic research. Bias usually produces deviations or distortions that tend to go in one direction. Bias becomes a problem when it weakens a true

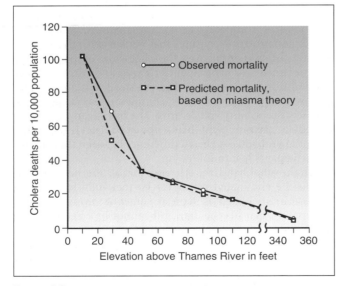

Figure 4-2 Predicted and observed cholera rates at various elevations above Thames River, London, 1849. (From Langmuir AD: *Bacteriol Rev* 24:173–181, 1961.)

Box 4-3	Common Pitfalls in Causal Research

Bias: A differential error that produces findings consistently distorted in one direction as a result of nonrandom factors.
Random error: A nondifferential error that produces findings that are too high and too low in approximately equal frequency because of random factors.
Confounding: The confusion of two supposedly causal variables, so that part or all of the purported effect of one variable is actually caused by the other.
Synergism: The interaction of two or more presumably causal variables, so that the total effect is greater than the sum of the individual effects.
Effect modification (interaction): A phenomenon in which a third variable alters the direction or strength of association between two other variables.

association, produces a false association, or distorts the apparent direction of the association between variables.

So many sources of bias in research have been identified that to list them can be overwhelming. It is easiest to think of the chronologic sequence of a clinical trial (see Chapter 5) and categorize biases in terms of assembly bias or detection bias.

1. Assembly Bias

The first step in a clinical trial involves assembling the groups of participants to be studied. If the characteristics of the intervention group and those of the control group are not comparable at the start, any differences between the two groups that appear in results (outcomes) might be caused by assembly bias instead of the intervention itself. Assembly bias in turn may take the form of selection bias or allocation bias.

SELECTION BIAS

Selection bias results when *participants* are allowed to select the study group they want to join. If subjects are allowed to choose, those who are more educated, more adventuresome, or more health conscious may want to try a new therapy or preventive measure. Any differences subsequently noted may be partly or entirely caused by differences among subjects rather than to the effect of the intervention. Almost any nonrandom method of allocation of subjects to study groups may produce bias.

Selection bias may be found in studies of treatment methods for terminal diseases. The most severely ill patients are often those most willing to try a new treatment, despite its known or unknown dangers, presumably because these patients believe that they have little to lose. Because of self-selection, a new treatment might be given to the patients who are sickest, with relatively poor results. These results could not be fairly compared with the results among patients who were not as sick.

ALLOCATION BIAS

Allocation bias may occur if *investigators* choose a nonrandom method of assigning participants to study groups. It also may occur if a random method is chosen, but not followed, by staff involved in conducting a clinical trial. In one study the investigators thought that patients were being randomly assigned to receive care from either the teaching service or the nonteaching service of a university-affiliated hospital. When early data were analyzed, however, it was clear that the randomization process tended to be bypassed, particularly during the hospital's night shift, to ensure that *interesting* patients were allocated to the teaching service.[15] In clinical trials, maintaining the integrity of the randomization process also requires resisting the pressures of study participants who prefer to be placed in a group who will receive a new form of treatment or preventive care.[16]

ASSOCIATED PROBLEMS OF VALIDITY

According to the ethics of scientific research, randomized clinical trials must allow potential study subjects to participate or not, as they choose. This requirement introduces an element of self-selection into the participant pool before randomization into individual study groups even takes place. Because of the subsequent randomization process, study results are presumed to have **internal** validity (i.e., validity for participants in the study). However, the degree to which results may be generalized to people who did not participate in the study may be unclear, because a self-selected study group is not really representative of any population. In other words, such a study may lack **external** validity (i.e., validity for the general population).

A good illustration of these problems occurred in the 1954 polio vaccine trials, which involved one intervention group and two control groups.[17] Earlier studies of paralytic poliomyelitis had shown that the rates of this disease were higher in upper socioeconomic groups than in lower socioeconomic groups. Children in lower socioeconomic groups were more likely to be exposed to the virus at a young age when the illness was generally milder and lifetime immunity (natural protection) was acquired. When a polio vaccine was first developed, some parents (usually those with more education) wanted their children to have a chance to receive the vaccine, so they agreed to let their children be randomly assigned to either the intervention group (the group to be immunized) or the primary control group (control group I), who received a placebo injection. Other parents (usually those with less education) did not want their children to be guinea pigs and receive the vaccine; their children were followed as a secondary control group (control group II). The investigators correctly predicted that the rate of poliomyelitis would be higher in control group I, whose socioeconomic status was higher, than in control group II, whose socioeconomic status was lower. During the study period, the rate of paralytic poliomyelitis was in fact 0.057% in control group I but only 0.035% in control group II.

Questions of *generalizability* (i.e., external validity) have arisen in regard to the Physicians' Health Study, a costly but well-performed field trial involving the use of aspirin to reduce cardiovascular events and beta carotene to prevent cancer.[18] All the approximately 22,000 participants in the study were male U.S. physicians, age 40 to 75, who met the exclusion criteria (also known as *baseline criteria*) of never having had heart disease, cancer, gastrointestinal disease, a bleeding tendency, or an allergy to aspirin. Early participants agreed to take part in the study, but after a trial period, the investigators dropped participants with poor compliance from the study group. To what group of people in the U.S. population can investigators generalize results obtained from a study of predominantly white, exclusively male, compliant, middle-aged or older physicians who were in good health at the start? Specifically, such results may not be generalizable to women or young men, and are probably not generalizable to people of color, those of lower socioeconomic status, or those with the excluded health problems. The unusually healthy character of these highly select research participants became evident only when their mortality rate, at one point in the study, was shown to be just 16% of the rate expected for men the same age in the United States. As a result, the investigators were forced to extend the study to obtain sufficient outcome events.

2. Detection Bias

When a clinical study is underway, the investigators focus on detecting and measuring possibly causal factors (e.g., high-fat diet or smoking) and outcomes of interest (e.g., disease or death) in the study groups. Care must be taken to ensure that the differences observed in the groups are not attributable to measurement bias or recall bias or other forms of detection bias.

Detection bias may be the result of failure to detect a case of disease, a possible causal factor, or an outcome of interest. In a study of a certain type of lung disease, if the case group consists of individuals receiving care in the pulmonary service of a hospital, whereas the control group consists of individuals in the community, early disease among the controls may be missed because they did not receive the intensive medical evaluation that the hospitalized patients received. The true difference between the cases and controls might be less than the apparent difference.

Detection bias may also occur if two groups of study subjects have large differences in their rates of loss to follow-up. In some clinical trials, the subjects who are lost to follow-up may be responding more poorly than the subjects who remain under observation, and they may leave to try other therapies. In other clinical trials, the subjects who are lost to follow-up may be those who respond the best, and they may feel well and thus lose interest in the trial.

MEASUREMENT BIAS

Measurement bias may occur during the collection of baseline or follow-up data. Bias may result from something as simple as measuring the height of patients with their shoes on, in which case all heights would be too large, or measuring their weight with their clothes on, in which case all weights would be too large. Even this situation is actually rather complicated, because the heels of men's shoes may differ systematically in height from those of women's shoes, while further variation in heel size may occur within each gendered group.

In the case of blood pressure values, bias can occur if some investigators or some study sites have blood pressure cuffs that measure incorrectly and cause the measurements to be higher or lower than the true values. Data from specific medical laboratories can also be subject to measurement bias. Some laboratories consistently report higher or lower values than others because they use different methods. Clinical investigators who collect laboratory data over time in the same institution or who compare laboratory data from different institutions must obtain the normal standards for each laboratory and adjust their analyses accordingly. Fortunately, differences in laboratory standards are a potential source of bias that can be corrected by investigators.

RECALL BIAS

Recall bias takes many forms. It may occur if people who have experienced an adverse event, such as a disease, are more likely to recall previous risk factors than people who have never experienced that event. Although all study subjects may forget some information, bias results if members of one study group are collectively more likely to remember events than are members of the other study group. Recall bias is a major problem in research into causes of congenital anomalies. Mothers who give birth to abnormal infants tend to think more about their pregnancy and are more likely to remember infections, medications, and injuries. This attentiveness may produce a *spurious* (falsely positive) association between a risk factor (e.g., respiratory infections) and the outcome (congenital abnormality).

B. Random Error

Random (chance) error, also known as **nondifferential error,** produces findings that are too high and too low in approximately equal amounts. Although a serious problem, random error is usually less damaging than bias because it is less likely to distort findings by reversing their overall direction. Nonetheless, random error decreases the probability of finding a real association by reducing the statistical power of a study.[19]

C. Confounding

Confounding (from Latin roots meaning "to pour together") is the confusion of two supposedly causal variables, so that part or all of the purported effect of one variable is actually caused by the other. For example, the percentage of gray hairs on the heads of adults is associated with the risk of myocardial infarction, but presumably that association is not causal. Age itself increases both the proportion of gray hairs and the risk of myocardial infarction.

Confounding can obscure a true causal relationship, as illustrated by this example. In the early 1970s, James F. Jekel and a colleague were researching the predictors for educational success among teenage mothers. Analysis of the data on these women revealed that both their age and their grade level were positively associated with their ultimate educational success: The older a young mother and the higher her grade level in school, the more likely she was to stay in school and graduate. However, age itself was also strongly associated with grade level in school, such that older teenagers were more likely to be in higher grades. When the effect of age was studied within each grade level, age was actually shown to be negatively associated with educational success. That is, the older a teenage mother was for a given grade level, the less successful she was likely to be.[20] This result evidently was obtained because a woman who was older than average at a given grade level might have been kept back because of academic or social difficulties, which were negative predictors of success. Thus an important aspect of the association of age and educational success was obscured by the confounding of age with grade level.

By convention, when a third variable masks or weakens a true association between two variables, this is **negative confounding.** When a third variable produces an association that does not actually exist, this is **positive confounding.** To be clear, neither type of confounding is a "good thing" (i.e., neither is a positive factor); both are "bad" (i.e., negative in terms of effect). The type of confounding illustrated with the example of predictors for educational success among teenage mothers is **qualitative confounding** (when a third variable causes the reversal of direction of effect).

D. Synergism

Synergism (from Greek roots meaning "work together") is the interaction of two or more presumably causal variables, so that the combined effect is clearly greater than the sum of the individual effects. For example, the risk of lung cancer is greater when a person has exposure to both asbestos and cigarette smoking than would be expected on the basis of summing the observed risks from each factor alone.[21]

Figure 4-3 shows how adverse medical factors interact synergistically to produce low-birth-weight infants.[22] Low birth weight in this study was defined as 2500 grams or less, and examples of adverse factors were teenage pregnancy and maternal smoking. For infants of white mothers, the risk of low birth weight was about 5% if one adverse factor was present and increased to slightly more than 15% if two adverse factors were present. Similarly, for infants of black mothers, the figure shows how adverse factors interacted synergistically to produce low-birth-weight infants.

E. Effect Modification (Interaction)

Sometimes the direction or strength of an association between two variables differs according to the value of a third variable. This is usually called **effect modification** by epidemiologists and **interaction** by biostatisticians.

A biologic example of effect modification can be seen in the ways in which Epstein-Barr virus (EBV) infection manifests in different geographic areas. Although EBV usually results in infectious mononucleosis in the United States, it often produces Burkitt's lymphoma in African regions where malaria is endemic. In the 1980s, to test whether malaria modifies the effects of EBV, investigators instituted a malaria suppression program in an African region where Burkitt's

lymphoma was usually found and followed the number of new cases. They reported that the incidence of Burkitt's lymphoma decreased after malaria was suppressed, although other factors seemed to be involved as well.[23]

A quantitative example of effect modification can be seen in the reported rates of hypertension among white men and women surveyed in the United States in 1991.[24] In both men and women, the probability of hypertension increased with age. In those 30 to 44 years, however, men were more likely than women to have hypertension, whereas in older groups, the reverse was true. In the age group 45 to 64, women were more likely than men to have hypertension, and in those 65 and older, women were much more likely to have hypertension. Gender did not reverse the trend of increasing rates of hypertension with increasing age, but the rate of increase did depend on gender. Thus we can say that gender modified the effect of age on blood pressure. Statistically, there was an interaction between age and gender as predictors of blood pressure.

IV. IMPORTANT REMINDERS ABOUT RISK FACTORS AND DISEASE

Although it is essential to avoid the pitfalls described previously, it is also necessary to keep two important concepts in mind. First, *one causal factor may increase the risk for several different diseases.* Cigarette smoking is a risk factor for cancer of the lung, larynx, mouth, and esophagus, as well as for chronic bronchitis and chronic obstructive pulmonary disease (COPD). Second, *one disease may have several different causal factors.* Although a strong risk factor for COPD, smoking may be only one of several contributing factors in a given case. Other factors may include occupational exposure to dust (e.g., coal dust, silicon) and genetic factors (e.g., α_1-antitrypsin deficiency). Similarly, the risk of myocardial infarction is influenced not only by a person's genes, diet, exercise, and smoking habits, but also by other medical conditions, such as high blood pressure and diabetes. A key task for epidemiologists is to determine the relative contribution of each causal factor to a given disease. This contribution, called the **attributable risk,** is discussed in Chapter 6.

The possibility of confounding and effect modification often makes the interpretation of epidemiologic studies difficult. Age, whether young or old, may be a confounder because it has a direct effect on the risk of death and of many diseases, so its impact must be removed before the causal effect of other variables can be known. Advancing age may also be an effect modifier, because it can change the magnitude of the risk of other variables.[25] The risk of myocardial infarction (MI) increases with age and with increasing levels of cholesterol and blood pressure—yet cholesterol and blood pressure also increase with age. To determine whether an association exists between cholesterol levels and MI, the effects of age and blood pressure must be controlled. Likewise, to determine the association between blood pressure and MI, the effects of age and cholesterol levels must be controlled. Although control can sometimes be achieved by research design and sample selection (e.g., by selecting study subjects in a narrow range of age and blood pressure), it is usually accomplished through statistical analysis (see Chapter 13).

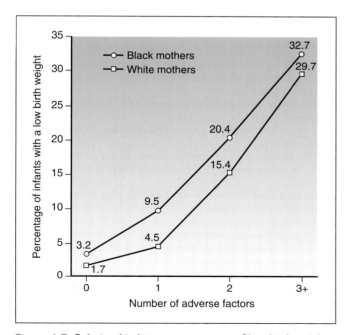

Figure 4-3 Relationship between percentage of low-birth-weight infants and number of adverse factors present during the pregnancy. Low birth weight was defined as 2500 g or less, and examples of adverse factors were teenage pregnancy and maternal smoking. (Data from Miller HC, Jekel JF: *Yale J Biol Med* 60:397–404, 1987.)

V. SUMMARY

Epidemiologists are concerned with discovering the causes of disease in the environment, nutrition, lifestyle, and genes of individuals and populations. Causes are factors that, if removed or modified, would be followed by a change in disease burden. In a given population, smoking and obesity would increase the disease burden, whereas vaccines would increase health, by reducing the disease burden. Research to determine causation is complicated, particularly because epidemiologists often do not have experimental control and must rely on observational methods.

Several criteria must be met to establish a causal relationship between a factor and a disease. First, a statistical association must be shown, and the association becomes more impressive if it is strong and consistent. Second, the factor must precede the disease. Third, there should be no alternative explanations that fit the data equally well. Demonstrating that these criteria are met is complicated by the hazards of bias, random error, confounding, synergism, and effect modification. Internal validity defines whether a study's results may be trusted, whereas external validity defines the degree to which the results may be considered relevant to individuals other than the study participants themselves.

References

1. *The New York Times*. 1991.
2. Doll R, Peto R: *The causes of cancer*, New York, 1981, Oxford University Press.
3. Bauman KE: *Research methods for community health and welfare*, New York, 1980, Oxford University Press.
4. US Surgeon General: *Smoking and health. Public Health Service Pub No 1103*, Washington, DC, 1964, US Government Printing Office.
5. Anderson G, et al. Chapter 17. In *Communicable disease control*, ed 4, New York, 1962, Macmillan.
6. Susser M: *Causal thinking in the health sciences*, New York, 1973, Oxford University Press.
7. Doll R, Hill AB: Lung cancer and other causes of death in relation to smoking: a second report on the mortality of British doctors. *BMJ* 2:1071–1081, 1956.
8. Suerbaum S, Michetti P: *Helicobacter pylori* infection. *N Engl J Med* 347:1175–1186, 2002.
9. Langmuir AD: Epidemiology of airborne infection. *Bacteriol Rev* 24:173–181, 1961.
10. Sullivan JL: Iron and the sex difference in heart disease risk. *Lancet* 1:1293–1294, 1981.
11. Salonen JT, Nyyssönen K, Korpela H, et al: High stored iron levels are associated with excess risk of myocardial infarction in Eastern Finnish men. *Circulation* 86:803–811, 1992.
12. Danesh J, Collins R, Peto R: Chronic infections and coronary heart disease: is there a link? *Lancet* 350:430–436, 1997.
13. Fabricant CG, Fabricant J, Litrenta MM, et al: Virus-induced atherosclerosis. *J Exp Med* 148:335–340, 1978.
14. Gurfinkel E, Bozovich G, Daroca A, et al: Randomized trial of roxithromycin in non-Q-wave coronary syndromes: ROXIS pilot study. *Lancet* 350:404–407, 1997.
15. Garrell M, Jekel JF: A comparison of quality of care on teaching and non-teaching services in a university-affiliated community hospital. *Conn Med* 43:659–663, 1979.
16. Lam JA, Hartwell SW, Jekel JF, et al: "I prayed real hard, so I know I'll get in": living with randomization in social research. *New Dir Program Eval* 63:55–66, 1994.
17. Francis T, Jr, Korns RF, Voight RB, et al: An evaluation of the 1954 poliomyelitis vaccine trials. *Am J Public Health* 45(pt 2):1–63, 1955.
18. Physicians' Health Study Steering Committee: Final report on the aspirin component of the ongoing Physicians' Health Study. *N Engl J Med* 321:129–135, 1989.
19. Kelsey JL, Whitemore AS, Evans AS, Thompson WD. Chapter 9. In *Methods in observational epidemiology*, ed 2, New York, 1996, Oxford University Press.
20. Klerman LV, Jekel JF: *School-age mothers: problems, programs, and policy*, Hamden, Conn, 1973, Linnet Books.
21. Hammond EC, Selikoff IJ, Seidman H: Asbestos exposure, cigarette smoking, and death rates. *Ann NY Acad Sci* 330:473–490, 1979.
22. Miller HC, Jekel JF: Incidence of low birth weight infants born to mothers with multiple risk factors. *Yale J Biol Med* 60:397–404, 1987.
23. Geser A, Brubaker G, Draper CC: Effect of a malaria suppression program on the incidence of African Burkitt's lymphoma. *Am J Epidemiol* 129:740–752, 1989.
24. National Center for Health Statistics: Health promotion and disease prevention: United States, 1990. *Vital and Health Statistics*, Series 10, No 185, Atlanta, 1993, Centers for Disease Control and Prevention.
25. Jacobsen SJ, Freedman DS, Hoffmann RG, et al: Cholesterol and coronary artery disease: age as an effect modifier. *J Clin Epidemiol* 45:1053–1059, 1992.

Select Readings

Greenland S, editor: Issues in causal inference. Part I. In *Evolution of epidemiologic ideas*, Chestnut Hill, Mass, 1987, Epidemiology Resources.

Haynes RB, et al: *Clinical epidemiology*, ed 3, Boston, 2006, Little, Brown.

Gordis L: *Epidemiology*, ed 3, Philadelphia, 2005, Saunders-Elsevier.

Mill JS: *A system of logic (1856)*. Summarized in Last JM: *A dictionary of epidemiology*, ed 2, New York, 1988, Oxford University Press.

Susser M: *Causal thinking in the health sciences*, New York, 1973, Oxford University Press.

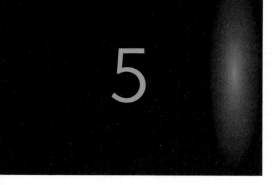

5

Common Research Designs and Issues in Epidemiology

I. FUNCTIONS OF RESEARCH DESIGN

Research is the process of answering a question that can be answered by appropriately collected data. The question may simply be, "What is (or was) the frequency of a disease in a certain place at a certain time?" The answer to this question is *descriptive*, but contrary to a common misperception, this does not mean that obtaining the answer (**descriptive research**) is a simple task. All research, whether quantitative or qualitative, is descriptive, and no research is better than the quality of the data obtained. To answer a question correctly, the data must be obtained and described appropriately. The rules that govern the process of collecting and arranging the data for analysis are called **research designs.**

Another research question may be, "What caused this disease?" **Hypothesis generation** is the process of developing a list of possible candidates for the *causes* of the disease and obtaining initial evidence that supports one or more of these candidates. When one or more hypotheses are generated, the hypothesis must be tested (**hypothesis testing**) by making predictions from the hypotheses and examining new data to

determine if the predictions are correct (see Chapters 6 and 10). If a hypothesis is not supported, it should be discarded or modified and tested again. Some research designs are appropriate for hypothesis generation, and some are appropriate for hypothesis testing. Some designs can be used for either, depending on the circumstances. No research design is perfect, however, because each has its advantages and disadvantages.

The basic function of most epidemiologic research designs is either to describe the pattern of health problems accurately or to enable a fair, unbiased comparison to be made between a group with and a group without a risk factor, a disease, or a preventive or therapeutic intervention. A good epidemiologic research design should perform the following functions:

- Enable a comparison of a variable (e.g., disease frequency) between two or more groups at one point in time or, in some cases, within one group before and after receiving an intervention or being exposed to a risk factor.
- Allow the comparison to be quantified in absolute terms (as with a risk difference or rate difference) or in relative terms (as with a relative risk or odds ratio; see Chapter 6).
- Permit the investigators to determine when the risk factor and the disease occurred, to determine the temporal sequence.
- Minimize biases, confounding, and other problems that would complicate interpretation of the data.

The research designs discussed in this chapter are the primary designs used in epidemiology. Depending on design choice, research designs can assist in developing hypotheses, testing hypotheses, or both. All designs can be used to generate hypotheses; and a few designs can be used to test them—with the caveat that hypothesis development and testing of the same hypothesis can never occur in a single study. Randomized clinical trials or randomized field trials are usually the best designs for testing hypotheses when feasible to perform.

II. TYPES OF RESEARCH DESIGN

Because some research questions can be answered by more than one type of research design, the choice of design depends on a variety of considerations, including the clinical topic (e.g., whether the disease or condition is rare or common) and the cost and availability of data. Research designs are often described as either observational or experimental.

In **observational studies** the investigators simply observe groups of study participants to learn about the possible effects of a treatment or risk factor; the assignment of participants to a treatment group or a control group remains outside the investigators' control. Observational studies can be either descriptive or analytic. In *descriptive* observational studies, no hypotheses are specified in advance, preexisting data are often used, and associations may or may not be causal. In *analytic* observational studies, hypotheses are specified in advance, new data are often collected, and differences between groups are measured.

In an **experimental study** design the investigator has more control over the assignment of participants, often placing them in treatment and control groups (e.g., by using a randomization method before the start of any treatment). Each type of research design has advantages and disadvantages, as discussed subsequently and summarized in Table 5-1 and Figure 5-1.

A. Observational Designs for Generating Hypotheses

1. Qualitative Studies

Qualitative research involves an investigation of clinical issues by using anthropologic techniques such as ethnographic observation, open-ended semistructured interviews, focus groups, and key informant interviews. The investigators attempt to listen to the participants without introducing their own bias as they gather data. They then review the results and identify patterns in the data in a structured and sometimes quantitative form. Results from qualitative research are often invaluable for informing and making sense of quantitative results and providing greater insights into clinical questions and public health problems. The two approaches (quantitative and qualitative) are complementary, with qualitative research providing rich, narrative information that tells a story beyond what reductionist statistics alone might reveal.

2. Cross-Sectional Surveys

A cross-sectional survey is a survey of a population at a single point in time. Surveys may be performed by trained interviewers in people's homes, by telephone interviewers using random-digit dialing, or by mailed, e-mailed, or Web-based questionnaires. Telephone surveys or e-mail questionnaires are often the quickest, but they typically have many nonresponders and refusals, and some people do not have telephones or e-mail access, or they may block calls or e-mails even if they do. Mailed surveys are also relatively inexpensive, but they usually have poor response rates, often 50% or less, except in the case of the U.S. Census, where

Table 5-1   Advantages and Disadvantages of Common Types of Studies Used in Epidemiology

Studies	Advantages	Disadvantages
Qualitative research	Generates hypotheses and initial exploration of issues in participants' own language without bias of investigator	Cannot test study hypotheses Can explore only what is presented or stated Has potential for bias
Cross-sectional surveys	Are fairly quick and easy to perform Are useful for hypothesis generation	Do not offer evidence of a temporal relationship between risk factors and disease Are subject to late-look bias Are not good for hypothesis testing
Ecological studies	Are fairly quick and easy to perform Are useful for hypothesis generation	Do not allow for causal conclusions to be drawn because the data are not associated with individual persons Are subject to ecological fallacy Are not good for hypothesis testing
Cohort studies	Can be performed retrospectively or prospectively Can be used to obtain a true (absolute) measure of risk Can study many disease outcomes Are good for studying rare risk factors	Are time-consuming and costly (especially prospective studies) Can study only the risk factors measured at the beginning Can be used only for common diseases May have losses to follow-up
Case-control studies	Are fairly quick and easy to perform Can study many risk factors Are good for studying rare diseases	Can obtain only a relative measure of risk Are subject to recall bias Selection of controls may be difficult Temporal relationships may be unclear Can study only one disease outcome at a time
Randomized controlled trials	Are the "gold standard" for evaluating treatment interventions (clinical trials) or preventive interventions (field trials) Allow investigator to have extensive control over research process	Are time-consuming and usually costly Can study only interventions or exposures that are controlled by investigator May have problems related to therapy changes and dropouts May be limited in generalizability Are often unethical to perform at all
Systematic reviews and meta-analysis	Decrease subjective element of literature review Increase statistical power Allow exploration of subgroups Provide quantitative estimates of effect	Mixing poor quality studies together in a review or meta-analysis does not improve the underlying quality of studies.
Cost-effectiveness analysis	Clinically important	Difficult to identify costs and payments in many health care systems

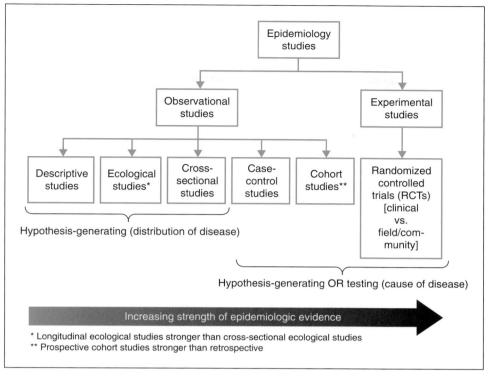

Figure 5-1 **Epidemiologic study designs and increasing strength of evidence.**

response is required by law, and follow-up of all nonresponders is standard.

Cross-sectional surveys have the advantage of being fairly quick and easy to perform. They are useful for determining the prevalence of risk factors and the frequency of prevalent cases of certain diseases for a defined population. They also are useful for measuring current health status and planning for some health services, including setting priorities for disease control. Many surveys have been undertaken to determine the knowledge, attitudes, and health practices of various populations, with the resulting data increasingly being made available to the general public (e.g., healthy-americans.org). A major disadvantage of using cross-sectional surveys is that data on the exposure to risk factors and the presence or absence of disease are collected simultaneously, creating difficulties in determining the temporal relationship of a presumed cause and effect. Another disadvantage is that cross-sectional surveys are biased in favor of longer-lasting and more indolent (mild) cases of diseases. Such cases are more likely to be found by a survey because people live longer with mild cases, enabling larger numbers of affected people to survive and to be interviewed. Severe diseases that tend to be rapidly fatal are less likely to be found by a survey. This phenomenon is often called **Neyman bias** or **late-look bias.** It is known as **length bias** in screening programs, which tend to find (and select for) less aggressive illnesses because patients are more likely to be found by screening (see Chapter 16).

Repeated cross-sectional surveys may be used to determine changes in risk factors and disease frequency in populations over time (but not the nature of the association between risk factors and diseases). Although the data derived from these surveys can be examined for such associations in order to generate hypotheses, cross-sectional surveys are not appropriate for testing the effectiveness of interventions. In such surveys, investigators might find that participants who reported immunization against a disease had fewer cases of the disease. The investigators would not know, however, whether this finding actually meant that people who sought immunization were more concerned about their health and less likely to expose themselves to the disease, known as **healthy participant bias.** If the investigators randomized the participants into two groups, as in a randomized clinical trial, and immunized only one of the groups, this would exclude self-selection as a possible explanation for the association.

Cross-sectional surveys are of particular value in infectious disease epidemiology, in which the prevalence of antibodies against infectious agents, when analyzed according to age or other variables, may provide evidence about when and in whom an infection has occurred. Proof of a recent acute infection can be obtained by two serum samples separated by a short interval. The first samples, the **acute sera,** are collected soon after symptoms appear. The second samples, the **convalescent sera,** are collected 10 to 28 days later. A significant increase in the serum titer of antibodies to a particular infectious agent is regarded as proof of recent infection.

Even if two serum samples are not taken, important inferences can often be drawn on the basis of titers of IgG and IgM, two immunoglobulin classes, in a single serum sample. A high IgG titer without an IgM titer of antibody to a particular infectious agent suggests that the study participant has been infected, but the infection occurred in the distant past. A high IgM titer with a low IgG titer suggests a current or very recent infection. An elevated IgM titer in the presence of a high IgG titer suggests that the infection occurred fairly recently.

3. Cross-Sectional Ecological Studies

Cross-sectional ecological studies relate the frequency with which some characteristic (e.g., smoking) and some outcome of interest (e.g., lung cancer) occur in the same geographic area (e.g., a city, state, or country). In contrast to all other epidemiologic studies, the unit of analysis in ecological studies is *populations,* not individuals. These studies are often useful for suggesting hypotheses but cannot be used to draw causal conclusions. Ecological studies provide no information as to whether the people who were exposed to the characteristic were the same people who developed the disease, whether the exposure or the onset of disease came first, or whether there are other explanations for the observed association. Concerned citizens are sometimes unaware of these weaknesses (sometimes called the **ecological fallacy**) and use findings from cross-sectional ecological surveys to make such statements as, "There are high levels of both toxic pollution and cancer in northern New Jersey, so the toxins are causing the cancer." Although superficially plausible, this conclusion may or may not be correct. For example, what if the individuals in the population who are exposed to the toxins are universally the people not developing cancer? Therefore the toxic pollutants would be exerting a protective effect for individuals despite the ecological evidence that may suggest the opposite conclusion.

In many cases, nevertheless, important hypotheses initially suggested by cross-sectional ecological studies were later supported by other types of studies. The rate of dental caries in children was found to be much higher in areas with low levels of natural fluoridation in the water than in areas with high levels of natural fluoridation.[1] Subsequent research established that this association was causal, and the introduction of water fluoridation and fluoride treatment of

teeth has been followed by striking reductions in the rate of dental caries.[2]

4. Longitudinal Ecological Studies

Longitudinal ecological studies use ongoing surveillance or frequent repeated cross-sectional survey data to measure trends in disease rates over many years in a defined population. By comparing the trends in disease rates with other changes in the society (e.g., wars, immigration, introduction of a vaccine or antibiotics), epidemiologists attempt to determine the impact of these changes on disease rates.

For example, the introduction of the polio vaccine resulted in a precipitous decrease in the rate of paralytic poliomyelitis in the U.S. population (see Chapter 3 and Fig. 3-9). In this case, because of the large number of people involved in the immunization program and the relatively slow rate of change for other factors in the population, longitudinal ecological studies were useful for determining the impact of this public health intervention. Nevertheless, confounding with other factors can distort the conclusions drawn from ecological studies, so if time is available (i.e., it is not an epidemic situation), investigators should perform field studies, such as randomized controlled field trials (see section II.C.2), before pursuing a new, large-scale public health intervention.

Another example of longitudinal ecological research is the study of rates of malaria in the U.S. population since 1930. As shown in Figure 5-2, the peaks in malaria rates can be readily related to social events, such as wars and immigration. The use of a logarithmic scale in the figure visually minimizes the relative decrease in disease frequency, making it less impressive to the eye, but this scale enables readers to see in detail the changes occurring when rates are low.

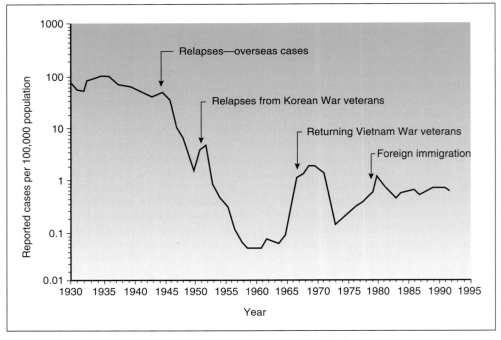

Figure 5-2 Incidence rates of malaria in the United States, by year of report, 1930-1992. (From Centers for Disease Control and Prevention: Summary of notifiable diseases, United States, 1992. *MMWR* 41:38, 1992.)

Important causal associations have been suggested by longitudinal ecological studies. About 20 years after an increase in the smoking rates in men, the lung cancer rate in the male population began increasing rapidly. Similarly, about 20 years after women began to smoke in large numbers, the lung cancer rate in the female population began to increase. The studies in this example were longitudinal ecological studies in the sense that they used only national data on smoking and lung cancer rates, which did not relate the individual cases of lung cancer to individual smokers. The task of establishing a causal relationship was left to cohort and case-control studies.

B. Observational Designs for Generating or Testing Hypotheses

I. Cohort Studies

A cohort is a clearly identified group of people to be studied. In cohort studies, investigators begin by assembling one or more cohorts, either by choosing persons specifically because they were or were not exposed to one or more risk factors of interest, or by taking a random sample of a given population. Participants are assessed to determine whether or not they develop the diseases of interest, and whether the risk factors predict the diseases that occur. The defining characteristic of cohort studies is that groups are typically defined on the basis of exposure and are followed for outcomes. This is in contrast to case-control studies (see section II.B.2), in which groups are assembled on the basis of outcome status and are queried for exposure status. There are two general types of cohort study, prospective and retrospective; Figure 5-3 shows the time relationships of these two types.

PROSPECTIVE COHORT STUDIES

In a prospective cohort study, the investigator assembles the study groups in the present, collects baseline data on them, and continues to collect data for a period that can last many years. Prospective cohort studies offer three main advantages, as follows:

1. The investigator can control and standardize data collection as the study progresses and can check the outcome events (e.g., diseases and death) carefully when these occur, ensuring the outcomes are correctly classified.
2. The estimates of risk obtained from prospective cohort studies represent true (absolute) risks for the groups studied.
3. Many different disease outcomes can be studied, including some that were not anticipated at the beginning of the study.

However, any disease outcomes that were not preplanned—or supported by evidence that was available a priori (before start of the study)—would be hypothesis generating only. Sometimes studies have **secondary outcomes** that are determined a priori, but for which the study is not adequately powered (see Chapter 12) and thus can only be hypothesis generating.

Cohort studies also have disadvantages. In such studies, only the risk factors defined and measured at the beginning of the study can be used. Other disadvantages of cohort studies are their high costs, the possible loss of study participants to follow-up, and the long wait until results are obtained.

The classic cohort study is the Framingham Heart Study, initiated in 1950 and continuing today.[3] Table 5-2 shows the

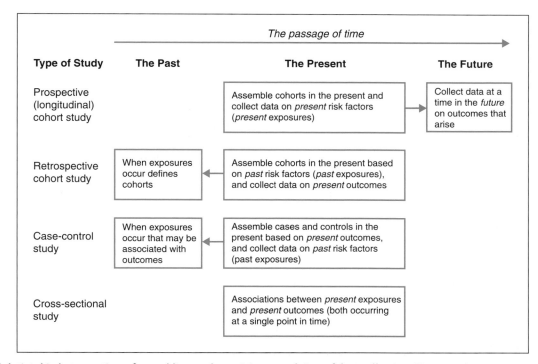

Figure 5-3 Relationship between time of assembling study participants and time of data collection. Illustration shows prospective cohort study, retrospective cohort study, case-control study, and cross-sectional study.

Table 5-2   Risk that 45-year-old Man Will Have Cardiovascular Disease within 8 Years

Risk Group	Characteristics of Risk Group	Risk (%)	Ratio
Lowest	All the following factors: Nonsmoker No glucose intolerance No hypertrophy of left ventricle Low systolic blood pressure (≤105 mm Hg) Low cholesterol level (≤185 mg/dL)	2.2	—
Highest	All the factors listed below	77.8	35.4
Intermediate	One of the following factors:		
	Smoker	3.8	1.7
	Glucose intolerance	3.9	1.8
	Hypertrophy of left ventricle	6	2.7
	Severe hypertension (systolic blood pressure ≥195 mm Hg)	8.4	3.8
	High cholesterol level (≥335 mg/dL)	8.5	3.8

Data from Pearson T, Becker D: Cardiovascular risk: computer program for IBM-compatible systems, using the Framingham Study 8-year risk equations, Johns Hopkins University; and Breslow L: *Science* 200:908–912, 1978.
http://hp2010.nhlbihin.net/atpiii/calculator.asp

8-year risk of heart disease as calculated from the Framingham Study's equations.[4] Although these risk ratios are not based on the most recent study data, the length of follow-up and the clarity of the message still make them useful for sharing with patients. Examples of other, more recent, large cohort studies are the Nurses' Health Study, begun in 1976 and continuing to track more than 120,000 nurses in the United States (www.nhs3.org), and the National Child Development Study, initiated after the Second World War and continuing to follow a large birth cohort in the United Kingdom.[5]

RETROSPECTIVE COHORT STUDIES

The time and cost limitations of prospective cohort studies can be mitigated in part by conducting retrospective cohort studies. In this approach the investigator uses historical data to define a risk group (e.g., people exposed to the Hiroshima atomic bomb in August 1945) and follows group members up to the present to see what outcomes (e.g., cancer and death) have occurred. This type of study has many of the advantages of a prospective cohort study, including the ability to calculate an absolute risk. However, it lacks the ability to monitor and control data collection that characterizes a prospective cohort study.

A retrospective cohort study in 1962 investigated the effects of prenatal x-ray exposure.[6] In prior decades, radiographs were often used to measure the size of the pelvic outlet of pregnant women, thus exposing fetuses to x-rays in utero. The investigators identified one group of participants who had been exposed in utero and another group who had not. They determined how many participants from each group had developed cancer during childhood or early adulthood (up to the time of data collection).

The individuals who had been exposed to x-rays in utero had a 40% increase in the risk of childhood cancers, or a risk ratio of 1.4, after adjustments for other factors.

2. Case-Control Studies

The investigator in a case-control study selects the case group and the control group on the basis of a defined outcome (e.g., having a disease of interest versus not having a disease of interest) and compares the groups in terms of their frequency of past exposure to possible risk factors (see Fig. 5-3). This strategy can be understood as comparing "the risk of having the risk factor" in the two groups. However, the actual risk of the outcome cannot be determined from such studies because the underlying population remains unknown. Instead, case-control studies can estimate the **relative risk** of the outcome, known as the **odds ratio.**

In the case-control study the cases and controls are assembled and then questioned (or their relatives or medical records are consulted) regarding past exposure to risk factors. For this reason, case-control studies were often called "retrospective studies" in previous decades; this term does not distinguish them from retrospective cohort studies and thus is no longer preferred. The time relationships in a case-control study are similar to those in a cross-sectional study in that investigators learn simultaneously about the current disease state and any past risk factors. In terms of assembling the participants, however, a case-control study differs from a cross-sectional study because the sample for the case-control study is chosen specifically from groups with and without the disease of interest. Often, everyone with the disease of interest in a given geographic area and time period can be selected as cases. This strategy reduces bias in case selection.

Case-control studies are especially useful when a study must be performed quickly and inexpensively or when the disease under study is rare (e.g., prevalence <1%). In a cohort study a huge number of study participants would need to be followed to find even a few cases of a rare disease, and the search might take a long time even if funds were available. If a new cancer were found in 1 of 1000 people screened per year (as does occur), an investigator would have to study 50,000 people to find just 100 cases over a typical follow-up time of 2 years. Although case-control studies can consider only one outcome (one disease) per study, many risk factors may be considered, a characteristic that makes such studies useful for generating hypotheses about the causes of a disease. Methodologic standards have been developed so that the quality of information obtained from case-control studies can approximate that obtained from much more difficult, costly, and time-consuming randomized clinical trials.

Despite these advantages, the use of case-control studies has several drawbacks. In determining risk factors, a major problem is the potential for *recall bias* (see Chapter 4). Also, it is not easy to know the correct control group for cases. Members of a control group are usually matched individually to members of the case group on the basis of age, gender, and often race. If possible, the investigator obtains controls from the same diagnostic setting in which cases were found, to avoid potential bias (e.g., if the disease is more likely to be detected in one setting than in another). If the controls were drawn from the same hospital and were examined for a disease of the same organ system (e.g., pulmonary disease), presumably a similar workup (including chest radiograph and spirometry) would be performed, so that asymptomatic cases of the disease would be less likely to be missed and incorrectly classified as controls. Similarly, in a study of birth defects, the control for each case might be the next infant who was born at the same hospital, of the same gender and race, with a mother of similar age from the same location. This strategy would control for season, location, gender, race, and age of mother. Given the difficulties of selecting a control group with no bias whatsoever, investigators often assemble two or more control groups, one of which is drawn from the general population.

A potential danger of studies that use matching is **overmatching.** If cases and controls were inadvertently matched on some characteristic that is potentially causal, that *cause* would be missed. For example, if cases and controls in early studies of the causes of lung cancer had been matched on smoking status, smoking would not appear as a potentially causal factor.

A case-control study was successful in identifying the risk associated with taking a synthetic hormone, diethylstilbestrol (DES), during pregnancy. In 1971 the mothers of seven of eight teenage girls diagnosed with clear cell adenocarcinoma of the vagina in Boston claimed to have taken DES while the child was in utero.[7] For controls, the authors identified girls without vaginal adenocarcinoma who were born in the same hospital and date of birth as the cases. None of the mothers of the 32 (control) girls without vaginal adenocarcinoma had taken DES during the corresponding pregnancy.

3. Nested Case-Control Studies

In a cohort study with a nested case-control study, a cohort of participants is first defined, and the baseline characteristics of the participants are obtained by interview, physical examination, and pertinent laboratory or imaging studies. The participants are then followed to determine the outcome. Participants who develop the condition of interest become cases in the nested case-control study; participants who do not develop the condition become eligible for the control group of the nested case-control study. The cases and a representative (or matched) sample of controls are studied, and data from the two groups are compared by using analytic methods appropriate for case-control studies.

A nested case-control design was used in a study of meningitis. Participants were drawn from a large, prospective cohort study of patients admitted to the emergency department because of suspected meningitis.[8,9] In the nested case-control study the *cases* were all the patients with a diagnosis of *nonbacterial* meningitis, and the *controls* represented a sample of patients not diagnosed with meningitis. The goal was to determine whether there was an association between the prior use of nonsteroidal antiinflammatory drugs and the frequency of nonbacterial meningitis. Using patients from the larger cohort study, for whom data had already been obtained, made the nested case-control study simpler and less costly.

A variant of the nested case-control design is the **case-cohort study.**[10] In this approach the study also begins with a cohort study, and the controls are similarly drawn from the cohort study but are identified *before* any cases develop, so some may later become cases. The analysis for case-cohort studies is more complex than for other case-control studies.

C. Experimental Designs for Testing Hypotheses

Two types of randomized controlled trials (RCTs) are discussed here: randomized controlled *clinical trials* (RCCTs) and randomized controlled *field trials* (RCFTs). Both designs follow the same series of steps shown in Figure 5-4 and have many of the same advantages and disadvantages. The major difference between the two is that clinical trials are typically used to test *therapeutic* interventions in *ill* persons, whereas field trials are typically used to test *preventive* interventions in *well* persons in the community.

1. Randomized Controlled Clinical Trials

In an RCCT, often referred to simply as a randomized controlled trial (RCT), patients are enrolled in a study and randomly assigned to one of the following two groups:

- Intervention or treatment group, who receives the experimental treatment
- Control group, who receives the nonexperimental treatment, consisting of either a placebo (inert substance) or a standard treatment method

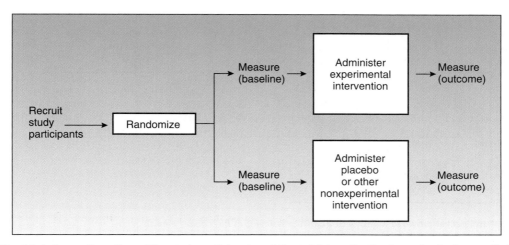

Figure 5-4 Relationship between time of recruiting study participants and time of data collection in randomized controlled trial (RCT; clinical or field).

The RCCT is considered the "gold standard" for studying interventions because of the ability to minimize bias in the information obtained from participants. Nevertheless, RCCTs do not entirely eliminate bias, and these trials pose some challenges and ethical dilemmas for investigators.

To be enrolled in an RCCT, patients must agree to participate without knowing whether they will receive the experimental or the nonexperimental treatment. When this condition is met, and patients are kept unaware of which treatment they receive during the trial, it establishes a **single-blind study** (or single-blinded; the participant is blind to the treatment). If possible, the observers who collect the data and those who are doing the analyses are also prevented from knowing which type of treatment each patient is given. When both participants and investigators are blinded, the trial is said to be a **double-blind study** (or double-blinded). Unfortunately, there is some ambiguity in the way blinding is described in the literature, thus we recommend including descriptions that clearly communicate which of the relevant groups were unaware of allocation.[11]

Ideally, trials should have a third level of blinding, sometimes known as **allocation concealment.** This third type of blinding means that the investigators delivering the intervention are also blinded as to whether they are providing experimental or control treatment (i.e., they are blinded to the allocation of participants to the experimental or control group). When participants, investigators who gather the data, and analysts are all blinded, this is functionally a **triple-blind study** (or triple-blinded), and this is optimal. To have true blinding, the nonexperimental treatment must appear identical (e.g., in size, shape, color, taste) to the experimental treatment.

Figure 5-5 shows the pill packet from a trial of two preventive measures from a famous RCT, the Physicians' Health Study (see Chapter 4). The round tablets were either aspirin or a placebo, but the study participants (and investigators) could not tell which. The elongated capsules were either beta carotene or a placebo, but again, the study participants (and investigators) could not tell which.

It is usually impossible and unethical to have patients participate blindly in a study involving a surgical intervention, because blinding would require a sham operation (although sometimes this is done). In studies involving nonsurgical interventions, investigators often can develop an effective placebo. For example, when investigators designed a computer game to teach asthmatic children how to care for themselves, with the goal of reducing hospitalizations, they distributed similar-looking computer games to children in the intervention group and the control group, but the games for the control group were without asthma content.[12]

Undertaking an RCCT is difficult, and potentially unethical, if the intervention is already well established in practice and strongly believed to be the best available, whether or not that belief had been confirmed scientifically by carefully designed and controlled studies. Because no RCCTs have compared prenatal care versus no prenatal care, there is no conclusive proof that prenatal care is valuable, and questions about its value are raised from time to time. The standard of

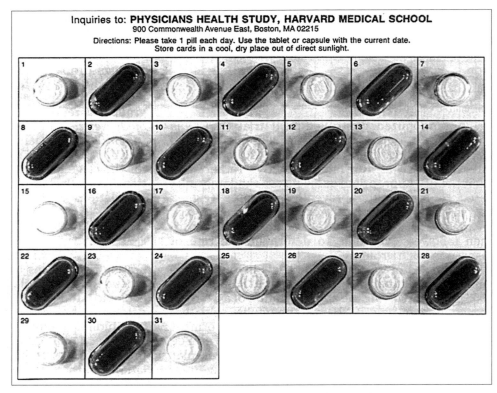

Figure 5-5 **"Bubble" pill packet provided monthly to 22,000 physicians in Physicians' Health Study.** In this simultaneous trial of aspirin to reduce cardiovascular disease and beta carotene to prevent cancer, the round white tablets contained either aspirin or placebo and the elongated capsules either beta carotene or placebo. The participants did not know which substances they were taking. (Courtesy Dr. Charles Hennekens, Director, Physicians' Health Study, Boston.)

practice might preclude a RCCT in which one arm involved no prenatal care. However, studies in which variations in the frequency, duration, and content of prenatal care were compared would likely avoid the ethical dilemma, while generating useful information. At a time when both medical ethics and evidence-based practice are salient concerns, there are new challenges involved in putting time-honored practices to the rigorous test of randomized trials.

In RCCTs, many biases remain possible, although some biases have been minimized by the randomized, prospective design and by double-blinding. For example, two groups under comparison may exhibit different rates at which patients drop out of the study or become lost to follow-up, and this difference could produce a greater change in the characteristics of the remaining study participants in one group than in the other.

Therapy changes and dropouts are special problems in RCCTs involving severe diseases, such as advanced cancer. The patients receiving the new treatment may continue to fail to respond, and either they or their physicians may decide to try a different treatment, which they must be allowed to do. Patients also may leave a study if the new treatment has unpleasant side effects, even though the treatment may be effective. In the past, some medications for hypertension reduced male potency, and many men discontinued their medication when this happened, despite its beneficial effect on their hypertension.

An apparent selection bias, called **publication bias,** makes it difficult to arrive at an overall interpretation of the results of clinical trials reported in the literature. For various reasons, pharmaceutical companies or investigators, or both, may not want to publish RCTs with *negative* results (i.e., results that do not favor the intervention being tested). Even journal editors may not be enthusiastic about publishing negative trials because they may not be interesting to their readers (i.e., unless they contradict established dogma and would be paradigm challenging and news generating). Published RCCTs on a new intervention, as a group, may therefore give a more favorable impression of the intervention than would be likely if all trials of that intervention (including trials that returned negative results) had been published.

To reduce this problem, a group of editors joined together to create a policy whereby their journals would consider publication only of results of RCCTs that had been registered with a clinical trial registry "before the onset of patient enrollment."[13] This requirement that all trials be registered before they begin is important if the sponsors and investigators want to be eligible to publish in a major medical journal. It is now possible to explore the clinical trial registry to find out what studies remain unpublished (http://clinicaltrials.gov).

2. Randomized Controlled Field Trials

An RCFT is similar to an RCCT (see Fig. 5-4), except that the intervention in an RCFT is usually preventive rather than therapeutic and conducted in the community. Appropriate participants are randomly allocated to receive the preventive measure (e.g., vaccine, oral drug) or to receive the placebo (e.g., injection of sterile saline, inert pill). They are followed over time to determine the rate of disease in each group. Examples of RCFTs include trials of vaccines to prevent paralytic poliomyelitis[14] and aspirin to reduce cardiovascular disease.[15]

The RCFTs and the RCCTs have similar advantages and disadvantages. One disadvantage is that results may take a long time to obtain, unless the effect of the treatment or preventive measure occurs quickly. The Physicians' Health Study cited earlier illustrates this problem. Although its trial of the preventive benefits of aspirin began in 1982, the final report on the aspirin component of the trial was not released until 7 years later.

Another disadvantage of RCFTs and RCCTs involves **external validity,** or the ability to generalize findings to other groups in the population (vs. **internal validity,** or the validity of results for study participants). After the study groups for an RCT have been assembled and various potential participants excluded according to the study's exclusion criteria, it may be unclear which population is actually represented by the remaining people in the trial.

D. Techniques for Data Summary, Cost-Effectiveness Analysis, and Postapproval Surveillance

Meta-analysis, decision analysis, and cost-effectiveness analysis are important techniques for examining and using data collected in clinical research. **Meta-analysis** is used to summarize the information obtained in many single studies on one topic. **Decision analysis** and **cost-effectiveness analysis** are used to summarize data and show how data can inform clinical or policy decisions. All three techniques are discussed in more detail in Chapter 8. One of the most important uses of summary techniques has been to develop recommendations for clinical preventive services (e.g., by the U.S. Preventive Services Task Force) and community preventive services (e.g., by the U.S. Community Services Task Force).[16,17] These task forces have used a hierarchy to indicate the quality of evidence, such that RCTs are at the apex (best internal validity), followed by designs with fewer protections against bias. Table 5-3 summarizes the hierarchy of evidence used by the

Table 5-3 Quality of Evidence Hierarchy Used by U.S. Preventive Services Task Force

Quality Rating*	Type of Study
I	Evidence obtained from at least one properly randomized controlled trial
II-1	Evidence obtained from well-designed controlled trials without randomization
II-2	Evidence obtained from well-designed cohort or case-control analytic studies, preferably from more than one center or research group
II-3	Evidence obtained from multiple time series with or without the intervention. Dramatic results in uncontrolled experiments (e.g., results of introduction of penicillin treatment in 1940s) also could be regarded as this type of evidence.
III	Opinions of respected authorities, based on clinical experience; descriptive studies and case reports; or reports of expert committees

*I = best.

U.S. Preventive Services Task Force (see Chapters 15-17). It was modified by the U.S. Community Services Task Force (see Chapter 18).

The usual drug approvals by the U.S. Food and Drug Administration (FDA) are based on RCTs of limited size and duration. Longer-term postapproval surveillance (now called Phase 4 clinical testing) is increasingly exhibiting its importance.[18] Such postapproval surveillance permits a much larger study sample and a longer observation time, so that side effects not seen in the earlier studies may become obvious. A much-publicized example of such findings was the removal of some cyclooxygenase-2 inhibitor medications from the market, because of an increase in cardiovascular events in these patients.

III. RESEARCH ISSUES IN EPIDEMIOLOGY

A. Dangers of Data Dredging

The common research designs described in this chapter are frequently used by investigators to gather and summarize data. Looking for messages in data carries the potential danger of finding those that do not really exist. In studies with large amounts of data, there is a temptation to use modern computer techniques to see which variables are related to which other variables and to make many associations. This process is sometimes referred to as "data dredging" and is often used in medical research, although this is sometimes not clarified in the published literature. Readers of medical literature should be aware of the special dangers in this activity.

The search for associations can be appropriate as long as the investigator keeps two points in mind. First, the scientific process requires that hypothesis development and hypothesis testing be based on *different* data sets. One data set is used to develop the hypothesis or model, which is used to make predictions, which are then tested on a new data set. Second, a **correlational study** (e.g., using Pearson correlation coefficient or chi-square test) is useful only for developing hypotheses, not for testing them. Stated in slightly different terms, a correlational study is only a form of screening method, to identify associations that might be real. Investigators who keep these points in mind are unlikely to make the mistake of thinking every association found in a data set represents a true association.

One celebrated example of the problem of data dredging was seen in the report of an association between coffee consumption and pancreatic cancer, obtained by looking at many associations in a large data set, without repeating the analysis on another data set to determine if it was consistent.[19] This approach was severely criticized at the time, and several subsequent studies failed to find a true association between coffee consumption and pancreatic cancer.[20]

How does this problem arise? Suppose there were 10 variables in a descriptive study, and the investigator wanted to try to associate each one with every other one. There would be 10×10 possible cells (Fig. 5-6). Ten of these would be each variable times itself, however, which is always a perfect correlation. That leaves 90 possible associations, but half of these would be "$x \times y$" and the other half "$y \times x$." Because the p values for bivariate tests are the same regardless of which is considered the independent variable and which the dependent one, there are only half as many truly independent associations, or 45. If the **$p = 0.05$ cutoff point** is used for defining a significant finding (alpha level) (see Chapter 10), 5 of 100 independent associations would be expected to occur by chance alone.[21] In the example, it means that slightly more than two "statistically significant" associations would be expected to occur just by chance.

The problem with multiple hypotheses is similar to that with multiple associations: the greater the number of

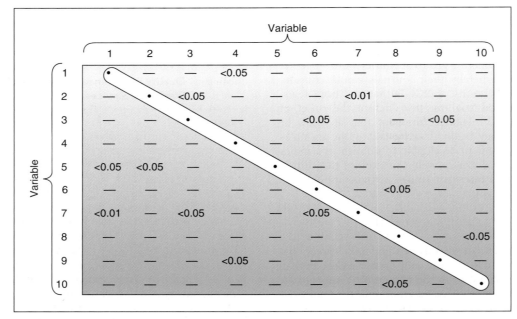

Figure 5-6 Matrix of possible statistical associations between 10 different variables from same research study. Perfect correlations of one variable with itself are shown by *dots*; nonstatistically significant relationships are shown by *dashes*; and statistically significant associations are shown by the *p* values. (Redrawn from Jekel JF: Should we stop using the p-value in descriptive studies? *Pediatrics* 60:124–126, 1977.)

hypotheses tested, the more likely that at least one of them will be found "statistically significant" by chance alone. One possible way to handle this problem is to lower the *p* value required before rejecting the null hypothesis (e.g., make *p* <0.05). This was done in a study testing the same medical educational hypothesis at five different hospitals.[21] If the alpha level in the study had been set at 0.05, there would have been an almost 25% probability of finding a statistically significant difference by chance alone in at least one of the five hospitals, because each hospital had a 5% (alpha = 0.05) probability of showing a difference from chance alone. To keep the risk of a false-positive finding in the entire study to no more than 0.05, the **alpha level chosen for rejecting the null hypothesis** was made more stringent by dividing alpha by 5 (number of hospitals) to make it 0.01. This method of adjusting for multiple hypotheses is called the **Bonferroni adjustment to alpha,** and it is quite stringent. Other possible adjustments are less stringent, but are more complicated statistically and used in different situations (e.g., Tukey, Scheffe, and Newman-Keuls procedures).[22]

B. Ethical Issues

Most research institutions have a committee specifically charged with the responsibility of reviewing all proposed research and ensuring that it is ethical. This type of committee is often called an **institutional review board** (IRB). IRBs have their foundation in the World Medical Association's Declaration of Helsinki, which was originally drafted in the 1960s. The primary goals of IRBs are to ensure the following:

- All research involving human subjects is of high quality so that any risks involved are justified.
- The potential benefits to the study participants or to society in general are greater than the potential harm from the research.
- Researchers obtain documented **informed consent** from study participants or their guardians.
- Researchers protect the confidentiality of their research data.
- Study participants are allowed to withdraw from the research at any time, without this action adversely affecting their care.

Most universities and hospitals now require that *all* **human research protocols** be approved by an IRB, whether or not the research is externally funded.

All scientists are bound by the obligations of honesty and integrity in their research. Investigators have a responsibility to protect human subjects, implement privacy and confidentiality protections, register clinical trials, interpret their data objectively and disclose all potential conflicts of interest in any reports and publications.[23] Industry-sponsored research is at greatest risk for conflicts of interest, and thus safeguards are helpful. With industry-sponsored research, ideally all the research data are available and analyzed independently of the sponsor.

Scientists have a professional responsibility to describe their study design and methods accurately and in sufficient detail and to assure readers that the work was carried out in accordance with ethical principles. Plagiarism, ghostwriting, and taking credit or payment for authorship of work written by another individual are unethical.

In this era of intense media and public interest in medical news, investigators need to be careful in the presentation of their research findings. Media coverage can be fraught with misinterpretation and unjustified extrapolation and conclusions.[24] Preliminary research results are frequently reported by the media as a critical new "breakthrough." Investigators therefore need to avoid raising false public expectations or providing misleading information.

IV. SUMMARY

Research is the attempt to answer questions with valid data. Epidemiologic research seeks to answer questions about the distribution of health, disease, or risk factors; to develop hypotheses about the causes of ill health and the effectiveness of preventive and curative interventions; and to test these hypotheses. Observational research designs suitable for generating hypotheses include qualitative studies, cross-sectional surveys, cross-sectional ecological studies, and longitudinal ecological studies. A cross-sectional study collects data about a population at one point in time, whereas a longitudinal study is conducted over a period of time. Cross-sectional surveys are useful in determining the prevalence of risk factors and diseases in the population but are weak in determining the temporal relationship between variables. Ecological studies obtain the rate of a disease and the frequency of exposure to a risk factor for an entire population, but the unit of study is the population and not the individuals within it, so exposure and disease cannot be linked in individual participants.

Observational research designs suitable for generating or testing hypotheses include prospective cohort studies, retrospective cohort studies, and case-control studies. In cohort studies, one study group consists of persons exposed to risk factors, and another group consists of persons not exposed. These groups are studied to determine and compare their rates of disease. Figure 5-3 illustrates the difference between a prospective and a retrospective cohort study. In case-control studies the case group consists of persons who have a particular disease, and the control group consists of persons who do not have the disease but are matched individually to the cases (e.g., in terms of age, gender, and type of medical workup). Each group is studied to determine the frequency of past exposure to possible risk factors. Based on this information, the relative odds that a disease is linked with a particular risk factor (odds ratio) can be calculated. The use of a cohort study with a nested case-control design may enable some hypotheses to be tested quickly and cost-effectively.

The experimental designs suitable for testing hypotheses are randomized controlled clinical trials (RCCTs, or RCTs) and randomized controlled field trials (RCFTs). Both types of trials follow the steps shown in Figure 5-4. The major difference between these two types is that clinical trials are generally used to test therapeutic interventions, whereas field trials are usually conducted to test preventive interventions. A trial is called a double-blind study if neither the participants nor the observers who collect the data know which type of intervention each participant receives.

Large data sets may contain associations by chance alone. Data dredging carries the greatest risk with analyses of large cohort data sets (i.e., when questions not part of the original basis for a study are appended). Institutional review boards evaluate study protocols before projects are undertaken to ensure that the research is of high quality with minimal and acceptable risk to study participants (human subjects).

References

1. Arnim S, et al: A study of dental changes in a group of Pueblo Indian children. *J Am Dent Assoc* 24:478–480, 1937.
2. US Centers for Disease Control and Prevention: Achievements in public health, 1900-1999: fluoridation of drinking water to prevent dental caries. *MMWR* 48:933–940, 1999.
3. Dawber TR, et al: Epidemiologic approaches to heart disease: the Framingham Study. *Am J Public Health* 41:279–286, 1951.
4. Breslow L: Risk factor intervention for health maintenance. *Science* 200:908–912, 1978.
5. http://www.cls.ioe.ac.uk/page.aspx?&sitesectionid=724&sitesectiontitle=National+Child+Development+Study.
6. MacMahon B: Prenatal x-ray exposure and childhood cancer. *J Natl Cancer Inst* 28:1173–1191, 1962.
7. Herbst AL, Ulfelder H, Poskanzer DC: Adenocarcinoma of the vagina: association of maternal stilbestrol therapy with tumor appearance in young women. *N Engl J Med* 284:878–881, 1971.
8. Hasbun R, Abrahams J, Jekel J, et al: Computed tomography of the head before lumbar puncture in adults with suspected meningitis. *N Engl J Med* 345:1727–1733, 2001.
9. Quagliarello VJ: Personal communication.
10. Last JM, editor: *A dictionary of epidemiology*, ed 4, New York, 2001, Oxford University Press.
11. Devereaux PJ, Manns BJ, Ghali WA, et al: Physician interpretations and textbook definitions of blinding terminology in randomized controlled trials. *JAMA* 285:2000–2003, 2001.
12. Rubin DH, Leventhal JM, Sadock RT, et al: Educational intervention by computer in childhood asthma. *Pediatrics* 77:1–10, 1986.
13. DeAngelis C, Drazen JM, Frizelle FA, et al: Clinical trial registration: a statement from the International Committee of Medical Journal Editors. *JAMA* 292:1363–1364, 2004.
14. Francis T, Jr, Korns RF, Voight RB, et al: An evaluation of the 1954 poliomyelitis vaccine trials. *Am J Public Health* 45(pt 2):1–63, 1955.
15. Physicians' Health Study Steering Committee: Final report on the aspirin component of the ongoing Physicians' Health Study. *N Engl J Med* 321:129–135, 1989.
16. US Preventive Services Task Force: *Guide to clinical preventive services,* ed 3, periodic updates, Agency for Healthcare Research and Quality. www.ahrq.gov/clinic/uspstfix.html.
17. Task Force on Community Preventive Services: *The guide to community preventive service: what works to promote health?* New York, 2005, Oxford University Press. www.thecommunityguide.org.
18. Vlahakes GJ: The value of Phase 4 clinical testing. *N Engl J Med* 354:413–415, 2006.
19. MacMahon B, Yen S, Trichopoulos D, et al: Coffee and cancer of the pancreas. *N Engl J Med* 304:630–633, 1981.
20. Feinstein AR, Horwitz RI, Spitzer WO, et al: Coffee and pancreatic cancer: the problems of etiologic science and epidemiologic case-control research. *JAMA* 246:957–961, 1981.
21. Jekel JF: Should we stop using the *p*-value in descriptive studies? *Pediatrics* 60:124–126, 1977.
22. Dawson B, Trapp RG: *Basic and clinical biostatistics*, ed 4, New York, 2004, Lange Medical Books/McGraw-Hill.
23. http://www.acponline.org/running_practice/ethics/manual/manual6th.htm#research.
24. http://www.healthnewsreview.org.

Select Readings

Friedman LM, Furberg CD, DeMets DL: *Fundamentals of clinical trials*, ed 3, St Louis, 1995, Mosby.
Gerstman BB: *Epidemiology kept simple*, New York, 1998, Wiley-Liss.
Gordis L: *Epidemiology*, ed 4, Philadelphia, 2009, Saunders-Elsevier.
Hennekens CH, Buring JE: *Epidemiology in medicine*, Boston, 1987, Little, Brown.
Kelsey JL, Whittemore AS, Evans AS, et al: *Methods in observational epidemiology*, ed 2, New York, 1996, Oxford University Press.
Koepsell T, Weiss NS: *Epidemiologic methods*, New York, 2003, Oxford University Press.
Schlesselman JJ: *Case-control studies: design, conduct, analysis*, New York, 1982, Oxford University Press. [A classic.]

Websites

http://healthyamericans.org/

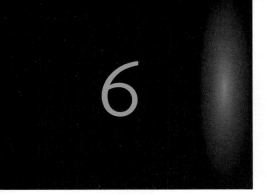

6

Assessment of Risk and Benefit in Epidemiologic Studies

Causal research in epidemiology requires that two fundamental distinctions be made. The first distinction is between people who have and people who do not have exposure to the risk factor (or protective factor) under study (the **independent variable**). The second distinction is between people who have and people who do not have the disease (or other outcome) under study (the **dependent variable**). These distinctions are seldom simple, and their measurements are subject to random errors and biases.

In addition, epidemiologic research may be complicated by other requirements. It may be necessary to analyze several independent (possibly causal) variables at the same time, including how they interact. For example, the frequency of hypertension is related to *age* and *gender,* and these variables interact in the following manner: before about age 50, men are more likely to be hypertensive; but after age 50, women are more likely to be hypertensive. Another complication involves the need to measure different degrees of *strength of exposure* to the risk factor, the *duration of exposure* to the risk factor, or both. Investigators study strength and duration in combination, for example, when they measure exposure to cigarettes in terms of *pack-years,* which is the average number of packs smoked per day times the number of years of smoking. Depending on the risk factor, it may be difficult to

determine the time of onset of exposure. This is true for risk factors such as sedentary lifestyle and excess intake of dietary sodium. Another complication of analysis is the need to measure different levels of *disease severity.* Exposure and outcome may vary across a range of values, rather than simply be *present* or *absent.*

Despite these complexities, much epidemiologic research still relies on the dichotomies of exposed/unexposed and diseased/nondiseased, which are often presented in the form of a **standard 2 × 2 table** (Table 6-1).

I. DEFINITION OF STUDY GROUPS

Causal research depends on the measurement of differences. In cohort studies the difference is between the frequency of disease in **persons exposed** to a risk factor and the frequency of disease in **persons not exposed** to the same risk factor. In case-control studies the difference is between the frequency of the risk factor in **case participants** (persons with the disease) and the frequency of the risk factor in **control participants** (persons without the disease).

The exposure may be to a *nutritional* factor (e.g., high–saturated fat diet), an *environmental* factor (e.g., radiation after Chernobyl disaster), a *behavioral* factor (e.g., cigarette smoking), a *physiologic* characteristic (e.g., high serum total cholesterol level), a *medical* intervention (e.g., antibiotic), or a *public health* intervention (e.g., vaccine). Other factors also play a role, and the categorization may vary (e.g., nutritional choices are often regarded as behavioral factors).

II. COMPARISON OF RISKS IN DIFFERENT STUDY GROUPS

Although differences in risk can be measured in absolute terms or in relative terms, the method used depends on the type of study performed. For reasons discussed in Chapter 5, case-control studies allow investigators to obtain only a relative measure of risk, whereas cohort studies and randomized controlled trials allow investigators to obtain absolute and relative measures of risk. Whenever possible, it is important to examine absolute and relative risks because they provide different information.

After the differences in risk are calculated by the methods outlined in detail subsequently, the level of statistical significance must be determined to ensure that any observed difference is probably real (i.e., not caused by chance). (Significance testing is discussed in detail in Chapter 10.)

Table 6-1   Standard 2 × 2 Table for Showing Association between a Risk Factor and a Disease

Risk Factor	Disease Status		Total
	Present	Absent	
Positive	a	b	$a + b$
Negative	c	d	$c + d$
TOTAL	$a + c$	$b + d$	$a + b + c + d$

Interpretation of the Cells

a = Participants with both the risk factor and the disease
b = Participants with the risk factor, but not the disease
c = Participants with the disease, but not the risk factor
d = Participants with neither the risk factor nor the disease
$a + b$ = All participants with the risk factor
$c + d$ = All participants without the risk factor
$a + c$ = All participants with the disease
$b + d$ = All participants without the disease
$a + b + c + d$ = All study participants

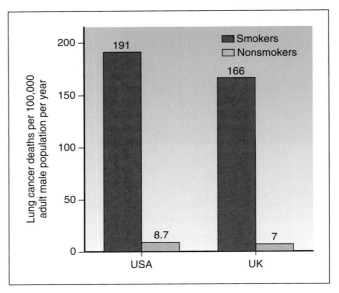

Figure 6-1   Risk of death from lung cancer. Comparison of the risks of death from lung cancer per 100,000 adult male population per year for smokers and nonsmokers in the United States (USA) and United Kingdom (UK). (Data from US Centers for Disease Control: *MMWR* 38:501–505, 1989; and Doll R, Hill AB: *BMJ* 2:1071–1081, 1956.)

When the difference is statistically significant, but not clinically important, it is real but trivial. When the difference appears to be clinically important, but is not statistically significant, it may be a false-negative (beta) error if the sample size is small (see Chapter 12), or it may be a chance finding.

A. Absolute Differences in Risk

Disease frequency usually is measured as a risk in cohort studies and clinical trials and as a rate when the disease and death data come from population-based reporting systems. An absolute difference in risks or rates can be expressed as a risk difference or as a rate difference. The **risk difference** is the risk in the exposed group minus the risk in the unexposed group. The **rate difference** is the rate in the exposed group minus the rate in the unexposed group (rates are defined in Chapter 2). The discussion in this chapter focuses on risks, which are used more often than rates in cohort studies.

When the level of risk in the exposed group is the same as the level of risk in the unexposed group, the risk difference is 0, and the conclusion is that the exposure makes no difference to the disease risk being studied. If an exposure is harmful (as in the case of cigarette smoking), the risk difference is expected to be greater than 0. If an exposure is protective (as in the case of a vaccine), the risk difference is expected to be less than 0 (i.e., a negative number, which in this case indicates a reduction in disease risk in the group exposed to the vaccine). The risk difference also is known as the **attributable risk** because it is an estimate of the amount of risk that *can be attributed to,* or *is attributable to* (is caused by), the risk factor.

In Table 6-1 the risk of disease in the exposed individuals is $a/(a + b)$, and the risk of disease in the unexposed individuals is $c/(c + d)$. When these symbols are used, the attributable risk (AR) can be expressed as the difference between the two:

$$AR = \text{Risk}_{(exposed)} - \text{Risk}_{(unexposed)}$$
$$= [a/(a+b)] - [c/(c+d)]$$

Figure 6-1 provides data on age-adjusted death rates for lung cancer among adult male smokers and nonsmokers in the U.S. population in 1986 and in the United Kingdom (UK) population.[1,2] For the United States in 1986, the lung cancer death rate in smokers was 191 per 100,000 population per year, whereas the rate in nonsmokers was 8.7 per 100,000 per year. Because the death rates for lung cancer in the population were low (<1% per year) in the year for which data are shown, the rate and the risk for lung cancer death would be essentially the same. The risk difference (attributable risk) in the United States can be calculated as follows:

$$191/100,000 - 8.7/100,000 = 182.3/100,000$$

Similarly, the attributable risk in the UK can be calculated as follows:

$$166/100,000 - 7/100,000 = 159/100,000$$

B. Relative Differences in Risk

Relative risk (RR) can be expressed in terms of a risk ratio (also abbreviated as RR) or estimated by an odds ratio (OR).

1. Relative Risk (Risk Ratio)

The **relative risk**, which is also known as the risk ratio (both abbreviated as RR), is the ratio of the risk in the exposed group to the risk in the unexposed group. If the risks in the exposed group and unexposed group are the same, RR = 1. If the risks in the two groups are not the same, calculating RR provides a straightforward way of showing in relative terms how much different (greater or smaller) the risks in the exposed group are compared with the risks in the unexposed group. The risk for the disease in the exposed group usually is greater if an exposure is harmful (as with cigarette smoking) or smaller if an exposure is protective (as with a

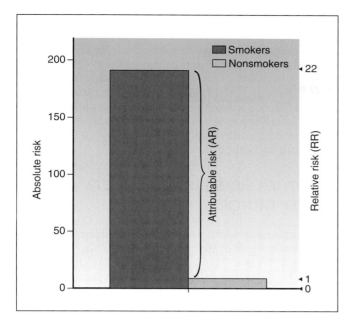

Figure 6-2 Risk of death from lung cancer. Diagram shows the risks of death from lung cancer per 100,000 adult male population per year for smokers and nonsmokers in the United States, expressed in absolute *terms (left axis)* and in relative terms *(right axis)*. (Data from US Centers for Disease Control: *MMWR* 38:501–505, 1989.)

vaccine). In terms of the groups and symbols defined in Table 6-1, relative risk (RR) would be calculated as follows:

$$RR = Risk_{(exposed)}/Risk_{(unexposed)}$$
$$= [a/(a+b)]/[c/(c+d)]$$

The data on lung cancer deaths in Figure 6-1 are used to determine the **attributable risk** (AR). The same data can be used to calculate the RR. For men in the United States, 191/100,000 divided by 8.7/100,000 yields an RR of 22. Figure 6-2 shows the conversion from absolute to relative risks. Absolute risk is shown on the left axis and relative risk on the right axis. In relative risk terms the value of the risk for lung cancer death in the unexposed group is 1. Compared with that, the risk for lung cancer death in the exposed group is 22 times as great, and the attributable risk is the difference, which is 182.3/100,000 in absolute risk terms and 21 in relative risk terms.

It also is important to consider the number of people to whom the relative risk applies. A large relative risk that applies to a small number of people may produce few excess deaths or cases of disease, whereas a small relative risk that applies to a large number of people may produce many excess deaths or cases of disease.

2. Odds Ratio

People may be unfamiliar with the concept of odds and the difference between "risk" and "odds." Based on the symbols used in Table 6-1, the **risk** of disease in the exposed group is $a/(a + b)$, whereas the **odds** of disease in the exposed group is simply a/b. If a is small compared with b, the odds would be similar to the risk. If a particular disease occurs in 1 person among a group of 100 persons in a given year, the

risk of that disease is 1 in 100 (0.0100), and the odds of that disease are 1 to 99 (0.0101). If the risk of the disease is relatively large (>5%), the odds ratio is not a good estimate of the risk ratio. The odds ratio can be calculated by dividing the odds of exposure in the diseased group by the odds of exposure in the nondiseased group. In the terms used in Table 6-1, the formula for the OR is as follows:

$$OR = (a/c)/(b/d)$$
$$= ad/bc$$

In mathematical terms, it would make no difference whether the odds ratio was calculated as $(a/c)/(b/d)$ or as $(a/b)/(c/d)$ because cross-multiplication in either case would yield ad/bc. In a case-control study, it makes no sense to use $(a/b)/(c/d)$ because cells a and b come from different study groups. The fact that the odds ratio is the same whether it is developed from a horizontal analysis of the table or from a vertical analysis proves to be valuable, however, for analyzing data from case-control studies. Although a risk or a risk ratio cannot be calculated from a case-control study, an odds ratio can be calculated. Under most real-world circumstances, the odds ratio from a carefully performed case-control study is a good estimate of the risk ratio that would have been obtained from a more costly and time-consuming prospective cohort study. The odds ratio may be used as an estimate of the risk ratio if the risk of disease in the population is low. (It can be used if the risk ratio is <1%, and probably if <5%.) The odds ratio also is used in logistic methods of statistical analysis (logistic regression, log-linear models, Cox regression analyses), discussed briefly in Chapter 13.

3. Which Side Is Up in the Risk Ratio and Odds Ratio?

If the risk for a disease is the same in the group exposed to a particular risk factor or protective factor as it is in the group not exposed to the factor, the risk ratio is expressed simply as 1.0. Hypothetically, the risk ratio could be 0 (i.e., if the individuals exposed to a protective factor have no risk, and the unexposed individuals have some risk), or it may be infinity (i.e., if the individuals exposed to a risk factor have some risk, and the unexposed individuals have no risk). In practical terms, however, because there usually is some disease in every large group, these extremes of the risk ratio are rare.

When risk factors are discussed, placing the exposed group in the numerator is a convention that makes intuitive sense (because the number becomes larger as the risk factor has a greater impact), and this convention is followed in the literature. However, the risk ratio also can be expressed with the exposed group in the denominator. Consider the case of cigarette smoking and myocardial infarction (MI), in which the risk of MI for smokers is greater than for nonsmokers. On the one hand, it is acceptable to put the smokers in the numerator and express the risk ratio as 2/1 (i.e., 2), meaning that the risk of MI is about twice as high for smokers as for nonsmokers of otherwise similar age, gender, and health status. On the other hand, it also is acceptable to put the smokers in the denominator and express the risk ratio as 1/2 (i.e., 0.5), meaning that nonsmokers have half the risk of smokers. Clarity simply requires that the nature of the comparison be explicit.

Another risk factor might produce 4 times the risk of a disease, in which case the ratio could be expressed as 4 or as 1/4, depending on how the risks are being compared. When the risk ratio is plotted on a logarithmic scale (Fig. 6-3), it is easy to see that, regardless of which way the ratio is expressed, the distance to the risk ratio of 1 is the same. Mathematically, it does not matter whether the risk for the exposed group or the unexposed group is in the numerator. Either way the risk ratio is easily interpretable. Almost always the risk of the exposed group is expressed in the numerator, however, so that the numbers make intuitive sense.

Although the equation for calculating the odds ratio differs from that for calculating the risk ratio, when the odds

ratio is calculated, the same principle applies: The ratio is usually expressed with the exposed group in the numerator, but mathematically it can be interpreted equally well if the exposed group is placed in the denominator.

When two risks or two rates are being compared, if there is no difference (i.e., the risks or rates are equal), the risk (rate) difference is expressed as 0. When the same two rates are compared by a relative risk or an odds ratio, however, the condition of no difference is represented by 1.0 because the numerator and denominator are equal.

III. OTHER MEASURES OF IMPACT OF RISK FACTORS

One of the most useful applications of epidemiology is to estimate how much disease burden is caused by certain modifiable risk factors. This is useful for policy development because the impact of risk factors or interventions to reduce risk factors can be compared with costs in cost-benefit and cost-effectiveness analyses (see Chapter 14). Also, health education is often more effective when educators can show how much impact a given risk factor has on individual risks. In addition to the risk difference, relative risk, and odds ratio, the most common measures of the impact of exposures are as follows (Box 6-1):

- Attributable risk percent in the exposed
- Population attributable risk
- Population attributable risk percent

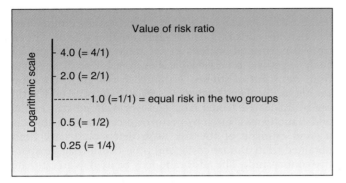

Figure 6-3 Possible risk ratios plotted on logarithmic scale. Scale shows that reciprocal risks are equidistant from the neutral point, where the risk ratio is equal to 1.0.

Box 6-1	Equations for Comparing Risks in Different Groups and Measuring Impact of Risk Factors
(1) Risk difference	= Attributable risk (AR)
	= $\text{Risk}_{(exposed)} - \text{Risk}_{(unexposed)}$
	= $[a/(a+b)]/[c/(c+d)]$
	where a represents subjects with both the risk factor and the disease; b represents subjects with the risk factor, but not the disease; c represents subjects with the disease, but not the risk factor; and d represents subjects with neither the risk factor nor the disease
(2) Relative risk (RR)	= Risk ratio (RR)
	= $\text{Risk}_{(exposed)}/\text{Risk}_{(unexposed)}$
	= $[a/(a+b)]/[c/(c+d)]$
(3) Odds ratio (OR)	= $(a/b)/(c/d)$
	= $(a/c)/(b/d)$
	= ad/bc
(4) Attributable risk percent in the exposed (AR% [exposed])	= $\dfrac{\text{Risk}_{(exposed)} - \text{Risk}_{(unexposed)}}{\text{Risk}_{(exposed)}} \times 100$
	= $\dfrac{RR-1}{RR} \times 100$
	$\approx \dfrac{OR-1}{OR} \times 100$
(5) Population attributable risk (PAR)	= $\text{Risk}_{(total)} - \text{Risk}_{(unexposed)}$
(6) Population attributable risk percent (PAR%)	= $\dfrac{\text{Risk}_{(total)} - \text{Risk}_{(unexposed)}}{\text{Risk}_{(total)}} \times 100$
	= $\dfrac{(Pe)(RR-1)}{1+(Pe)(RR-1)} \times 100$
	where Pe stands for the effective proportion of the population exposed to the risk factor

In the discussion of these measures, smoking and lung cancer are used as the examples of risk factor and disease, and the calculations are based on 1986 rates for the United States (see Fig. 6-1).

A. Attributable Risk Percent in the Exposed

If an investigator wanted to answer the question, "Among smokers, what percentage of the total risk for fatal lung cancer is caused by smoking?" it would be necessary to calculate the attributable risk percent in the exposed, which is abbreviated as $AR\%_{(exposed)}$. There are two methods of calculation, one based on absolute differences in risk and the other based on relative differences in risk. The following equation is based on absolute differences:

$$AR\%_{(exposed)} = \frac{Risk_{(exposed)} - Risk_{(unexposed)}}{Risk_{(exposed)}} \times 100$$

If the 1986 U.S. data on the lung cancer death rates (expressed as deaths per 100,000 per year) in adult male smokers and nonsmokers are used, the calculation is as follows:

$$AR\%_{(exposed)} = \frac{(191 - 8.7)}{191} \times 100 = \frac{182.3}{191} \times 100 = 95.4\%$$

If the absolute risk is unknown, the relative risk (RR) can be used instead to calculate the $AR_{(exposed)}$, with the following formula:

$$AR\%_{(exposed)} = \frac{(RR - 1)}{RR} \times 100$$

Earlier in this chapter, the RR for the U.S. data was calculated as 22, so this figure can be used in the equation:

$$AR\%_{(exposed)} = \frac{(22 - 1)}{22} \times 100 = 95.5\%$$

The percentage based on the formula using relative risk is the same as the percentage based on the formula using absolute risk (except for rounding errors). Why does this work? The important point to remember is that the relative risk for the unexposed group is always 1 because that is the group to whom the exposed group is compared. The attributable risk, which is the amount of risk in excess of the risk in the unexposed group, is RR = 1 (see Fig. 6-2). Because the odds ratio may be used to estimate the risk ratio if the risk of disease in the population is small, the $AR\%_{(exposed)}$ also can be estimated by using odds ratios obtained from case-control studies and substituting them for the RR in the previous formula.

B. Population Attributable Risk

The population attributable risk (PAR) allows an investigator to answer the question, "Among the general population, how much of the total risk for fatal disease X is caused by exposure to Y?" PAR is defined as the risk in the total population minus the risk in the unexposed population:

$$PAR = Risk_{(total)} - Risk_{(unexposed)}$$

Answers to this type of question are not as useful to know for counseling patients, but are of considerable value to policy makers. Using the U.S. data for 1986, the investigator would subtract the risk in the adult male nonsmokers (8.7/100,000 per year) from the risk in the total adult male population (72.5/100,000 per year) to find the population attributable risk (63.8/100,000 per year). It can be presumed that if there had never been any smokers in the United States, the total U.S. lung cancer death rate in men would be much lower, perhaps close to 8.7/100,000 per year. The excess over this figure—63.8/100,000 per year based on these data—could be attributed to smoking.

C. Population Attributable Risk Percent

The population attributable risk percent (PAR%) answers the question, "Among the general population, what percentage of the total risk for X (e.g., fatal lung cancer) is caused by the exposure Y (e.g., smoking)?" As with the $AR\%_{(exposed)}$, the PAR% can be calculated using either absolute or relative differences in risk. The following equation is based on absolute differences:

$$PAR\% = \frac{Risk_{(total)} - Risk_{(unexposed)}}{Risk_{(total)}} \times 100$$

When the U.S. data discussed earlier for men are used, the calculation is as follows:

$$PAR\% = \frac{(72.5 - 8.7)}{72.5} \times 100 = \frac{63.8}{72.5} \times 100 = 88\%$$

The PAR% instead could be calculated using the risk ratio (or the odds ratio if the data come from a case-control study). First, it is necessary to incorporate another measure into the formula—the proportion exposed, which is abbreviated as Pe and is defined as the effective proportion of the population exposed to the risk factor. The equation is as follows:

$$PAR\% = \frac{(Pe)(RR - 1)}{1 + (Pe)(RR - 1)} \times 100$$

In the case of smoking, the Pe would be the *effective* proportion of the adult population who smoked. This figure must be estimated, rather than being obtained directly, because of the long latent period from the start of smoking until the onset of lung cancer and the occurrence of death. The proportion of smokers has generally been decreasing over time in the United States, with recent prevalence at <25% of the population. Here, the Pe is assumed to be 0.35, or 35%.

As calculated earlier, the relative risk (RR) for lung cancer in the United States was 22. If this number is used, the calculation can be completed as follows:

$$PAR\% = \frac{(0.35)(22 - 1)}{1 + (0.35)(22 - 1)} \times 100 = \frac{7.35}{1 + 7.35} = 88\%$$

Figure 6-4 shows diagrammatically how the formula for PAR% works.

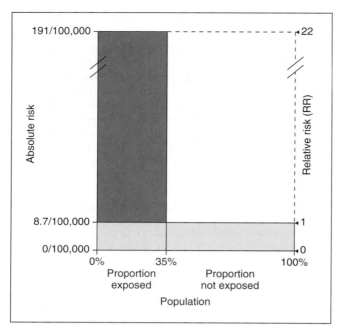

Figure 6-4 Population attributable risk percent (PAR%). Diagram shows how the equation for PAR% works. The x-axis shows the population, divided into two groups: the 35% of the population representing the proportion exposed *(Pe)* to the risk factor (i.e., the effective population of smokers), and the remaining 65% of the population, who are nonsmokers. The right side of the y-axis shows the relative risk (RR) of lung cancer death. For reference, the left side of the y-axis shows the absolute risk of lung cancer death. Dark-gray shading, light-gray shading, and a light blue are used to show the relationship between the risk factor (smoking) and the disease outcome (lung cancer death) in the smokers and nonsmokers. The light-blue part represents outcomes that are not attributable to the risk factor in nonsmokers. The dark-gray part represents the outcomes that are attributable to the risk factor in smokers. The light-gray part represents the outcomes that are not attributable to the risk factor in smokers (i.e., lung cancer deaths that are not attributable to smoking, although the deaths occurred in smokers). The equation is as follows:

$$PAR\% = \frac{(Pe)(RR-1)}{1+(Pe)(RR-1)} \times 100$$

$$= \frac{(0.35)(22-1)}{1+(0.35)(22-1)} \times 100$$

$$= \frac{7.35}{1+7.35} \times 100 = 88\%$$

IV. USES OF RISK ASSESSMENT DATA

After the various measures of the impact of smoking on lung cancer deaths have been calculated, the results can be used in policy analysis and in counseling patients.

A. Application of Risk Data to Policy Analysis

I. *Estimating Benefit of Interventions in Populations*

Population attributable risk (PAR) data often can be used to estimate the benefit of a proposed intervention, such as the number of lung cancer deaths that would be prevented by instituting a smoking reduction program in a

Table 6-2 Measures of Smoking and Lung Cancer Deaths in Men, United States, 1986

Measure	Amount
Lung cancer deaths among smokers*	191 per 100,000 per year
Lung cancer deaths among nonsmokers*	8.7 per 100,000 per year
Proportion exposed *(Pe)* to the risk factor (effective population of smokers, averaged over time)	35%, or 0.35
Population risk of lung cancer death†	72.5 per 100,000 per year
Relative risk (RR)†	22 [191/8.7 = 22]
Attributable risk (AR)†	182.3 per 100,000 per year [191 − 8.7 = 182.3]
Attributable risk percent in the exposed (AR%$_{(exposed)}$)†	95.4% [182.3/191 × 100 = 95.4]
Population attributable risk (PAR)†	63.8 per 100,000 per year [72.5 − 8.7 = 63.8]
Population attributable risk percent (PAR%)†	88% [63.8/72.5 × 100 = 88]

*Data from US Centers for Disease Control: *MMWR* 38:501–505, 1989.
†These rates were calculated from the data with asterisk and the assumption that an average of 35% of the adult male population smoked.

large population. For example, assume that in the United States the proportion of men who smoke has averaged about 25% for more than two decades (as it did during much of the 1990s). Also assume that the amount of smoking has been constant among men who smoke, and that the lung cancer death rate in this group remains constant (represented by lung cancer death rate in Table 6-2, which is 191 per 100,000 per year for smokers vs. 8.7 per 100,000 per year for nonsmokers). Given these assumptions, the rate of lung cancer deaths in the total adult male population would be a weighted average of the rates in smokers and nonsmokers:

$$Rate\ per\ 100,000\ male$$
$$population\ per\ year = (Weight_{smokers})(Rate_{smokers}) +$$
$$(Weight_{nonsmokers})(Rate_{nonsmokers})$$
$$= (0.25)(191) + (0.75)(8.7)$$
$$= 47.8 + 6.5 = 54.3$$

The PAR, also expressed as a rate per 100,000 male population, would be calculated as follows:

$$PAR = 54.3 - 8.7 = 45.6$$

If a major smoking reduction program (possibly financed by the tobacco settlement money) were to reduce the proportion of adult male smokers from 25% to 20% for an extended period, and if the lung cancer death rates for male smokers and nonsmokers remained constant, the revised rate of lung cancer deaths in the total adult male population would be calculated as follows:

$$Rate\ per\ 100,000\ male$$
$$population\ per\ year = (Weight_{smokers})(Rate_{smokers}) +$$
$$(Weight_{nonsmokers})(Rate_{nonsmokers})$$
$$= (0.20)(191) + (0.80)(8.7)$$
$$= 38.2 + 7.0 = 45.2$$

Under these conditions, per 100,000 male population:

$$PAR = 45.2 - 8.7 = 36.5$$

The difference between the first PAR (45.6) and the second PAR (36.5) is 9.1/100,000 adult men. This means that a smoking reduction program that was able to reduce the proportion of adult male smokers from 25% to 20% eventually would be expected to prevent about 9 lung cancer deaths per 100,000 men per year. If there were 100 million men, the intervention would be responsible for preventing 9100 deaths per year. If there were a similar number of women, and they had a similar reduction in smoking rate and lung cancer death rate, 9100 deaths per year would be prevented in women, bringing the total to 18,200 deaths prevented in the adult population per year.

2. Cost-Effectiveness Analysis

In cost-effectiveness analysis, investigators estimate the costs in dollars of an intervention along with the corresponding effects of that intervention. For health interventions, the *effects* are usually measured in terms of the number of injuries, illnesses, or deaths prevented. Although external factors may complicate the calculation of costs and effects, it is generally more difficult to measure effects, partly because many costs are known quickly, whereas effects may take a long time to measure.

In the previous example of a smoking reduction program, if the costs of the program were $1 billion per year, and if 18,200 lung cancer deaths were prevented per year, it would have cost about $54,945 to prevent each death. If the costs of the program were assigned to a hypothetical population of 200 million adults, instead of to the individuals whose deaths the program prevented, it would have cost $5 per adult per year. If the costs of the program were assigned to the adults who quit smoking (5%), it would have cost about $100 per *quitter* per year.

These amounts may seem high, but it is important to keep in mind that the cost estimates here are fictitious, and that the adult population size estimates are crude. It also is important to remember that in addition to preventing lung cancer deaths, a smoking reduction program would offer other benefits. These would include reductions in the rates of various nonfatal and fatal illnesses among smokers, including heart attacks, chronic obstructive pulmonary disease, and other cancers (nasopharyngeal, esophageal, bladder). If the assumptions were accurate, and if all the positive effects of smoking cessation were included in the analysis, the costs per health benefit would be much less than those shown previously. The cost-effectiveness of the program would vary depending on which segment of the population were assigned to pay the costs and how the outcomes of interest were defined.

3. Cost-Benefit Analysis

In cost-benefit analysis, costs and benefits are measured in dollars. To calculate the benefits of a smoking reduction program, investigators would have to convert the positive effects (e.g., reduction in lung cancer deaths) into dollar amounts before the comparison with costs were made. In their calculation of benefits, they would consider a variety of factors, including the savings in medical care and the increased productivity from added years of life. This approach would require them to estimate the average costs of care for one case of lung cancer; the dollar value (in terms of productivity) of adding 1 year of life; and the average number of productive years of life gained by preventing lung cancer. Investigators also would include the time value of money in their analysis by discounting benefits that would occur only in the future. (For more details on cost-effectiveness analysis, cost-benefit analysis, cost-utility analysis, and discounting, see Chapter 14.)

4. Other Methods of Describing the Value of Interventions

The anticipated value of an intervention—whether it is a vaccine, a type of treatment, or a change in nutrition or behavior—is frequently expressed in absolute terms (absolute risk reduction), in relative terms (relative risk reduction), or as the reduction in incidence density (e.g., reduction in risk per 100 person-years). These epidemiologic expressions, however, may not give patients or their physicians a clear sense of the impact of a particular intervention. Each method tends to communicate different factors, so a variety of measures are needed (Box 6-2).

ABSOLUTE AND RELATIVE RISK REDUCTION

The **absolute risk reduction** (ARR) and the **relative risk reduction** (RRR) are descriptive measures that are easy to calculate and understand.[3] For example, assume that the yearly risk of a certain disease is 0.010 in the presence of the risk factor and 0.004 in the absence of the risk factor. The ARR and RRR would be calculated as follows:

$$ARR = Risk_{(exposed)} - Risk_{(unexposed)} = 0.010 - 0.004$$
$$= 0.006$$

$$RRR = \frac{Risk_{(exposed)} - Risk_{(unexposed)}}{Risk_{(exposed)}} = \frac{0.010 - 0.004}{0.010}$$
$$= \frac{0.006}{0.010} = 0.6 = 60\%$$

In this example, an intervention that removed the risk factor would reduce the risk of disease by 0.006 in absolute terms (ARR) or produce a 60% reduction of risk in relative terms (RRR). When the RRR is applied to the effectiveness of vaccines, it is called the **vaccine effectiveness** or the **protective efficacy** (see Chapter 15).

REDUCTION IN INCIDENCE DENSITY

In estimating the effects of treatment methods used to eradicate or prevent a disease, it is important to incorporate the length of time that treatment is needed to obtain one **unit of benefit,** usually defined as the eradication or prevention of disease in one person.[4] The simplest way to incorporate length of time is to use incidence density, expressed in terms of the **number of person-years** of treatment. When warfarin treatment was given on a long-term basis to prevent cerebrovascular accidents (strokes) in patients who had

Box 6-2	Calculation of Risk Reduction and Other Measures to Describe the Practical Value of Treatment

PART 1 **Beginning Data and Assumptions**

(a) Treatment-Derived Benefit

Various studies have shown that the risk of stroke in patients with atrial fibrillation can be prevented by long-term treatment with warfarin, an anticoagulant. Baker[5] reviewed the results of five of these studies and reported the following:

Average number of strokes *without* warfarin treatment	**= 5.1 per 100 patient-years**
	= 0.051 per patient per year
Average number of strokes *with* warfarin treatment	**= 1.8 per 100 patient-years**
	= 0.018 per patient per year

(b) Treatment-Induced Harm

Patients who are treated with drugs are always at some risk of harm. Averages are not available for serious adverse events, such as cerebral and gastrointestinal hemorrhage, in the five studies analyzed by Baker.[5] Assume here that the average number of serious adverse events in patients with atrial fibrillation treated with warfarin is 1 per 100 patient-years = 0.01 per patient per year (fictitious data).

PART 2 **Measures of Treatment-Derived Benefit**

Risk difference
$$= \text{Risk}_{(exposed)} - \text{Risk}_{(unexposed)}$$
$$= 5.1 - 1.8 = \textbf{3.3 per 100 patient-years}$$

Absolute risk reduction (ARR)
$$= \text{Risk}_{(exposed)} - \text{Risk}_{(unexposed)}$$
$$= 0.051 - 0.018 = 0.033$$

Relative risk reduction (RRR)
$$= \frac{\text{Risk}_{(exposed)} - \text{Risk}_{(unexposed)}}{\text{Risk}_{(exposed)}}$$
$$= \frac{0.051 - 0.018}{0.051} = \frac{0.033}{0.051} = 0.65 = \textbf{65\%}$$

PART 3 **Measures of Treatment-Induced Harm (Fictitious Data)**

Absolute risk increase (ARI) $= \text{Risk}_{(exposed)} - \text{Risk}_{(unexposed)} = 0.01$

PART 4 **Calculation of NNT and NNH**

(a) NNT is the number of patients with atrial fibrillation who would need to be treated with warfarin for 1 year each to prevent one stroke.

$$\text{NNT} = 1/\text{ARR} = 1/0.033 = 30.3 = \sim\textbf{31 patients}$$

(b) NNH is the number of patients with atrial fibrillation who would need to be treated with warfarin for 1 year each to cause serious harm.

$$\text{NNH} = 1/\text{ARI} = 1/0.01 = \textbf{100 patients}$$

(c) Whenever the ARR is larger than the ARI (i.e., the NNH is larger than the NNT), more patients would be helped than would be harmed by the treatment. The ratio can be calculated in two different ways:

$$\text{ARR/ARI} = 0.033/0.01 = 3.3$$
$$\text{NNH/NNT} = 100/30.3 = 3.3$$

This means that the number of patients who would be helped is 3 times as large as the number who would be harmed. This result and the calculations on which it is based may be oversimplifications because the amount of benefit may be quantitatively and qualitatively different from the amount of harm derived from a treatment.

Data for the average number of strokes with and without warfarin treatment from Baker D: *Health Failure Quality Improvement Newsletter* 4, 1997.

atrial fibrillation, its benefits were reported in terms of the reduction in strokes per 100 patient-years. When one investigator reviewed five studies of warfarin versus placebo treatment in patients with atrial fibrillation, he found that the average number of strokes that occurred per 100 patient-years was 1.8 in patients treated with warfarin and 5.1 in patients treated with placebo.[5] As shown in Box 6-2, the risk difference between these groups is 3.3 per 100 patient-years; the ARR is 0.033 per patient-year; and the RRR is 65%.

NUMBER NEEDED TO TREAT OR HARM

An increasingly popular measure used to describe the practical value of treatment is called the **number needed to treat** (NNT), meaning the number of patients who would need to receive a specific type of treatment for one patient to benefit from the treatment.[4] The NNT is calculated as the number 1 divided by the ARR. In its simplest form, this is expressed as a proportion: NNT = 1/ARR. For example, a new therapy healed leg ulcers in one third of patients whose ulcers were resistant to all other forms of treatment. In this case the ARR is 0.333, and the NNT is 1/0.333 = 3. These results suggest that, on average, it would be necessary to give this new therapy to three patients with resistant leg ulcers to benefit one patient. The NNT is helpful for making comparisons of the effectiveness of different types of interventions.[6-8]

The basis for the **number needed to harm** (NNH) is similar to that for the NNT, but it is applied to the negative effects of treatment. In the NNH the fundamental item of data is the **absolute risk increase** (ARI), which is analogous to the ARR in the NNT. The NNH formula is similar to that of the NNT: NNH = 1/ARI. The results of one clinical trial can be used to illustrate the calculation of the NNH.[9] In this trial, infants in the intervention group were given iron-fortified formula, and infants in the control group were given formula without iron (regular formula). The mothers of all the infants were asked to report whether their babies had symptoms of colic. They reported colic in 56.8% of infants who received iron-fortified formula and in 40.8% of infants who received regular formula. In this case, ARI = 0.568 − 0.408 = 0.16, and NNH = 1/0.16 = 6.25. This calculation suggests that 1 of every 6 or 7 infants given iron-fortified formula would develop colic because of the formula, while another 2 or 3 infants would develop colic even without iron in the formula.

Although NNT and NNH are helpful for describing the effects of treatment, several points about their use should be emphasized. First, a complete analysis of NNT and NNH should provide confidence intervals for the estimates.[10] (For an introduction to confidence intervals, see Chapter 10.) Second, the length of time that treatment is needed to obtain a unit of benefit should also be incorporated (see previous discussion of incidence density). Third, the net benefit from an intervention should be reduced in some way to account for any harm done. This analysis becomes complicated if it is performed with maximum precision, because the investigator needs to calculate the proportion of treated patients who derive benefit only, the proportion who derive harm only, and the proportion who derive both benefit and harm.[11]

B. Application of Risk Measures to Counseling Patients

Suppose a patient is resistant to the idea of quitting smoking but is open to counseling about the topic. Or, suppose a physician has been asked to give a short talk summarizing the effect of smoking on death rates caused by lung cancer. In each of these situations, by using the measures of risk discussed here and summarized in Table 6-2, the physician could present the following estimates of the impact of smoking (although taken from studies in men, the data apply reasonably well to women as well):

- In the United States, smokers are about 22 times as likely as nonsmokers to die of lung cancer.
- About 95 of every 100 lung cancer deaths in people who smoke can be attributed to their smoking.
- About 158,000 deaths annually result from respiratory tract cancer, and because about 88% can be attributed to smoking, smoking is responsible for about 139,000 deaths per year from respiratory tract cancer in the United States.

Assuming that the risk of fatal lung cancer among smokers is 191/100,000 per year, this equals 0.00191 per year (absolute risk increase). If we consider fatal lung cancer as a *harm* and use the NNH approach, 1 divided by 0.00191 yields 523.6, or approximately 524. In round numbers, therefore, we would expect 1 in every 525 adult smokers to die of lung cancer each year.

V. SUMMARY

Epidemiologic research is usually designed to demonstrate one or more primary contrasts in risk, rate, or odds of disease or exposure. The most straightforward of these measures are the risk difference (attributable risk) and the rate difference, which show in absolute terms how much the risk of one group, usually the group exposed to a risk or preventive factor, differs from that of another group. This contrast can also be expressed as a ratio of risks, rates, or odds; the greater this ratio, the greater the difference resulting from the exposure. The impact of a risk factor on the total burden of any given disease can be measured in terms of an attributable risk percentage for the exposed group or for the population in general. If it is known by how much and in whom a preventive program can reduce the risk ratio, we can then calculate the total benefit of the program, including its cost-effectiveness. Measures such as the RRR, NNT, and NNH are used to determine the effect of interventions.

References

1. US Centers for Disease Control: Chronic disease reports: deaths from lung cancer—United States, 1986. *MMWR* 38:501–505, 1989.
2. Doll R, Hill AB: Lung cancer and other causes of death in relation to smoking; a second report on the mortality of British doctors. *BMJ* 2:1071–1081, 1956.
3. Haynes RB, Sackett DL, Guyatt GH, et al: *Clinical epidemiology*, ed 3, Philadelphia, 2006, Lippincott, Williams & Wilkins.
4. Laupacis A, Sackett DL, Roberts RS: An assessment of clinically useful measures of the consequences of treatment. *N Engl J Med* 318:1728–1733, 1988.

5. Baker D: Anticoagulation for atrial fibrillation. White Institute for Health Services Research. *Health Failure Quality Improvement Newsletter* 4(Sept 15):1997.

6. Kumana CR, Cheung BM, Lauder IJ: Gauging the impact of statins using number needed to treat. *JAMA* 282:1899–1901, 1999.

7. Woolf SH: The need for perspective in evidence-based medicine. *JAMA* 282:2358–2365, 1999.

8. Katz DL: *Clinical epidemiology and evidence-based medicine,* Thousand Oaks, Calif, 2001, Sage.

9. Syracuse Consortium for Pediatric Clinical Studies: Iron-fortified formulas and gastrointestinal symptoms in infants: a controlled study. *Pediatrics* 66:168–170, 1980.

10. Altman DG: Confidence intervals for the number needed to treat. *BMJ* 317:1309–1312, 1998.

11. Mancini GB, Schulzer JM: Reporting risks and benefits of therapy by use of the concepts of unqualified success and unmitigated failure. *Circulation* 99:377–383, 1999.

Select Readings

Gordis L: *Epidemiology,* ed 3, Philadelphia, 2001, Saunders.

Kelsey JL, Whittemore AS, Evans AS, et al: *Methods in observational epidemiology,* ed 2, New York, 1996, Oxford University Press.

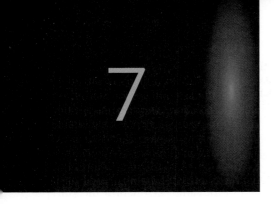

7

Understanding the Quality of Data in Clinical Medicine

I. GOALS OF DATA COLLECTION AND ANALYSIS

Clinical medicine requires the constant collection, evaluation, analysis, and use of quantitative and qualitative data. The data are used for diagnosis, prognosis, and choosing and evaluating treatments. The data may be accurate to varying degrees. To the extent that data are inaccurate, we say there is "error" in the data. It may be disquieting to talk about errors in medicine, but errors in data occur and are difficult to eliminate.

The term *error* is used in more than one way. It can be used to mean mistakes in the diagnosis and treatment of patients or to mean more egregious mistakes with clear negligence, such as removing the wrong body part. This meaning of *error* was emphasized in *To Err Is Human: Building a Safer Health System*, a report issued in 2000 by the U.S. Institute of Medicine.[1] The report caused a considerable stir nationally.[2] Methods for reducing medical mistakes are discussed in Chapters 15 and 29.

Medical histories, physical examinations, laboratory values, and imaging reports are never perfect because of the limitations of the human process. In clinical medicine and research, it is important to minimize errors in data so that these errors can be used to guide, rather than mislead, the individuals who provide the care. The emphasis in this chapter is on ways to measure and improve the quality of medical data.

A. Promoting Accuracy and Precision

Two distinct but related goals of data collection are accuracy and precision. **Accuracy** refers to the ability of a measurement to be correct on the average. If a measure is not accurate, it is *biased* because it deviates, on average, from the true value in one direction or the other, rather than equally in both directions. **Precision,** sometimes known as **reproducibility** or **reliability,** is the ability of a measurement to give the same result or a similar result with repeated measurements of the same factor. **Random error** is nondifferential error because it does not distort data consistently in any one direction. Random error alone, if large, results in lack of precision, but not bias, because distortions from truth may occur comparably in both directions (see discussion of bias in Chapter 4).

To ask whether accuracy or precision is more important in data collection would be like asking which wing of an airplane is more important. As shown in Figures 7-1 and 7-2, unless both qualities are present, the data would be generally useless. *Accuracy* is shown in the fact that the mean (average) is the true (correct) value, whereas *precision* (reliability) is evident in the fact that all values are close to the true value (Fig. 7-1, *A*). Figure 7-1, *B*, shows a measure that is accurate but not precise, meaning that it gives the correct answer only on the average. Such a measure might be useful for some types of research, but even so, it would not be reassuring to the investigator. For an individual patient, there is no utility in some factor being correct on the average if it is wrong for that patient. To guide diagnosis and treatment, each observation must be correct. Figure 7-1, *C*, shows data that are precise but are biased, rather than being accurate, and are misleading. Figure 7-1, *D*, shows data that are neither accurate nor precise and are useless or even dangerous. Figure 7-2 uses a target and bullet holes to show the same concepts.

B. Reducing Differential and Nondifferential Errors

As discussed in Chapter 4, there are several types of errors to avoid in the collection of data; this section focuses on errors associated with measurement. A **measurement bias** is a **differential error**—that is, a nonrandom, systematic, or consistent error in which the values tend to be inaccurate in a particular direction. Measurement bias results from measuring the heights of patients with their shoes on or from measuring patient blood pressures with a blood pressure cuff that reads too high or too low. Statistical analysis cannot

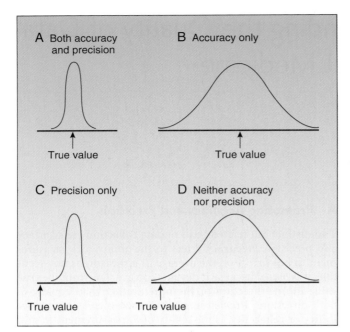

Figure 7-1 **Possible combinations of accuracy and precision in describing a continuous variable.** The x-axis is a range of values, with the arrow indicating the true value. **A** to **D,** The four curves are the probability distributions of observed values.

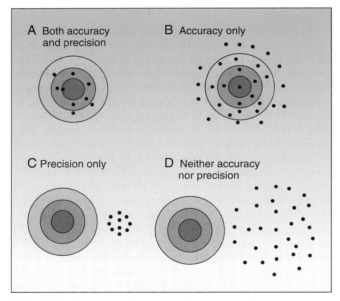

Figure 7-2 **Possible combinations of accuracy and precision in describing a continuous variable. A** to **D,** The targets are used with bullet holes to show the four concepts illustrated in Figure 7-1 with curves.

correct for bias, unless the amount of bias in each individual measurement is known. In the example of the patients' height measurements, bias could be corrected only if the height of each patient's shoe heel were known and subtracted from that patient's reported height.

Although measuring patients in their bare feet could eliminate bias, it would not eliminate **random errors**, or **nondifferential errors**. When data have only random errors, some observations are too high and some are too low. It is even possible for random errors to produce biased results.[3]

If there are enough observations, however, data with only random errors usually produce a correct estimate of the average value (see Chapter 9).

C. Reducing Intraobserver and Interobserver Variability

If the same clinician takes successive measurements of the blood pressure or height of the same person, or if the same clinician examines the same x-ray film several times without knowing that it is the same film, there usually are some differences in the measurements or interpretations obtained. This is known as **intraobserver** (*within* observer) **variability.** If two different clinicians measure the same person's blood pressure or examine the same x-ray film independently, there usually are some differences. This is called **interobserver** (*between* observers) **variability.** One goal of data collection is to reduce the amount of intraobserver and interobserver variability. Although much of medicine is still an art, there is also a science in collecting data and studying its quality.

II. STUDYING THE ACCURACY AND USEFULNESS OF SCREENING AND DIAGNOSTIC TESTS

One way to judge the usefulness of a screening or diagnostic test for a particular disease is to evaluate how often its results are correct in two groups of individuals: (1) a group in whom the disease is known to be *present* and in whom the test results should be positive and (2) a group in whom the disease is known to be *absent* and in whom the test results should be negative. This form of research is not as easy as it initially might appear because several factors influence whether the results for an individual subject would be accurate and whether the test in general would be useful in diagnosing or screening for a particular disease. These factors include the stage of the disease and the spectrum of disease in the study population. The population in whom the diagnostic or screening test is evaluated should have characteristics similar to the characteristics of the populations in whom the test would be used. Data derived from evaluating tests in men or young people may not be as useful in women or old people.[4]

A. False-Positive and False-Negative Results

In science, if something is said to be true when it actually is false, this is variously called a **type I error,** a **false-positive error,** or an **alpha error.** If something is said to be false when it actually is true, this is called a **type II error,** a **false-negative error,** or a **beta error.** The finding of a positive result in a patient in whom the disease is absent is called a **false-positive result,** and the finding of a negative result in a patient in whom the disease is present is called a **false-negative result.**

The **stage of disease** often influences the test results. Tests for infectious diseases, such as the blood test for human immunodeficiency virus (HIV) and the tuberculin skin test for tuberculosis, are likely to be accurate only after immunity has developed, which might be weeks after the initial infection. Very early in the course of almost any infection, a patient may have no immunologic evidence of infection, and tests done during this time may yield false-negative results.

False-negative results may also occur late in infections such as tuberculosis, when the disease is severe and the immune system is overwhelmed and unable to produce a positive skin test result. This inadequate immune system response is called **anergy** (from Greek, meaning "not working") and can develop with any illness or stress severe enough to cause depression of the immune system.[5] Advanced age also can be a cause of anergy.

The **spectrum of disease** in the study population is important when evaluating a test's potential usefulness in the real world. False-negative and false-positive results can be more of a problem than anticipated. In the case of the tuberculin skin test, false-positive results were formerly found in persons from the southeastern United States. Exposure to atypical mycobacteria in the soil was common in this region, and because there was some cross-reactivity between the atypical mycobacteria and the mycobacteria tested in the tuberculin skin test, equivocal and even false-positive test results were common among this population until standards were tightened. To accomplish this, the use of an antigen called "old tuberculin" was replaced by the use of a *purified protein derivative* (PPD) of mycobacteria at a standardized strength of 5 tuberculin units. The diameter of skin induration needed for a positive test result was increased from 5 to 10 mm. These tightened criteria worked satisfactorily for decades, until the appearance of acquired immunodeficiency syndrome (AIDS). Now, because of the possibility of anergy in HIV-infected individuals, it has been recommended that a smaller diameter of induration in the tuberculin skin test be considered positive for these patients.[6] However, lowering the *critical diameter* (the diameter of the area of induration after a PPD test) also increases the frequency of false-positive results, especially among individuals immunized with bacille Calmette-Guérin (BCG) vaccine and many individuals living in the southeastern United States. These trends show the inevitable tradeoff between **sensitivity** (i.e., reliably finding a disease when it is present and avoiding false negatives) and **specificity** (i.e., reliably excluding a disease when it is absent and avoiding false positives). We want the smoke detectors in our homes to go off every time there is a fire (i.e., we want them to be sensitive), but not to be constantly going off when there is no fire (i.e., we want them to be specific).

False-positive and false-negative results are not limited to tests of infectious diseases, as illustrated in the use of serum calcium values to rule out parathyroid disease, particularly hyperparathyroidism, in new patients seen at an endocrinology clinic. *Hyperparathyroidism* is a disease of calcium metabolism. In an affected patient the serum level of calcium is often elevated, but usually varies from time to time. When the calcium level is not elevated in a patient with hyperparathyroidism, the result would be considered "falsely negative." Conversely, when the calcium level is elevated in a patient without hyperparathyroidism (but instead with cancer, sarcoidosis, multiple myeloma, milk-alkali syndrome, or another condition that can increase calcium level), the result would be considered "falsely positive" for hyperparathyroidism, even though it revealed a different problem.

Figure 7-3 shows two possible frequency distributions of serum calcium values, one in a population of healthy people without parathyroid disease and the other in a population

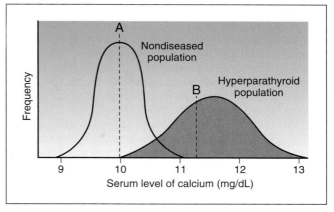

Figure 7-3 Overlap in values of randomly taken tests in a population mostly of healthy people *(curve on left)* **but with some diseased people** *(curve on right).* A person with a calcium level below point A would be unlikely to have hyperparathyroidism. A person with a calcium level above point B would be likely to have an abnormality of calcium metabolism, possibly hyperparathyroidism. A person with a calcium level between point A and point B may or may not have an abnormality of calcium metabolism. (*Note:* The normal range of calcium depends on the method used in a specific laboratory. In some laboratories, the range is 8.5 to 10.5 mg/dL. In others, as in this illustration, it is 9 to 11 mg/dL.)

of patients with hyperparathyroidism. If the calcium level were sufficiently low (e.g., below point A), the patient would be unlikely to have hyperparathyroidism. If the calcium level were sufficiently high (e.g., above point B), the patient would be likely to have an abnormality of calcium metabolism, possibly hyperparathyroidism. If the calcium level were in the intermediate range (between point A and point B in Fig. 7-3) in a single calcium test, although the patient probably would not have a disease of calcium metabolism, this possibility could not be ruled out, and if such disease were suspected, serial calcium values and other tests would be obtained.

Laboratories publish a range of "normal" values for substances that they measure, such as calcium. A calcium value beyond the *normal* range for that laboratory requires further diagnostic tests. For many laboratories, the upper limit of normal for serum calcium is 11 mg/dL. If the **cutoff point** for the upper limit of normal is set too low, considerable time and money would be wasted following up on false-positive results, but if it is set too high, persons with the disease might be missed. As discussed subsequently, determining the sensitivity, specificity, and predictive values of a test at different cutoff points would help investigators choose the best cutoff point for that test. It would be convenient if there were no overlaps between the test results in diseased and nondiseased persons. If this were true, the only source of error would be in the performance of the tests. In reality the distribution of test values in diseased persons often overlaps with the distribution of values in nondiseased persons.

It is easier to visualize the idea of a false-positive error where there is a clear distinction between the diagnosis of a diseased versus a nondiseased condition, as in the evaluation of a spot on a mammogram.[7,8] Even this situation, however, is not always simple. The area in question on a mammogram either does or does not represent breast cancer; a diagnosis of cancer is made only after breast tissue is obtained and reviewed by the pathologist. There may be a true abnormality on the mammogram (e.g., calcifications) without the presence of cancer. If only calcifications without cancer were present, a radiologist's reading of a positive (abnormal) exam would be falsely positive for cancer (the primary concern), but it would be correct about the presence of an abnormality (the calcifications). In contrast, a radiologist's reading of this mammogram as "normal" would be a true negative for cancer, but a false negative for calcifications. Radiologists frequently indicate uncertainty by reporting the results as "abnormality present—possibly/probably not cancer" and recommending that additional tests be done or that the exam be repeated after a defined number of months. Such readings are analogous to laboratory values in the indeterminate range.

B. Sensitivity and Specificity

Sensitivity and specificity are two important measures of test function. They are ways to report the performance of diagnostic tests when the true disease state is known. To calculate these measures, the data concerning the subjects studied and the test results can be put in a 2 × 2 table of the type shown in Table 7-1. The cells in this table are labeled a, b, c, and d, as in Table 6-1, but the measures to be calculated are different.

The first column under True Disease Status in Table 7-1 represents all the diseased participants, consisting of those with **true-positive results** (a) and those with **false-negative results** (c). The second disease status column represents all the nondiseased participants, consisting of those with **false-positive results** (b) and those with **true-negative results** (d). When the total in the disease column is divided by the total of all the participants studied, the result represents the **prevalence rate** (proportion) of the disease in the study population.

Sensitivity, which refers to the ability of a test to detect a disease when present, is calculated as $a/(a + c)$. If a test is not sensitive, it fails to detect disease in some of the diseased participants, and these participants appear in cell c. The rate at which this occurs is called the **false-negative error rate** and is calculated as $c/(a + c)$. The correct denominator for the false-negative error rate is all those who are diseased, because only those who are diseased are at risk for falsely being called "nondiseased." The sensitivity and the false-negative error rate add up to 1.0 (100%).

Specificity, which refers to the ability of a test to indicate nondisease when no disease is present, is calculated as $d/(b + d)$. If a test is not specific, it falsely indicates the presence of disease in nondiseased subjects, and these subjects appear in cell b. The rate at which this occurs is called the **false-positive error rate.** Because only nondiseased participants are at risk for falsely being called diseased, this rate is calculated as $b/(b + d)$. The specificity and the false-positive error rate add up to 1.0 (100%).

As an example to illustrate what the letters in Table 7-1 imply, suppose that 80 consecutive persons entering an endocrinology clinic have their serum calcium level checked and have a hyperparathyroidism workup to determine whether or not they have the disease. Also, assume that the upper cutoff point for "normal" serum calcium is 11 mg/dL, so that levels greater than 11 mg/dL are presumptively "test positive" and levels of 11 mg/dL or less are "test negative." Third, assume that the results are as shown in Table 7-2. The following observations could be made. Of the 80 persons tested, 20 ultimately were shown to have hyperparathyroidism (prevalence of 25%). Of these 20 persons, 12 had an elevated calcium level in initial calcium testing. The sensitivity of the initial test was 60%, and the false-negative error

---

Table 7-1 Standard 2 × 2 Table Comparing Test Results and True Disease Status of Participants Tested

| Test Result | True Disease Status | | Total |
	Diseased	Nondiseased	
Positive	a	b	$a + b$
Negative	c	d	$c + d$
TOTAL	$a + c$	$b + d$	$a + b + c + d$

Interpretation of the Cells

a = Participants with true-positive test result
b = Participants with false-positive test result
c = Participants with false-negative test result
d = Participants with true-negative test result
$a + b$ = All participants with positive test result
$c + d$ = All participants with negative test result
$a + c$ = All participants with the disease
$b + d$ = All participants without the disease
$a + b + c + d$ = All study participants

Formulas

$a/(a + c)$ = Sensitivity
$d/(b + d)$ = Specificity
$b/(b + d)$ = False-positive error rate (alpha error rate, type I error rate)
$c/(a + c)$ = False-negative error rate (beta error rate, type II error rate)
$a/(a + b)$ = Positive predictive value (PPV)
$d/(c + d)$ = Negative predictive value (NPV)
$[a/(a + c)]/[b/(b + d)] = (a/b)/[(a + c)/(b + d)]$ = Likelihood ratio positive (LR+)
$[c/(a + c)]/[d/(b + d)] = (c/d)/[(a + c)/(b + d)]$ = Likelihood ratio negative (LR−)
$(a + c)/(a + b + c + d)$ = Prevalence

Table 7-2 Serum Level of Calcium and True Disease Status of 80 Participants Tested (Fictitious Data)

| Serum Level of Calcium | True Disease Status | | Total |
	Diseased	Nondiseased	
Positive	12	3	15
Negative	8	57	65
TOTAL	20	60	80

Calculations Based on Formulas in Table 7-1

12/20 = 60% = Sensitivity
57/60 = 95% = Specificity
3/60 = 5% = False-positive error rate (alpha error rate, type I error rate)
8/20 = 40% = False-negative error rate (beta error rate, type II error rate)
12/15 = 80% = Positive predictive value (PPV)
57/65 = 88% = Negative predictive value (NPV)
(12/20)/(3/60) = 12.0 = Likelihood ratio positive (LR+)
(8/20)/(57/60) = 0.42 = Likelihood ratio negative (LR−)
12.0/0.42 = 28.6 = Ratio of LR+ to LR− = Odds ratio
20/80 = 25% = Prevalence of disease

rate was 40% (8/20). This is consistent with patients with hyperparathyroidism having serum calcium levels that alternate between the high-normal range and definite elevation, so more than one calcium test is needed. The specificity in Table 7-2 was higher than the sensitivity, with normal levels correctly identified in 57 of 60 nondiseased persons, indicating 95% specificity. The false-positive error rate was 5% (3/60).

C. Predictive Values

Sensitivity and specificity are helpful but do not directly answer two important clinical questions: If a participant's test result is positive, what is the probability that the person has the disease under investigation? If the result is negative, what is the probability that the person does not have the disease? These questions, which are influenced by sensitivity, specificity, and prevalence, can be answered by doing a horizontal analysis, rather than a vertical analysis, in Table 7-1.

In Table 7-1, the formula $a/(a + b)$ is used to calculate the **positive predictive value** (PPV). In a study population, this measure indicates what proportion of the subjects with positive test results had the disease. Likewise, the formula $d/(c + d)$ is used to calculate the **negative predictive value** (NPV), which indicates what proportion of the subjects with negative test results did not have the disease.

In Table 7-2, the positive predictive value is 80% (12/15), and the negative predictive value is 88% (57/65). Based on these numbers, the clinician could not be fully confident in either a positive or a negative test result. Why are the predictive values so low? The predictive values would have been 100% (completely correct) if there were no false-positive or false-negative errors. Medical tests are almost never perfect. This makes predictive values difficult to interpret because, in the presence of false-positive or false-negative findings, the predictive values are influenced profoundly by the prevalence of the condition being sought.[9] Predictive values can be influenced by the prevalence of the condition being assessed, unlike sensitivity and specificity, which are independent of prevalence.

As shown in Table 7-1, the prevalence is the total number of diseased persons $(a + c)$ divided by the total number of persons studied $(a + b + c + d)$. If there is a 1% prevalence of a condition (and most conditions are relatively rare), at most there could be an average of 1 true-positive test result out of each 100 persons examined. If there is a 5% false-positive rate (not unusual for many tests), however, 5% of 99 disease-free persons would have false-positive test results. This would mean almost 5 false-positive results of each 100 tests. In this example, almost 5 of every 6 positive test results could be expected to be falsely positive. It almost seems as though probability is conspiring against the use of screening and diagnostic tests in clinical medicine.

Whenever clinicians are testing for rare conditions, whether in routine clinical examinations or in large community screening programs, they must be prepared for most of the positive test results to be falsely positive. They must be prepared to follow up with additional testing in persons who have positive results to determine if the disease is really present. This does not mean that screening tests should be avoided for conditions that have a low prevalence. It still may be worthwhile to do a screening program because the persons who need follow-up diagnostic tests may represent a small

percentage of the total population. A crucial point to remember is that one test does not make a diagnosis, unless it is a **pathognomonic test,** a test that elicits a reaction synonymous with having the disease (a "gold standard"). Box 7-1 summarizes principles concerning **screening tests** and **confirmatory tests.**

D. Likelihood Ratios, Odds Ratios, and Cutoff Points

In contrast to predictive values, likelihood ratios are not influenced by the prevalence of the disease. The **likelihood ratio positive** (LR+) is the ratio of the sensitivity of a test to the false-positive error rate of the test. As shown in Table 7-1, the equation is as follows: $[a/(a + c)] \div [b/(b + d)]$. Because the LR+ is the ratio of something that clinicians do want in a test (sensitivity) divided by something they do not want (false-positive error rate), the higher the ratio, the better the test is. For a test to be good, the ratio should be much larger than 1. The sensitivity and the false-positive error rate are independent of the prevalence of the disease. Their ratio is also independent of the prevalence.

In a similar manner, the **likelihood ratio negative** (LR−) is the ratio of the false-negative error rate divided by the specificity, or $[c/(a + c)] \div [d/(b + d)]$. In this case, because the LR− is the ratio of something clinicians do not want (false-negative error rate) divided by something they do want (specificity), the smaller the LR− (i.e., the closer it is to

0), the better the test is. If the LR+ of a test is large and the LR− is small, it is probably a good test.

The LR+ can be calculated from the hypothetical data in Table 7-2. The sensitivity is 12/20, or 60%. The false-positive error rate (1 − specificity) is 3/60, or 5%. The ratio of these is the LR+, which equals 0.60/0.05, or 12.0. Although this looks good, the sensitivity data indicate that, on average, 40% of the diseased persons would be missed. The LR− here would be 8/20 divided by 57/60, or 0.421, which is much larger than acceptable.

Experts in test analysis sometimes calculate the **ratio of LR+ to LR−** to obtain a measure of separation between the positive and the negative test. In this example, LR+/LR− would be 12.0/0.421, which is equal to 28.5, a number not as large as acceptable (many consider values <50 indicate weak tests). If the data are from a 2 × 2 table, the same result could have been obtained more simply by calculating the **odds ratio** (*ad/bc*), which here equals [(12)(57)]/[(3)(8)], or 28.5. For a discussion of the concepts of proportions and odds, see Box 7-2.

The LR+ looks better if a high (more stringent) **cutoff point** is used (e.g., a serum calcium level of 13 mg/dL for hyperparathyroidism), although choosing a high cutoff also lowers the sensitivity. This improvement in the LR+ occurs because, as the cutoff point is raised, true-positive results are eliminated at a slower rate than are false-positive results, so the ratio of true positive to false positive increases. The ratio of LR+ to LR− increases, despite the fact that more of the diseased individuals would be missed. The high LR+ means that when clinicians do find a high calcium level in an individual being tested, they can be reasonably certain that hyperparathyroidism or some other disease of calcium metabolism is present. Similarly, if an extremely low cutoff point is used, when clinicians find an even lower value in a patient, they can be reasonably certain that the disease is absent.

Although these principles can be used to create value ranges that allow clinicians to be reasonably certain about a diagnosis in the highest and lowest groups, the results in the middle group or groups (e.g., between points *A* and *B* in Fig. 7-3) often remain problematic. Clinicians may be comfortable treating patients in the highest groups and deferring treatment for those in the lowest groups, but they may now need to pursue additional testing for patients whose values fall in the middle. These issues apply when interpreting medical tests such as a ventilation-perfusion scan, the results of which are reported as normal, low probability, indeterminate, or high probability.[10]

Three or more ranges can be used to categorize the values of any test whose results occur along a continuum. In Table 7-3 the results of a serum test formerly used to identify myocardial damage are divided into four ranges.[11] In this classic study, 360 patients who had symptoms suggesting myocardial infarction (MI) had an initial blood sample drawn to determine the level of creatine kinase (CK), an enzyme released into the blood of patients with MI. After the final diagnoses were made, the initial CK values were compared with these diagnoses, and four groups were created. Four levels are too many to measure the sensitivity and specificity in a 2 × 2 table (as in Tables 7-1 and 7-2), but likelihood ratios still can be calculated.

Likelihood ratios can be applied to multiple levels of a test because of a unique characteristic of odds: The result is the same regardless of whether the analysis in a table is done vertically or horizontally. The LR+ is the ratio of two probabilities: the ratio of sensitivity to (1 − specificity). This also can be expressed as [*a*/(*a* + *c*) ÷ [*b*/(*b* + *d*)]. When rearranged algebraically, this equation can be rewritten as follows:

$$LR+ = (a/b)/[(a+c)/(b+d)]$$

which is the odds of disease among persons in whom the test yielded positive results, divided by the odds of disease in the

Box 7-2	Concepts of Proportions and Odds

Most people are familiar with *proportions* (percentages), which take the form *a*/(*a* + *b*). Some may be less familiar, however, with the idea of an *odds,* which is simply *a*/*b*. In a mathematical sense, a proportion is less pure because the term *a* is in the numerator and the denominator of a proportion, which is not true of an odds. The odds is the probability that something will occur divided by the probability that it will not occur (or the number of times it occurs divided by the number of times it does not occur). Odds can only describe a variable that is *dichotomous* (i.e., has only two possible outcomes, such as success and failure).

The *odds* of a particular outcome (outcome *X*) can be converted to the *probability* of that outcome, and vice versa, using the following formula:

$$\text{Probability of outcome } X = \frac{\text{Odds of outcome } X}{1 + \text{Odds of outcome } X}$$

Suppose that the proportion of successful at-bats of a baseball player on a certain night equals 1/3 (a batting average of 0.333). That means there was one success (*X*) and two failures (*Y*). The odds of success (number of successes to number of failures) is 1:2, or 0.5. To convert back to a proportion from the odds, put the odds of 0.5 into the above equation, giving 0.5/(1 + 0.5) = 0.5/1.5 = 0.333.

If the player goes 1 for 4 another night, the proportion of success is 1/4 (a batting average of 0.250), and the odds of success is 1:3, or 0.333. The formula converts the odds (0.333) back into a proportion: 0.333/(1 + 0.333) = 0.333/1.333 = 0.250.

Table 7-3   **Calculation of Likelihood Ratios for Myocardial Infarction (MI) in Analyzing Performance of a Serum Test with Multiple Cutoff Points (Multiple and Calculable Ranges of Results)**

Serum CK Value*	Diagnosis of MI		Likelihood Ratio
	MI Present	MI Absent	
≥280 IU/L	97	1	(97/1)/(230/130) = 54.8
80-279 IU/L	118	15	(118/15)/(230/130) = 4.45
40-79 IU/L	13	26	(13/26)/(230/130) = 0.28
0-39 IU/L	2	88	(2/88)/(230/130) = 0.013
TOTALS	230	130	

Data from Smith AF: *Lancet* 2:178, 1967.
*The methods of determining serum creatine kinase (CK) values have changed since the time of this report, so these values cannot be applied directly to patient care at present. Troponins are currently used more often than CK, but the data used illustrate the likelihood ratio principle well.

entire population. The LR+ indicates how much the odds of disease were *increased* if the test result was *positive*.

Similarly, the LR− is the ratio of two probabilities: the ratio of (1 − sensitivity) to specificity. Alternatively, this can be expressed as $[c/(a + c)] \div [d/(b + d)]$, and the formula can be rearranged algebraically as follows:

$$LR- = (c/d)/[(a+c)/(b+d)]$$

which is the odds of missed disease among persons in whom the test yielded negative results, divided by the odds of disease in the entire population. The LR− shows how much the odds of disease were *decreased* if the test result was *negative*.

Does this new way of calculating the likelihood ratio really work? Compare Table 7-2, in which the LR+ can be calculated as follows and yields exactly the same result as previously obtained:

$$LR+ = (12/3)/(12+8)/(3+57)$$
$$= (12/3)/(20/60)$$
$$= 4/0.333 = 12.0$$

Likewise, the LR− can be calculated as follows and yields the same result as before:

$$LR- = (8/57)/(12+8)/(3+57)$$
$$= (8/57)/(20/60)$$
$$= 0.140/0.333 = 0.42$$

The likelihood ratio (without specifying positive or negative) can be described as the odds of disease given a specified test value divided by the odds of disease in the study population. This general definition of LR can be used for numerous test ranges, as shown for the four ranges of CK result in Table 7-3. If the CK value was 280 IU/L or more, the LR was large (54.8), making it highly probable that the patient had an MI. If the CK was 39 IU/L or less, the LR was small (0.013), meaning that MI was probably absent. The LRs for the two middle ranges of CK values do not elicit as much confidence in the test, however, so additional tests would be needed to make a diagnosis in patients whose CK values were between 40 and 279 IU/L.

In Tables 7-2 and 7-3 the **posttest odds** of disease (*a/b*) equals the **pretest odds** multiplied by the LRs. In Table 7-2 the pretest odds of disease were 20/60, or 0.333, because this is all that was known about the distribution of disease in the study population before the test was given (i.e., 20/60 is the prevalence). The LR+, as calculated previously, turned out to be 12.0. When 0.333 is multiplied by 12.0, the result is 4. This is the same as the posttest odds, which was found to be 12/3, or 4. (See also Bayes theorem in Chapter 8.)

E. Receiver Operating Characteristic Curves

In clinical tests used to measure continuous variables such as serum calcium, blood glucose, or blood pressure, the choice of the best cutoff point is often difficult. As discussed earlier, there are few false-positive results and many false-negative results if the cutoff point is very high, and the reverse occurs if the cutoff point is very low. Because calcium, glucose, blood pressure, and other values can fluctuate in any

individual, whether healthy or diseased, there is some overlap of values in the "normal" population and values in the diseased population (see Fig. 7-3).

To decide on a good cutoff point, investigators could construct a **receiver operating characteristic** (ROC) **curve**. Beginning with new or previously published data that showed the test results and the true status for *every person tested in a study*, the investigators could calculate the sensitivity and false-positive error rate for several possible cutoff points and plot the points on a square graph. Increasingly seen in the medical literature, ROC curves originated in World War II in evaluating the performance of radar receiver operators: a "true positive" was a correct early warning of enemy planes crossing the English Channel; a "false positive" occurred when a radar operator sent out an alarm but no enemy planes appeared; and a "false-negative" when enemy planes appeared without previous warning from the radar operators.

An example of an ROC curve for blood pressure screening is shown in Figure 7-4 (fictitious data). The *y*-axis shows the **sensitivity** of a test, and the *x*-axis shows the **false-positive error rate** (1 − specificity). Because the LR+ of a test is defined as the sensitivity divided by the false-positive error rate, *the ROC curve can be considered a graph of the LR+.*

If a group of investigators wanted to determine the best cutoff for a blood pressure screening program, they might begin by taking a single initial blood pressure measurement in a large population and then performing a complete workup for persistent hypertension in all of the individuals. Each person would have data on a single screening blood pressure value and an ultimate diagnosis concerning the presence or absence of hypertension. Based on this information, an ROC curve could be constructed. If the cutoff for identifying individuals with suspected high blood pressure were set at 0 mm Hg (an extreme example to illustrate the

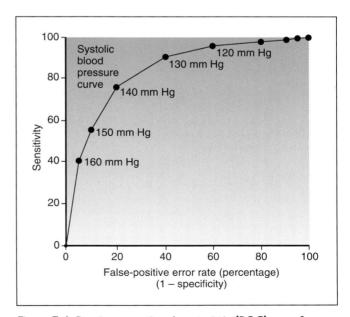

Figure 7-4 Receiver operating characteristic (ROC) curve for blood pressure. ROC curve from a study to determine the best cutoff point for a blood pressure screening program (fictitious data). Numbers beside the points on the curve are the cutoffs of systolic blood pressure that gave the corresponding sensitivity and false-positive error rate.

procedure), *all living* study participants would be included in the group suspected to have hypertension. This means that all of the persons with hypertension would be detected, and the sensitivity would be 100%. However, all of the normal persons also would screen positive for hypertension, so the false-positive error rate would be 100%, and the point would be placed in the upper right (100%-100%) corner of the graph. By similar reasoning, if an extremely high blood pressure, such as 500 mm Hg, was taken as the cutoff, nobody would be detected with hypertension, so sensitivity would be 0%. There would be no false-positive results either, however, so the false-positive error rate also would be 0%. This point would be placed in the lower left (0%-0%) corner of the graph.

Next, the investigators would analyze the data for the lowest reasonable cutoff point—for example, a systolic blood pressure of 120 mm Hg—and plot the corresponding sensitivity and false-positive error rate on the graph. Then they could use 130 mm Hg as the cutoff, determine the new sensitivity and false-positive error rate, and plot the data point on the graph. This would be repeated for 140 mm Hg and for higher values. It is unlikely that the cutoff point for the diagnosis of hypertension would be a systolic blood pressure of less than 120 mm Hg or greater than 150 mm Hg. When all are in place, the points can be connected to resemble Figure 7-4. Ordinarily, the best cutoff point would be the point closest to the upper left corner, the corner representing a sensitivity of 100% and a false-positive error rate of 0%.

The ideal ROC curve for a test would rise almost vertically from the lower left corner and move horizontally almost along the upper line, as shown in the uppermost ROC curve in Figure 7-5, the *excellent curve*. If the sensitivity always equaled the false-positive error rate, the result would be a diagonal straight line from the lower left to the upper right corner, the *no benefit line*. The ROC curve for most clinical tests is somewhere between these two extremes, similar to either the *good curve* or the *fair curve*.

The ROC curve in Figure 7-6 shows the sensitivity and false-positive error rates found in a study of patients with follicular thyroid tumors.[12] The investigator sought to use the diameter of the tumors as measured at surgery to determine the probability of malignancy. Initially, when the ROC curve was plotted using the tumor diameters of patients of all ages, the curve was disappointing (not shown in Fig. 7-6). When the patients were divided into two age groups (patients <50 and patients ≥50 years old), the diameter of the tumors was found to be strongly predictive of cancer in the older group, but not in the younger group. It is unusual for the curve to hug the axes as it does for the older group, but this was caused by the relatively small number of patients involved (96 patients). In Figure 7-6 the curve for the older age group can be compared with that for the younger age group. At a tumor diameter of **4.5 cm,** the sensitivity in older patients was approximately 75%, in contrast to about 35% in the younger patients, and the corresponding false-positive error rates were 0% and 25%. At a tumor diameter of **3.5 cm,** the sensitivities were not greatly different from each other, about 75% in the older patients and 65% in the younger patients, but the corresponding false-positive error rates were very different, about 15% and 45%. At a tumor diameter of **3 cm,** the corresponding sensitivities for the older and the younger patients were 100% and 65%, and the false-positive error rates were 35% and 60%, respectively.

Analysis of ROC curves is becoming more sophisticated and popular in fields such as radiology. One method of comparing different tests is to determine the *area under the ROC curve* for each test and to use a statistical test of significance to decide if the area under one curve differs significantly from the area under the other curve. The greater the area under the curve, the better the test is.[13] In Figure 7-6 the diagonal line from the lower left to the upper right represents the area of *no benefit*, where the sensitivity and false-positive error rate are the same; the area under this line is 50%. The

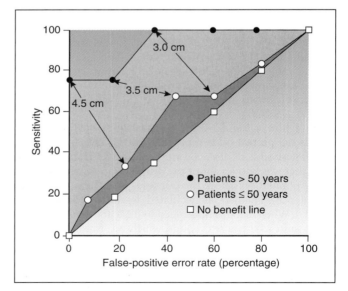

Figure 7-6 ROC curves for a test to determine malignancy status of follicular thyroid tumor based on its diameter. *Upper curve,* Results in patients 50 years or older; *middle curve,* results in patients younger than 50; *bottom curve,* line of no benefit from the test. Numbers beside the points on the curves are the tumor diameters that gave the corresponding sensitivity and false-positive error rate. (Data courtesy Dr. Barbara Kinder, formerly Department of Surgery, Yale University School of Medicine, New Haven, Conn.)

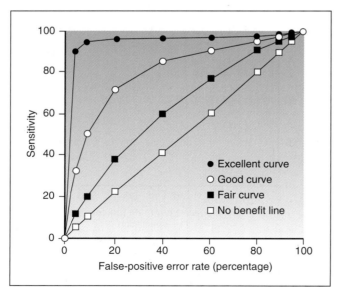

Figure 7-5 ROC curves for four tests. The uppermost curve is the best of the four.

area under the curve for younger patients is close to 60%, whereas the area under the curve for older patients is near 90%. These data suggest that for older patients, the size of this type of thyroid tumor can help the surgeon decide whether or not to remove the tumor before receiving a pathology assessment. For younger patients, the tumor diameter does not help in this decision.

III. MEASURING AGREEMENT

An important question in clinical medicine and in research is the extent to which different observations of the same phenomenon differ. If there is intraobserver agreement and interobserver agreement, as defined at the beginning of this chapter, the data in a study are considered highly reliable and elicit more confidence than if they lack either type of agreement. Reliability is not proof of validity, however. Two observers can report the same readings (i.e., show reliability), but both observers could be wrong.

It is not unusual to find imperfect agreement between observers, and a clinician looking again at the same data (e.g., heart or knee examination, interpretation of x-ray film or pathology slide) may disagree with his or her own previous reading. A study of variability in radiologists' interpretations found that different readers frequently disagreed about the interpretation of a specific mammogram. In two independent readings of the same mammogram, radiologists disagreed with their own previous readings almost as frequently.[8]

A. Overall Percent Agreement

If a test uses a *dichotomous variable* (i.e., two categories of results, such as positive and negative), the results can be placed in a standard 2×2 table so that observer agreement can be calculated (Table 7-4). Cells a and d represent agreement, whereas cells b and c represent disagreement.

A common way to measure agreement is to calculate the **overall percent agreement.** If 90% of the observations are in cells a and d, the overall percent agreement would be 90%. Nevertheless, merely reporting the overall percent agreement is considered inadequate for numerous reasons. First, the overall percent agreement does not indicate the prevalence of the finding in the participants studied. Second, it does not show how the disagreements occurred; were the positive and negative results distributed evenly between the two observers, or did one observer consistently find more positive results than the other? Third, considerable agreement would be expected by chance alone, and the overall percent agreement does not define the extent to which the agreement improves on chance. The prevalence of positive findings and the direction of disagreement between two observers can be reported easily from tables such as Table 7-4. Measuring the extent to which agreement exceeds that expected by chance requires a measurement statistic called the **kappa.**

B. Kappa Test Ratio

Two clinicians have examined the same 100 patients during the same hour and record either the presence of a heart murmur or the absence of a heart murmur in each patient. For 7 patients, the first clinician reports the absence of a

Table 7-4 Standard 2 × 2 Table Comparing Test Results Reported by Two Observers

Observer No. 2	Observer No. 1		Total
	Positive	Negative	
Positive	a	b	$a + b$
Negative	c	d	$c + d$
TOTAL	$a + c$	$b + d$	$a + b + c + d$

Interpretation of the Cells

a = Positive/positive observer agreement
b = Negative/positive observer disagreement
c = Positive/negative observer disagreement
d = Negative/negative observer agreement

Formulas

$a + d$ + Observed agreement (A_o)
$a + b + c + d$ = Maximum possible agreement (N)
$(a + d)/(a + b + c + d)$ = Overall percent agreement
$[(a + b)(a + c)]/(a + b + c + d)$ = Cell a agreement expected by chance
$[(c + d)(b + d)]/(a + b + c + d)$ = Cell d agreement expected by chance
Cell a agreement expected by chance + Cell d agreement expected by chance = Total agreement expected by chance (A_c)
$(A_o - A_c)/(N - A_c)$ = kappa

Table 7-5 Clinical Agreement between Two Clinicians on Presence or Absence of Cardiac Murmur on Physical Examination of 100 Patients (Fictitious Data)

Clinician No. 2	Clinician No. 1		Total
	Murmur Present	Murmur Absent	
Murmur present	30	7	37
Murmur absent	3	60	63
TOTAL	33	67	100

Calculations Based on Formulas in Table 7-4

$30 + 60 = 90$ = Observed agreement (A_o)
$30 + 7 + 3 + 60 = 100$ = Maximum possible agreement (N)
$(30 + 60)/(30 + 7 + 3 + 60) = 90/100 = 90\%$ = Overall percent agreement
$[(30 + 7)(30 + 3)]/100 = [(37)(33)]/100 = 12.2$ = Cell a agreement expected by chance
$[(3 + 60)(7 + 60)]/100 = [(63)(67)]/100 = 42.2$ = Cell d agreement expected by chance
$12.2 + 42.2 = 54.4$ = Total agreement expected by chance (A_c)
$(90 - 54.4)/(100 - 54.4) = 35.6/45.6 = 0.78 = 78\%$ = kappa

murmur and the second clinician reports the presence of a murmur, and for 3 patients the second clinician reports the absence and the first clinician reports the presence of a murmur. For 30 patients the clinicians agree on the presence of a heart murmur, and for 60 patients the clinicians agree on the absence of a murmur. These results could be arranged in a 2×2 table (Table 7-5). In addition to calculating the overall percent agreement (90%), the kappa test could be performed to determine the extent to which the agreement between the two clinicians improved on chance agreement alone. Even if the two clinicians only guessed about the presence or absence of a murmur, they sometimes would agree by chance.

As shown in Tables 7-4 and 7-5, the **observed agreement** (A_o) is the sum of the actual number of observations in cells a and d. The **maximum possible agreement** is the total number of observations (N). The **agreement expected by chance** (A_c) is the sum of the expected number of observations in cells a and d. The method used to calculate the expected agreement for the kappa test is the same method used for the chi-square test (see Chapter 11). For a given cell, such as cell a, the cell's row total is multiplied by the cell's column total, and the product is divided by the grand total. For cell a, the agreement expected by chance is calculated as $[(a + b)(a + c)] \div (a + b + c + d)$.

Kappa is a ratio. The numerator is the observed improvement over chance agreement ($A_o - A_c$), and the denominator is the maximum possible improvement over chance agreement ($N - A_c$). The kappa ratio is a proportion that can take on values from -1 (indicating perfect disagreement) through 0 (representing the agreement expected by chance) to $+1$ (indicating perfect agreement). Frequently, the results of the kappa test are expressed as a percentage. The following arbitrary divisions for interpreting the results are often used: less than 20% is negligible improvement over chance, 20% to 40% is minimal, 40% to 60% is fair, 60% to 80% is good, and greater than 80% is excellent.[14] In the example of cardiac murmurs, the kappa test yielded a result of 0.78, or 78%, indicating that the clinician ratings were a "good" improvement on the chance expectation.

The reliability of most tests in clinical medicine that require human judgment seems to fall in the fair or good range. Although the kappa test described here provides valuable data on observer agreement for diagnoses recorded as "present" or "absent," some studies involve three or more outcome categories (e.g., negative, suspicious, or probable). For such data, a **weighted kappa test** must be used. The weighted test is similar in principle to the unweighted test described here, but it is more complex.[15] The weighted test gives partial credit for agreement that is close but not perfect.

In the evaluation of the accuracy and usefulness of a laboratory assay, imaging procedure, or any other clinical test, comparing the findings of one observer with the findings of another observer is not as useful as comparing the findings of an observer with the true disease status in the patients being tested. The **true disease status,** which is used to determine the sensitivity and specificity of tests, is considered to be the "gold standard," and its use is preferable whenever such data are available. Gold standards seldom exist in clinical medicine, however, and even a small error in the gold standard can create the appearance of considerable error in a test.[16] Studies of the errors of new diagnostic tests are urgently needed; in addition, new studies are needed for many of the older diagnostic tests.

IV. SUMMARY

Three important goals of data collection and analysis are the promotion of accuracy and precision (see Figs. 7-1 and 7-2), the reduction of differential and nondifferential errors (nonrandom and random errors), and the reduction in interobserver and intraobserver variability (variability between findings of two observers or between findings of one observer on two occasions). Various statistical methods are available to study the accuracy and usefulness of screening tests and diagnostic (confirmatory) tests in clinical medicine. In general, tests with a high degree of sensitivity and a corresponding low false-negative error rate are helpful for screening patients (for ruling out), whereas tests with a high degree of specificity and a corresponding low false-positive error rate are useful for confirming (ruling in) the diagnosis in patients suspected to have a particular disease. Tables 7-1, 7-2, and 7-3 provide definitions of and formulas for calculating sensitivity, specificity, error rates, predictive values, and likelihood ratios. Tables 7-4 and 7-5 define measures of intraobserver and interobserver agreement and provide formulas for calculating the overall percent agreement and the kappa test ratio.

References

1. Kohn LT, Corrigan JM, Donaldson MS, editors: *To err is human: building a safer health system.* Report of the Institute of Medicine, Washington, DC, 2000, National Academy Press.
2. Brennan T: The Institute of Medicine report on medical errors: could it do harm? *N Engl J Med* 342:1123–1125, 2000.
3. Dosemeci M, Wacholder S, Lubin JH: Does nondifferential misclassification of exposure always bias a true effect toward the null value? *Am J Epidemiol* 132:746–748, 1990.
4. Ransohoff DF, Feinstein AR: Problems of spectrum and bias in evaluating the efficacy of diagnostic tests. *N Engl J Med* 299:926–930, 1978.
5. Abbas AA, et al: *Cellular and molecular immunology,* Philadelphia, 1991, Saunders.
6. Rose DN, Schechter CB, Adler JJ: Interpretation of the tuberculin skin test. *J Gen Intern Med* 10:635–642, 1995.
7. Elmore JG, Barton MB, Moceri VM, et al: Ten-year risk of false-positive screening mammograms and clinical breast examinations. *N Engl J Med* 338:1089–1096, 1998.
8. Elmore JG, Wells CK, Lee CH, et al: Variability in radiologists' interpretations of mammograms. *N Engl J Med* 331:1493–1499, 1994.
9. Jekel JF, Greenberg RA, Drake BM: Influence of the prevalence of infection on tuberculin skin testing programs. *Public Health Rep* 84:883–886, 1969.
10. Stein PD: Diagnosis of pulmonary embolism. *Curr Opin Pulm Med* 2:295–299, 1996.
11. Smith AF: Diagnostic value of serum-creatine-kinase in a coronary-care unit. *Lancet* 2:178, 1967.
12. Kinder B: Personal communication. 1994.
13. Pepe MS: *The statistical evaluation of medical tests for classification and prediction,* Oxford, 2003, Oxford University Press.
14. Sackett DL, Tugwell P, Haynes RB, et al: *Clinical epidemiology: a basic science for clinical medicine,* ed 2, Boston, 1991, Little, Brown.
15. Cicchetti DV, Sharma Y, Cotlier E: Assessment of observer variability in the classification of human cataracts. *Yale J Biol Med* 55:81–88, 1982.
16. Greenberg RA, Jekel JF: Some problems in the determination of the false-positive and false-negative rates of tuberculin tests. *Am Rev Respir Dis* 100:645–650, 1969.

Select Reading

Haynes RB, Sackett DL, Guyatt GH, et al: *Clinical epidemiology,* ed 3, Philadelphia, 2006, Lippincott, Williams & Wilkins.
Ransohoff DF, Feinstein AR: Problems of spectrum and bias in evaluating the efficacy of diagnostic tests. *N Engl J Med* 299:926–930, 1978. [Use of diagnostic tests to rule in or rule out a disease.]
Sackett DL, Tugwell P, Haynes RB, et al: *Clinical epidemiology: a basic science for clinical medicine,* ed 2, Boston, 1991, Little, Brown. [Clinical agreement.]

Biostatistics

2

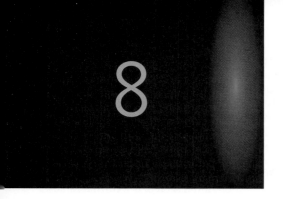

8 Statistical Foundations of Clinical Decisions

There is an increasing demand for clinical decisions to be based on the best available clinical research. This approach to clinical practice has come to be widely referred to as **evidence-based medicine** (EBM). Since early in the 20th century, medical decisions have been based on a combination of clinical experience and judgment gained from research. More recently, with the rapid increase in the accessibility of the literature through Internet searches, and with the steady improvements in the methods of clinical epidemiology and biostatistics, it has become possible to base more diagnostic and therapeutic decisions on quantitative information provided by clinical research. EBM requires that clinicians do the following:

- Access the most relevant research data.
- Decide which studies are most trustworthy and applicable to the clinical question under consideration.
- Use appropriate methods available to determine the best diagnostic and therapeutic approaches to each problem.

Many methods described in this text, especially some of the tools discussed in this chapter, such as Bayes theorem, clinical decision analysis, and meta-analysis, may be considered tools for the practice of EBM.

There is no controversy about the need to improve clinical decision making and maximize the quality of care. Opinions do differ, however regarding the extent to which the tools discussed in this chapter are likely to help in actual clinical decision making. Some individuals and medical centers already use these methods to guide the care of individual patients. Others acknowledge that the tools can help to formulate policy and analyze the cost-effectiveness of medical interventions, such as immunizations,[1,2] but they may not use the techniques for making decisions about individual patients. Even when the most highly regarded means are used to procure evidence, such as double-blind, placebo-controlled clinical trials, the applicability of that evidence to an individual patient is uncertain and a matter of judgment.

Regardless of the clinician's philosophic approach to using these methods for actual clinical care, they can help clinicians to understand the quantitative basis for making clinical decisions in the increasingly complex field of medicine.

I. BAYES THEOREM

Although it is useful to know the sensitivity and specificity of a test, when a clinician decides to use a certain test on a patient, the following two clinical questions require answers (see Chapter 7):

- If the test results are positive, what is the probability that the patient has the disease?
- If the test results are negative, what is the probability that the patient does not have the disease?

Bayes theorem provides a way to answer these questions. Bayes theorem, first described centuries ago by the English clergyman after whom it is named, is one of the most imposing statistical formulas in medicine. Put in symbols more meaningful in medicine, the formula is as follows:

$$p(D+\,|\,T+) = \frac{p(T+\,|\,D+)p(D+)}{[p(T+\,|\,D+)p(D+) + p(T+\,|\,D-)p(D-)]}$$

where p denotes probability, D+ means that the patient has the disease in question, D− means that the patient does not have the disease, T+ means that a certain diagnostic test for the disease is positive, T− means that the test is negative, and the vertical line (|) means *conditional on* what immediately follows.

Many clinicians, even those who understand sensitivity, specificity, and predictive values, throw in the towel when it comes to Bayes theorem. A close look at the previous equation reveals, however, that Bayes theorem is merely the formula for the **positive predictive value** (PPV), a value discussed in Chapter 7 and illustrated there in a standard 2 × 2 table (see Table 7-1).

The **numerator of Bayes theorem** merely describes **cell *a*** (the true-positive results) in Table 7-1. The probability of being in cell *a* is equal to the prevalence times the sensitivity, where $p(D+)$ is the prevalence (expressed as the probability of being in the diseased column) and where $p(T+ \mid D+)$ is the sensitivity (the probability of being in the top, test-positive, row, *given the fact of being in the diseased column*). The **denominator of Bayes theorem** consists of two terms, the first of which describes **cell *a*** (the true-positive results), and the second of which describes **cell *b*** (the false-positive results) in Table 7-1. In the second term of the denominator, the probability of the false-positive error rate, or $p(T+ \mid D-)$, is multiplied by the prevalence of nondiseased persons, or $p(D-)$. As outlined in Chapter 7, the true-positive results (a) divided by the true-positive plus false-positive results ($a + b$) gives $a/(a + b)$, which is the positive predictive value.

In genetics, a simpler-appearing formula for Bayes theorem is sometimes used. The numerator is the same, but the denominator is merely $p(T+)$. This makes sense because the denominator in $a/(a + b)$ is equal to all those who have positive test results, whether they are true-positive or false-positive results.

Now that Bayes theorem has been demystified, its uses in community screening and in individual patient care can be discussed.

A. Community Screening Programs

In a population with a low prevalence of a particular disease, most of the positive results in a screening program for the disease likely would be falsely positive (see Chapter 7). Although this fact does not automatically invalidate a screening program, it raises some concerns about cost-effectiveness, which can be explored using Bayes theorem.

A program employing the tuberculin tine test to screen children for tuberculosis (TB) is discussed as an example (based on actual experience).[3] This test uses small amounts of tuberculin antigen on the tips of tiny prongs called *tines*. The tines pierce the skin on the forearm and leave some antigen behind. The skin is examined 48 hours later, and the presence of an inflammatory reaction in the area where the tines entered is considered a positive result. If the sensitivity and specificity of the test and the prevalence of TB in the community are known, Bayes theorem can be used to predict what proportion of the children with positive test results will have true-positive results (i.e., will actually be infected with *Mycobacterium tuberculosis*).

Box 8-1 shows how the calculations are made. Suppose a test has a sensitivity of 96% and a specificity of 94%. If the prevalence of TB in the community is 1%, only 13.9% of those with a positive test result would be likely to be infected with TB. Clinicians involved in community health programs can quickly develop a table that lists different levels of test sensitivity, test specificity, and disease prevalence that shows how these levels affect the proportion of positive results that are likely to be true-positive results. Although this calculation is fairly straightforward and extremely useful, it is not used often in the early stages of planning for screening programs. Before a new test is used, particularly for screening a large population, it is best to apply the test's sensitivity and

specificity to the anticipated prevalence of the condition in the population. This helps avoid awkward surprises and is useful in the planning of appropriate follow-up for test-positive individuals. If the primary concern is simply to determine the overall performance of a test, however, likelihood ratios, which are independent of prevalence, are recommended (see Chapter 7).

There is another important point to keep in mind when planning community screening programs. The first time a previously unscreened population is screened, a considerable number of cases of disease may be found, but a repeat screening program soon afterward may find relatively few cases of new disease. This is because the first screening would detect cases that had their onset over *many* years (**prevalent cases**), whereas the second screening primarily would detect cases that had their onset during the interval since the last screening (**incident cases**).

B. Individual Patient Care

Suppose a clinician is uncertain about a patient's diagnosis, obtains a test result for a certain disease, and the test is positive. Even if the clinician knows the sensitivity and specificity of the test, this does not solve the problem, because to calculate the positive predictive value, whether using Bayes theorem or a 2 × 2 table (e.g., Table 7-1), it is necessary to know the *prevalence of the disease*. In a *clinical* setting, the prevalence can be considered the *expected prevalence* in the population of which the patient is part. The actual prevalence is usually unknown, but often a reasonable estimate can be made.

For example, a clinician in a general medical clinic sees a male patient who complains of easy fatigability and has a history of kidney stones, but no other symptoms or signs of parathyroid disease on physical examination. The clinician considers the probability of hyperparathyroidism and decides that it is low, perhaps 2% (reflecting that in 100 similar patients, probably only 2 of them would have the disease). This probability is called the **prior probability**, reflecting that it is estimated *before* the performance of laboratory tests and is based on the estimated prevalence of a particular disease among patients with similar signs and symptoms. Although the clinician believes that the probability of hyperparathyroidism is low, he or she orders a serum calcium test to "rule out" the diagnosis. To the clinician's surprise, the results of the test come back positive, with an elevated level of 12.2 mg/dL. The clinician could order more tests for parathyroid disease, but even here, some test results might come back positive and some negative.

Under the circumstances, Bayes theorem could be used to help interpret the positive test. A second estimate of disease probability in this patient could be calculated. It is called the **posterior probability,** reflecting that it is made *after* the test results are known. Calculation of the posterior probability is based on the sensitivity and specificity of the test that was performed and on the prior probability of disease before the test was performed, which in this case was 2%. Suppose the serum calcium test had 90% sensitivity and 95% specificity (which implies it had a false-positive error rate of 5%; specificity + false-positive error rate = 100%). When this information is used in the Bayes equation, as shown in Box 8-2, the result is a posterior probability of 27%. This means that the patient is now in a group of patients with a substantial

Box 8-1	Use of Bayes Theorem or 2 × 2 Table to Determine Positive Predictive Value of Hypothetical Tuberculin Screening Program

PART 1 Beginning Data

Sensitivity of tuberculin tine test	= 96%	= 0.96
False-negative error rate of test	= 4%	= 0.04
Specificity of test	= 94%	= 0.94
False-positive error rate of test	= 6%	= 0.06
Prevalence of tuberculosis in community	= 1%	= 0.01

PART 2 Use of Bayes Theorem

$$p(D+\,|\,T+) = \frac{p(T+\,|\,D+)p(D+)}{[p(T+\,|\,D+)p(D+) + p(T+\,|\,D-)p(D-)]}$$

$$= \frac{(\text{Sensitivity})(\text{Prevalence})}{[(\text{Sensitivity})(\text{Prevalence}) + (\text{False-positive error rate})(1 - \text{Prevalence})]}$$

$$= \frac{(0.96)(0.01)}{[(0.96)(0.01) + (0.06)(0.99)]} = \frac{0.0096}{[0.0096 + 0.0594]} = \frac{0.0096}{0.0690} = 0.139 = \mathbf{13.9\%}$$

PART 3 Use of 2 × 2 Table, with Numbers Based on Study of 10,000 Persons

Test Result	True Disease Status (No.)		
	Diseased	Nondiseased	Total
Positive	96 (96%)	594 (6%)	690 (7%)
Negative	4 (4%)	9306 (94%)	9310 (93%)
TOTAL	100 (100%)	9900 (100%)	10,000 (100%)

Positive predictive value = 96/690 = 0.139 = **13.9%**

Data from Jekel JF, Greenberg RA, Drake BM: Influence of the prevalence of infection on tuberculin skin testing programs. *Public Health Reports* 84:883–886, 1969.

possibility, but still far from certainty, of parathyroid disease. In Box 8-2, the result is the same (i.e., 27%) when a 2 × 2 table is used. This is true because, as discussed previously, the probability based on the Bayes theorem is identical to the positive predictive value.

In light of the 27% posterior probability, the clinician decides to order a serum parathyroid hormone concentration test with simultaneous measurement of serum calcium, even though this test is expensive. If the parathyroid hormone test had a sensitivity of 95% and a specificity of 98%, and the results turned out to be positive, the Bayes theorem could be used again to calculate the probability of parathyroid disease in this patient. This time, however, the *posterior* probability for the *first* test (27%) would be used as the *prior* probability for the *second* test. The result of the calculation, as shown in Box 8-3, is a new probability of 94%. The patient likely does have hyperparathyroidism, although lack of true, numerical certainty even at this stage is noteworthy.

Why did the posterior probability increase so much the second time? One reason was that the *prior probability was considerably higher* in the second calculation than in the first (27% versus 2%), based on the first test yielding positive results. Another reason was that the *specificity of the second test was assumed to be quite high* (98%), which greatly reduced the false-positive error rate and increased the PPV. A highly specific test is useful for "ruling in" disease, which in essence is what has happened here.

C. Influence of the Sequence of Testing

With an increasing number of diagnostic tests available in clinical medicine, the clinician now needs to consider whether to do many tests simultaneously or to do them sequentially. As outlined in Chapter 7, tests used to "rule out" a diagnosis should have a high degree of sensitivity, whereas tests used to "rule in" a diagnosis should have a high degree of specificity (see Box 7-1). The *sequential approach* is best done as follows:

1. Starting with the most sensitive test.
2. Continuing with increasingly specific tests if the previous test yields positive results.
3. Stopping when a test yields negative results.

Compared with the simultaneous approach, the sequential approach to testing is more conservative and is more economical in the care of outpatients. The sequential

Box 8-2   Use of Bayes Theorem or 2 × 2 Table to Determine Posterior Probability and Positive Predictive Value in Clinical Setting (Hypothetical Data)

PART 1   **Beginning Data (Before Performing First Test)**

Sensitivity of first test	= 90%	= 0.90
Specificity of first test	= 95%	= 0.95
Prior probability of disease	= 2%	= 0.02

PART 2   **Use of Bayes Theorem to Calculate First Posterior Probability**

$$p(D+|T+) = \frac{p(T+|D+)p(D+)}{[p(T+|D+)p(D+) + p(T+|D-)p(D-)]}$$

$$= \frac{(0.90)(0.02)}{[(0.90)(0.02) + (0.05)(0.98)]}$$

$$= \frac{0.018}{[0.018 + 0.049]} = \frac{0.018}{0.067} = 0.269 = \mathbf{27\%}$$

PART 3   **Use of a 2 × 2 Table to Calculate First Positive Predictive Value**

	True Disease Status (No.)		
Test Result	Diseased	Nondiseased	Total
Positive	18 (90%)	49 (5%)	67 (6.7%)
Negative	2 (10%)	931 (95%)	933 (93.3%)
TOTAL	20 (100%)	980 (100%)	1000 (100%)

Positive predictive value = 18/67 = **27%**

Box 8-3   Use of Bayes Theorem or 2 × 2 Table to Determine Second Posterior Probability and Second Positive Predictive Value in Clinical Setting

PART 1   **Beginning Data (Before Performing the Second Test)**

Sensitivity of second test	= 95%	= 0.95
Specificity of second test	= 98%	= 0.98
Prior probability of disease (see Box 8-2)	= **27%**	= 0.27

PART 2   **Use of Bayes Theorem to Calculate First Posterior Probability**

$$p(D+|T+) = \frac{p(T+|D+)p(D+)}{[p(T+|D+)p(D+) + p(T+|D-)p(D-)]}$$

$$= \frac{(0.95)(0.27)}{[(0.95)(0.27) + (0.02)(0.73)]}$$

$$= \frac{0.257}{[0.257 + 0.0146]} = \frac{0.257}{0.272} = 0.9449^* = \mathbf{94\%}$$

PART 3   **Use of 2 × 2 Table to Calculate First Positive Predictive Value**

	True Disease Status (No.)		
Test Result	Diseased	Nondiseased	Total
Positive	256 (95%)	15 (2%)	271 (27.1%)
Negative	13 (5%)	716 (98%)	729 (72.9%)
TOTAL	269 (100%)	731 (100%)	1000 (100%)

Positive predictive value = 256/271 = 0.9446* = **94%**

*The slight difference in the results for the two approaches is caused by rounding errors. It is not important clinically.

approach may increase the length of stay for a hospitalized patient, however, so the cost implications may be unclear.

The sequence of testing may have implications for the overall accuracy. If multiple diagnostic tests are performed at the same time, the natural tendency is to ignore the negative results, while seriously considering the positive results. This approach to establishing a diagnosis may not be ideal, however. Even if the tests are performed simultaneously, it is probably best to consider first the results of the most sensitive test. If a negative result is reported for that test, the result is probably a true-negative one (the patient probably does not have the disease). Why? Highly sensitive tests are reliably positive when disease is present and tend to deliver negative results only when disease is truly absent. Simultaneous testing may produce conflicting results, but a careful consideration of each test's result in light of the test's sensitivity and specificity should improve the chances of making the correct diagnosis.

II. DECISION ANALYSIS

A decision-making tool that has come into the medical literature from management science is called **decision analysis.** Its purpose is to improve decision making under conditions of uncertainty. In clinical medicine, decision analysis can be used for an individual patient or for a general class of patients. As a technique, decision analysis is more popular clinically than Bayes theorem, and it is being used with increasing frequency in the literature, particularly to make judgments about a class of patients or clinical problems.

The primary value of decision analysis is to help health care workers understand the following:

- The types of data that must go into a clinical decision
- The sequence in which decisions need to be made

- The personal values of the patient that must be considered before major decisions are made

As a general rule, decision analysis is more important as a tool to help clinicians take a disciplined approach to decision making than as a tool for making the actual clinical decisions. Nevertheless, as computer programs for using decision analysis become more available, some clinicians are using decision analysis in their clinical work.

A. Steps in Creating a Decision Tree

There are five logical steps to setting up a decision tree, as follows[4]:

1. Identify and set limits to the problem.
2. Diagram the options.
3. Obtain information on each option.
4. Compare the utility values.
5. Perform sensitivity analysis.

1. Identify the Problem

When identifying a course of clinical action, the clinician must determine the possible alternative clinical decisions, the sequence in which the decisions must be made, and the possible patient outcomes of each decision. The clinical problem illustrated here is whether or not to remove a gallbladder in a patient with silent gallstones.[5]

2. Diagram the Options

Figure 8-1 provides a simple example of how to diagram the options. The beginning point of a decision tree is the patient's current clinical status. **Decision nodes,** defined as points where clinicians need to make decisions, are represented by

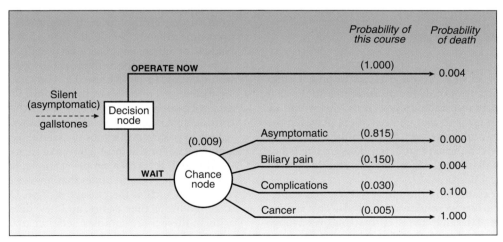

Figure 8-1 Decision tree on treatment for silent (asymptomatic) gallstones. The *decision node,* defined as a point where the clinician has to make a decision, is represented by a *square.* The *chance node,* defined as a point where the clinician must wait to see the outcome, is represented by a *circle.* If the clinician decides to operate now, the probability of surgery is 100% (1.000), and the probability of death (the negative utility value) from complications of surgery is 0.04% (0.004, or 1 of every 250 patients undergoing surgery). If the clinician decides to wait, there are four possible outcomes, each with a different probability and negative utility value: (1) 81.5% (0.815) probability of remaining asymptomatic, in which case the probability of dying from gallstones would be 0% (0.000); (2) 15% (0.150) probability of developing biliary pain, which would lead to surgery and a 0.4% (0.004) risk of death; (3) 3% (0.030) probability of biliary complications (e.g., acute cholecystitis, common duct obstruction), with a 10% (0.100) risk of death; or (4) 0.5% (0.005) probability of gallbladder cancer, with a 100% (1.000) risk of death. The probabilities of the possible outcomes at the chance node add up to 1 (here, 0.815 + 0.150 + 0.030 + 0.005 = 1.000). (From Rose DN, Wiesel J: *N Engl J Med* 308:221–222, 1983. © Massachusetts Medical Society. All rights reserved. Adapted with permission in 1996, 1999, 2006, 2011.)

squares or rectangles. **Chance nodes,** defined as points where clinicians need to wait to see the outcomes, are represented by circles. Time goes from left to right, so the first decision is at the left, and subsequent decisions are progressively to the right. In Figure 8-1 the beginning point is the presence of asymptomatic gallstones, and the primary decision at the decision node is whether to operate immediately or to wait.[5]

3. Obtain Information on Each Option

First, the **probability of each possible outcome** must be obtained from published studies or be estimated on the basis of clinical experience. In Figure 8-1, if the clinician waits rather than operating, the probability is 81.5% (0.815) that the patient will remain asymptomatic, 15% that the patient will have periodic biliary pain, 3% that the patient will develop complications such as acute cholecystitis or common duct obstruction from gallstones, and 0.5% that the patient eventually will develop cancer of the gallbladder. The probabilities of the possible outcomes for a chance node must add up to 100%, as they do in this case.

Second, the **utility of each final outcome** must be obtained. In decision analysis the term *utility* is used to mean the value of a chosen course of action. Utility may be expressed as a **desirable outcome** (e.g., years of disease-free survival), in which case larger values have greater utility, or it may be expressed as an **undesirable outcome** (e.g., death, illness, high cost), in which case smaller values have greater utility. Clinical decision analysis seeks to show which clinical decision would maximize utility. In Figure 8-1, each final outcome is expressed in terms of a negative utility (i.e., probability of death). If surgery is performed now, the probability of death is 0.4% (0.004). If the surgeon waits, and the patient remains asymptomatic for life, the probability of a gallbladder-related death is 0%. The probabilities of death for biliary pain, complications, and cancer are 0.4%, 10%, and 100%.

4. Compare Utility Values and Perform Sensitivity Analysis

The decision tree can show how a given set of probabilities and utilities would turn out. If the decision tree shows that one choice is clearly preferable to any other, this would be strong evidence in favor of that choice. Often, however, the decision analysis would give two or more outcomes with similar utilities, which means that better data are needed or that factors other than the decision analysis should be used to make the clinical decision.

In addition to comparing the utility values, it is sometimes helpful to perform a **sensitivity analysis.** This is done to see if the results of the analysis are fairly stable over a range of assumptions. It might consist of varying the estimated probabilities of occurrence of a particular outcome at various points in the decision tree to see how the overall outcomes and clinical decisions would be affected by these changes. This helps the clinician and the patient to see which assumptions and decisions have the largest impact on the outcomes through a reasonable range of values. Figure 8-1 can be used to show how to compare utility values and to discuss the rationale for performing a sensitivity analysis. (Note that the use of the word *sensitivity* here is quite different from the

way the term was used up to this point. This use of the term was probably developed because the objective of the analysis is to see how *sensitive* the conclusions are to changes in assumptions.)

In the decision tree in Figure 8-1, there are two branches from the decision node, one labeled "operate now" and the other labeled "wait." As discussed earlier, the probability of death from operating immediately is 0.004, whereas there are four different probabilities of death from waiting, depending on what happens during the waiting period (the patient remains asymptomatic or develops pain, complications, or cancer). Before the utility of operating now versus waiting can be compared, it is necessary to **average out** the data associated with the four possible outcomes of waiting. First, the probability of each outcome from waiting is multiplied by the probability that death would ensue following that particular outcome. Then, the four products are summed. In Figure 8-1, for the choice to wait, the calculation for averaging out is $(0.815 \times 0.000) + (0.150 \times 0.004) + (0.030 \times 0.100) + (0.005 \times 1.000) = 0.0086 = 0.009$, or slightly more than twice the risk of operating now. This probability of death from the gallbladder and its treatment results from the decision to wait.

Based on the previous calculations, the best option would seem to be to operate now. Because these two outcome probabilities are fairly close to each other (0.004 vs. 0.009, a difference of only 0.005, which equals 0.5%, or 1 in 200 cases), however, the decision analysis does not lead strongly to either conclusion, and the balance might be changed by newer assumptions. It would be a good idea to perform a sensitivity analysis on these data. If the same conclusion remains for a wide range of data assumptions, the clinician would be relatively confident in the decision. If small changes in the data changed the direction of the decision, the decision analysis is probably unhelpful. However, other issues must be considered as well.

Factors other than probability of death influence patient preference in the real world. Most of the deaths that occur from surgery in the decision tree under discussion would occur immediately, but deaths caused by cancer of the gallbladder or other complications usually would occur many years later. Given the timing of the deaths, many patients would choose to avoid immediate surgery (e.g., because they are feeling well or have family responsibilities), preferring to deal with complications if and when they arise, or have a considerable risk of death. Some patients, however, who are willing to risk everything for the sake of a cure, might express a preference for the most aggressive treatment possible.

Although this was a simple example, other decision trees have multiple decision nodes that involve complicated issues and factors such as the passage of time. Decision trees need to be redone as time passes, and new data and assumptions arise. In these more complex decision analyses, the objective is to find decisions that are clearly less satisfactory than others and to cut off or *prune* these branches because they are not rational alternatives. The process of choosing the best branch at each decision node, working backward from the right to the left, is called **folding back.** Decision trees can be used only in problems that do not have a repetitive outcome, such as recurring embolic strokes in patients with atrial fibrillation. Such problems are better evaluated with Markov models or Monte Carlo simulations, which are beyond the scope of this text.[6,7]

B. Applications of Decision Trees

Decision trees can be used in the clinical setting, as discussed earlier in the case of patients with asymptomatic gallstones, but are increasingly being applied to public health problems. When considering what strategy would be most cost-effective in eliminating the problem of hepatitis B virus (HBV), some authors used a decision tree to analyze data concerning several possible options: no routine HBV vaccination, a screening program followed by HBV vaccination for persons meeting certain criteria, and HBV vaccination for specific populations (newborns, 10-year-olds, high-risk adults, general adult U.S. population).[2]

III. DATA SYNTHESIS

One of the best ways to reach reliable and generalizable conclusions from the medical literature is to base such judgments on very large data sets. For example, if a particular treatment were applied to everyone in the world, statistical testing of its effects would be moot. Whatever the effects of a given treatment, or exposure, in the entire population would simply be fact. The reason for p values, confidence intervals, and error bars is to indicate the degree to which a sample population is likely to reflect the "real world" experience in the population at large. When the test sample is the population at large, the tools of extrapolated inference are not required.

Although trials involving the entire population are not conducted, for obvious reasons, an important concept is revealed by this *reductio ad absurdum*: large test populations are apt to approximate truth for the population at large better than small populations. This is almost self-evident. A study conducted in some small, select group is much less likely to generalize to other groups than a comparable study in a large, diverse group. Large samples provide the advantages of both statistical power (see Chapter 12) and external validity/generalizability (see Chapter 10), assuming that the population is clearly defined and the sample represents it well (i.e., a large trial of breast cancer screening in men would provide little useful information about screening in women, given the marked differences in vulnerability and incidence).

One way to generate data based on large, diverse samples is to conduct a large, multisite intervention trial. This is routinely done with funding from large pharmaceutical companies testing the utility of a proprietary drug and at times from federal agencies, notably the U.S. National Institutes of Health (NIH). The Diabetes Prevention Program[8] and the Women's Health Initiative[9] are examples of extremely large, extremely costly, federally funded intervention trials. In both cases, thousands of participants were involved.

Often, however, logistical constraints, related to recruitment, time, money, and other resources, preclude conducting such large trials. Trials from individual laboratories involving small samples are much more common. The aggregation of findings from multiple smaller trials thus becomes an efficient, cost-effective means of approximating the statistical power and generalizability of much larger trials. The aggregation of findings may be qualitative (**systematic review**) or quantitative (**meta-analysis**). At times, data aggregation may pertain to a whole domain of medicine, rather than a narrowly framed question, for which a method known as **evidence mapping** is of specific utility.

A. Systematic Review

A systematic review is an aggregation from multiple studies addressing a similar research question in a similar way. The review of the literature is systematic in that prespecified criteria are imposed for inclusion, generally pertaining to methods, measures, and population(s). According to the Cochrane Collaborative's *Cochrane Handbook for Systematic Review of Interventions*, the salient characteristics of a systematic review include the following:

- A clearly stated set of objectives with predefined eligibility criteria for studies
- Explicit, reproducible methodology
- Systematic search that attempts to identify all studies that would meet the eligibility criteria
- Assessment of the validity of the findings of the included studies, as through the assessment of risk of bias
- Systematic presentation and synthesis of the characteristics and findings of the included studies

Systematic reviews may be purely qualitative. This is appropriate either when qualitative studies are being aggregated[10] or when trials addressing a given research question differ substantially in measures, methods, or both and are not amenable to data pooling.[11,12] Such differences may preclude quantitative data synthesis, which depends on reasonable comparability. Quantitative synthesis allows for formal statistical analysis and is thus referred to as *meta-analysis* (i.e., "analysis among many"). A systematic review may include or exclude meta-analysis. A meta-analysis, in contrast, requires a systematic review of the literature to aggregate the studies that serve as the data sources. Generally, when a quantitative synthesis is included, the entire project is referred to as a meta-analysis, because this presupposes a systematic review was conducted. When such aggregative approaches exclude quantitative data synthesis, they tend to be called systematic reviews. However, some articles refer explicitly to the application of both methodologies.[13]

There are standard approaches to adjudicating the quality and inclusion of articles for a systematic review. The details of the process are beyond the scope of this text. Two sources of systematic reviews that provide details regarding quality assessment online are the Cochrane Collaborative (http://www.cochrane-handbook.org/) and the U.S. Centers for Disease Control and Prevention (CDC) *Guide to Community Preventive Services* (www.thecommunityguide.org/index.html).

B. Meta-Analysis

Meta-analyses aggregate the results of studies to establish a composite impression (qualitative) or measure (quantitative) of the strength of a particular association. The approximation of randomized controlled trial (RCT) results with the aggregated results of observational studies has been described[14,15] but also challenged.[16]

A **qualitative meta-analysis** is essentially a systematic review of the literature on a particular topic. In any truly systematic review, standardized criteria are employed for study selection, and only those studies with prestipulated methods and study populations are included.[17] All pertinent articles are reviewed, and the strengths and weaknesses of each are described. Usually the analysis indicates the number of controlled studies of the outcome in question and provides an impression, although not a statistical measure, of the weight of evidence. If anything differentiates a "garden variety" systematic review from a qualitative meta-analysis, it is the commitment in the latter to expressing a summary judgment about the overall weight of evidence, rather than stopping with a description of the various studies meeting criteria. The terms are used interchangeably more often than not, although the distinctions generate debate.[18]

Quantitative meta-analysis takes one of two forms: the data are analyzed as reported in the literature, or the raw data from multiple studies are obtained and aggregated.[17] The former approach is less demanding and time-consuming than the latter and does not require the same degree of cooperation from other investigators. A meta-analysis in which raw data are aggregated requires that access to such data be accorded by the investigators responsible for each pertinent trial, because it depends on information not routinely included in publications.

In either variety of quantitative meta-analysis, strict criteria are employed for the selection of pertinent studies as in systematic reviews. In essence, a meta-analysis begins with a systematic review. Despite these criteria, some variability in methods among studies is inevitable. This is generally measured in a **test of homogeneity;** details of the test method are readily available[19] and are beyond the scope of this discussion.

The less variation in the trials included, the more meaningful the aggregation of findings tends to be. Typically, when only the published data are used, trials are displayed on plots that show whether or not they support an association, and if so, with what degree of statistical significance. This is shown by setting a vertical line at a **relative risk** of 1 (no association), then plotting the 95% confidence intervals for the results of each study included. The generation of such plots, called **forest plots,** requires the conversion of study specific data into a unit-free, standardized effect size,

typically the Cohen's D.[20] The Cochrane Collaborative, which provides meta-analytic software called RevMan, uses a comparable measure called "Hedge's adjusted g" (http://www.cochrane.org/). Figure 8-2 provides an example of a plot of effect sizes.

Would such a figure be a sufficient basis to draw conclusions about the preferred intervention methods? No. Information about the individual trials is still needed. A quantitative meta-analysis is of use when it provides information on individual trial strengths and weaknesses, the comparability of the trials assessed, and the distribution of results.

The most rigorous form of meta-analysis is fully quantitative, aggregating raw data from multiple trials after ensuring the comparability of subjects and methods among the trials included. Such meta-analyses are relatively rare because they are dependent on the availability of multiple, highly comparable trials. If such trials are convincing, a meta-analysis is generally unneeded. If such trials are unconvincing, the probability of the trials having comparable subjects and methods is often low.

Despite these limitations, such analyses are occasionally done. An example is an analysis of angioplasty in acute myocardial infarction, in which the data from 23 separate trials were pooled together and reanalyzed.[21]

Because meta-analyses are typically limited to published data, they often assess the potential influence of **publication bias** by use of a **funnel plot.**[17,22] In essence, a funnel plot attempts to populate a "funnel" of expected effect sizes around a mean; significant gaps in the funnel, particularly missing studies with null or "negative" effects, are interpreted to suggest publication bias (a relative reluctance to publish negative findings). Figure 8-3 shows an example of a funnel plot.

Meta-analysis is predicated on either a **fixed effects** or a **random effects** model. In the fixed effects model the pooled data of the available studies are used to answer the question, Is there evidence here of an outcome effect? The data from the selected trials are considered to comprise the entire study sample. In random effects modeling the data from the

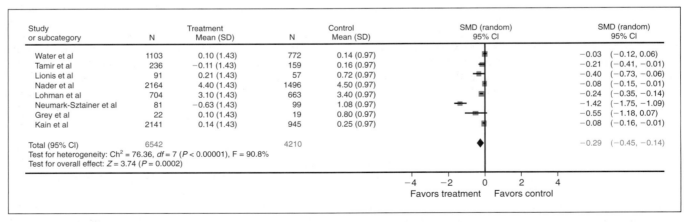

Figure 8-2 Plot of standardized effects sizes. Each point is the mean effect for a given study, and the lines to either side of it represent the 95% confidence interval (CI). The vertical line is the *line of unity* and represents a null effect; those estimates with 95% CI crossing the null line do not support a significant effect; those studies with estimates that do not cross the null line do. The *diamond* represents the pooled effects size estimate and its CI. *SMD,* Standardized mean difference. This particular figure is a comparison of nutrition plus physical activity interventions versus control for prevention and treatment of childhood obesity in schools. (Modified from Katz DL, O'Connell M, Njike VY, et al: Strategies for the prevention and control of obesity in the school setting: systematic review and meta-analysis, *Int J Obes Lond* 32:1780–1789, 2008.)

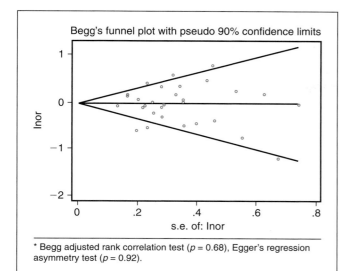

Begg's funnel plot with pseudo 90% confidence limits

* Begg adjusted rank correlation test ($p = 0.68$), Egger's regression asymmetry test ($p = 0.92$).

Figure 8-3 Funnel plot showing distribution of trial results around a line of mean effect. Larger trials should cluster near the mean effect, and smaller trials to either side of it. If one side of the funnel is relatively vacant of trials compared with the other, publication bias is likely. A symmetric funnel plot argues against an important influence of publication bias, supporting that the results of the meta-analysis are reliable. *lnor*, natural log of the odds ratio; *s.e.*, standard error. (From Botelho F, Lunet N, Barros H: Coffee and gastric cancer: systematic review and meta-analysis, *Cad Saude Publica* 22:889–900, 2006.)

selected trials are presumed to represent a representative sample of a larger population of studies. This approach is used to answer the question, Do the available data indicate that the larger population of data from which they were drawn provides evidence of an outcome effect?[17]

Although filling a niche among options for medical investigation, meta-analysis is itself subject to important limitations. Aggregated data invariably compound the errors intrinsic to the original sources. Heterogeneity of methods or of study participants may result in the proverbial comparison between "apples and oranges." The pitfalls of meta-analysis are revealed because the results may be different from the results of large RCTs.[23,24]

The Cochrane Collaborative is an organization devoted to the performance and dissemination of systematic reviews and meta-analyses based on consistent application of state-of-the-art methods. The organization supports a large number of study groups charged with the generation and updating of reviews in specific content areas. Cochrane reviews are accessible at www.Cochrane.org.

C. Evidence Mapping

When the question of interest is whether there is evidence pertaining to a given broad topic in medicine, methods of systematic review and meta-analysis are too narrow. Both help answer a specific question, but neither provides the "view from altitude" of an expanse of related literature. An example of a relevant but broad question might be, Is there evidence to support the therapeutic efficacy of acupuncture for any condition? Such a question might generate an overview of relevant evidence, which in turn might be used to guide the articulation of specific, more narrowly framed

questions (e.g., is traditional Chinese acupuncture superior to placebo in the treatment of migraine headache?).

The term *evidence mapping* has been applied to the characterization of the quantity and quality of evidence in a topical domain too broad to warrant a systematic review. Specific methods of evidence mapping have been described and adopted as a support in health care policy development by the World Health Organization (WHO).[25]

IV. ELEMENTARY PROBABILITY THEORY

Because clinicians need to deal frequently with probabilities and risks, it is important to be able to detect *fallacies*, even if the clinician might not choose to calculate probabilities. A newsletter from a New Haven insurance agent made the following argument in an effort to sell long-term care insurance:

> Statistics indicate that if you are fortunate enough to reach age 65, the odds are ... 50/50 you will spend time in a nursing home ... Ergo (our logic): If there are two of you, it would seem the odds are 100% that one of you will need nursing home care.

Is this writer's logic correct when he states that if two married people reach the age of 65, there is essentially a 100% chance that at least one member of the couple will require nursing home care? Although common sense indicates this is not true because at least some couples are certain to escape, it is better to know *where* the fallacy in the writer's reasoning lies. Three basic rules of probability should be kept in mind when considering arguments such as used in this example: the independence rule, the product rule, and the addition rule.

A. Independence Rule

The independence rule, as in the case of the null hypothesis, states that one probability (e.g., husband's chance of needing to spend time in a nursing home) is not influenced by the outcome of another probability (wife needing to spend time in a nursing home). If these two probabilities are independent of each other, the correct probabilities can be obtained by many trials of flipping an unbiased coin, twice in a row, repeated many times. Assume that the first flip of a trial is the probability that the husband would need nursing home care, and that the second flip is the probability that the wife would. Two successive heads would mean both husband and wife would need such care (not necessarily at the same time), one head and one tail would mean that one partner would need care and one would not, and two tails would mean that neither would need care. Heads could be recorded as a plus sign (+), meaning that nursing home care is necessary; tails could be recorded as a minus sign (−), meaning that nursing home care is unnecessary; and the symbols H and W could be used for husband and wife.

In statistical terms, the independence rule for the husband can be expressed as follows: $p\{H+ \mid W+\} = p\{H+ \mid W-\}$. Here, p denotes probability; H+ denotes confinement of the husband; the vertical line means "given that" or "conditional on" what immediately follows; W+ denotes confinement of the wife; and W− denotes no confinement for the wife. The independence rule does not mean that the husband and wife must have an equal probability of being confined to a nursing home; it requires only that the probability of one partner (whatever that probability is) is not influenced by what happens to the other.

B. Product Rule

The product rule is used to determine the probability of *two* things being true. The manner of calculation depends on whether the two things are independent.

In the example of the husband and wife, if independence is assumed, this simplifies the calculation because the probability that *both* the husband and the wife will be confined to a nursing home is simply the product of their independent probabilities. The easiest way to illustrate this is to flip a coin. If the probability for each was 50%, repeated trials of two flips would show the following: a 25% chance of getting two heads in a row (H+ and W+), a 25% chance of getting first a head and then a tail (H+ and W−), a 25% chance of getting first a tail and then a head (H− and W+), and a 25% chance of getting two tails (H− and W−). If each member of a couple has a 50% probability of requiring nursing home care at some time, and if these probabilities are independent, the chances that at least one member of the couple would require nursing home care at some time would be 75%, not 100%. The quick way to calculate the probability of one or both being confined is to say that it is 100% minus the probability of neither being confined, which is 25% (calculated in the second part of the next paragraph).

Putting this in statistical symbols, the probability that both the husband and the wife would spend time in a nursing home is:

$$p\{H+ \text{ and } W+\} = p\{+\} \times p\{W+\} = 0.5 \times 0.5 = 0.25$$

Likewise, the probability that *neither* the husband nor the wife will be confined to a nursing home is the product of the probabilities of not being in a nursing home:

$$p\{H- \text{ and } W-\} = p\{H-\} \times p\{W-\} = (1 - p\{H+\}) \times (1 - p\{W+\})$$
$$= (1 - 0.5) \times (1 - 0.5) = 0.25$$

These answers are the same answers that were derived from flipping coins.

If independence *cannot* be assumed, a more general product rule must be used. In calculating the probability that *neither* the husband nor the wife would be confined to a nursing home, the general product rule says that:

$$p\{H- \text{ and } W-\} = p\{H- \mid W-\} \times p\{W-\}$$

The answer would be the same if the rule was expressed as:

$$p\{H- \text{ and } W-\} = p\{W- \mid H-\} \times p\{H-\}$$

In this example, the probability of the husband not being confined if the wife is not confined is 0.5, and the probability that the wife will not be confined is 0.5. The $p\{H- \text{ and } W-\}$ = 0.5 × 0.5 = 0.25, again the same answer as derived from flipping coins.

Although the insurance agent assumed that the probabilities for the husband and wife were each 50%, a detailed study estimated that the probability of confinement in a nursing home after age 65 was 33% for the husband and 52% for the wife.[11] If independence between these probabilities is assumed, the probability that they both will be confined to a nursing home would be calculated as the product of the separate probabilities:

$$0.33 \times 0.52 = 0.17 = \textbf{17\%}$$

C. Addition Rule

One of the insurance agent's errors was in adding the probabilities when he should have multiplied them. A quick way to know that adding the probabilities was incorrect would have been to say, "Suppose each partner had a 90% chance of being confined." If adding were the correct approach, the total probability would be 180%, which is impossible. According to the addition rule, all the possible different probabilities in a situation must add up to 1 (100%), no more and no less. The addition rule is used to determine the probability of one thing being true under all possible conditions. It may be used to determine the lifetime probability that the husband will be confined to a nursing home, taking into consideration that the wife may or may not be confined. In this case, the equation would be as follows:

$$p\{H+\} = p\{H+ \mid W+\} \times p\{W+\} + p\{H+ \mid W-\} \times p\{W-\}$$

Box 8-4 shows the calculations for this formula, based on probabilities discussed here. Husbands have a lower probability of being in a nursing home than do wives, partly because wives are often younger and may take care of the husband at home, removing his need for a nursing home, and partly because women live longer and are more likely to reach the age at which many people require nursing home care. The numerator and the denominator of Bayes theorem are based on the general product rule and the addition rule.

V. SUMMARY

Although there is general agreement about the need to improve clinical decision making, there is controversy about the methods to be used to achieve this goal. Among the tools available for decision analysis are Bayes theorem and decision trees. These tools can be applied to individual patient care and to community health programs. Bayes theorem can be used to calculate positive predictive values and posterior probabilities (see Boxes 8-1, 8-2, and 8-3). Decision trees can help health care workers pursue a logical, step-by-step approach to exploring the possible alternative clinical decisions, the sequence in which these decisions must be made, and the probabilities and utilities of each possible outcome (see Fig. 8-1). The aggregation of findings from multiple studies can enhance statistical power and support external validity (generalizability). When study findings are aggregated using clearly defined methods to assess suitability and quality, the approach is called systematic review. When data can be aggregated to calculate a mean effect size, the method is meta-analysis. When the quantity and quality of evidence for a broad content area is of interest, a method called evidence mapping may prove useful.

In the calculation of probabilities, three basic rules should be kept in mind: the independence rule, the product rule,

| Box 8-4 | Calculation of All Possible Probabilities of Husband and Wife Requiring or Not Requiring Care in a Nursing Home |

PART 1 Definitions

H+ = Probability that the husband will require care in a nursing home at some time
H− = Probability that the husband will not require care in a nursing home at some time
W+ = Probability that the wife will require care in a nursing home at some time
W− = Probability that the wife will not require care in a nursing home at some time

PART 2 Assumptions on Which Calculations Are Based

(1) The following holds true if the wife does not require care in a nursing home: H+ = 0.3 *and* H− = 0.7
(2) The following holds true if the wife does require care in a nursing home: H+ = 0.4 *and* H− = 0.6
(3) The following holds true whether or not the husband requires care in a nursing home: W+ = 0.52 *and* W− = 0.48

PART 3 Calculations

(1) Probability that neither the husband nor the wife will require care in a nursing home:

$$p\{H-\text{ and }W-\} = p\{H-\,|\,W-\} \times p\{W-\} = 0.7 \times 0.48 = \textbf{0.336}$$

(2) Probability that both the husband and the wife will require care in a nursing home:

$$p\{H+\text{ and }W+\} = p\{H+\,|\,W+\} \times p\{W-\} = 0.4 \times 0.52 = \textbf{0.208}$$

(3) Probability that the husband will require care and the wife will not require care in a nursing home:

$$p\{H+\text{ and }W-\} = p\{H+\,|\,W-\} \times p\{W-\} = 0.3 \times 0.48 = \textbf{0.144}$$

(4) Probability that the husband will not require care and the wife will require care in a nursing home:

$$p\{H-\text{ and }W+\} = p\{H-\,|\,W+\} = p\{W+\} = 0.6 \times 0.52 = \textbf{0.312}$$

(5) Sum of the above probabilities (must always equal 1.00):

$$0.336 + 0.208 + 0.144 + 0.312 = \textbf{1.00}$$

As it should, the sum of (1) and (3) equals the probability that the wife will not require care in a nursing home (0.336 + 0.144 = 0.48). Likewise, the sum of (1) and (4) equals the probability that the husband will not require care in a nursing home (0.336 + 0.312 = 0.648), on average.

Data on which probability estimates are based from Kemper P, Murtaugh CM: Lifetime use of nursing home care, *N Engl J Med* 324:595–600, 1991.

and the addition rule. If the independence of two events can be assumed, the probability of both events occurring jointly is the product of their separate probabilities. This is true whether the probability is that something will happen or that something will not happen.

References

1. Koplan JP, Schoenbaum SC, Weinstein MC, et al: Pertussis vaccine: an analysis of benefits, risks, and costs. *N Engl J Med* 301:906–911, 1979.
2. Bloom BS, Hillman AL, Fendrick AM, et al: A reappraisal of hepatitis B virus vaccination strategies using cost-effectiveness analysis. *Ann Intern Med* 118:298–306, 1993.
3. Jekel JF, Greenberg RA, Drake BM: Influence of the prevalence of infection on tuberculin skin testing programs. *Public Health Rep* 84:883–886, 1969.
4. Weinstein MC, Fineberg HV: *Clinical decision analysis*, Philadelphia, 1980, Saunders.
5. Rose DN, Wiesel J: [Letter to the editor]. *N Engl J Med* 308:221–222, 1983.
6. Sonnenberg FA, Beck JR: Markov models in medical decision making: a practical guide. *Med Decis Making* 13:322–338, 1993.
7. Munink M, Glasziou P, Siegel J, et al: *Decision making in health and medicine: integrating evidence and values*, Cambridge, 2001, Cambridge University Press.
8. Knowler WC, Barrett-Connor E, Fowler SE, et al: Reduction in the incidence of type 2 diabetes with lifestyle intervention or metformin. *N Engl J Med* 346:393–403, 2002.
9. Howard BV, Van Horn L, Hsia J, et al: Low-fat dietary pattern and risk of cardiovascular disease. The Women's Health Initiative Randomized Controlled Dietary Modification Trial. *JAMA* 295:655–666, 2006.
10. Irving MJ, Tong A, Jan S, et al: Factors that influence the decision to be an organ donor: a systematic review of the qualitative literature. *Nephrol Dial Transplant* 27:2526–2533, 2011.
11. Lehnert T, Sonntag D, Konnopka A, et al: The long-term cost-effectiveness of obesity prevention interventions: systematic literature review. *Obes Rev* 13:537–553, 2012.

12. Man SC, Chan KW, Lu JH, et al: Systematic review on the efficacy and safety of herbal medicines for vascular dementia. *Evid Based Complement Altern Med* 2012:426215, 2012.

13. Tan CJ, Dasari BV, Gardiner K: Systematic review and meta-analysis of randomized clinical trials of self-expanding metallic stents as a bridge to surgery versus emergency surgery for malignant left-sided large bowel obstruction. *Br J Surg* 99:469–476, 2012.

14. Benson K, Hartz J: A comparison of observational studies and randomized, controlled trials. *N Engl J Med* 342:1878–1886, 2000.

15. Concato J, Shah N, Horwitz RI: Randomized, controlled trials, observational studies, and the hierarchy of research designs. *N Engl J Med* 342:1887–1892, 2000.

16. Pocock SJ, Elbourne DR: Randomized trials or observational tribulations? *N Engl J Med* 342:1907–1909, 2000.

17. Petitti DB: *Meta-analysis, decision analysis, and cost-effectiveness analysis*, ed 2, New York, 2000, Oxford University Press.

18. http://www.leeds.ac.uk/educol/documents/00001724.htm.

19. Kulinskaya E, Dollinger MB, Bjørkestøl K: Testing for homogeneity in meta-analysis. I. The one-parameter case: standardized mean difference. *Biometrics* 67:203–212, 2011.

20. Fortier-Brochu E, Beaulieu-Bonneau S, Ivers H, et al: Insomnia and daytime cognitive performance: a meta-analysis. *Sleep Med Rev* 16:83–94, 2012.

21. Michels KB, Yusuf S: Does PTCA in acute myocardial infarction affect mortality and reinfarction rates? A quantitative overview (meta-analysis) of the randomized clinical trials. *Circulation* 91:476–485, 1995.

22. Copas J, Shi JQ: Meta-analysis, funnel plots and sensitivity analysis. *Biostatistics* 1:247–262, 2000.

23. LeLorier J, Grégoire G, Benhaddad A, et al: Discrepancies between meta-analyses and subsequent large, randomized controlled trials. *N Engl J Med* 337:536–542, 1997.

24. Bailar JC 3rd: The promise and problems of meta-analysis. *N Engl J Med* 337:559–561, 1997.

25. Katz DL, Williams AL, Girard C, et al: The evidence base for complementary and alternative medicine: methods of evidence mapping with application to CAM. *Altern Ther Health Med* 9:22–30, 2003. http://www.evidencemap.org/about.

Select Readings

Blettner M, Sauerbrei W, Schlehofer B, et al: Traditional reviews, meta-analysis, and pooled analyses in epidemiology. *Int J Epidemiol* 28:1–9, 1999.

Friedland DJ, editor: *Evidence-based medicine: a framework for clinical practice*, Stamford, Conn, 1998, Appleton & Lange.

Kemper P, Murtaugh CM: Lifetime use of nursing home care. *N Engl J Med* 324:595–600, 1991.

Petitti DB: *Meta-analysis, decision analysis, and cost-effectiveness analysis: methods for quantitative synthesis in medicine*, New York, 1994, Oxford University Press.

Sackett DL, Richardson WS, Rosenberg W, et al: *Evidence-based medicine: how to practice and teach EBM*, Edinburgh, 1997, Churchill Livingstone.

Weinstein MC, Fineberg HV: *Clinical decision analysis*, Philadelphia, 1980, Saunders.

Whitehead A: *Meta-analysis of controlled clinical trials*, West Sussex, UK, 2002, Wiley & Sons.

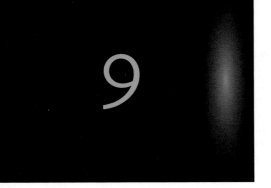

9

Describing Variation in Data

Variation is evident in almost every characteristic of patients, including their blood pressure and other physiologic measurements, diseases, environments, diets, and other aspects of their lifestyle. A measure of a single characteristic that can vary is called a **variable.** Statistics enables investigators to do the following:

■ Describe the patterns of variation in single variables, as discussed in this chapter.
■ Determine when observed differences are likely to be real differences, as discussed in Chapters 10 and 11.
■ Determine the patterns and strength of association between variables, as discussed in Chapters 11 and 13.

I. SOURCES OF VARIATION IN MEDICINE

Although variation in clinical medicine may be caused by biologic differences or the presence or absence of disease, it also may result from differences in the techniques and conditions of measurement, errors in measurement, and random variation. Some variation distorts data systematically in one direction, such as measuring and weighing patients while wearing shoes. This form of distortion is called **systematic error** and can introduce bias. Bias in turn may obscure or distort the *truth* being sought in a given study. Other variation is random, such as slight, inevitable inaccuracies in obtaining any measure (e.g., blood pressure). Because **random error** makes some readings too high and others too low, it is not systematic and does not introduce bias. However, by increasing variation in the data, random error increases the noise amidst which the *signal* of association, or cause and effect, must be discerned. The "louder" the noise, the more difficult it is to detect a signal and the more likely to miss an actual signal. All these issues are revisited here and in subsequent chapters. The sources of variation are illustrated in this chapter using the measurement of blood pressure in particular.

Biologic differences include factors such as differences in genes, nutrition, environmental exposures, age, gender, and race. Blood pressure tends to be higher among individuals with high salt intake, in older persons, and in persons of African descent. Tall parents usually have tall children. Extremely short people may have specific genetic conditions (e.g., achondroplasia) or a deficiency of growth hormone. Although poor nutrition slows growth, and starvation may stop growth altogether, good nutrition allows the full genetic growth potential to be achieved. Polluted water may cause intestinal infections in children, which can retard growth, partly because such infections exacerbate malnutrition.

Variation is seen not only in the **presence or absence of disease**, but also in the **stages or extent of disease**. Cancer of the cervix may be in situ, localized, invasive, or metastatic. In some patients, multiple diseases may be present (comorbidity). For example, insulin-dependent diabetes mellitus may be accompanied by coronary artery disease or renal disease.

Different conditions of measurement often account for the variations observed in medical data and include factors such as time of day, ambient temperature or noise, and the presence of fatigue or anxiety in the patient. Blood pressure is higher with anxiety or following exercise and lower after sleep. These differences in blood pressure are not errors of measurement, but of standardizing the conditions under which the data are obtained. Standardizing such conditions is important to avoid variation attributable to them and the introduction of bias.

Different techniques of measurement can produce different results. A blood pressure (BP) measurement derived from the use of an intra-arterial catheter may differ from a measurement derived from the use of an arm cuff. This may result from differences in the measurement site (e.g., central or distal arterial site), thickness of the arm (which influences reading from BP cuff), rigidity of the artery (reflecting degree of atherosclerosis), and interobserver differences in the interpretation of BP sounds.

Some variation is caused by **measurement error.** Two different BP cuffs of the same size may give different measurements in the same patient because of defective performance by one of the cuffs. Different laboratory instruments or methods may produce different readings from the same sample. Different x-ray machines may produce films of varying quality. When two clinicians examine the same patient or the same specimen (e.g., x-ray film), they may report different results[1] (see Chapter 7). One radiologist may read a mammogram as abnormal and recommend further tests, such as a biopsy, whereas another radiologist may read the same mammogram as normal and not recommend further workup.[2] One clinician may detect a problem such as a retinal hemorrhage or a heart murmur, and another may fail to detect it. Two clinicians may detect a heart murmur in the same patient but disagree on its characteristics. If two clinicians are asked to characterize a dark skin lesion, one may call it a "nevus," whereas the other may say it is "suspicious for malignant melanoma." A pathologic specimen would be used to resolve the difference, but that, too, is subject to interpretation, and two pathologists might differ.

Variation seems to be a ubiquitous phenomenon in clinical medicine and research. Statistics can help investigators to interpret data despite biologic variation, but statistics cannot correct for errors in the observation or recording of data. Stated differently, statistics can compensate for random error in a variety of ways, but statistics cannot fix, "after the fact" (post hoc), bias introduced by systematic error.

II. STATISTICS AND VARIABLES

Statistical methods help clinicians and investigators understand and explain the variation in medical data. The first step in understanding variation is to *describe* it. This chapter focuses on how to describe variation in medical observations. Statistics can be viewed as a set of tools for working with data, just as brushes are tools used by an artist for painting. One reason for the choice of a specific tool over another is the type of material with which the tool would be used. One type of brush is needed for oil paints, another for tempera paints, and another type for watercolors. The artist must know the materials to be used to choose the correct tools. Similarly, a person who works with data must understand the different types of variables that exist in medicine.

A. Quantitative and Qualitative Data

The first question to answer before analyzing data is whether the data describe a quantitative or a qualitative characteristic. A **quantitative characteristic,** such as a systolic blood pressure or serum sodium level, is characterized using a rigid, continuous measurement scale. A **qualitative characteristic,** such as coloration of the skin, is described by its features, generally in words rather than numbers. Normal skin can vary in color from pinkish white through tan to dark brown or black. Medical problems can cause changes in skin color,

with *white* denoting pallor, as in anemia; *red* suggesting inflammation, as in a rash or a sunburn; *blue* denoting cyanosis, as in cardiac or lung failure; *bluish purple* occurring when blood has been released subcutaneously, as in a bruise; and *yellow* suggesting the presence of jaundice, as in common bile duct obstruction or liver disease.

Examples of disease manifestations that have quantitative and qualitative characteristics are heart murmurs and bowel sounds. Not only does the loudness of a heart murmur vary from patient to patient (and can be described on a 5-point scale), but the sound also may vary from blowing to harsh or rasping in quality. The timing of the murmur in the cardiac cycle also is important.

Information on any characteristic that can vary is called a **variable.** The qualitative information on colors just described could form a qualitative variable called *skin color.* The quantitative information on blood pressure could be contained in variables called *systolic* and *diastolic* blood pressure.

B. Types of Variables

Variables can be classified as nominal variables, dichotomous (binary) variables, ordinal (ranked) variables, continuous (dimensional) variables, ratio variables, and risks and proportions (Table 9-1).

I. Nominal Variables

Nominal variables are "naming" or categorical variables that have no measurement scales and no rank order. Examples are blood groups (O, A, B, and AB), occupations, food groups, and skin color. If skin color is the variable being examined, a different number can be assigned to each color (e.g., 1 is bluish purple, 2 is black, 3 is white, 4 is blue, 5 is tan) before the information is entered into a computer data

Table 9-1 Examples of the Different Types of Data

Information Content	Variable Type	Examples
Higher	Ratio	Temperature (Kelvin); blood pressure*
	Continuous (dimensional)	Temperature (Fahrenheit)*
	Ordinal (ranked)	Edema = 3+ out of 5
		Perceived quality of care = good/fair/poor
	Binary (dichotomous)	Gender; heart murmur = present/absent
	Nominal	Blood type; color = cyanotic or jaundiced; taste = bitter or sweet
Lower		

*For most types of data analysis, the distinction between continuous data and ratio data is unimportant. Risks and proportions sometimes are analyzed using the statistical methods for continuous variables, and sometimes observed counts are analyzed in tables, using nonparametric methods (see Chapter 11).

Note: Variables with higher information content may be collapsed into variables with less information content. For example, *hypertension* could be described as "165/95 mm Hg" (continuous data), "absent/mild/moderate/severe" (ordinal data), or "present/absent" (binary data). One cannot move in the other direction, however. Also, knowing the type of variables being analyzed is crucial for deciding which statistical test to use (see Table 11-1).

system. Any number could be assigned to any color, and that would make no difference to the statistical analysis. This is because the number is merely a numerical name for a color, and size of the number used has no inherent meaning; the number given to a particular color has nothing to do with the quality, value, or importance of the color.

2. Dichotomous (Binary) Variables

If all skin colors were included in one nominal variable, there is a problem: the variable does not distinguish between *normal* and *abnormal* skin color, which is usually the most important aspect of skin color for clinical and research purposes. As discussed, abnormal skin color (e.g., pallor, jaundice, cyanosis) may be a sign of numerous health problems (e.g., anemia, liver disease, cardiac failure). Researchers might choose to create a variable with only two levels: normal skin color (coded as a 1) and abnormal skin color (coded as a 2). This new variable, which has only two levels, is said to be *dichotomous* (Greek, "cut into two").

Many dichotomous variables, such as well/sick, living/dead, and normal/abnormal, have an implied direction that is favorable. Knowing that direction would be important for interpreting the data, but not for the statistical analysis. Other dichotomous variables, such as female/male and treatment/placebo, have no a priori qualitative direction.

Dichotomous variables, although common and important, often are inadequate by themselves to describe something fully. When analyzing cancer therapy, it is important to know not only whether the patient survives or dies (a dichotomous variable), but also *how long* the patient survives (time forms a *continuous* variable). A survival analysis or life table analysis, as described in Chapter 11, may be done. It is important to know the *quality of patients' lives* while they are receiving the therapy; this might be measured with an *ordinal* variable, discussed next. Similarly, for a study of heart murmurs, various types of data may be needed, such as *dichotomous* data concerning a murmur's timing (e.g., systolic or diastolic), *nominal* data on its location (e.g., aortic valve area) and character (e.g., rough), and *ordinal* data on its loudness (e.g., grade III). Dichotomous variables and nominal variables sometimes are called **discrete variables** because the different categories are completely separate from each other.

3. Ordinal (Ranked) Variables

Many types of medical data can be characterized in terms of three or more qualitative values that have a clearly implied direction from better to worse. An example might be "satisfaction with care" that could take on the values of "very satisfied," "fairly satisfied," or "not satisfied." These data are not measured on a measurement scale. They form an ordinal (i.e., ordered or ranked) variable.

There are many clinical examples of ordinal variables. The amount of swelling in a patient's legs is estimated by the clinician and is usually reported as "none" or 1+, 2+, 3+, or 4+ pitting edema (puffiness). A patient may have a systolic murmur ranging from 1+ to 6+. Respiratory distress is reported as being absent, mild, moderate, or severe. Although pain also may be reported as being absent, mild, moderate, or severe, in most cases, patients are asked to describe their pain on a scale from 0 to 10, with 0 being no pain and 10

the worst imaginable pain. The utility of such scales to quantify subjective assessments such as pain intensity is controversial and is the subject of ongoing research.

Ordinal variables are not measured on an exact measurement scale, but more information is contained in them than in nominal variables. It is possible to see the relationship between two ordinal categories and know whether one category is more desirable than another. Because they contain more information than nominal variables, ordinal variables enable more informative conclusions to be drawn. As described in Chapter 11, ordinal variables often require special techniques of analysis.

4. Continuous (Dimensional) Variables

Many types of medically important data are measured on continuous (dimensional) measurement scales. Patients' heights, weights, systolic and diastolic blood pressures, and serum glucose levels all are examples of data measured on continuous scales. Even more information is contained in continuous data than in ordinal data because continuous data not only show the position of the different observations relative to each other, but also show the extent to which one observation differs from another. Continuous data often enable investigators to make more detailed inferences than do ordinal or nominal data.

Relationships between continuous variables are not always linear (in a straight line). The relationship between the birth weight and the probability of survival of newborns is not linear.[3] As shown in Figure 9-1, infants weighing less than 3000 g and infants weighing more than 4500 g are historically at greater risk for neonatal death than are infants weighing 3000 to 4500 g (~6.6-9.9 lb).

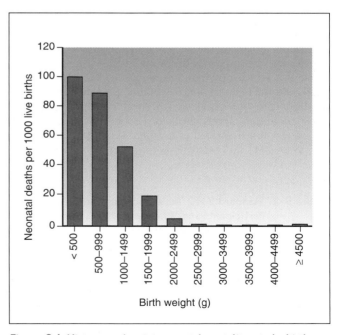

Figure 9-1 **Histogram showing neonatal mortality rate by birth weight group, all races, United States, 1980.** (Data from Buehler JW et al: *Public Health Rep* 102:151–161, 1987.)

5. Ratio Variables

If a continuous scale has a true 0 point, the variables derived from it can be called ratio variables. The Kelvin temperature scale is a ratio scale because 0 degrees on this scale is absolute 0. The centigrade temperature scale is a continuous scale, but not a ratio scale because 0 degrees on this scale does not mean the absence of heat. For some purposes, it may be useful to know that 200 units of something is twice as large as 100 units, information provided only by a ratio scale. For most statistical analyses, however, including significance testing, the distinction between continuous and ratio variables is not important.

6. Risks and Proportions as Variables

As discussed in Chapter 2, a risk is the conditional probability of an event (e.g., death or disease) in a defined population in a defined period. Risks and proportions, which are two important types of measurement in medicine, share some characteristics of a discrete variable and some characteristics of a continuous variable. It makes no conceptual sense to say that a "fraction" of a death occurred or that a "fraction" of a person experienced an event. It does make sense, however, to say that a discrete event (e.g., death) or a discrete characteristic (e.g., presence of a murmur) occurred in a fraction of a population. Risks and proportions are variables created by the ratio of counts in the numerator to counts in the denominator. Risks and proportions sometimes are analyzed using the statistical methods for continuous variables (see Chapter 10), and sometimes observed counts are analyzed in tables, using statistical methods for analyzing discrete data (see Chapter 11).

C. Counts and Units of Observation

The unit of observation is the person or thing from which the data originated. Common examples of units of observation in medical research are persons, animals, and cells. Units of observation may be arranged in a **frequency table,** with one characteristic on the x-axis, another characteristic on the y-axis, and the appropriate counts in the cells of the table. Table 9-2, which provides an example of this type of 2×2 table, shows that among 71 young professional persons studied, 63% of women and 57% of men previously had their cholesterol levels checked. Using these data and the chi-square test described in Chapter 11, one can determine whether or not the difference in the percentage of women and men with cholesterol checks was likely a result of chance variation (in this case the answer is "yes").

D. Combining Data

A continuous variable may be converted to an ordinal variable by grouping units with similar values together. For example, the individual birth weights of infants (a continuous variable) can be converted to ranges of birth weights (an ordinal variable), as shown in Figure 9-1. When the data are presented as categories or ranges (e.g., <500, 500-999, 1000-1499 g), information is lost because the individual weights of infants are no longer apparent. An infant weighing 501 g is in the same category as an infant weighing 999 g, but the infant weighing 999 g is in a different category from an infant weighing 1000 g, just 1 g more. The advantage is that now percentages can be created, and the relationship of birth weight to mortality is easier to show.

Three or more groups must be formed when converting a continuous variable to an ordinal variable. In the example of birth weight, the result of forming several groups is that it creates an ordinal variable that progresses from the heaviest to the lightest birth weight (or vice versa). If a continuous variable such as birth weight is divided into only two groups, however, a *dichotomous* variable is created. Infant birth weight often is divided into two groups, creating a dichotomous variable of infants weighing less than 2500 g (low birth weight) and infants weighing 2500 g or more (normal birth weight). The fewer the number of groups formed from a continuous variable, however, the greater is the amount of information that is lost.

III. FREQUENCY DISTRIBUTIONS

A. Frequency Distributions of Continuous Variables

Observations on one variable may be shown visually by putting the variable's values on one axis (usually the horizontal axis or x-axis) and putting the frequency with which that value appears on the other axis (usually the vertical axis or y-axis). This is known as a **frequency distribution.** Table 9-3 and Figure 9-2 show the distribution of the levels of total cholesterol among 71 professional persons. The figure is shown in addition to the table because the data are easier to interpret from the figure.

1. Range of a Variable

A frequency distribution can be described, although imperfectly, using only the lowest and highest numbers in the data set. For example, the cholesterol levels in Table 9-3 vary from a low value of 124 mg/dL to a high value of 264 mg/dL. The distance between the lowest and highest observations is called the **range** of the variable.

2. Real and Theoretical Frequency Distributions

Real frequency distributions are those obtained from actual data, and theoretical frequency distributions are calculated using certain assumptions. When theoretical distributions

---

Table 9-2 **Standard 2 × 2 Table Showing Gender of 71 Participants and Whether or Not Serum Total Cholesterol Was Checked**

| Gender | Cholesterol Level (No. of Participants) | | |
	Checked	Not Checked	Total
Female	17 (63%)	10 (37%)	27 (100%)
Male	25 (57%)	19 (43%)	44 (100%)
TOTAL	42 (59%)	29 (41%)	71 (100%)

Data from unpublished findings in a sample of 71 professional persons in Connecticut.

Table 9-3 Serum Levels of Total Cholesterol Reported in 71 Participants*

Cholesterol Value (mg/dL)	No. Observations	Cholesterol Value (mg/dL)	No. Observations	Cholesterol Value (mg/dL)	No. Observations
124	1	164	3	196	2
128	1	165	1	197	2
132	1	166	1	206	1
133	1	169	1	208	1
136	1	171	4	209	1
138	1	175	1	213	1
139	1	177	2	217	1
146	1	178	2	220	1
147	1	179	1	221	1
149	1	180	4	222	1
151	1	181	1	226	1
153	2	184	2	227	1
158	3	186	1	228	1
160	1	188	2	241	1
161	1	191	3	264	1
162	1	192	2	—	—
163	2	194	2	—	—

Data from unpublished findings in a sample of 71 professional persons in Connecticut.
*In this data set, the mean is 179.1 mg/dL, and the standard deviation is 28.2 mg/dL.

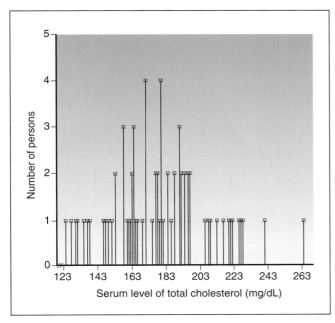

Figure 9-2 **Histogram showing frequency distribution of serum levels of total cholesterol.** As reported in a sample of 71 participants; data shown here are same data listed in Table 9-3; see also Figures 9-4 and 9-5. (Data from unpublished findings in a sample of 71 professional persons in Connecticut.)

are used, they are assumed to describe the underlying populations from whom data are obtained. Most measurements of continuous data in medicine and biology tend to approximate the particular theoretical distribution known as the **normal distribution.** It is also called the **gaussian distribution** (after Johann Karl Gauss, who best described it).

The normal (gaussian) distribution looks something like a bell seen from the side (Fig. 9-3). In statistical texts, smooth, bell-shaped curves are drawn to describe normal distributions. Real samples of data, however, are seldom (if ever) perfectly smooth and bell-shaped. The frequency distribution of total cholesterol values among the 71 young professionals shows peaks and valleys when the data are presented in the manner shown in Figure 9-2. This should not cause concern, however, if partitioning the same data into reasonably narrow ranges results in a bell-shaped frequency distribution. When the cholesterol levels from Table 9-3 and Figure 9-2 are partitioned into seven groups with narrow ranges (ranges of 20-mg/dL width), the resulting frequency distribution appears almost perfectly normal (gaussian) (Fig. 9-4). If the sample size had been much larger than 71, the distribution of raw data also might have looked more gaussian (see Fig. 9-2).

In textbooks, smooth, bell-shaped curves are often used to represent the **expected frequency of observations** (the height of the curve on the *y*-axis) for the different possible values on a measurement scale (on the *x*-axis) (see Fig. 9-3). When readers see a perfectly smooth, bell-shaped gaussian distribution, they should remember that the *y*-axis is usually describing the frequency with which the corresponding values in the *x*-axis are expected to be found. With an intuitive feeling for the meaning of Figure 9-3, it is easier to understand the medical literature, statistical textbooks, and problems presented on examinations.

Although the term "normal" distribution is used in this book and frequently in the literature, there is no implication that data that do not conform strictly to this distribution are somehow "abnormal." Even when data do not have perfectly normal distributions, it is possible to draw inferences (tentative conclusions) about the data by using statistical tests that assume the observed data came from a normal (gaussian) distribution. If the sample size is sufficiently large, this assumption usually works well, even if the underlying distribution is skewed (see later, and central limit theorem in Chapter 10).

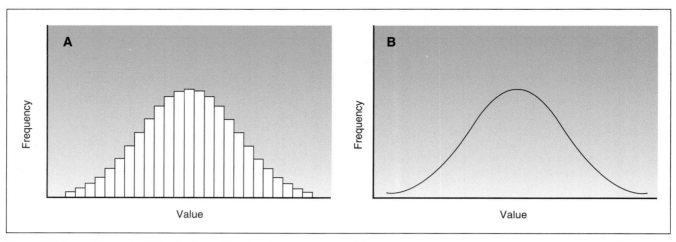

Figure 9-3 Normal (gaussian) distribution, with value shown on x-axis and frequency on y-axis. A, Probability distribution of (fictitious) data, plotted as a histogram with narrow ranges of values on the x-axis. **B,** The way this idea is represented, for simplicity, in textbooks, articles, and tests.

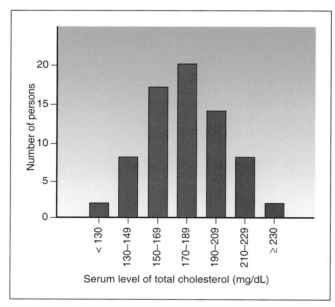

Figure 9-4 Histogram showing frequency distribution of serum levels of total cholesterol. As reported in a sample from the 71 participants in Table 9-3, grouped in ranges of 20 mg/dL. The individual values for the 71 participants are reported in Table 9-3 and shown in Figure 9-2. The mean is 179.1 mg/dL, and the median is 178 mg/dL. The original data are needed to be able to calculate these and determine the range. The value of this histogram is to show how these data form a normal distribution, although the N is relatively small.

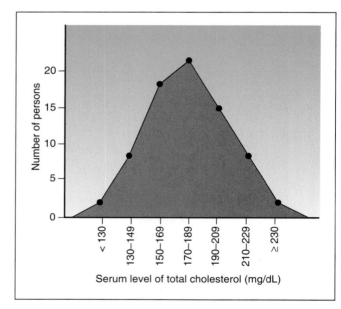

Figure 9-5 Frequency polygon showing the frequency distribution of serum levels of total cholesterol. As reported in a sample from the 71 participants in Table 9-3, grouped in ranges of 20 mg/dL. Data for this polygon are the same as the data for histogram in Figure 9-4. Individual values for the 71 participants are reported in Table 9-3 and Figure 9-2.

3. Histograms, Frequency Polygons, and Line Graphs

Figures in the medical literature show data in several ways, including histograms, frequency polygons, and line graphs. A **histogram** is a bar graph in which the number of units of observation (e.g., persons) is shown on the y-axis, the measurement values (e.g., cholesterol levels) are shown on the x-axis, and the frequency distribution is illustrated by a series of vertical bars. In a histogram the area of each bar represents the relative proportion of all observations that fall in the range represented by that bar. Figure 9-2 is a histogram in which each bar represents a single numerical value for the cholesterol level. An extremely large number of observations would be needed to obtain a smooth curve for such single values. A smoother distribution is obtained by combining data into narrow ranges on the x-axis (see Fig. 9-4).

A **frequency polygon** is a shorthand way of presenting a histogram by putting a dot at the center of the top of each bar and connecting these dots with a line. In this way, a graph called a **frequency polygon** is created. Figure 9-5 shows a frequency polygon that was constructed from the histogram shown in Figure 9-4. Although histograms generally are recommended for presenting frequency distributions, the shape of the distribution is seen more easily in a frequency polygon than in a histogram.

Chapter 3 provides many examples of **line graphs** depicting relationships between *incidence rates* on the *y*-axis and time on the *x*-axis (see Figs. 3-1 and 3-2). An **epidemic time curve** is a histogram in which the *x*-axis is time and the *y*-axis is the number of *incident cases* in each time interval (see Fig. 3-11).

Figure 3-1, which shows the incidence rates of reported salmonellosis in the United States during several decades, is an example of an **arithmetic line graph,** meaning the *x*-axis and *y*-axis use an arithmetic scale. Figure 3-2 illustrates the impact that diphtheria vaccine (and perhaps other factors) had on the incidence rates of disease and death from diphtheria during several decades. It is an example of a **semilogarithmic line graph** in which the *x*-axis uses an arithmetic scale, but the *y*-axis uses a logarithmic scale to amplify the lower end of the scale. Although having the disadvantage of making the absolute magnitude of the changes appear less dramatic, semilogarithmic line graphs have the advantages of (1) enabling the detail of changes in very low rates of disease to be seen (difficult on an arithmetic graph comparing current rates with rates from previous decades) and (2) depicting proportionately similar changes as parallel lines (see Fig. 3-2). The decline in diphtheria deaths was proportionately similar to the decline in reported cases of disease, so the case fatality ratio (~10%) remained fairly constant over time. Semilogarithmic line graphs also allow for a wide range of values to be plotted in a single graph without using an inordinately large sheet of paper. Although unusual, data on both the *x*-axis and the *y*-axis might be displayed on logarithmic scales; such a plot would be *fully* logarithmic.

4. Parameters of a Frequency Distribution

Frequency distributions from continuous data are defined by two types of descriptors, known as **parameters:** measures of central tendency and measures of dispersion. The **measures of central tendency** locate observations on a measurement scale and are similar to a street address for the variable. The **measures of dispersion** suggest how widely the observations are spread out, as with indicating the property lines for a given address. In the case of a normal (gaussian) distribution, the bell-shaped curve can be fully described using only the mean (a measure of central tendency) and the standard deviation (a measure of dispersion).

MEASURES OF CENTRAL TENDENCY

The first step in examining a distribution is to look for the central tendency of the observations. Most types of medical data tend to clump in such a way that the *density* of observed values is greatest near the center of the distribution. In the case of the observed cholesterol values listed in Table 9-3 and depicted graphically in Figure 9-2, there appears to be some tendency for the values to cluster near the center of the distribution, but this tendency is much clearer visually when the values from Table 9-3 and Figure 9-2 are grouped in ranges of 20 mg/dL, as shown in Figure 9-4. The next step is to examine the distribution in greater detail and look for the mode, the median, and the mean, which are the three measures of central tendency.

Mode The most commonly observed value (i.e., the value that occurs most frequently) in a data set is called the mode. The mode is of some clinical interest, but seldom of statistical utility. A distribution typically has a mode at more than one value. For example, in Figure 9-2, the most commonly observed cholesterol levels (each with four observations) are 171 mg/dL and 180 mg/dL. In this case, although technically the figure shows a bimodal distribution, the two modes are close enough together to be considered part of the same central cluster. In other cases, distributions may be truly bimodal, usually because the population contains two subgroups, each of which has a different distribution that peaks at a different point. More than one mode also can be produced artificially by what is known as *digit preference,* when observers tend to favor certain numbers over others. For example, persons who measure blood pressure values tend to favor even numbers, particularly numbers ending in 0 (e.g., 120 mm Hg).

Median The median is the middle observation when data have been arranged in order from the lowest value to the highest value. The median value in Table 9-3 is 178 mg/dL. When there is an even number of observations, the median is considered to lie halfway between the two middle observations. For example, in Table 9-4, which shows the high-density lipoprotein (HDL) cholesterol values for 26 persons, the two middle observations are the 13th and 14th observations. The corresponding values for these are 57 and 58 mg/dL, so the median is 57.5 mg/dL.

Table 9-4 Raw Data and Results of Calculations in Study of Serum Levels of High-Density Lipoprotein (HDL) Cholesterol in 26 Participants

Parameter	Raw Data or Results of Calculation
No. observations, or N	26
Initial HDL cholesterol values (mg/dL) of participants	31, 41, 44, 46, 47, 47, 48, 48, 49, 52, 53, 54, 57, 58, 58, 60, 60, 62, 63, 64, 67, 69, 70, 77, 81, and 90
Highest value (mg/dL)	90
Lowest value (mg/dL)	31
Mode (mg/dL)	47, 48, 58, and 60
Median (mg/dL)	$(57 + 58)/2 = 57.5$
Sum of the values, or sum of x_i (mg/dL)	1496
Mean, or $\bar{x}$ (mg/dL)	$1496/26 = 57.5$
Range (mg/dL)	$90 - 31 = 59$
Interquartile range (mg/dL)	$64 - 48 = 16$
Sum of $(x_i - \bar{x})^2$, or TSS	4298.46 mg/dL squared*
Variance, or s^2	171.94 mg/dL†
Standard deviation, or s	$\sqrt{171.94} = 13.1$ mg/dL

*For a discussion and example of how statisticians measure the total sum of the squares (TSS), see Box 9-3.
†Here, the following formula is used:

$$\text{Variance} = s^2 = \frac{\sum (x_i^2) - \dfrac{\left(\sum x_i\right)^2}{N}}{N-1} = \frac{90{,}376 - \dfrac{2{,}238{,}016}{26}}{26-1}$$

$$= \frac{90{,}376 - 86{,}077.54}{25} = \frac{4298.46}{25} = 171.94$$

The median HDL value also is called the 50th percentile observation because 50% of the observations lie at that value or below. Percentiles frequently are used in educational testing and in medicine to describe normal growth standards for children. They also are used to describe the LD_{50} for experimental animals, defined as the dose of an agent (e.g., a drug) that is lethal for 50% of the animals exposed to it. The median length of survival may be more useful than the mean (average) length of survival because the median is not strongly influenced by a few study participants with unusually short or unusually long survival periods. The median gives a better sense of the survival of a typical study participant. The median is seldom used to make complicated inferences from medical data, however, because it does not lend itself to the development of advanced statistics. The median is used frequently in health care utilization and economics because many of the variables in these areas of study are skewed (see *skewness* definition later).

Mean   The mean is the average value, or the sum (Σ) of all the observed values (x_i) divided by the total number of observations (N):

$$\text{Mean} = \bar{x} = \frac{\Sigma(x_i)}{N}$$

where the subscript letter i means "for each individual observation." The mean ($\bar{x}$) has practical and theoretical advantages as a measure of central tendency. It is simple to calculate, and the sum of the deviations of observations from the mean (expressed in terms of negative and positive numbers) should equal 0, which provides a simple check of the calculations. The mean also has mathematical properties that enable the development of advanced statistics (Box 9-1). Most descriptive analyses of continuous variables and even advanced statistical analyses use the mean as the measure of central tendency. Table 9-4 gives an example of the calculation of the mean.

MEASURES OF DISPERSION

After the central tendency of a frequency distribution is determined, the next step is to determine how spread out (dispersed) the numbers are. This can be done by calculating measures based on percentiles or measures based on the mean.

Box 9-1	Properties of the Mean

1. The mean of a random sample is an unbiased estimator of the mean of the population from which it came.
2. The mean is the mathematical expectation. As such, it is different from the mode, which is the value observed most often.
3. For a set of data, the sum of the squared deviations of the observations from the mean is smaller than the sum of the squared deviations from any other number.
4. For a set of data, the sum of the squared deviations from the mean is fixed for a given set of observations. (This property is not unique to the mean, but it is a necessary property of any good measure of central tendency.)

Measures of Dispersion Based on Percentiles   Percentiles, which are sometimes called *quantiles,* are the percentage of observations below the point indicated when all the observations are ranked in descending order. The median, discussed previously, is the 50th percentile. The 75th percentile is the point at or below which 75% of the observations lie, whereas the 25th percentile is the point at or below which 25% of the observations lie.

In Table 9-4 the overall range of HDL cholesterol values is 59 mg/dL, reflecting the distance between the highest value (90 mg/dL) and the lowest value (31 mg/dL) in the data set. After data are ranked from highest to lowest, the data can be divided into quarters *(quartiles)* according to their rank. In the same table, the 75th and 25th percentiles are 64 mg/dL and 48 mg/dL, and the distance between them is 16 mg/dL. This distance is called the *interquartile range,* sometimes abbreviated Q3-Q1. Because of central clumping, the interquartile range is usually considerably smaller than half the size of the overall range of values, as in Table 9-4. (For more on these measures, see later discussion of quantiles.)

The advantage of using percentiles is that they can be applied to any set of continuous data, even if the data do not form any known distribution. Because few tests of statistical significance have been developed for use with medians and other percentiles, the use of percentiles in medicine is mostly limited to description, but in this role, percentiles are often useful clinically and educationally.

Measures of Dispersion Based on the Mean   Mean deviation, variance, and standard deviation are three measures of dispersion based on the mean.

Mean Deviation   Mean deviation is seldom used but helps define the concept of dispersion. Because the mean has many advantages, it might seem logical to measure dispersion by taking the average deviation from the mean. That proves to be useless, however, because the sum of the deviations from the mean is 0. This inconvenience can be solved easily by computing the mean deviation, which is the average of the absolute value of the deviations from the mean, as shown in the following formula:

$$\text{Mean deviation} = \frac{\Sigma(|x_i - \bar{x}|)}{N}$$

Because the mean deviation does not have mathematical properties on which to base many statistical tests, the formula has not come into popular use. Instead, the variance has become the fundamental measure of dispersion in statistics that are based on the normal distribution.

Variance   The variance for a set of observed data is the sum of the squared deviations from the mean, divided by the number of observations minus 1:

$$\text{Variance} = s^2 = \frac{\Sigma(x_i - \bar{x})^2}{N-1}$$

The symbol for a variance calculated from observed data (a sample variance) is s^2. In the previous formula, squaring solves the problem that the deviations from the mean add up to 0. Dividing by $N-1$ (called **degrees of freedom;** see Box 10-2), instead of dividing by N, is necessary for the sample variance to be an unbiased estimator of the population variance. A simple explanation for this denominator is

Box 9-2	Properties of the Variance

1. For an observed set of data, when the denominator of the equation for variance is expressed as the number of observations minus 1 (i.e., $N - 1$), the variance of a random sample is an unbiased estimator of the variance of the population from which it was taken.
2. The variance of the sum of two independently sampled variables is equal to the sum of the variances.
3. The variance of the difference between two independently sampled variables is equal to the sum of their individual variances as well. (The importance of this should become clear when the t-test is considered in Chapter 10.)

that when the mean is known, and all observations except the last one have been established, the value of the final observation becomes fixed and is not free to vary, so it does not contribute to the variance.

The *numerator of the variance* (i.e., sum of squared deviations of observations from the mean) is an extremely important measure in statistics. It is usually called either the **sum of squares** (SS) or the **total sum of squares** (TSS). The TSS measures the total amount of variation in a set of observations. Box 9-2 lists the mathematical properties of variance that permit the development of statistical tests, and Box 9-3 explains how statisticians measure variation. Understanding the concept of variation makes statistics easier to understand.

Box 9-3	How Do Statisticians Measure Variation?

In statistics, variation is measured as the sum of the squared deviations of the individual observations from an expected value, such as the mean. The mean is the mathematical expectation (expected value) of a continuous frequency distribution. The quantity of variation in a given set of observations is the numerator of the variance, which is known as the sum of the squares (SS). The sum of the squares of a dependent variable sometimes is called the total sum of the squares (TSS), which is the total amount of variation that needs to be explained.

For illustrative purposes, assume the data set consists of these six numbers: 1, 2, 4, 7, 10, and 12. Assume that x_i denotes the individual observations, $\bar{x}$ is the mean, N is the number of observations, s^2 is the variance, and s is the standard deviation.

PART 1 Tabular Representation of the Data

	x_i	$(x - \bar{x})$	$\bar{x}$
	1	−5	25
	2	−4	16
	4	−2	4
	7	+1	1
	10	+4	16
	12	+6	36
Sum, or Σ	36	0	98

PART 2 Graphic Representation of Data Shown in Third Column of Above Table, $(x_i - \bar{x})^2$, for Each of the Six Observations

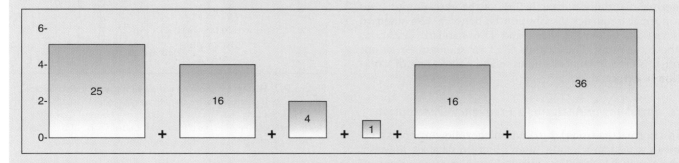

PART 3 Calculation of Numbers that Describe a Distribution (i.e., the Parameters)

$\Sigma(x_i) = 36$

$N = 6$

$\bar{x} = 6$

$\Sigma(x_i - \bar{x})^2 = \text{TSS} = 98$

$s^2 = \text{TSS}/(N - 1) = 98/5 = 19.6$

$s = \sqrt{19.6} = 4.43$

For simplicity of calculation, another (but algebraically equivalent) formula is used to calculate the variance. It is the sum of the squared values for each observation minus a correction factor (to correct for the fact that the deviations from zero, rather than the deviations from the mean, are being squared), all divided by $N - 1$:

$$\text{Variance} = s^2 = \frac{\sum (x_i^2) - \left[\frac{\left(\sum x_i\right)^2}{N}\right]}{N - 1}$$

Table 9-4 illustrates the calculation of a variance using this second formula.

Standard Deviation The variance tends to be a large and unwieldy number, and its value falls outside the range of observed values in a data set. The **standard deviation,** which is the square root of the variance, usually is used to describe the amount of spread in the frequency distribution. Conceptually, the standard deviation is an average of the deviations from the mean. The symbol for the standard deviation of an observed data set is s, and the formula is as follows:

$$\text{Standard deviation} = s = \sqrt{\frac{\sum (x_i - \bar{x})^2}{N - 1}}$$

In an observed data set, the term $\bar{x} \pm s$ represents 1 standard deviation above and below the mean, and the term $\bar{x} \pm 2s$ represents 2 standard deviations above and below the mean. One standard deviation falls well within the range of observed numbers in most data sets and has a known relationship to the normal (gaussian) distribution. This relationship often is useful in drawing inferences in statistics.

In a theoretical normal (gaussian) distribution, as shown in Figure 9-6, the area under the curve represents the probability of all the observations in the distribution. One standard deviation above and below the mean, represented by the distance from point A to point B, encompasses 68% of the area under the curve, and 68% of the observations in a normal distribution are expected to fall within this range. Two standard deviations above and below the mean include 95.4% of the area (i.e., 95.4% of the observations) in a normal distribution. Exactly 95% of the observations from a normal frequency distribution lie between 1.96 standard deviations below the mean and 1.96 standard deviations above the mean. The formula $\bar{x} \pm 1.96$ standard deviations often is used in clinical studies to show the extent of variation in clinical data.

5. Problems in Analyzing a Frequency Distribution

In a normal (gaussian) distribution, the following holds true: mean = median = mode. In an observed data set, however, there may be skewness, kurtosis, and extreme values, in which case the measures of central tendency may not follow this pattern.

SKEWNESS AND KURTOSIS

A horizontal stretching of a frequency distribution to one side or the other, so that one tail of observations is longer

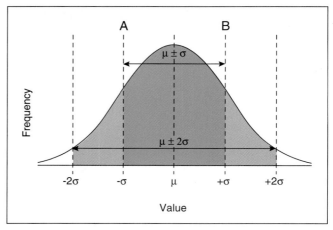

Figure 9-6 Theoretical normal (gaussian) distribution showing where I and 2 standard deviations above and below the mean would fall. Lowercase Greek letter mu (μ) stands for the mean in the theoretical distribution, and Greek sigma (σ) stands for the standard deviation in the theoretical population. (The italic Roman letters *x* and *s* apply to an observed [sample] population.) The area under the curve represents all the observations in the distribution. One standard deviation above and below the mean, shown in dark blue and represented by the distance from point A to point B, encompasses 68% of the area under the curve, and 68% of the observations in a normal distribution fall within this range. Two standard deviations above and below the mean, represented by the areas shown in dark and light blue, include 95.4% of the area under the curve and 95.4% of the observations in a normal distribution.

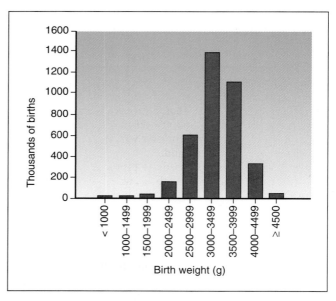

Figure 9-7 Histogram showing a skewed frequency distribution. Values are for thousands of births by birth weight group, United States, 1987. Note the long "tail" on the left. (Data from National Center for Health Statistics: *Trends in low birth weight: United States, 1975-85.* Series 21, No 48, Washington, DC, 1989, Government Printing Office.)

and has more observations than the other tail, is called **skewness.** When a histogram or frequency polygon has a longer tail on the left side of the diagram, as in Figure 9-7 and Figure 9-8, *A,* the distribution is said to be "skewed to the left." If a distribution is skewed, the mean is found farther in the direction of the long tail than the median because the mean is more heavily influenced by extreme values.

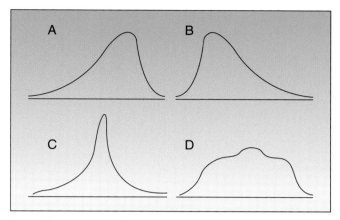

Figure 9-8 Examples of skewed and kurtotic frequency distributions. Distribution **A** is skewed to the left; distribution **B** is skewed to the right; they have the long tail to the left **(A)** and to the right **(B)** of the peak. Distribution **C** is kurtotic, with abnormal peaking; distribution **D** is kurtotic, with abnormal flattening compared with the normal distribution.

A quick way to obtain an approximate idea of whether or not a frequency distribution is skewed is to compare the mean and the median. If these two measures are close to each other, the distribution is probably not skewed. In the data from Table 9-3, the mean equals 179.1 mg/dL, and the median equals 178 mg/dL. These two values are very close, and as Figure 9-4 shows, the distribution also does not appear to be skewed.

Kurtosis is characterized by a vertical stretching or flattening of the frequency distribution. As shown in Figure 9-8, a kurtotic distribution could appear more peaked or more flattened than the normal bell-shaped distribution.

Significant skewness or kurtosis can be detected by statistical tests. Many statistical tests require the data to be normally distributed, and the tests may not be valid if used to compare extremely abnormal distributions. The statistical tests discussed in this book are relatively robust, meaning that as long as the data are not overly skewed or kurtotic, the results can be considered valid.

Kurtosis is seldom discussed as a problem in the statistical or medical literature, although skewness is observed frequently, and adjustments for skewness are made when needed.

EXTREME VALUES (OUTLIERS)

One of the most perplexing problems for the analysis of data is how to treat a value that is abnormally far above or below the mean. This problem is suggested in the data set of cholesterol values shown in Table 9-3 and Figure 9-2. The standard deviation of the distribution in the data set is 28.2 mg/dL, so that if the distribution were normal, 95% of the cholesterol values would be expected to be between 123.8 and 234.4 mg/dL (i.e., the mean ± 1.96 standard deviations = 179.1 mg/dL ± the product of 1.96 × 28.2). Ninety-nine percent of the values would be expected to be found within the range of the mean ± 2.58 standard deviations, which in this case would be between 106.3 and 251.9 mg/dL.

When the data are observed visually in Figure 9-2, everything looks normal below the mean; the lowest value is 124 mg/dL, which is within the 95% limits. The upper value is 264 mg/dL, however, which is beyond the 99% limits of

expectation and looks suspiciously far from the other values. Because many people have these high total cholesterol values, and because the observation is almost within the 99% limits, there is probably no reason to believe that the value is erroneous (although there might be a reason to be clinically concerned with such a high cholesterol value in a young person). Plausibility is a gauge to be used when considering the reliability of outlying data. Before analyzing the data set, the investigator should check the original source of data, to ensure this value is what the laboratory reported.

6. Methods of Depicting a Frequency Distribution

In the medical literature, histograms and line graphs are used to illustrate frequency distributions, as defined earlier with frequency polygons. There are advantages to displaying data visually. Other methods of visually displaying data include stem and leaf diagrams, quantiles, and boxplots, which can be printed out by computer programs such as the Statistical Analysis System (SAS), or SPSS (http://www.spss.com/). Figure 9-9 plots the HDL cholesterol values for 26 young adults provided in Table 9-4.

STEM AND LEAF DIAGRAMS

As shown in Figure 9-9, the stem and leaf diagram has three components. The **stem,** which is the vertical column of numbers on the left, represents the value of the left-hand digit (in this case, the 10s digit). The **leaf** is the set of numbers immediately to the right of the stem and is separated from the stem by a space (as here) or by a vertical line. Each of the numbers in the leaf represents the single number digit in one of the 26 observations in the data set of HDL cholesterol values. The stem and leaf value shown on the top line of the diagram represents 90 mg/dL. The **# symbol** to the right of the leaf tells how many observations were seen in the range indicated (in this case, 1 observation of 90 mg/dL). Observations that can be made quickly from viewing the stem and leaf diagram include the following (Fig. 9-9):

1. The highest value in the data set was 90 mg/dL.
2. The lowest value was 31 mg/dL.
3. There were eight observations in the range of the 40s, consisting of 41, 44, 46, 47, 47, 48, 48, and 49.
4. When the diagram is viewed with the left side turned to the bottom, the distribution looks fairly normal, although it has a long tail to the left (i.e., it is skewed to the left).

QUANTILES

Below the stem and leaf diagram in Figure 9-9 is a display of the quantiles (percentiles). The data include the *maximum* (100% of the values were at this level or below) and *minimum* (0% of the values were below this level); the 99%, 95%, 90%, 10%, 5%, and 1% values; the *range;* the *mode;* and the *interquartile range* (from the 75th percentile to the 25th percentile, abbreviated Q3-Q1).

BOXPLOTS

The modified boxplot is shown to the right of the stem and leaf diagram in Fig. 9-9 and provides an even briefer way of summarizing the data.

```
        Stem Leaf                          #                    Boxplot
          9 0                               1                       0
          8 1                               1                       |
          7 07                              2                       |
          6 0023479                         7                   +-----+
          5 234788                          6                   *--+--*
          4 14677889                        8                   +-----+
          3 1                               1                       |
            ----+----+----+----+                                   |
        Multiply Stem.Leaf by 10**+ 1


                          Quantiles (Percentiles)

        100% Max          90              99%               90
         75% Q3           64              95%               81
         50% Med          57.5            90%               77
         25% Q1           48              10%               44
          0% Min          31              5%                41
                                          1%                31

        Range             59
        Q3 - Q1           16
        Mode              47
```

Figure 9-9 **Stem and leaf diagram, boxplot, and quantiles (percentiles).** For the data shown in Table 9-4, as printed out by the Statistical Analysis System (SAS). See the text for a detailed description of how to interpret these data.

In the boxplot the rectangle formed by four plus signs (+) and the horizontal dashes (—) depicts the interquartile range. The two asterisks (*) connected by dashes depict the median. The mean, shown by the smaller plus sign (+), is very close to the median. Outside the rectangle, there are two vertical lines, called the "whiskers" of the boxplot. The whiskers extend as far as the data, but no more than 1.5 times the interquartile range above the 75th percentile and 1.5 times the interquartile range below the 25th percentile. They show the range where most of the values would be expected, given the median and interquartile range of the distribution. Values beyond the whiskers but within 3 interquartile ranges of the box are shown as a 0, and values more extreme than this are shown with an asterisk. In Figure 9-9, all the observed data values except the value of 90 mg/dL might reasonably have been expected; this value may be an outlier observation, however, as indicated by the 0 near the top, just above the top of the upper whisker.

It takes only a quick look at the boxplot to see how wide the distribution is, whether or not it is skewed, where the interquartile range falls, how close the median is to the mean, and how many (if any) observations might reasonably be considered outliers.

7. Use of Unit-Free (Normalized) Data

Data from a normal (gaussian) frequency distribution can be described completely by the mean and the standard deviation. Even the same set of data, however, would provide a different value for the mean and standard deviation depending on the choice of **units of measurement**. For example, the same person's height may be expressed as 66 inches or 167.6 cm, and an infant's birth weight may be recorded as 2500 g or 5.5 lb. Because the units of measurement differ, so do the numbers, although the true height and weight are the same. To eliminate the effects produced by the choice of units, the data can be put into a unit-free form (normalized).

The result is that each item of data is measured as the number of standard deviations above or below the mean for that set of data.

The first step in normalizing data is to calculate the mean and standard deviation. The second step is to set the mean equal to 0 by subtracting the mean from each observation in whatever units have been used. The third step is to measure each observation in terms of the number of standard deviations it is above or below the mean. The normalized values obtained by this process are called **z values**, which are sometimes used in clinical medicine (e.g., bone density measurements to test for osteoporosis). The formula for creating individual z values (z_i) is as follows:

$$z_i = \frac{x_i - \bar{x}}{s}$$

Where x_i represents individual observations, $\bar{x}$ represents the mean of the observations, and s is the standard deviation. Suppose that the goal is to standardize blood pressure values for a group of patients whose systolic blood pressures were observed to have a mean of 120 mm Hg and a standard deviation of 10 mm Hg. If two of the values to be standardized were 140 mm Hg and 115 mm Hg, the calculations would be as follows:

$$\frac{140-120}{10} = +2.0 \qquad \frac{115-120}{10} = -0.5$$

A distribution of z values always has a mean of 0 and a standard deviation of 1. These z values may be called by various names, often **standard normal deviates.**

Clinically, z values are useful for determining how extreme an observed test result is. For example, in Table 9-3 the highest total cholesterol value observed among 71 persons was 264 mg/dL, 23 points higher than the next highest value. Is this cholesterol value suspect? When the previous formula is used, the z value is (264 − 179.1)/28.2 = +3.0. This means that it is 3 standard deviations above the mean. Usually, about 1% of observed values are 2.58 standard deviations or more away from the mean. Because this is the only one of the 71 observed values this high, and such values are often seen clinically, there is no reason to suppose it is an error. Plausibility is important when evaluating outliers, as noted earlier. A height of 10 feet for a person would be suspect because it falls outside of human experience.

B. Frequency Distributions of Dichotomous Data and Proportions

Dichotomous data can be seen in terms of flipping a coin. If the coin is flipped in an unbiased manner, on the average it would be expected to land with the heads side up for half the flips and with the tails side up for half the flips, so the probability of heads would equal 0.5, and the probability of tails would equal 0.5. The sum of all the probabilities for all the possible outcomes must equal 1.0. If a coin is flipped 10 times, the result would rarely be 10 heads or 10 tails, would less rarely be a combination of 9 heads plus 1 tail, and would most frequently be a combination of 5 heads and 5 tails.

The probabilities of obtaining various combinations of heads and tails from flipping a coin can be calculated by **expanding the binomial formula**, $(a + b)^n$, as shown in Box 9-4. In this formula, a is the probability of heads, b is the probability of tails, and n is the number of coin tosses in a trial. If n is large (e.g., hundreds of tosses of the coin), and if the coin is thrown in an unbiased manner, the distribution of the binomial toss would look much like a normal (gaussian) distribution. If n were infinite, a were 0.5, and b were 0.5, the **binomial distribution** would be *identical* to the normal distribution. A mean and standard deviation can be calculated for the binomial distribution.

If the probability of heads does not equal 0.5, the binomial distribution would look like a skewed distribution, and the earlier cautions concerning statistical analysis would apply. Because of the close relationship between the binomial and the normal distributions, binary data expressed as **proportions** can be analyzed using theory based on the normal distribution.

C. Frequency Distributions of Other Types of Data

Data from nominal (categorical) and ordinal (ranked) variables are not properly analyzed using tests based on the normal (gaussian) distribution. These data should be analyzed using statistical methods that make no assumptions about an underlying frequency distribution. Because they are not based on normal or binomial distribution (for which parameters such as means and standard deviations can be calculated), statistical tests for nominal and ordinal variables are called **nonparametric tests.** Of particular importance in medicine, the analysis of the counts in frequency tables (e.g., Table 9-2) depends on a different distribution, known as the *chi-square distribution* (see Chapter 11). Because the chi-square analysis does not require that the data themselves follow any particular distribution, it is also a nonparametric test.

Ordinal data sometimes are analyzed in the medical literature as though they were continuous data, and means and standard deviations are reported. This is usually satisfactory for describing ordinal data, but it is generally not appropriate for significance testing. The preferred tests are discussed in Chapter 11 and include the Wilcoxon test, the Mann-Whitney U test, and other tests for ordinal data. These tests do not require that the data follow any particular distribution; they require only that the data be ordinal.

The **Poisson distribution** is used to describe uncommon events occurring in time or in space or in both. It has the convenient property that the mean equals the variance.[4] It is especially useful in evaluating the clustering of rare events, such as suspected "cancer clusters."[5] Further discussion of the Poisson distribution is beyond the scope of this text.*

IV. SUMMARY

Although variation in clinical medicine may be caused by biologic differences or the presence or absence of disease, it also may result from differences in measurement techniques and conditions, errors in measurement, and random variation. Statistics is an aid to describing and understanding variation. Statistics cannot correct for measurement errors or bias, however, and the analysis can only *adjust* for random error in the sense that it can estimate how much of the total variation is caused by random error and how much by a particular factor being investigated.

Fundamental to any analysis of data is an understanding of the types of variables or data being analyzed. Data types include nominal, dichotomous, ordinal, continuous, and ratio data as well as risks, rates, and proportions. Continuous (measurement) data usually show a frequency distribution that can be described in terms of two parameters: a measure of central tendency (of which median and mean are the most important) and a measure of dispersion based on the mean (of which variance and standard deviation are the most important). The most common distribution is called the normal (gaussian) bell-shaped distribution; the mean and the median coincide, and 95% of the observations are within 1.96 standard deviations above and below the mean. Frequently, the normal distribution appears pulled to one side or the other (has a long tail), called a skewed distribution; the mean is farther in the direction of the long tail than is the median.

Data may be made unit free (may be *normalized*) by creating z values. This is accomplished by subtracting the mean from each value and dividing the result by the standard deviation. This expresses the value of each observation as the number of standard deviations the value is above or below the mean. The probability distribution for dichotomous data may be described by the binomial distribution. If the probability of success and failure are the same (0.5 each), and if the number of trials is large, the binomial distribution approximates the normal distribution. For studying rare events, the Poisson distribution is most helpful. When the normal (gaussian) distribution cannot be assumed, nonparametric statistics can be used to study differences and associations among variables.

*For those interested, a useful overview is available: http://www.umass.edu/wsp/statistics/lessons/poisson/index.html.

| Box 9-4 | How to Determine Probabilities by Expanding the Binomial |

The basic binomial formula is $(a + b)^n$. The probabilities of getting various combinations of heads and tails from flipping an unbiased coin can be calculated by expanding this formula. Although the example of heads/tails is used here, the formula and concepts described can also be applied to the probabilities of life/death associated with particular diagnoses, success/failure in treatment, and other clinically relevant dichotomous data.

When the binomial formula is applied to flipping a coin in an unbiased manner, a is the probability of obtaining heads, b is the probability of obtaining tails, and n is the number of trials (coin tosses). The process of calculating the probabilities is called **expanding the binomial,** and the distribution of probabilities for each combination is the **binomial** distribution.

With **one** flip of the coin, there is a 0.5 (50%) chance of heads and a 0.5 (50%) chance of tails, with the sum of 1.0.

Two flips of the coin could produce the following outcomes: two heads, one head and one tail (in either the head/tail or tail/head order), or two tails. What are the probabilities of these possible outcomes? The answer is given by the previous formula, with $n = 2$. It is $(a + b)$ times itself:

$$(a+b)^2 = a^2 + 2ab + b^2$$
$$= (0.5)(0.5) + (2)(0.5)(0.5) + (0.5)(0.5)$$
$$= 0.25 + 0.50 + 0.25$$

In other words, with two flips of a coin, the probabilities of the various possible outcomes are as follows:
Two heads = 0.25
One head and one tail (in either order) = 0.25 + 0.25 + 0.50
Two tails = 0.25
The sum of the probabilities = 1.0

Three flips of a coin could produce the following outcomes: three heads, two heads and one tail, two tails and one head, or three tails. The probabilities, calculated by using the formula $(a + b)^3$, are as follows:
Three heads = $a^3 = (0.5)^3 = 0.125$
Two heads and one tail = $3(a^2)(b) = (3)(0.25)(0.5) = 0.375$
One head and two tails = $3(a)(b^2) = (3)(0.5)(0.25) = 0.375$
Three tails = $b^3 = (0.5)^3 = 0.125$
The sum of the probabilities = 1.0

If a **biased** coin (e.g., $a = 0.4$ and $b = 0.6$) were tossed three times, the probabilities would be as follows:
Three heads = $a^3 = (0.4)^3 = 0.064$
Two heads and one tail = $3(a^2)(b) = (3)(0.16)(0.6) = 0.288$
One head and two tails = $3(a)(b^2) = (3)(0.4)(0.36) = 0.432$
Three tails = $b^3 = (0.6)^3 = 0.216$
The sum of the probabilities = 1.0

The coefficients for expanding $(a + b)^n$ can be found easily using a Pascal triangle*, in which each coefficient is the sum of the two above.

$n =$	Coefficients	Examples
1	1 1	$1a + 1b$
2	1 2 1	$1a^2 + 2ab + 1b^2$
3	1 3 3 1	$1a^3 + 3(a^2)(b) + 3(a)(b^2) + 1b^3$
4	1 4 6 4 1	$1a^4 + 4(a^3)(b) + 6(a^2)(b^2) + 4(a)(b^3) + 1b^4$

If the probabilities from tossing an unbiased coin are plotted as histograms, as the number of coin tosses becomes greater, the probabilities look more and more like a normal (gaussian) distribution.

---

*http://mathworld.wolfram.com/PascalsTriangle.html.

References

1. Yerushalmy J, et al: The role of dual reading in mass radiography. *Am Rev Respir Dis* 61:443–464, 1950.
2. Elmore JG, Wells CK, Lee CH, et al: Variability in radiologists' interpretations of mammograms. *N Engl J Med* 331:1493–1499, 1994.
3. Buehler JW, Kleinman JC, Hogue CJ, et al: Birth weight–specific infant mortality, United States, 1960 and 1980. *Public Health Rep* 102:151–161, 1987.
4. Gerstman BB: *Epidemiology kept simple*, New York, 1998, Wiley-Liss.
5. Reynolds P, Smith DF, Satariano E, et al: The Four-County Study of Childhood Cancer: clusters in context. *Stat Med* 15:683–697, 1996.

Select Reading

Dawson-Saunders B, Trapp RG: *Basic and clinical biostatistics*, ed 4, New York, 2004, Lange Medical Books/McGraw-Hill.

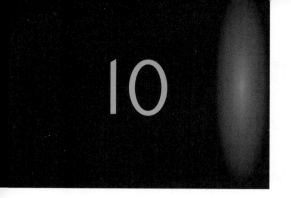

10 Statistical Inference and Hypothesis Testing

With the nature of variation, types of data and variables, and characteristics of data distribution reviewed in Chapter 9 as background, we now explore how to make inferences from data.

I. NATURE AND PURPOSE OF STATISTICAL INFERENCE

Inference means the drawing of conclusions from data. *Statistical inference* can be defined as the drawing of conclusions from quantitative or qualitative information using the methods of statistics to describe and arrange the data and to test suitable hypotheses.

A. Differences between Deductive and Inductive Reasoning

Because data do not come with their own interpretation, the interpretation must be put into the data by **inductive reasoning** (from Latin, meaning "to lead into"). This approach to reasoning is less familiar to most people than **deductive reasoning** (Latin, "to lead out from"), which is learned from mathematics, particularly from geometry.

Deductive reasoning proceeds *from the general* (i.e., from assumptions, propositions, or formulas considered true) *to the specific* (i.e., to specific members belonging to the general category). Consider the following two propositions:

- All Americans believe in democracy.
- This person is an American.

If both propositions are true, then the following deduction must be true:

- This person believes in democracy.

Deductive reasoning is of special use in science after hypotheses are formed. Using deductive reasoning, an investigator can say, "*If* the following hypothesis is true, *then* the following prediction or predictions also should be true." If a prediction can be tested empirically, the hypothesis may be rejected or not rejected on the basis of the findings. If the data are inconsistent with the predictions from the hypothesis, the hypothesis must be rejected or modified. Even if the data are consistent with the hypothesis, however, they cannot prove that the hypothesis is true, as shown in Chapter 4 (see Fig. 4-2).

Clinicians often proceed from formulas accepted as true and from observed data to determine the values that variables must have in a certain clinical situation. For example, if the amount of a medication that can be safely given per kilogram of body weight is known, it is simple to calculate how much of that medication can be given to a patient weighing 50 kg. This is deductive reasoning because it proceeds from the general (a formula) to the specific (the patient).

Inductive reasoning, in contrast, seeks to find valid generalizations and general principles from data. Statistics, the quantitative aid to inductive reasoning, proceeds *from the specific* (i.e., from data) *to the general* (i.e., to formulas or conclusions about the data). By sampling a population and determining the age and the blood pressure of the persons in the sample (the specific data), an investigator, using statistical methods, can determine the general relationship between age and blood pressure (e.g., that, on average, blood pressure increases with age).

B. Differences between Mathematics and Statistics

The differences between mathematics and statistics can be illustrated by showing that they approach the same basic equation in two different ways:

$$y = mx + b$$

This equation is the formula for a straight line in analytic geometry. It is also the formula for simple regression analysis in statistics, although the letters used and their order customarily are different.

In the mathematical formula the b is a constant and stands for the *y-intercept* (i.e., value of y when the variable x equals 0). The value m also is a constant and stands for the *slope* (amount of change in y for a unit increase in the value of x). The important point is that in mathematics, one of the variables (x or y) is unknown and needs to be calculated, whereas the formula and the constants are known. In statistics the *reverse* is true. The variables x and y are known for all persons in the sample, and the investigator may want to determine the linear relationship between them. This is done by *estimating* the slope and the intercept, which can be done using the form of statistical analysis called *linear regression* (see Chapter 11).

As a general rule, *what is known in statistics is unknown in mathematics,* and vice versa. In statistics the investigator starts from specific observations (data) to induce (estimate) the general relationships between variables.

II. PROCESS OF TESTING HYPOTHESES

Hypotheses are predictions about what the examination of appropriately collected data will show. This discussion introduces the basic concepts underlying common tests of statistical significance, such as *t*-tests. These tests determine the probability that an observed difference between means, for example, represents a true, statistically significant difference (i.e., a difference probably not caused by chance). They do this by determining if the observed difference is convincingly different from what was expected from the *model*. In basic statistics the model is usually a *null hypothesis* that there will be no difference between the means.

The discussion in this section focuses on the justification for, and interpretation of, the **p value**, which is the **probability** that a difference as large as one observed might have occurred by chance. The p value is obtained from calculating one of the standard statistical tests. It is designed to minimize the likelihood of making a false-positive conclusion. False-negative conclusions are discussed more fully in Chapter 12 in the section on sample size.

A. False-Positive and False-Negative Errors

Science is based on the following set of principles:

- Previous experience serves as the basis for developing hypotheses.
- Hypotheses serve as the basis for developing predictions.
- Predictions must be subjected to experimental or observational testing.

- If the predictions are consistent with the data, they are retained, but if they are inconsistent with the data, they are rejected or modified.

When deciding whether data are consistent or inconsistent with the hypotheses, investigators are subject to two types of error. An investigator could assert that the data support a hypothesis, when in fact the hypothesis is false; this would be a **false-positive error,** also called an **alpha error** or a **type I error.** Conversely, they could assert that the data do *not* support the hypothesis, when in fact the hypothesis is true; this would be a **false-negative error,** also called a **beta error** or a **type II error.**

Based on the knowledge that scientists become attached to their own hypotheses, and the conviction that the proof in science (as in courts of law) must be "beyond a reasonable doubt," investigators historically have been particularly careful to avoid false-positive error. This is probably best for theoretical science in general. It also makes sense for hypothesis testing related specifically to medical practice, where the greatest imperative is "first, do no harm" (Latin *primum non nocere*). Although it often fails in practice to avoid harm, medicine is dedicated to this principle, and the high standards for the avoidance of type I error reflect this. However, medicine is subject to the harms of error in either direction. False-negative error in a diagnostic test may mean missing a disease until it is too late to institute therapy, and false-negative error in the study of a medical intervention may mean overlooking an effective treatment. Therefore, investigators cannot feel comfortable about false-negative errors in either case.

Box 10-1 shows the usual sequence of statistical testing of hypotheses; analyzing data using these five basic steps is discussed next.

1. Develop Null Hypothesis and Alternative Hypothesis

The first step consists of stating the null hypothesis and the alternative hypothesis. The **null hypothesis** states that there is no real (true) difference between the means (or proportions) of the groups being compared (or that there is no real association between two continuous variables). For example, the null hypothesis for the data presented in Table 9-2 is that, based on the observed data, there is no true difference between the percentage of men and the percentage of women who had previously had their serum cholesterol levels checked.

Box 10-1	Process of Testing a Null Hypothesis for Statistical Significance

1. Develop the null and alternative hypotheses.
2. Establish an appropriate alpha level.
3. Perform a suitable test of statistical significance on appropriately collected data.
4. Compare the p value from the test with the alpha level.
5. Reject or fail to reject the null hypothesis.

It may seem strange to begin the process by asserting that something is *not* true, but it is much easier to disprove an assertion than to prove that something is true. If the data are not consistent with a hypothesis, the hypothesis should be rejected and the **alternative hypothesis** accepted instead. Because the null hypothesis stated there was *no* difference between means, and that was rejected, the alternative hypothesis states that there *must be* a true difference between the groups being compared. (If the data are consistent with a hypothesis, this still does not prove the hypothesis, because other hypotheses may fit the data equally well or better.)

Consider a hypothetical clinical trial of a drug designed to reduce high blood pressure among patients with essential hypertension (hypertension occurring without an organic cause yet known, such as hyperthyroidism or renal artery stenosis). One group of patients would receive the experimental drug, and the other group (the control group) would receive a placebo. The null hypothesis might be that, after the intervention, the average change in blood pressure in the treatment group will not differ from the average change in blood pressure in the control group. If a test of significance (e.g., *t*-test on average change in systolic blood pressure) forces rejection of the null hypothesis, the alternative hypothesis—that there was a true difference in the average change in blood pressure between the two groups—would be accepted. As discussed later, there is a statistical distinction between hypothesizing that a drug will or will not *change* blood pressure, versus hypothesizing whether a drug will or will not *lower* blood pressure. The former does not specify a directional inclination a priori (before the fact) and suggests a "two-tailed" hypothesis test. The latter does suggest a directional inclination and suggests a "one-tailed" test.

2. Establish Alpha Level

Second, before doing any calculations to test the null hypothesis, the investigator must establish a criterion called the **alpha level**, which is the highest risk of making a false-positive error that the investigator is willing to accept. By custom, the level of alpha is usually set at $p = 0.05$. This says that the investigator is willing to run a 5% risk (but no more) of being in error when rejecting the null hypothesis and asserting that the treatment and control groups truly differ. In choosing an arbitrary alpha level, the investigator inserts value judgment into the process. Because that is done before the data are collected, however, it avoids the post hoc (after the fact) bias of adjusting the alpha level to make the data show statistical significance after the investigator has looked at the data.

An everyday analogy may help to simplify the logic of the alpha level and the process of significance testing. Suppose that a couple were given instructions to buy a silver bracelet for a friend during a trip, *if* one could be bought for $50 or less. Any more would be too high a price to pay. Alpha is similar to the price limit in the analogy. When alpha has been set (e.g., at $p \leq 0.05$, analogous to $\leq \$50$ in the illustration), an investigator would *buy* the alternative hypothesis of a true difference if, but only if, the cost (in terms of the probability of being wrong in rejecting the null hypothesis) were no greater than 1 in 20 (0.05). The alpha is analogous to the amount an investigator is willing to pay, in terms of the risk of being wrong, if he or she rejects the null hypothesis and accepts the alternative hypothesis.

3. Perform Test of Statistical Significance

When the alpha level is established, the next step is to obtain the **p value** for the data. To do this, the investigator must perform a suitable statistical test of significance on appropriately collected data, such as data obtained from a randomized controlled trial (RCT). This chapter and Chapter 11 focus on some suitable tests. The p value obtained by a statistical test (e.g., *t*-test, described later) gives the probability of obtaining the observed result by chance rather than as a result of a true effect. When the probability of an outcome being caused by chance is sufficiently remote, the null hypothesis is rejected. The p value states specifically just how remote that probability is.

Usually, if the observed p value in a study is ≤ 0.05, members of the scientific community who read about an investigation accept the difference as being real. Although setting alpha at ≤ 0.05 is arbitrary, this level has become so customary that it is wise to provide explanations for choosing another alpha level or for choosing not to perform tests of significance at all, which may be the best approach in some descriptive studies. Similarly, two-tailed tests of hypothesis, which require a more extreme result to reject the null hypothesis than do one-tailed tests, are the norm; a one-tailed test should be well justified. When the directional effect of a given intervention (e.g., it can be neutral or beneficial, but is certain not to be harmful) is known with confidence, a one-tailed test can be justified (see later discussion).

4. Compare p Value Obtained with Alpha

After the p value is obtained, it is compared with the alpha level previously chosen.

5. Reject or Fail to Reject Null Hypothesis

If the p value is found to be *greater* than the alpha level, the investigator *fails to reject* the null hypothesis. Failing to reject the null hypothesis is *not* the same as accepting the null hypothesis as true. Rather, it is similar to a jury's finding that the evidence did not prove guilt (or in the example here, did not prove the difference) beyond a reasonable doubt. In the United States a court trial is not designed to prove innocence. The defendant's innocence is assumed and must be disproved beyond a reasonable doubt. Similarly, in statistics, a lack of difference is assumed, and it is up to the statistical analysis to show that the null hypothesis is unlikely to be true. The rationale for using this approach in medical research is similar to the rationale in the courts. Although the courts are able to convict the guilty, the goal of exonerating the innocent is an even higher priority. In medicine, confirming the benefit of a new treatment is important, but avoiding the use of ineffective therapies is an even higher priority (first, do no harm).

If the p value is found to be less than or equal to the alpha level, the next step is to reject the null hypothesis and to accept the **alternative hypothesis,** that is, the hypothesis that there is in fact a real difference or association. Although it may seem awkward, this process is now standard in medical science and has yielded considerable scientific benefits.

B. Variation in Individual Observations and in Multiple Samples

Most tests of significance relate to a difference between two means or proportions of a variable (e.g., a decrease in blood pressure). The two groups are often a treatment group and a control group. They help investigators decide whether an observed difference is real, which in statistical terms is defined as *whether the difference is greater than would be expected by chance alone.* In the example of the experimental drug to reduce blood pressure in hypertensive patients, the experimenters would measure the blood pressures of the study participants under experimental conditions before and after the new drug or placebo is given. They would determine the average change seen in the treatment group and the average change seen in the control group and pursue tests to determine whether the difference was large enough to be unlikely to have occurred by chance alone. The fundamental process in this particular test of significance would be to see if the mean blood pressure changes in the two study groups were different from each other.

Why not just inspect the means to see if they were different? This is inadequate because it is unknown whether the observed difference was unusual or whether a difference that large might have been found frequently if the experiment were repeated. Although the investigators examine the findings in particular patients, their real interest is in determining whether the findings of the study could be generalized to other, similar hypertensive patients. To generalize beyond the participants in the single study, the investigators must know the extent to which the differences discovered in the study are reliable. The estimate of reliability is given by the standard error, which is not the same as the standard deviation discussed in Chapter 9.

1. Standard Deviation and Standard Error

Chapter 9 focused on *individual observations* and the extent to which they differed from the mean. One assertion was that a normal (gaussian) distribution could be completely described by its mean and standard deviation. Figure 9-6 showed that, for a truly normal distribution, 68% of observations fall within the range described as the mean ± 1 standard deviation, 95.4% fall within the range of the mean ± 2 standard deviations, and 95% fall within the range of the mean ± 1.96 standard deviations. This information is useful in describing individual observations (raw data), but it is not directly useful when comparing means or proportions.

Because most research is done on samples, rather than on complete populations, we need to have some idea of how close the mean of our study sample is likely to come to the real-world mean (i.e., mean in underlying population from whom the sample came). If we took 100 samples (such as might be done in multicenter trials), the means in our samples would differ from each other, but they would cluster around the true mean. We could plot the *sample means* just as we could plot individual observations, and if we did so, these means would show their own distribution. This distribution of means is also a normal (gaussian) distribution, with its own mean and standard deviation. The standard deviation of the distribution of *means* is called something different, the **standard error,** because it helps us to estimate the probable error of our sample mean's estimate of the true

population mean. The standard error is an unbiased estimate of the standard error in the entire population from whom the sample was taken. (Technically, the variance is an unbiased estimator of the population variance, and the standard deviation, although not quite unbiased, is close enough to being unbiased that it works well.)

The standard error is a parameter that enables the investigator to do two things that are central to the function of statistics. One is to estimate the probable amount of error around a quantitative assertion (called "confidence limits"). The other is to perform tests of statistical significance. If the standard deviation and sample size of one research sample are known, the standard error can be estimated.

The data shown in Table 10-1 can be used to explore the concept of standard error. The table lists the systolic and diastolic blood pressures of 26 young, healthy, adult subjects. To determine the range of expected variation in the estimate of the mean blood pressure obtained from the 26 subjects, the investigator would need an unbiased estimate of the variation in the underlying population. How can this be done with only one small sample?

Although the proof is not shown here, an unbiased estimate of the standard error can be obtained from the standard deviation of a single research sample if the standard deviation was originally calculated using the degrees of freedom ($N - 1$) in the denominator (see Chapter 9). The formula for converting this standard deviation (SD) to a standard error (SE) is as follows:

$$\text{Standard error} = \text{SE} = \frac{\text{SD}}{\sqrt{N}}$$

Table 10-1 **Systolic and Diastolic Blood Pressure Values of 26 Young, Healthy, Adult Participants**

Participant	Blood Pressure (mm Hg) Systolic	Blood Pressure (mm Hg) Diastolic	Gender
1	108	62	F
2	134	74	M
3	100	64	F
4	108	68	F
5	112	72	M
6	112	64	F
7	112	68	F
8	122	70	M
9	116	70	M
10	116	70	M
11	120	72	M
12	108	70	F
13	108	70	F
14	96	64	F
15	114	74	M
16	108	68	M
17	128	86	M
18	114	68	M
19	112	64	M
20	124	70	F
21	90	60	F
22	102	64	F
23	106	70	M
24	124	74	M
25	130	72	M
26	116	70	F

Data from unpublished findings in a sample of 26 professional persons in Connecticut.

The larger the sample size (N), the smaller is the standard error, and the better the estimate of the population mean. At any given point on the x-axis, the height of the bell-shaped curve for the distribution of the sample means represents the relative probability that a single sample mean would have that value. Most of the time, the sample mean would be near the true mean, which would be estimated closely by the mean of the means. Less often, it would be farther away from the average of the sample means.

In the medical literature, means are often reported either as the mean ± 1 SD or as the mean ± 1 SE. Reported data must be examined carefully to determine whether the SD or the SE is shown. Either is acceptable in theory because an SD can be converted to an SE, and vice versa, if the sample size is known. Many journals have a policy, however, stating whether the SD or SE must be reported. The sample size should always be shown.

2. Confidence Intervals

The SD shows the variability of individual observations, whereas the SE shows the variability of means. The mean ± 1.96 SD estimates the range in which 95% of individual observations would be expected to fall, whereas the mean ± 1.96 SE estimates the range in which 95% of the means of repeated samples of the same size would be expected to fall. If the value for the mean ± 1.96 SE is known, it can be used to calculate the 95% confidence interval, which is the range of values in which the investigator can be 95% confident that the true mean of the underlying population falls. Other confidence intervals, such as the 99% confidence interval, also can be determined easily. Box 10-2 shows the calculation of the SE and the 95% confidence interval for the systolic blood pressure data in Table 10-1.

Confidence intervals alone can be used as a test to determine whether a mean or proportion differs significantly from a **fixed value.** The most common situation for this is

testing to see whether a risk ratio or an odds ratio differs significantly from the ratio of 1.0 (which means no difference). If a risk ratio of 1.7 had a 95% confidence interval between 0.92 and 2.70, it would not be statistically significantly different from 1.0, if the alpha was chosen to be 0.05, because the confidence interval includes 1.0. If the same risk ratio had a 95% confidence interval between 1.02 and 2.60, however, it would be statistically significantly different from a risk ratio of 1.0 because 1.0 does not fall within the 95% confidence interval shown.

When a confidence interval does include the relevant fixed value, such as 1.0 for a risk ratio, it means that one cannot *exclude* the possibility that the intervention of interest differs in its effects from the control with 95% confidence. Within the *bounds* of 95% confidence is the possibility that the two interventions exert identical effects, that is, a risk ratio of 1.0.

A confidence interval thus provides the same service as a *p* value, indicating statistical significance. It goes beyond the *p* value, however, by showing what *range* of values, with 95% confidence, is likely to contain the value representing the "true" effect of the intervention. When a confidence interval is narrow, it defines the true effect within a small range of possible values; when the interval is wide, even if significant, it suggests the true effect lies within a wide range of possible values.

III. TESTS OF STATISTICAL SIGNIFICANCE

The tests described in this section allow investigators to compare two parameters, such as means or proportions, and to determine whether the difference between them is statistically significant. The various **t-tests** (one-tailed or two-tailed Student's *t*-test and paired *t*-test) compare differences between **means,** while **z-tests** compare differences between **proportions.** All these tests make comparisons possible by calculating the appropriate form of a ratio, called a **critical ratio** because it permits the investigator to make a decision. This is done by comparing the observed ratio (critical ratio) obtained from whatever test is performed (e.g., value of *t* from a *t*-test) with the values in the appropriate statistical table (e.g., table of *t* values) for the observed number of degrees of freedom.

Before individual tests are discussed in detail, the concepts of critical ratios and degrees of freedom are defined. The statistical tables of *t* values and *z* values are included at the end of the book (see Appendix, Tables B and C).

A. Critical Ratios

Critical ratios are the means by which tests of statistical significance enable clinicians to obtain a *p* value that is used to make a decision on the null hypothesis. A critical ratio is the ratio of some parameter in the numerator (e.g., a difference between means from two sets of data) divided by the **standard error** (SE) of that parameter (the standard error of the difference between the means). The general formula for tests of significance is as follows:

Box 10-2	Calculation of Standard Error and 95% Confidence Interval for Systolic Blood Pressure Values of 26 Subjects

PART 1 Beginning Data (see Table 10-1)

Number of observations, or N = 26
Mean, or x- = 113.1 mm Hg
Standard deviation, or SD = 10.3 mm Hg

PART 2 Calculation of Standard Error (SE)

$$SE = SD/\sqrt{N} = 10.3/\sqrt{26} = 10.3/5.1 = \textbf{2.02 mm Hg}$$

PART 3 Calculation of 95% Confidence Interval (95% CI)

$$95\% \ CI = mean \pm 1.96 \ SE$$
$$= 113.1 \pm (1.96)(2.02)$$
$$= 113.1 \pm 3.96$$
$$= between \ 113.1 - 3.96 \ and \ 113.1 + 3.96$$
$$= \textbf{109.1, 117.1 mm Hg}$$

$$\text{Critical ratio} = \frac{\text{Parameter}}{\text{SE of that parameter}}$$

When applied to the Student's *t*-test, the formula becomes:

$$\text{Critical ratio} = t = \frac{\text{Difference between two means}}{\text{SE of the difference between the two means}}$$

When applied to a *z*-test, the formula becomes:

$$\text{Critical ratio} = z = \frac{\text{Difference between two proportions}}{\text{SE of the difference between the two proportions}}$$

The value of the critical ratio (e.g., *t* or *z*) is looked up in the appropriate table (of *t* or *z* values; Appendix Tables B and C) to determine the corresponding value of *p*. (Note that statistical software packages [e.g., SAS, STATA, SPSS] generate the *p* value automatically.) For any critical ratio, the larger the ratio, the more likely it is that the difference between means or proportions is caused by more than just random variation (i.e., the more likely the difference can be considered statistically significant and real). Unless the total sample size is small (e.g., <30), the finding of a critical ratio of greater than about 2 usually indicates that the difference is statistically significant. This enables the investigator to reject the null hypothesis. The statistical tables adjust the critical ratios for the sample size by means of the degrees of freedom (see later).

The reason that a critical ratio works is complex and can best be explained using an illustration. Assume that an investigator conducted 1000 different clinical trials of the same *ineffective* antihypertensive drug, and each trial had the same large sample size. In each trial, assume that the investigator obtained an average value for the change in blood pressure in the experimental group ($\overline{x}_E$) and an average value for the change in blood pressure in the control group ($\overline{x}_C$). For each trial, there would be two means, and the difference between the means could be expressed as $\overline{x}_E - \overline{x}_C$. In this study the null hypothesis would be that the difference between the means was not a real difference.

If the null hypothesis were true (i.e., no true difference), chance variation would still cause $\overline{x}_E$ to be greater than $\overline{x}_C$ about half the time, despite the drug's lack of effect. The reverse would be true, also by chance, about half the time. In a rare trial, $\overline{x}_E$ would exactly equal $\overline{x}_C$. On the average, however, the differences between the two means would be near 0, reflecting the drug's lack of effect.

If the values representing the difference between the two means in each of the 1000 clinical trials were plotted on a graph, the distribution curve would appear normal (i.e., gaussian), with an average difference of 0, as in Figure 10-1, *A*. Chance variation would cause 95% of the values to fall within the large central zone, which covers the area of 0 ± 1.96 SE and is colored light blue. This is the zone for *failing to reject* the null hypothesis. Outside this zone is the zone for *rejecting* the null hypothesis, which consists of two areas colored dark blue (Fig. 10-1, *A*).

If only one clinical trial was performed, and if the ratio of the difference between the means of the two groups was outside the area of 0 ± 1.96 SE of the difference, either the study was a rare (i.e., ≤0.05) example of a false-positive difference, or there was a true difference between the groups. By setting alpha at 0.05, the investigator is willing to take a 5% risk (i.e., a 1-in-20 risk) of a false-positive assertion, but is not willing to take a higher risk. This implies that if alpha is set at 0.05, and if 20 data sets of two research samples that

are *not* truly different are compared, one "statistically significant" difference would be expected by chance alone. Some false-positive results are to be expected in the medical literature. They are inevitable, which is why follow-up studies are performed to confirm the findings.

B. Degrees of Freedom

The term *degrees of freedom* refers to the number of observations that are free to vary. Box 10-3 presents the idea behind this important statistical concept. For simplicity, the degrees of freedom for any test are considered to be the total sample size − 1 degree of freedom for each mean that is calculated. In Student's *t*-test, 2 degrees of freedom are lost because two means are calculated (one mean for each group whose means are to be compared). The general formula for the degrees of freedom for Student's two-group *t*-test is $N_1 + N_2 - 2$, where N_1 is the sample size in the first group, and N_2 is the sample size in the second group.

C. Use of *t*-Tests

Formerly, *t*-tests were among the three or four most frequently used statistical tests in medical research, and they still are often found.[1,2] The purpose of a *t*-test is to compare the means of a continuous variable in two research samples, such as a treatment group and a control group. This is done by determining whether the difference between the two observed means exceeds the difference that would be expected by chance from the two random samples.

I. Sample Populations and Sizes

If the two research samples come from two different groups (e.g., a group of men and a group of women), Student's *t*-test

---

Box 10-3	Idea behind the Degrees of Freedom

The term *degrees of freedom* refers to the number of observations *(N)* that are free to vary. A degree of freedom is lost every time a mean is calculated. Why should this be?

Before putting on a pair of gloves, a person has the freedom to decide whether to begin with the left or right glove. When the person puts on the first glove, however, he or she loses the freedom to decide which glove to put on last. If centipedes put on shoes, they would have a choice to make for the first 99 shoes, but not for the 100th shoe. Right at the end, the freedom to choose (vary) is restricted.

In statistics, if there are two observed values, only one estimate of the variation between them is possible. Something has to serve as the basis against which other observations are compared. The mean is the most *solid* estimate of the expected value of a variable, so it is assumed to be *fixed*. This implies that the numerator of the mean (the sum of individual observations, or the sum of x_i), which is based on *N* observations, is also fixed. When *N* − 1 observations (each of which was, presumably, free to vary) have been added up, the last observation is not free to vary because the total values of the *N* observations must add up to the sum of x_i. For this reason, 1 degree of freedom is lost each time a mean is calculated. When estimating the variance of a sample, the proper variance is the sum of squares divided by the degrees of freedom (*N* − 1).

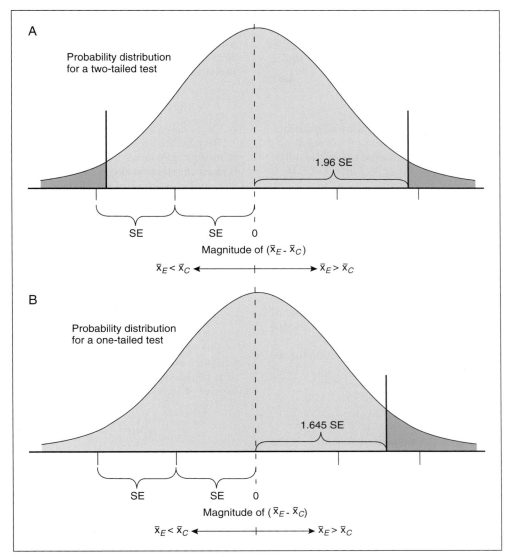

Figure 10-1 Probability distribution of difference between two means when null hypothesis is actually true (i.e., when there is no real difference between the two means). *Dark blue,* Zone for rejecting the null hypothesis; *light blue,* zone for failing to reject the null hypothesis. **A,** When a two-tailed test is used, there is a rejection zone on each side of the distribution. **B,** When a one-tailed test is used, there is a rejection zone on only one side. *SE,* Standard error; $\bar{x}_E$, mean for experimental group; $\bar{x}_C$, mean for control group.

is used. If the two samples come from the same group (e.g., pretreatment and posttreatment values for the same study participants), the paired *t*-test is used.

The two-sample (Student's) *t*-test and the paired *t*-test depend on certain assumptions, including the assumption that the data being studied are normally distributed in the larger population from which the sample came. Very seldom, however, are observed data perfectly normally distributed. This does not invalidate the *t*-test because there is a convenient theorem that rescues the *t*-test (and much of statistics as well). The **central limit theorem** can be derived theoretically or observed by experimentation. According to the theorem, for reasonably large samples (e.g., ≥30 observations of blood pressure in each sample), the distribution of the means of many samples is *normal* (gaussian), although the data in individual samples may have skewness, kurtosis, or unevenness. Because the critical theoretical requirement for the *t*-test is that the sample means be *normally distributed,* a

t-test may be computed on almost any set of continuous data, if the observations can be considered a random sample, and if the sample size is reasonably large.

2. t Distribution

The *t* distribution was described by Gosset, who used the pseudonym "Student" when he wrote the description. Salsburg gives one explanation of how the *t*-test received its name and other humorous perspectives on statistics.[3] The normal distribution is also called the *z* distribution. The *t* distribution looks similar to the *z* distribution except that its tails are wider and its peak is slightly less high, depending on the sample size. The *t* distribution is needed because when the sample sizes of studies are small, the observed estimates of the mean and variance are subject to considerable error. The larger the sample size, the smaller are the errors, and the more the *t* distribution looks like the normal distribution. If the sample size were infinite, the two distributions would be identical. For practical purposes, when the combined sample size of the two groups being compared is larger than 120, the difference between the normal distribution and the *t* distribution is negligible.

3. *Student's t-Test*

Student's *t*-test can be one-tailed or two-tailed. The calculations are the same, but the interpretation of the resulting *t* differs. The common features are discussed before the differences are outlined.

CALCULATION OF THE VALUE OF *T*

In both types of Student's *t*-test, *t* is calculated by taking the observed difference between the means of the two groups (the numerator) and dividing this difference by the standard error of the difference between the means of the two groups (the denominator). Before *t* can be calculated, the **standard error of the difference between the means** (SED) must be determined. The basic formula for this is the square root of the sum of the respective population variances, each divided by its own sample size.

For a theoretical distribution, the correct equation for the SED would be as follows:

$$\text{SED of } \mu_E - \mu_C = \sqrt{\frac{\sigma_E^2}{N_E} + \frac{\sigma_C^2}{N_C}}$$

where the Greek letter μ is the population mean, E is the experimental population, C is the control population, σ^2 is the variance of the population, and N is the number of observations in the population. The rationale behind this formula is discussed in Box 10-4.

The theoretical formula requires that the population variances be known, which usually is not true with experimental data. Nevertheless, if the sample sizes are large enough (e.g., if the total of the two samples is ≥ 30), the previous formula

can be used with the sample variances substituted for the population variances. When dealing with samples, instead of using Greek letters in the formulas, the italic Roman symbol $\bar{x}$ is used to indicate the mean of the sample, and the italic Roman symbol s^2 is used to indicate the variance:

$$\text{Estimate of the SED of } \bar{x}_E - \bar{x}_C = \sqrt{\frac{s_E^2}{N_E} + \frac{s_C^2}{N_C}}$$

Because the *t*-test typically is used to test a null hypothesis of *no difference between two means*, the assumption generally is made that there is also no difference between the variances, so a **pooled estimate of the SED** (SED_P) may be used instead. In this case, if the sample sizes are approximately equal in the two groups, and if the combined sample size is large enough (e.g., >30 in the combined sample), the previous formula for the estimate of the standard error of the difference becomes:

$$\text{SED}_p \text{ of } \bar{x}_E - \bar{x}_C = \sqrt{s_P^2\left(\frac{1}{N_E} + \frac{1}{N_C}\right)}$$
$$= \sqrt{s_P^2[(1/N_E) + (1/N_C)]}$$

The s_P^2, called the **pooled estimate of the variance,** is a weighted average of s_E^2 and s_C^2. The s_P^2 is calculated as the sum of the two sums of squares divided by the combined degrees of freedom:

$$s_P^2 = \frac{\sum(x_1 - \bar{x}_E)^2 + \sum(x_C - \bar{x}_C)^2}{N_E + N_C - 2}$$

If one sample size is much greater than the other, or if the variance of one sample is much greater than the variance of the other, more complex formulas are needed.[4] When Student's *t*-test is used to test the null hypothesis in research involving an experimental group and a control group, it usually takes the general form of the following equation:

$$t = \frac{\bar{x}_E + \bar{x}_C - 0}{\sqrt{s_P^2[(1/N_E) + (1/N_C)]}}$$
$$df = N_E + N_C - 2$$

The 0 in the numerator of the equation for *t* was added for correctness because the *t*-test determines if the difference between the means is significantly different from 0. Because the 0 does not affect the calculations in any way, however, it is usually omitted from *t*-test formulas.

The same formula, recast in terms to apply to any two independent samples (e.g., samples of men and women), is as follows:

$$t = \frac{\bar{x}_1 - \bar{x}_2 - 0}{\sqrt{s_P^2[(1/N_1) + (1/N_2)]}}$$
$$df = N_1 + N_2 - 2$$

in which $\bar{x}_1$ is the mean of the first sample, $\bar{x}_2$ is the mean of the second sample, s_P^2 is the pooled estimate of the variance, N_1 is the size of the first sample, N_2 is the size of the second sample, and *df* is the degrees of freedom. The 0 in the numerator indicates that the null hypothesis states the

---

Box 10-4	**Formula for Standard Error of Difference between Means**

The standard error equals the standard deviation (σ) divided by the square root of the sample size *(N)*. Alternatively, this can be expressed as the square root of the variance (σ^2) divided by *N*:

$$\text{Standard error} = \text{SE} = \frac{\sigma}{\sqrt{N}} = \sqrt{\frac{\sigma^2}{N}}$$

As mentioned in Chapter 9 (see Box 9-2), the variance of a difference is equal to the sum of the variances. The variance of the difference between the mean of an experimental group (μ_E) and the mean of a control group (μ_C) could be expressed as follows: $\sigma_E^2 + \sigma_C^2$.

As shown above, a standard error can be written as the square root of the variance divided by the sample size, allowing the equation to be expressed as:

$$\text{Standard error of } \mu_E - \mu_C = \sqrt{\frac{\sigma_E^2}{N_E} + \frac{\sigma_C^2}{N_C}}$$

Box 10-5	Calculation of Results from Student's *t*-Test Comparing Systolic Blood Pressure of 14 Male Participants with 12 Female Participants

PART 1 Beginning Data (see Table 10-1)

Number of observations, or $N = 14$ for males, or M; 12 for females, or F
Mean, or $\bar{x} = 118.3$ mm Hg for males; 107.0 mm Hg for females
Variance, or $s^2 = 70.1$ mm Hg for males; 82.5 mm Hg for females
Sum of $(\bar{x}_i - \bar{x})^2$, or TSS $= 911.3$ mm Hg for males; 907.5 mm Hg for females
Alpha value for the *t*-test = 0.05

PART 2 Calculation of *t* Value Based on Pooled Variance (s_P^2) and Pooled Standard Error of the Difference (SED$_P$)

$$s_P^2 = \frac{TSS_M + TSS_F}{N_M + N_F - 2} = \frac{911.3 + 907.5}{14 + 12 - 2} = \frac{1818.8}{24} = 75.78 \text{ mm Hg}$$

$$SED_P = \sqrt{s_P^2[(1/N_M) + (1/N_F)]}$$

$$= \sqrt{75.78[(1/14) + (1/12)]}$$

$$= \sqrt{75.78(0.1548)} = \sqrt{11.73} = 3.42 \text{ mm Hg}$$

$$t = \frac{\bar{x}_M - \bar{x}_F - 0}{\sqrt{s_P^2[(1/N_M) + (1/N_F)]}} = \frac{\bar{x}_M - \bar{x}_F - 0}{SED_P}$$

$$= \frac{118.3 + 107.0 - 0}{3.42} = \frac{11.30}{3.42} = \textbf{3.30}$$

PART 3 Alternative Calculation of *t* Value Based on SED Equation Using Observed Variances for Males and Females, Rather than Based on SED$_P$ Equation Using Pooled Variance

$$SED = \sqrt{\frac{s_M^2}{N_M} + \frac{s_F^2}{N_M}} = \sqrt{\frac{70.1}{14} + \frac{82.5}{12}}$$

$$= \sqrt{5.01 + 6.88} = \sqrt{11.89} = 3.45 \text{ mm}$$

$$t = \frac{\bar{x}_M - \bar{x}_F - 0}{SED}$$

$$= \frac{118.3 + 107.0 - 0}{3.45} = \frac{11.30}{3.45} = \textbf{3.28}$$

Compared with the equation in Part 2, the equation in Part 3 usually is easier to remember and to calculate, and it adjusts for differences in the variances and the sample sizes. The result here ($t = 3.28$) is almost identical to that above ($t = 3.30$), even though the sample size is small.

PART 4 Calculation of Degrees of Freedom (*df*) for *t*-test and Interpretation of *t* value

$$df = N_M + N_F - 2 = 14 + 12 - 2 = 24$$

For a *t* value of 3.30, with 24 degrees of freedom, *p* value is less than 0.01, as indicated in the table of the values of *t* (see Appendix). This means that the male participants have a significantly different (higher) systolic blood pressure than do the female participants in this data set.

difference between the means would not be significantly different from 0.* The *df* is needed to enable the investigator to refer to the correct line in the table of the values of *t* and their relationship to the *p* value (see Appendix, Table C).

Box 10-5 shows the use of a *t*-test to compare the mean systolic blood pressures of the 14 men and 12 women whose

---

*The value stated in the null hypothesis could be different from 0. In that case, the test would determine whether the observed difference between means was greater than the number in the null hypothesis, which might be a minimum goal. Because the 0—or other number—does not contribute to the variance, it does not alter the denominator. Because the hypothesis still asserts there is "no difference" in the numerator, it is still a null hypothesis.

data were given in Table 10-1. Box 10-6 presents a different and more visual way of understanding the *t*-test.

The *t*-test is designed to help investigators distinguish *explained variation* from *unexplained variation* (random error, or chance). These concepts are similar to the concepts of *signal* and *background noise* in radio broadcast engineering. Listeners who are searching for a particular station on their radio dial find background noise on almost every radio frequency. When they reach the station they want to hear, they may not notice the background noise because the signal is much stronger than the noise. Because the radio can amplify a weak signal greatly, the critical factor is the ratio of the strength of the signal to the strength of the background noise. The greater the ratio, the clearer is the station's

Box 10-6   Does the Eye Naturally Perform ± t-Tests?

The paired diagrams in this box show three patterns of overlap between two frequency distributions (e.g., a treatment group and a control group). These distributions can be thought of as the frequency distributions of systolic blood pressure values among hypertensive patients after randomization and treatment either with an experimental drug or with a placebo. The treatment group's distribution is shown in *gray,* the control group's distribution is shown in *blue,* and the area of overlap is shown with gray and blue hatch marks. The means are indicated by the vertical dotted lines. The three different pairs show variation in the spread of systolic blood pressure values.

Examine the three diagrams. Then try to guess whether each pair was sampled from the same universe (i.e., was not significantly different) or was sampled from two different universes (i.e., was significantly different).

Most observers believe that the distributions in pair A look as though they were sampled from different universes. When asked why they think so, they usually state that there is little overlap between the two frequency distributions. Most observers are not convinced that the distributions in either pair B or pair C were sampled from different universes. They say that there is considerable overlap in each of these

pairs, and this makes them doubt that there is a real difference. Their visual impressions are indeed correct.

It is not the absolute distance between the two means that leads most observers to say "different" for pair A and "not different" for pair B, because the distance between the means was drawn to be exactly the same in pairs A and B. It is also not the absolute amount of dispersion that causes them to say "different" for pair A and "not different" for pair C, because the dispersions were drawn to be the same in pairs A and C. The essential point, which the eye notices, is the ratio of the distance between the means to the variation around the means. The greater the distance between the means for a given amount of dispersion, the less likely it is that the samples were from the same universe. This ratio is exactly what the *t*-test calculates:

$$t = \frac{\text{Distance between the means}}{\text{Variation around the means}}$$

where the variation around the means is expressed as the standard error of the difference between the means. The eye naturally does a *t*-test, although it does not quantify the relationship as precisely as does the *t*-test.

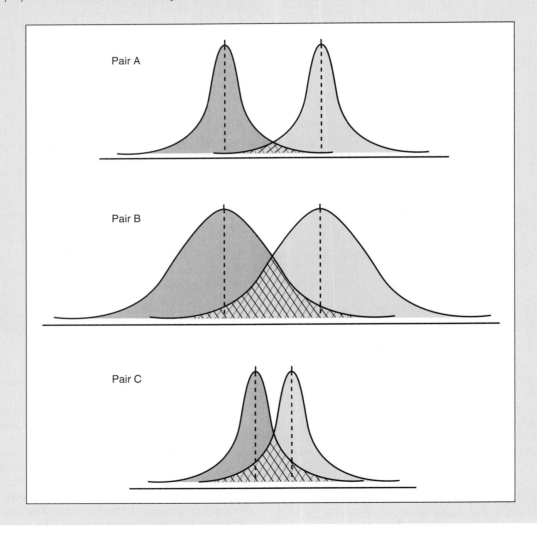

Pair A

Pair B

Pair C

sound. The closer the ratio is to 1.0 (i.e., the point at which the magnitude of the noise equals that of the signal), the less satisfactory is the sound the listener hears.

In medical studies the particular factor being investigated is similar to the radio signal, and random error is similar to background noise. Statistical analysis helps distinguish one from the other by comparing their strength. If the variation caused by the intervention is considerably larger than the variation caused by random factors (i.e., in the t-test the ratio is >1.96), the effect of the intervention becomes detectable above the statistical *noise* of random factors.

INTERPRETATION OF THE RESULTS

If the value of t is large, the p value is small because it is unlikely that a large t ratio would be obtained by chance alone. If the p value is ≤0.05, it is customary to accept the difference as real. Such findings are called "statistically significant."

Conceptually, the p value is the probability of being in error if the null hypothesis of no difference between the means is rejected (and the alternative hypothesis of a true difference is accepted).

ONE-TAILED AND TWO-TAILED ±t-TESTS

The conceptual diagram in Figure 10-1 shows the theory behind the acceptance and rejection regions for the one-tailed and two-tailed types of Student's t-test. These tests are also sometimes called a *one-sided test* or a *two-sided test*.

In the two-tailed test the alpha (e.g., of 0.05) is equally divided at the ends of the two tails of the distribution (see Fig. 10-1, *A*). The two-tailed test is generally recommended because differences in either direction are usually important to document. For example, it is important to know if a new treatment is significantly better than a standard or placebo treatment, but it is also important to know if a new treatment is significantly worse and should be avoided. In this situation the two-tailed test provides an accepted criterion for when a difference shows the new treatment to be better or worse.

Sometimes, only a one-tailed test is appropriate. Suppose that a new therapy is known to cost much more than the currently used treatment. It would not be used if it were worse than the current therapy, but it also would not be used if it were merely as good as the current therapy. It would be used only if it were significantly better than the current therapy. Under these circumstances, some investigators consider it acceptable to use a one-tailed test because they are concerned only with whether the new treatment is *better*; if it is not better, it will not be recommended. In this situation the 5% rejection region for the null hypothesis is all at one tail of the distribution (see Fig. 10-1, *B*), instead of being evenly divided between the extremes of the two tails.

In the one-tailed test the null hypothesis nonrejection region extends only to 1.645 standard errors above the "no difference" point of 0. In the two-tailed test, it extends to 1.96 SE above and below the "no difference" point. This makes the one-tailed test more robust, that is, more able to detect a significant difference, if it is in the expected direction. Many investigators dislike one-tailed tests because they believe that if an intervention is significantly worse than the standard therapy, that fact should be documented

scientifically. Most reviewers and editors require that the use of a one-tailed significance test be justified. The two-tailed test is more *conservative*, making it more difficult to reject the null hypothesis when the outcome is in the expected direction. The implications of choosing a one-tailed or two-tailed test are explored further in Box 10-7.

4. Paired t-Test

In many medical studies, individuals are followed over time to see if there is a change in the value of some continuous variable. Typically, this occurs in a "before and after" experiment, such as one testing to see if there was a decrease in average blood pressure after treatment or to see if there was a reduction in weight after the use of a special diet. In this type of comparison, an individual patient serves as his or her own control. The appropriate statistical test for this type of data is the paired t-test. The paired t-test is more robust than Student's t-test because it considers the variation from only one group of people, whereas Student's t-test considers variation from two groups. Variation that is detected in the paired t-test is presumably attributable to the intervention or to changes over time in the same person.

Box 10-7	**Implications of Choosing a One-Tailed or Two-Tailed Test of Significance**

For students who are confused by the implications of choosing a one-tailed or two-tailed test, a football analogy may be helpful. The coach of a football team wants to assess the skill of potential quarterbacks. He is unwilling to allow mere completion of a pass to serve as evidence of throwing accuracy because he knows that a pass could be completed by chance, even if the football did not go where the quarterback intended. Because the coach is an amateur statistician, he further infers that if the quarterback were to throw randomly, the ball would often land near the center of the field and would less often land way off toward one sideline or the other. The distribution of random throws on the 100-foot-wide field might even be gaussian (thinks the coach).

The coach asks quarterback applicants to throw to a receiver along the sideline. The coach announces that each applicant has a choice: (1) he may pick one side ahead of time and complete a pass to that side within 5 feet of the sideline, or (2) he may throw to either side, but then must complete the pass within 2.5 feet of the sideline. The coach's null hypothesis is simply that the quarterback would not be able to complete a pass within the specified zone. In either case, a complete pass outside the specified zone would be attributed to chance because it is not what was intended.

The coach does not give applicants the option of throwing to either side and completing the pass within 5 feet of the sideline. If the coach were to allow applicants to elect this option, the coach would "reject" his null hypothesis on the basis of chance 10% of the time, and he is unwilling to take so great a risk of selecting a lucky but unskillful quarterback.

The quarterback has more room to work with if he prefers to throw to one side (one-tailed test) and can count on throwing in only that direction. If he is unsure in which direction he may wish to throw, he can get credit for a completed pass in either direction (two-tailed test), but has only a narrow zone for which to aim.

CALCULATION OF THE VALUE OF *T*

To calculate a paired *t*-test, a new variable must be created. This variable, called *d*, is the difference between the values before and after the intervention for each individual studied. The paired *t*-test is a test of the null hypothesis that, on the average, the difference is equal to 0, which is what would be expected if there were no change over time. Using the symbol $\bar{d}$ to indicate the mean observed difference between the before and after values, the formula for the paired *t*-test is as follows:

$$t_{\text{paired}} = t_p = \frac{\bar{d}_1 - 0}{\text{Standard error of } \bar{d}}$$

$$= \frac{\bar{d} - 0}{\sqrt{\dfrac{s_d^2}{N}}}$$

$$df = N - 1$$

The numerator contains a 0 because the null hypothesis says that the observed difference will not differ from 0; however, the 0 does not enter into the calculation and can be omitted. Because the 0 in this formula is a constant, it has no variance, and the only error in estimating the mean difference is its own standard error.

The formulas for Student's *t*-test and the paired *t*-test are similar: the ratio of a difference to the variation around that difference (the standard error). In Student's *t*-test, each of the two distributions to be compared contributes to the variation of the difference, and the two variances must be added. In the paired *t*-test, there is only one frequency distribution, that of the before-after difference in each person. In the paired *t*-test, because only one mean is calculated $(\bar{d})$, only 1 degree of freedom is lost; the formula for the degrees of freedom is $N - 1$.

INTERPRETATION OF THE RESULTS

The values of *t* and their relationship to *p* are shown in a statistical table in the Appendix (see Table C). If the value of *t* is large, the *p* value will be small because it is unlikely that a large *t* ratio would be obtained by chance alone. If the *p* value is 0.05 or less, it is customary to assume that there is a real difference (i.e., that the null hypothesis of no difference can be rejected).

D. Use of *z*-Tests

In contrast to *t*-tests, which compare differences between means, *z*-tests compare differences between proportions. In medicine, examples of proportions that are frequently studied are sensitivity; specificity; positive predictive value; risks; and percentages of people with symptoms, illness, or recovery. Frequently, the goal of research is to see if the proportion of patients surviving in a treated group differs from that in an untreated group. This can be evaluated using a *z*-test for proportions.

CALCULATION OF THE VALUE OF *Z*

As discussed earlier (see Critical Ratios), *z* is calculated by taking the observed difference between the two proportions

(the numerator) and dividing it by the standard error of the difference between the two proportions (the denominator). For purposes of illustration, assume that research is being conducted to see if the proportion of patients surviving in a treated group is greater than that in an untreated group. For each group, if *p* is the proportion of successes (survivals), then $1 - p$ is the proportion of failures (nonsurvivals). If *N* represents the size of the group on whom the proportion is based, the parameters of the proportion could be calculated as follows:

$$\text{Variance (proportion)} = \frac{p(1-p)}{N}$$

$$\text{Standard error (proportion)} = \text{SE}_p = \sqrt{\frac{p(1-p)}{N}}$$

$$95\% \text{ Confidence interval} = 95\% \text{ CI} = p \pm 1.96 \, \text{SE}_p$$

If there is a 0.60 (60%) survival rate after a given treatment, the calculations of SE_p and the 95% CI (confidence interval) of the proportion, based on a sample of 100 study subjects, would be as follows:

$$\text{SE}_p = \sqrt{(0.6)(0.4)/100}$$

$$= \sqrt{0.24/100}$$

$$= 0.049$$

$$95\% \text{ CI} = 0.6 \pm (1.96)(0.049)$$

$$= 0.6 \pm 0.096$$

$$= \text{between } 0.6 - 0.096 \text{ and } 0.6 + 0.096$$

$$= 0.504, 0.696$$

The result of the CI calculation means that in 95% of cases, the "true" proportion surviving in the universe is expected to be between 50.4% and 69.6%.

Now that there is a way to obtain the standard error of a proportion, the **standard error of the difference between proportions** also can be obtained, and the equation for the *z*-test can be expressed as follows:

$$z = \frac{p_1 - p_2 - 0}{\sqrt{\bar{p}(1-\bar{p})[(1/N_1) + (1/N_2)]}}$$

in which p_1 is the proportion of the first sample, p_2 is the proportion of the second sample, N_1 is the size of the first sample, N_2 is the size of the second sample, and $\bar{P}$ is the mean proportion of successes in all observations combined. The 0 in the numerator indicates that the null hypothesis states that the difference between the proportions will not be significantly different from 0.

INTERPRETATION OF THE RESULTS

The previous formula for *z* is similar to the formula for *t* in Student's *t*-test, as described earlier (see the pooled variance formula). Because the variance and the standard error of the proportion are based on a theoretical distribution (binomial approximation to *z* distribution), however, the *z* distribution is used instead of the *t* distribution in determining whether the difference is statistically significant. When the *z* ratio is large, as when the *t* ratio is large, the difference is more likely to be real.

The computations for the z-test appear different from the computations for the chi-square test (see Chapter 11), but when the same data are set up as a 2 × 2 table, the results are identical. Most people find it easier to do a chi-square test than to do a z-test for proportions, but they both accomplish the same goal.

E. Use of Other Tests

Chapter 11 discusses other statistical significance tests used in the analysis of two variables (bivariate analysis), and Chapter 13 discusses tests used in the analysis of multiple independent variables (multivariable analysis).

IV. SPECIAL CONSIDERATIONS

A. Variation between Groups versus Variation within Groups

If the differences between two groups are found to be statistically significant, it is appropriate to ask why the groups are different and how much of the total variation is explained by the variable defining the two groups, such as treatment versus control. A straightforward comparison of the heights of men and women can be used to illustrate the considerations involved in answering the following question: Why are men taller than women? Although biologists might respond that genetic, hormonal, and perhaps nutritional factors explain the differences in height, a biostatistician would take a different approach. After first pointing out that individual men are not always taller than individual women, but that the average height of men is greater than that of women, the biostatistician would seek to determine the amount of the total variation in height that is explained by the gender

difference and whether or not the difference is more than would be expected by chance.

For purposes of this discussion, suppose that the heights of 200 randomly selected university students were measured, that 100 of these students were men and 100 were women, and that the unit of measure was centimeters. As discussed in Chapter 9, the **total variation** would be equal to the sum of the squared deviations, which is usually called the **total sum of squares** (TSS) but sometimes referred to simply as the **sum of squares** (SS). In the total group of 200 students, suppose that the total SS (the sum of the squared deviations from the average height for all 200 students) was found to be 10,000 cm². This number is the total amount of variation that needs to be explained in the data set. The biostatistician would begin by seeking to determine how much of this variation was caused by gender and how much was caused by other factors.

Figure 10-2 shows a hypothetical frequency distribution of the heights of a sample of women (black marks) and a sample of men (blue marks), indicating the density of observations at the different heights. An approximate normal curve is drawn over each of the two distributions, and the overall mean *(grand mean)* is indicated by the vertical dotted line, along with the mean height for women (a *gender mean*) and the mean height for men (a gender mean).

Measuring the TSS (the total unexplained variation) from the grand mean yielded a result of 10,000 cm². Measuring the SS for men from the mean for men and the SS for women from the mean for women would yield a smaller amount of unexplained variation, about 6000 cm². This leaves 60% of the variation still to be explained. The other 40% of the variation is explained, however, by the variable *gender*. From a statistical perspective, *explaining variation* implies reducing the unexplained SS. If more explanatory variables (e.g., age, height of father, height of mother, nutritional status) are

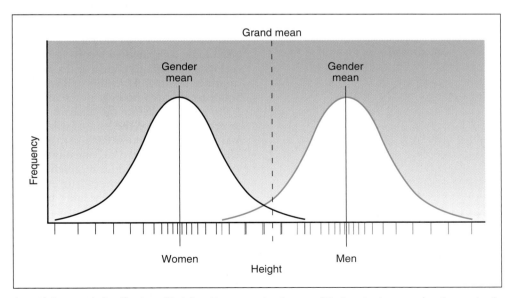

Figure 10-2 Hypothetical frequency distribution of heights. From a sample of women (*black marks* along x-axis) and a sample of men (*blue marks* along x-axis), indicating the density of observations at the different heights. An approximate normal curve is drawn over each of the two distributions, and the overall mean (grand mean) is indicated by the *vertical dashed line*, along with the mean height for women (a gender mean) and the mean height for men (a gender mean).

analyzed, the unexplained SS may be reduced still further, and even more of the variation can be said to be *explained.*

The following question is even more specific: Why is the shortest woman shorter than the tallest man? Statistically, there are two parts to the explanation:

■ She is a member of the class (group) of individuals (women) who have a shorter mean height than do men.
■ She is the shortest of her group of women, and the man selected is the tallest of the group of men, so they are at the opposite extremes of height within their respective groups.

The greater the distance between the means for men and women, the greater is the proportion of the variation likely to be explained by **variation between groups.** The larger the standard deviation of heights of women and men, the greater is the proportion of the variation likely to be explained by **variation within groups.** The within-groups variation might be reduced still further, however, if other independent variables were added.

Suppose that all women were of equal height, all men were of equal height, and men were taller than women (Fig. 10-3, *A*). What percentage of the variation in height would be explained by gender, and what percentage would be

unexplained? The answer is that all the variation would be caused by gender (between-groups variation), and because there is no within-groups variation, no variation would be left unexplained.

Alternatively, suppose that women varied in height, that men varied in height, and that the mean heights of the men and women were the same (Fig. 10-3, *B*). Now what percentage of the variation in height would be explained by gender, and what percentage would be unexplained? None of the variation would be caused by gender, and all of it would be left unexplained.

This simple example shows what statistics ultimately tries to do: divide the total variation into a part that is explained by the independent variables (called the "model") and a part that is still unexplained. This activity is called **analyzing variation** or analyzing the TSS. A specific method for doing this under certain circumstances and testing hypotheses at the same time is called **analysis of variance** (ANOVA) (see Chapter 13).

B. Clinical Importance and External Validity versus Statistical Significance

A frequent error made by investigators has been to find a statistically significant difference, reject the null hypothesis, and recommend the finding as being useful for determining disease etiology, making a clinical diagnosis, or treating disease, without considering whether the finding is clinically important or whether it has external validity. Testing for statistical significance is important because it helps investigators reject assertions that are not true. Even if a finding is **statistically significant,** however, it may not be **clinically or scientifically important.** For example, with a very large sample size, it is possible to show that an average decrease of 2 mm Hg in blood pressure with a certain medication is statistically significant. Such a small decrease in blood pressure would not be of much clinical use, however, and would not be clinically important in a single patient. However, an average reduction in blood pressure by this amount in a large population might prevent some heart attacks and strokes and have some value, although the limited benefits would need to be compared with costs and side effects. Sometimes a clinician treating a patient and a public health practitioner considering an intervention with wide population impact interpret research findings differently.

In addition, before the findings of a study can be put to general clinical use, the issue of whether the study has **external validity,** or **generalizability,** must be addressed. In a clinical trial of a new drug, one must ask whether the **sample** of patients in the study is representative of the **universe** of patients for whom the new drug eventually might be used. Studies can lack external validity because the **spectrum of disease** in the sample of patients is different from the spectrum of disease in the universe of patients. Types, stages, and severity of disease can vary. The spectrum must be defined clearly in terms of the criteria for including or excluding patients, and these criteria must be reported with the findings. If patients with a severe form of the disease were excluded from the study, this **exclusion criterion** must be reported because the results of the study would not be generalizable to patients with severe disease. (See the discussion of the Physicians' Health Study in Chapter 4; the results from

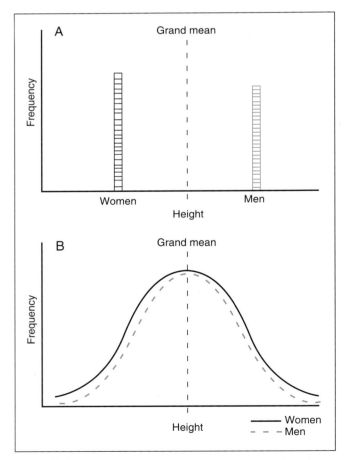

Figure 10-3 Two hypothetical frequency distributions of heights.
From a sample of women *(black lines)* and a sample of men *(blue lines).* **A,** How the distribution would appear if all women were of equal height, all men were of equal height, and men were taller than women. **B,** How the distribution would appear if women varied in height, men varied in height, but the mean heights of men and women were the same.

a study of healthy, compliant physicians might not be generalizable to all adults.)

The study also can lack external validity because the **spectrum of individual characteristics** in the sample of patients was different from the spectrum of individual characteristics in the universe of patients. The sample could differ from most patients on the basis of age, gender, income or educational level, ethnic background, and many other characteristics.

V. SUMMARY

Statistics is an aid to inductive reasoning, which is the effort to find generalizable relationships and differences in observed data. It is the reverse process from mathematics, which is the attempt to apply known formulas to specific data to predict an outcome. Statistics helps investigators reach reasonable conclusions and estimations from observed data and provide approximate limits to the probability of being in error when making conclusions and estimations from the data. Significance testing starts with the statement of a null hypothesis, such as the hypothesis that there is no true difference between the mean found in an experimental group and the mean found in the control group. The test of statistical significance (a critical ratio) provides a p value that gives the probability of being wrong if the null hypothesis is rejected. If the results

of the significance test allow the investigator to reject the null hypothesis, the investigator can accept the alternative hypothesis that a true difference exists.

Student's t-test enables the investigator to compare the means of a continuous variable (e.g., weight) from two different groups of study subjects to determine whether the difference between the means is greater than would be expected by chance alone. The paired t-test enables the investigator to evaluate the average in a continuous variable in a group of study participants before and after some intervention is given. In contrast to t-tests, which compare the difference between means, z-tests compare the difference between proportions.

References

1. Emerson JD, Colditz GA: Use of statistical analysis. *N Engl J Med* 309:709–713, 1983.
2. Horton NJ, Switzer SS: Statistical methods in the *Journal*. *N Engl J Med* 353:1977–1979, 2005.
3. Salsburg D: *The lady tasting tea,* New York, 2001, Holt.
4. Moore DS, McCabe GP: *Introduction to the practice of statistics,* New York, 1993, Freeman.

Select Reading

Dawson-Saunders B, Trapp RG: *Basic and clinical biostatistics,* ed 4, New York, 2004, Lange Medical Books/McGraw-Hill.

Bivariate Analysis

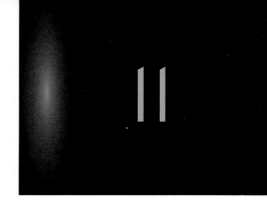

A variety of statistical tests can be used to analyze the relationship between two or more variables. Similar to Chapter 10, this chapter focuses on **bivariate analysis,** which is the analysis of the relationship between one independent (possibly causal) variable and one dependent (outcome) variable. Chapter 13 focuses on **multivariable analysis,** or the analysis of the relationship of more than one independent variable

to a single dependent variable. (The term *multivariate* technically refers to analysis of multiple independent *and* multiple dependent variables, although it is often used interchangeably with *multivariable*). Statistical tests should be chosen only after the types of clinical data to be analyzed and the basic research design have been established. Steps in developing a research protocol include posing a good question; establishing a research hypothesis; establishing suitable measures; and deciding on the study design. The selection of measures in turn indicates the appropriate methods of statistical analysis. In general, the analytic approach should begin with a study of the individual variables, including their distributions and outliers, and a search for errors. Then bivariate analysis can be done to test hypotheses and probe for relationships. Only after these procedures have been done, and if there is more than one independent variable to consider, should multivariable analysis be conducted.

I. CHOOSING AN APPROPRIATE STATISTICAL TEST

Among the factors involved in choosing an appropriate statistical test are the goals and research design of the study and the type of data being collected. Statistical testing is not required when the results of interest are purely descriptive, such as percentages, sensitivity, or specificity. Statistical testing is required whenever the quantitative difference in a measure between groups, or a change in a measure over time, is of interest. A contrast or change in a measure may be caused by random factors or a meaningful association; statistical testing is intended to make this distinction.

Table 11-1 shows the numerous tests of statistical significance that are available for bivariate (two-variable) analysis. The types of variables and the research design set the limits to statistical analysis and determine which test or tests are appropriate. The four **types of variables** are *continuous* data (e.g., levels of glucose in blood samples), *ordinal* data (e.g., rankings of very satisfied, satisfied, and unsatisfied), *dichotomous* data (e.g., alive vs. dead), and *nominal* data (e.g., ethnic group). An investigator must understand the types of variables and how the type of variable influences the choice of statistical tests, just as a painter must understand types of media (e.g., oils, tempera, watercolors) and how the different media influence the appropriate brushes and techniques to be used.

The type of research design also is important when choosing a form of statistical analysis. If the **research design** involves *before-and-after comparisons* in the same study

Table 11-1 Choice of Appropriate Statistical Significance Test in Bivariate Analysis (Analysis of One Independent Variable and One Dependent Variable)

First Variable	Second Variable	Examples	Appropriate Test or Tests of Significance
Continuous (C)	Continuous (C)	Age (C) and systolic blood pressure (C)	Pearson correlation coefficient (r); linear regression
Continuous (C)	Ordinal (O)	Age (C) and satisfaction (O)*	Group the continuous variable and calculate Spearman correlation coefficient (rho)†
Continuous (C)	Dichotomous unpaired (DU)	Systolic blood pressure (C) and gender (DU)	Student's t-test
Continuous (C)	Dichotomous paired (DP)	Difference in systolic blood pressure (C) before vs. after treatment (DP)	Paired t-test
Continuous (C)	Nominal (N)	Hemoglobin level (C) and blood type (N)	ANOVA (*F*-test)
Ordinal (O)	Ordinal (O)	Correlation of care (O)* and severity of satisfaction with illness (O)	Spearman correlation coefficient (rho); Kendall correlation coefficient (tau)
Ordinal (O)	Dichotomous unpaired (DU)	Satisfaction (O) and gender (DU)	Mann-Whitney U test
Ordinal (O)	Dichotomous paired (DP)	Difference in satisfaction (O) before vs. after a program (DP)	Wilcoxon matched-pairs signed-ranks test
Ordinal (O)	Nominal (N)	Satisfaction (O) and ethnicity (N)	Kruskal-Wallis test
Dichotomous (D)	Dichotomous unpaired (DU)	Success/failure (D) in treated/untreated groups (DU)	Chi-square test; Fisher exact probability test
Dichotomous (D)	Dichotomous paired (DP)	Change in success/failure (D) before vs. after treatment (DP)	McNemar chi-square test
Dichotomous (D)	Nominal (N)	Success/failure (D) and blood type (N)	Chi-square test
Nominal (N)	Nominal (N)	Ethnicity (N) and blood type (N)	Chi-square test

*The following is an example of satisfaction described by an ordinal scale: *very satisfied, somewhat satisfied, neither satisfied nor dissatisfied, somewhat dissatisfied,* and *very dissatisfied*. When such scales ask respondents to indicate how strongly they agree or disagree with a given statement, they are referred to as "Likert scales."
†Possibly use one-way analysis of variance (ANOVA, or *F*-test).

participants, or involves comparisons of matched pairs of study participants, a *paired* test of statistical significance (e.g., the paired *t*-test if one variable is continuous and one dichotomous) would be appropriate. If the sampling procedure in a study is not random, statistical tests that assume random sampling, such as most of the parametric tests, may not be valid.

II. MAKING INFERENCES (PARAMETRIC ANALYSIS) FROM CONTINUOUS DATA

Studies often involve one variable that is continuous (e.g., blood pressure) and another variable that is not (e.g., treatment group, which is dichotomous). As shown in Table 11-1, a *t*-test is appropriate for analyzing these data. A *one-way* analysis of variance (ANOVA) is appropriate for analyzing the relationship between one continuous variable and one nominal variable. Chapter 10 discusses the use of Student's and paired *t*-tests in detail and introduces the concept of ANOVA (see Variation between Groups versus Variation within Groups).

If a study involves two continuous variables, such as systolic blood pressure and diastolic blood pressure, the following questions may be answered:

1. Is there a real relationship between the variables or not?
2. If there is a real relationship, is it a positive or negative linear relationship (a straight-line relationship), or is it more complex?
3. If there is a linear relationship, how strongly linear is it—do the data points almost lie along a straight line?

4. Is the relationship likely to be true and not just a chance relationship?
5. Can the findings be generalized to other populations?

The best way to begin to answer these questions is to plot the continuous data on a joint distribution graph for visual inspection and then to perform correlation analysis and simple linear regression analysis.

The distribution of continuous variables can usually be characterized in terms of the mean and standard deviation. These are referred to as **parameters,** and data that can be characterized by these parameters can generally be analyzed by methods that rely on them. All such methods of analysis are referred to as *parametric,* in contrast to *nonparametric* methods, for which assumptions about the mean and standard deviation cannot be made and are not required. Parametric methods are applicable when the data being analyzed may be assumed to approximate a normal distribution.

A. Joint Distribution Graph

The raw data concerning the systolic and diastolic blood pressures of 26 young, healthy, adult participants were introduced in Chapter 10 and listed in Table 10-1. These same data can be plotted on a joint distribution graph, as shown in Figure 11-1. The data lie generally along a straight line, going from the lower left to the upper right on the graph, and all the observations except one are fairly close to the line.

As indicated in Figure 11-2, the correlation between two variables, labeled *x* and *y,* can range from nonexistent to strong. If the value of *y* increases as *x* increases, the correlation is positive; if *y* decreases as *x* increases, the correlation

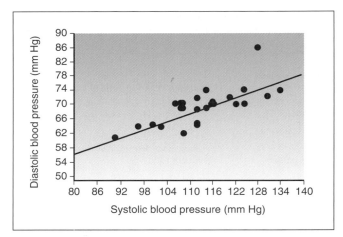

Figure 11-1 **Joint distribution graph of systolic (*x*-axis) and diastolic (*y*-axis) blood pressure values of 26 young, healthy, adult participants.** The raw data for these participants are listed in Table 10-1. The correlation between the two variables is strong and is positive.

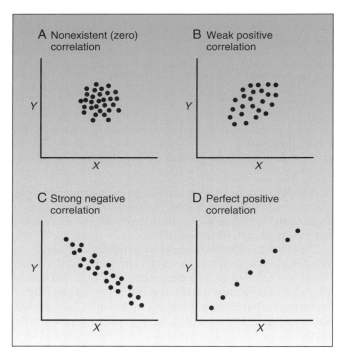

Figure 11-2 **Four possible patterns in joint distribution graphs.** As seen in examples **A** to **D**, the correlation between two continuous variables, labeled *X* and *Y*, can range from nonexistent to perfect. If the value of *y* increases as *x* increases, the correlation is positive. If *y* decreases as *x* increases, the correlation is negative.

is negative. It appears from the graph in Figure 11-1 that the correlation between diastolic and systolic blood pressure is strong and positive. Based on Figure 11-1, the answer to the first question posed previously is that there is a real relationship between diastolic and systolic blood pressure. The answer to the second question is that the relationship is positive and is almost linear. The graph does not provide quantitative information about how strong the association is

(although it looks strong to the eye), and the graph does not reveal the probability that such a relationship could have occurred by chance. To answer these questions more precisely, it is necessary to use the techniques of correlation and simple linear regression. Neither the graph nor these statistical techniques can answer the question of how general the findings are to other populations, however, which depends on research design, especially the method of sampling.

B. Pearson Correlation Coefficient

Even without plotting the observations for two continuous variables on a graph, the strength of their linear relationship can be determined by calculating the **Pearson product-moment correlation coefficient.** This coefficient is given the symbol r, referred to as the *r* **value,** which varies from −1 to +1, going through 0. A finding of −1 indicates that the two variables have a perfect negative linear relationship, +1 indicates that they have a perfect positive linear relationship, and 0 indicates that the two variables are totally independent of each other. The *r* value is rarely found to be −1 or +1, but frequently there is an imperfect correlation between the two variables, resulting in *r* values between 0 and 1 or between 0 and −1. Because the Pearson correlation coefficient is strongly influenced by extreme values, the value of *r* can be trusted only when the distribution of each of the two variables to be correlated is approximately normal (i.e., without severe skewness or extreme outlier values).

The formula for the correlation coefficient *r* is shown here. The numerator is the sum of the covariances. The **covariance** is the product of the deviation of an observation from the mean of the *x* variable multiplied by the same observation's deviation from the mean of the *y* variable. (When marked on a graph, this usually gives a rectangular area, in contrast to the sum of squares, which are squares of the deviations from the mean.) The denominator of *r* is the square root of the sum of the squared deviations from the mean of the *x* variable multiplied by the sum of the squared deviations from the mean of the *y* variable:

$$r = \frac{\sum (x_i - \bar{x})(y_i - \bar{y})}{\sqrt{\sum (x_i - \bar{x})^2 \sum (y_i - \bar{y})^2}}$$

Using statistical computer programs, investigators can determine whether the value of *r* is greater than would be expected by chance alone (i.e., whether the two variables are statistically associated). Most statistical programs provide the *p* value along with the correlation coefficient, but the *p* value of the correlation coefficient can be calculated easily. Its associated *t* can be calculated from the following formula, and the *p* value can be determined from a table of *t* (see Appendix, Table C)[1]:

$$t = \frac{\sqrt{N-2}}{\sqrt{1-r^2}} \quad df = N - 2$$

As with every test of significance, for any given level of strength of association, the larger the sample size, the more likely it is to be statistically significant. A weak correlation in a large sample might be statistically significant, despite that it was not etiologically or clinically important (see later and Box 11-5). The converse may also be true; a result that is statistically weak still may be of public health and clinical importance if it pertains to a large portion of the population.

There is no perfect statistical way to estimate clinical importance, but with continuous variables, a valuable concept is the **strength of the association,** measured by the square of the correlation coefficient, or r^2. The r^2 **value** is the proportion of variation in y explained by x (or vice versa). It is an important parameter in advanced statistics. Looking at the strength of association is analogous to looking at the size and clinical importance of an observed difference, as discussed in Chapter 10.

For purposes of showing the calculation of r and r^2, a small set of data is introduced in Box 11-1. The data, consisting of the observed heights (variable x) and weights (variable y) of eight participants, are presented first in tabular form and then in graph form. When r is calculated, the result is

---

Box 11-1	Analysis of Relationship between Height and Weight (Two Continuous Variables) in Eight Study Participants

PART 1   Tabular and Graphic Representation of the Data

Participant	Variable x (Height, cm)	Variable y (Weight, kg)
1	182.9	78.5
2	172.7	60.8
3	175.3	68.0
4	172.7	65.8
5	160.0	52.2
6	165.1	54.4
7	172.7	60.3
8	162.6	52.2

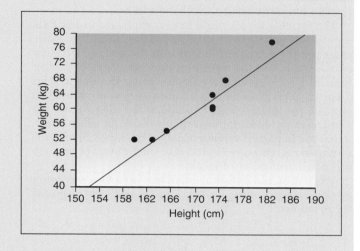

PART 2   Calculation of Moments

$\Sigma(x_i) = 1364$ cm

$\Sigma(y_i) = 492.2$ kg

$N = 8$

$\bar{x} = 1364/8 = 170.50$ cm

$\bar{y} = 492.2/8 = 61.53$ kg

$\Sigma(x_i - \bar{x})(y_i - \bar{y}) = 456.88$

$\Sigma(x_i - \bar{x})^2 = 393.1$

$\Sigma(y_i - \bar{y})^2 = 575.1$

Note: Moments are various descriptors of a distribution, including the number of observations, the sum of their values, the mean, the variance, the standard deviation, and tests of normality.

PART 3   Calculation of Pearson Correlation Coefficient (r) and Strength of Association of Variables (r^2)

$$r = \frac{\sum(x_i - \bar{x})(y_i - \bar{y})}{\sqrt{\sum(x_i - \bar{x})^2 \sum(y_i - \bar{y})^2}}$$

$$= \frac{456.88}{\sqrt{(393.1)(575.1)}} = \frac{456.88}{\sqrt{226,071.8}} = \frac{456.88}{475.47} = 0.96$$

$$r^2 = (0.96)^2 = 0.92 = 92\%$$

Interpretation: The two variables are highly correlated. The association between the two variables is strong and positive with 92% of variation in weight (y) explained by variation in height (x).

PART 4   Calculation of the Slope (b) for a Regression of Weight (y) on Height (x)

$$b = \frac{\sum(x_i - \bar{x})(y_i - \bar{y})}{\sum(x_i - \bar{x})^2} = \frac{456.88}{393.1} = 1.16$$

Interpretation: There is a 1.16-kg increase in weight (y) for each 1-cm increase in height (x). The y-intercept, which indicates the value of x when y is 0, is not meaningful in the case of these two variables, and it is not calculated here.

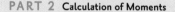

Data from unpublished findings in a sample of eight professional persons in Connecticut.

0.96, which indicates a strong positive linear relationship and provides quantitative information to confirm what is visually apparent in the graph. Given that r is 0.96, r^2 is $(0.96)^2$, or 0.92. A 0.92 strength of association means that 92% of the variation in weight is *explained* by height. The remaining 8% of the variation in this sample is presumed to be caused by factors other than height.

C. Linear Regression Analysis

Linear regression is related to correlation analysis, but it produces two parameters that can be directly related to the data: the slope and the intercept. Linear regression seeks to quantify the linear relationship that may exist between an independent variable x and a dependent variable y, whereas correlation analysis seeks to measure the strength of correlation. More specifically, regression specifies how much y would be expected to change (and in what direction) for a unit change in x. Correlation analysis indicates whether y changes proportionately with changes in x.

The formula for a straight line, as expressed in statistics, is $y = a + bx$ (see Chapter 10). The y is the value of an observation on the y-axis; x is the value of the same observation on the x-axis; a is the regression constant (value of y when value of x is 0); and b is the slope (change in value of y for a unit change in value of x). Linear regression is used to estimate two parameters: the slope of the line (b) and the y-intercept (a). Most fundamental is the slope, which determines the impact of variable x on y. The slope can tell how much weight is expected to increase, on the average, for each additional centimeter of height.

When the usual statistical notation is used for a regression of y on x, the formulas for the slope (b) and y-intercept (a) are as follows:

$$b = \frac{\sum(x_i - \bar{x})(y_i - \bar{y})}{\sum(x_i - \bar{x})^2}$$
$$a = \bar{y} - b\bar{x}$$

Box 11-1 shows the calculation of the slope (b) for the observed heights and weights of eight participants. The graph in Box 11-1 shows the linear relationship between the height and weight data, with the regression line inserted. In these eight participants, the slope was 1.16, meaning that there was an average increase of 1.16 kg of weight for every 1-cm increase in height.

Linear regression analysis enables investigators to predict the value of y from the values that x takes. The formula for linear regression is a form of statistical modeling, where the adequacy of the model is determined by how closely the value of y can be predicted from the other variable. It is of interest to see how much the systolic blood pressure increases, on the average, for each added year of age. Linear regression is useful in answering routine questions in clinical practice, such as, "How much exercise do I need to do to raise my HDL 10 points, or lose 10 pounds?" Such questions involve the magnitude of change in a given factor, y, for a specific change in behavior, or exposure, x.

Just as it is possible to set confidence intervals around parameters such as means and proportions (see Chapter 10), it is possible to set confidence intervals around the parameters of the regression, the slope, and the intercept, using computations based on linear regression formulas. Most statistical computer programs perform these computations, and moderately advanced statistics books provide the formulas.[2] Multiple linear regression and other methods involved in the analysis of more than two variables are discussed in Chapter 13.

III. MAKING INFERENCES (NONPARAMETRIC ANALYSIS) FROM ORDINAL DATA

Many medical data are ordinal, meaning the observations can be ranked from the lowest value to the highest value, but they are not measured on an exact scale. In some cases, investigators assume that ordinal data meet the criteria for continuous (measurement) data and analyze these variables as though they had been obtained from a measurement scale. If patients' satisfaction with the care in a given hospital were being studied, the investigators might assume that the conceptual distance between "very satisfied" (e.g., coded as a 3) and "fairly satisfied" (coded as a 2) is equal to the difference between "fairly satisfied" (coded as a 2) and "unsatisfied" (coded as a 1). If the investigators are willing to make these assumptions, the data might be analyzed using the parametric statistical methods discussed here and in Chapter 10, such as t-tests, analysis of variance, and analysis of the Pearson correlation coefficient. This assumption is dubious, however, and seldom appropriate for use in publications.

If the investigator is not willing to assume an ordinal variable can be analyzed as though it were continuous, many bivariate statistical tests for ordinal data can be used[1,3] (see Table 11-1 and later description). Hand calculation of these tests for ordinal data is extremely tedious and invites errors. No examples are given here, and the use of a computer for these calculations is customary.

Tests specific for ordinal data are **nonparametric** because they do not require assumptions about the mean and standard deviation of the data, known as parameters, and are not dependent on them.

A. Mann-Whitney *U* Test

The test for ordinal data that is similar to the Student's t-test is the Mann-Whitney U test. U, similar to t, designates a probability distribution. In the Mann-Whitney test, all the observations in a study of two samples (e.g., experimental and control groups) are ranked numerically from the smallest to the largest, without regard to whether the observations came from the experimental group or from the control group. Next, the observations from the experimental group are identified, the values of the ranks in this sample are summed, and the average rank and the variance of those ranks are determined. The process is repeated for the observations from the control group. If the null hypothesis is true (i.e., if there is no real difference between the two samples), the average ranks of the two samples should be similar. If the average rank of one sample is considerably greater than that of the other sample, the null hypothesis probably can be rejected, but a test of significance is needed to be sure. Because the U-test method is tedious, a t-test can be done instead (considering the ranks as though they were continuous data), and often this yields similar results.[1]

The Mann-Whitney U test was applied, for example, in a study comparing lithotripsy to ureteroscopy in the treatment of renal calculi.[4]

B. Wilcoxon Matched-Pairs Signed-Ranks Test

The rank-order test that is comparable to the paired t-test is the Wilcoxon matched-pairs signed-ranks test. In this test, all the observations in a study of two samples are ranked numerically from the largest to the smallest, without regard to whether the observations came from the first sample (e.g., pretreatment sample) or from the second sample (e.g., posttreatment sample). After pairs of data are identified (e.g., pretreatment and posttreatment observations are linked), the pretreatment-posttreatment difference in rank is identified for each pair. For example, if for a given pair the pretreatment observation scored 7 ranks higher than the posttreatment observation, the difference would be noted as -7. If in another pair the pretreatment observation scored 5 ranks lower than the posttreatment observation, the difference would be noted as $+5$. Each pair would be scored in this way. If the null hypothesis were true (i.e., if there were no real difference between the samples), the sum of the positive and negative scores should be close to 0. If the average difference is considerably different from 0, the null hypothesis can be rejected.

The Wilcoxon test, for example, was used to compare knowledge, attitude, and practice measures between groups in an educational program for type 1 diabetes.[5]

C. Kruskal-Wallis Test

If the investigators in a study involving continuous data want to compare the means of three or more groups simultaneously, the appropriate test is a one-way analysis of variance (a one-way ANOVA), usually called an F-test. The comparable test for ordinal data is called the Kruskal-Wallis test or the **Kruskal-Wallis one-way ANOVA.** As in the Mann-Whitney U test, for the Kruskal-Wallis test, all the data are ranked numerically, and the rank values are summed in each of the groups to be compared. The Kruskal-Wallis test seeks to determine if the average ranks from three or more groups differ from one another more than would be expected by chance alone. It is another example of a critical ratio (see Chapter 10), in which the magnitude of the difference is in the numerator, and a measure of the random variability is in the denominator. If the ratio is sufficiently large, the null hypothesis is rejected.

The Kruskal-Wallis test was used, for example, in an analysis of the effects of electronic medical record systems on the quality of documentation in primary care.[6]

D. Spearman and Kendall Correlation Coefficients

When relating two *continuous* variables to each other, investigators can use regression analysis or correlation analysis. For *ordinal* variables, there is no test comparable to regression because it is difficult to see how a *slope* could be measured without an underlying measurement scale. For ordinal data, however, several tests are comparable to correlation, the two most common of which are briefly defined here. The first is the **Spearman rank correlation coefficient,** whose symbol is the Greek letter **rho**; it is similar to r. The second is the **Kendall rank correlation coefficient,** which is symbolized by the Greek letter **tau.** (Actually, tau comes in three forms, depending on whether the test makes use of or ignores ties in the data, and whether the table being analyzed is symmetric or not. Most tables to which tau is applied are symmetric and may have ties in the data—for this, Kendall's **tau-b** is used.) The tests for rho and tau usually give similar results, but the rho is usually used in the medical literature, perhaps because of its conceptual similarity to the Pearson r. The tau may give better results with small sample sizes.

The Spearman rank test was used, for example, in a validation study of a tool to address the preservation, for example, dignity at end of life.[7]

E. Sign Test

Sometimes an experimental intervention produces positive results on most of many different measurements, but few, if any, of the individual outcome variables show a difference that is statistically significant. In this case, the sign test can be extremely helpful to compare the results in the experimental group with those in the control group. If the null hypothesis is true (i.e., there is no real difference between the groups), by chance, the experimental group should perform better on about half the measurements, and the control group should perform better on about half.

The only data needed for the sign test are the records of whether, on the average, the experimental participants or the control participants scored "better" on each outcome variable (by what amount is not important). If the average score for a given variable is better in the experimental group, the result is recorded as a plus sign ($+$); if the average score for that variable is better in the control group, the result is recorded as a minus sign ($-$); and if the average score in the two groups is exactly the same, no result is recorded, and the variable is omitted from the analysis. For the sign test, "better" can be determined from a continuous variable, ordinal variable, dichotomous variable, clinical score, or component of a score. Because under the null hypothesis the expected proportion of plus signs is 0.5 and of minus signs is 0.5, the test compares the observed proportion of successes with the expected value of 0.5.

The sign test was employed, for example, in a study of the effect of an electronic classroom communication device on medical student examination scores.[8]

IV. MAKING INFERENCES (NONPARAMETRIC ANALYSIS) FROM DICHOTOMOUS AND NOMINAL DATA

As indicated in Table 11-1, the chi-square test, Fisher exact probability test, and McNemar chi-square test can be used in the analysis of dichotomous data, although they use different statistical theory. Usually, the data are first arranged in a 2×2 table, and the goal is to test the null hypothesis that the variables are independent.

A. 2 × 2 Contingency Table

Data arranged as in Box 11-2 form what is known as a *contingency table* because it is used to determine whether the distribution of one variable is conditionally dependent (contingent) on the other variable. More specifically, Box 11-2 provides an example of a 2 × 2 contingency table, meaning that it has two cells in each direction. In this case, the table shows the data for a study of 91 patients who had a myocardial infarction.[9] One variable is treatment (propranolol vs. a placebo), and the other is outcome (survival for at least 28 days vs. death within 28 days).

A cell is a specific location in a contingency table. In this case, each cell shows the observed number, the expected number, and the percentage of study participants in each treatment group who lived or died. In Box 11-2 the top left cell indicates that 38 patients who were treated with propranolol survived the first 28 days of observation, that they represented 84% of all patients who were treated with propranolol, and that 33.13 patients treated with propranolol were expected to survive the first 28 days of observation, based on the null hypothesis. The methods for calculating the percentages and expected counts are discussed subsequently.

The other three cells indicate the same type of data (observed number, expected number, and percentage) for patients who died after propranolol treatment, patients who survived after placebo treatment, and patients who died after placebo treatment. The bottom row shows the column totals, and the right-hand column shows the row totals.

If there are more than two cells in each direction of a contingency table, the table is called an $R \times C$ table, where R stands for the number of rows and C stands for the number of columns. Although the principles of the chi-square test

---

Box 11-2   Chi-Square Analysis of Relationship between Treatment and Outcome (Two Nonparametric Variables, Unpaired) in 91 Participants

PART 1 Beginning Data, Presented in a 2 × 2 Contingency Table, Where *O* Denotes Observed Counts and *E* Denotes Expected Counts

| | Outcome | | | | Total | |
| | Survival for at Least 28 Days | | Death | | | |
Treatment	No.	(%)	No.	(%)	No.	(%)
Propranolol (*O*)	38	(84)	7	(16)	45	(100)
Propranolol (*E*)	33.13		11.87		45	
Placebo (*O*)	29	(63)	17	(37)	46	(100)
Placebo (*E*)	33.87		12.13		46	
Total	67	(74)	24	(26)	91	(100)

PART 2 Calculation of the Chi-Square (χ^2) Value

$$\chi^2 = \sum \left[\frac{(O-E)^2}{E} \right]$$

$$= \frac{(38-33.13)^2}{33.13} + \frac{(7-11.87)^2}{11.87} + \frac{(29-33.87)^2}{33.87} + \frac{(17-12.13)^2}{12.13}$$

$$= \frac{(4.87)^2}{33.13} + \frac{(-4.87)^2}{11.87} + \frac{(-4.87)^2}{33.87} + \frac{(4.87)^2}{12.13}$$

$$= \frac{23.72}{33.13} + \frac{23.72}{11.87} + \frac{23.72}{33.87} + \frac{23.72}{12.13}$$

$$= 0.72 + 2.00 + 0.70 + 1.96 = \textbf{5.38}$$

PART 3 Calculation of Degrees of Freedom (*df*) for Contingency Table, Based on Number of Rows (*R*) and Columns (*C*)

$$df = (R-1)(C-1) = (2-1)(2-1) = 1$$

PART 4 Determination of the *p* Value

Value from the chi-square table for 5.38 on 1 *df*: $0.01 < p < 0.025$ (statistically significant)

Exact *p* from a computer program: 0.0205 (statistically significant)

Interpretation: The results noted in this 2 × 2 table are statistically significant. That is, it is highly probable (only 1 chance in about 50 of being wrong) that the investigator can reject the null hypothesis of independence and accept the alternative hypothesis that propranolol does affect the outcome of myocardial infarction (the effect observed to be in a positive direction).

Data from Snow PJ: Effect of propranolol in myocardial infarction. *Lancet* 2:551–553, 1965.

are valid for $R \times C$ tables, the subsequent discussion focuses on 2×2 tables for the sake of simplicity.

B. Chi-Square Test of Independence

Along with *t*-tests, the other commonly used basic form of statistical analysis in the medical literature is the chi-square test of the independence of two variables in a contingency table.[10] The chi-square test is another example of a common approach to statistical analysis known as **statistical modeling,** which seeks to develop a statistical expression (the model) that predicts the behavior of a dependent variable on the basis of knowledge of one or more independent variables. The process of comparing the **observed counts** with the **expected counts**—that is, of comparing O with E—is called a **goodness-of-fit test** because the goal is to see how well the observed counts in a contingency table *fit* the counts expected on the basis of the model. Usually, the model in such a table is the null hypothesis that the two variables are independent of each other. If the chi-square value is small, the null hypothesis provides a good fit, and it is not rejected. If the chi-square value is large, however, the data do not fit the hypothesis well, and the null hypothesis is rejected.

Box 11-2 is used here to illustrate the steps and considerations involved in constructing a 2×2 contingency table and in calculating the chi-square value. For the data presented in Box 11-2, the null hypothesis is that treating the myocardial infarction patients with propranolol did not influence the percentage of patients who survived for at least 28 days. Treatment is the independent variable, and outcome is the dependent variable. The alternative hypothesis is that the outcome (survival or death) depended on the treatment.

I. Calculation of Percentages

Each of the four cells of Box 11-2 shows an observed count and a percentage. The percentage in the first cell of the contingency table was calculated by dividing the number of propranolol-treated patients who survived (38) by the total number of propranolol-treated patients (45), which equals 84%. This percentage was calculated as the frequency distribution of the dependent variable (survival) within the propranolol-treated group.

If treatment depended on survival, rather than vice versa, the percentage would be calculated by dividing the number of propranolol-treated patients who survived (38) by the total number of survivors (67), but this arrangement does not make sense. The way the percentages are calculated affects the way people think about and interpret the data, but it does not influence the way the chi-square test is calculated. The appropriate way to calculate the percentages in a contingency table is to calculate the frequency distribution of the dependent variable within each category of the independent variable.

2. Calculation of Expected Counts

In Box 11-2, the propranolol-treated group consists of 45 patients, the placebo-treated group consists of 46 patients, and the total for the study is 91 patients. The observed counts indicate how many of each group actually survived, whereas the expected counts indicate how many of each group would be expected to survive if the method of treatment made no difference (i.e., if survival were independent of treatment). The formula for calculating the expected count in one cell of the table (here the top left cell) is as follows:

$$E_{1,1} = \frac{\text{Row}_1 \text{ total}}{\text{Study total}} \times \text{Column}_1 \text{ total}$$

where $E_{1,1}$ is defined as the cell in row$_1$, column$_1$. The same is done for each cell in the table.

In Box 11-2, if survival were independent of the treatment group, 45 of 91 (or 49.45%) of the observations in each column would be expected to be in the top row because that is the overall proportion of patients who received propranolol. It follows that 0.4945×67 (or 33.13) observations (the total in column$_1$) would be expected in the left upper cell, whereas 0.4945×24 (or 11.87) observations (the total in column$_2$) would be expected in the right upper cell. The *expected* counts may include fractions, and the sum of the expected counts in a given row should equal the sum of the observed counts in that row (33.13 + 11.87 = 45). By the same logic, 50.55% of observations would be expected to be in the bottom row, with 33.87 in the left lower cell and 12.13 in the right lower cell, so that the row total equals the sum of the observed counts (33.87 + 12.13 = 46). Finally, as shown in Box 11-2, the column totals for expected counts should add up to the column totals for observed counts.

The *expected* counts in *each cell* of a 2×2 contingency table should equal 5 or more, or the assumptions and approximations inherent in the chi-square test may break down. For a study involving a larger contingency table (an $R \times C$ table), the investigator usually can compromise on this slightly by allowing 20% of the expected counts to be less than 5, but at the same time ensuring that none of the expected counts is less than 2. If these conditions are not met in a 2×2 table, the Fisher exact probability test (see later) should be used instead of the chi-square test.

3. Calculation of the Chi-Square Value

When the observed (O) and expected (E) counts are known, the chi-square (χ^2) value can be calculated. One of two methods can be used, depending on the size of the counts.

METHOD FOR LARGE NUMBERS

In Box 11-2, the investigators begin by calculating the chi-square value for each cell in the table, using the following formula:

$$\frac{(O - E)^2}{E}$$

The numerator is the square of the deviation of the observed count in a given cell from the count that would be expected in that cell if the null hypothesis were true. This is similar to the numerator of the variance, which is expressed as $\sum (x_i - \bar{x})^2$, where x_i is the *observed* value and $\bar{x}$ (the mean) is the *expected* value (see Chapter 9). The denominator for variance is the degrees of freedom ($N - 1$), however, whereas the denominator for chi-square is the expected number (E).

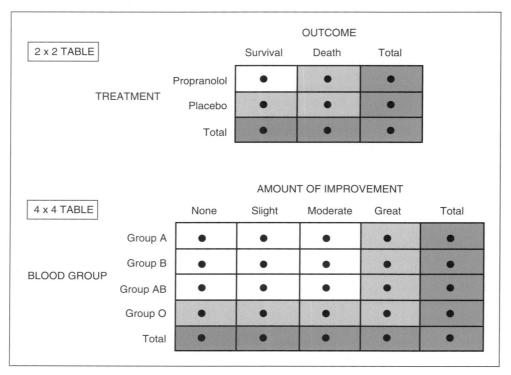

Figure 11-3 Conceptualization of the calculation of the degrees of freedom (*df*) in a 2 × 2 contingency table (*top*) and in a 4 × 4 contingency table (*bottom*). A *white* cell is free to vary, a *light-blue* cell is not free to vary, and a *dark-blue* cell is a row or column total. The formula is *df*=(*R*−1)(*C*−1), where *R* denotes the number of rows and *C* denotes the number of columns. For 2 × 2 table, *df*= 1; for 4 × 4 table, *df*= 9.

To obtain the total chi-square value for a 2 × 2 table, the investigators add up the chi-square values for the four cells:

$$\chi^2 = \sum \left[\frac{(O-E)^2}{E} \right]$$

The basic statistical method for measuring the total amount of variation in a data set, the total sum of squares (TSS), is rewritten for the chi-square test as the sum of $(O - E)^2$.

Box 11-2 shows how chi-square is calculated for the study of 91 patients with myocardial infarction. Before the result ($\chi^2 = 5.38$) can be interpreted, the degrees of freedom must be determined.

4. Determination of Degrees of Freedom

As discussed in Chapter 10 and Box 10-3, the term *degrees of freedom* refers to the number of observations that can be considered to be free to vary. A statistician needs some solid (nonvarying) place to begin. According to the null hypothesis, the best estimate of the expected counts in the cells of a contingency table is given by the row and column totals, so they are considered to be fixed (in the same way as is the mean when calculating a variance). An observed count can be entered freely into one of the cells of a 2 × 2 table (e.g., top left cell), but when that count is entered, none of the other three cells are free to vary. This means that a 2 × 2 table has only 1 degree of freedom.

Another look at Box 11-2 helps explain why there is only 1 degree of freedom in a table with two rows and two columns. If 38 is entered freely in the top left cell, the only possible number that can go in the cell immediately to the

right of it is 7 because the two numbers in the top row must equal the *fixed* row total of 45. Similarly, the only possible number that can go in the cell directly below is 29 because the column must add up to 67. Finally, the only possible number for the remaining cell is 17 because the row total must equal 46 and the column total must equal 24. This is illustrated in Figure 11-3, where the cells that are free to vary are shown in white, the cells that are not free to vary are shown in light blue, and the fixed row and column totals are shown in dark blue. The top table in the figure corresponds to the table in Box 11-2.

The same principle applies to contingency tables with more than two rows and columns. In $R \times C$ contingency tables, imagine that the right-hand column and the bottom row are never free to vary because they must contain the numbers that make the totals come out right (see the bottom table in Fig. 11-3). The formula for degrees of freedom in a contingency table of any size is as follows:

$$df = (R-1)(C-1)$$

where *df* denotes degrees of freedom, *R* is the number of rows, and *C* is the number of columns.

5. Interpretation of Results

After the chi-square value and the degrees of freedom are known, a standard table of chi-square values (see Appendix, Table D) can be consulted to determine the corresponding *p* value. The *p* value indicates the probability that a chi-square value that large would have resulted from chance alone. For data shown in Box 11-2, the chi-square value was 5.38 on 1 degree of freedom, and the *p* value listed for that chi-square value in the standard table for a two-tailed test was between 0.01 and 0.025 (0.01 < p < 0.025). Most computer programs provide the exact p value when calculating a chi-square; for the data in Box 11-2, the p value was 0.0205. Because the observed p was less than alpha (alpha = 0.05), the results were considered statistically significant, the null hypothesis that propranolol made no difference was rejected, and the alternative hypothesis that propranolol made a difference was accepted.

The alternative hypothesis does not state whether the effect of the treatment would be to increase or decrease survival. This is because the null hypothesis was only that there would be no difference. In other words, the null hypothesis as stated required a two-tailed test of statistical significance (see Chapter 10). The investigator could have tested the null hypothesis that the propranolol-treated group would show a higher survival rate than the placebo-treated group, but this would have required interpreting the chi-square value as a one-tailed test of statistical significance. The choice of a one-tailed test versus a two-tailed test does not affect the way a statistical test is performed, but it does affect how the critical ratio obtained is converted to a p value in a statistical table.

C. Chi-Square Test for Paired Data (McNemar Test)

The chi-square test as just described is useful for comparing the distribution of a categorical variable in two or more groups, but a different test is needed to compare *before-and-after* findings in the *same individuals* or to compare findings in a matched analysis. The appropriate test for this situation for dichotomous variables is the McNemar chi-square test.

1. McNemar Test of Before-and-After Comparisons

The discussion of t-tests in Chapter 10 noted that when doing a before-and-after study, a research participant serves as his or her own control. Here it was appropriate to use the *paired t-test*, instead of the Student's *t*-test. In the case of a matched 2 × 2 table, it would similarly be appropriate to use the **McNemar test**, which is a type of paired chi-square test of data with 1 degree of freedom.[1]

Suppose that an investigator wanted to see how attitudes about visiting Salt Lake City changed among audience members attending a particular Broadway show (fictitious scenario). The researcher enrolls 200 willing audience members who complete questionnaires indicating their interest in visiting Salt Lake City both before and after the show, and their responses are recorded as either positive or negative (i.e., dichotomous responses). The data could be set up in a 2 × 2 table with the preshow opinion on the left axis and the postshow opinion at the top, as shown in Box 11-3. Each of the four cells represents one of the following four possible combinations:

- Cell a = Positive opinion before and after (no change)
- Cell b = Change from positive to negative opinion
- Cell c = Change from negative to positive opinion
- Cell d = Negative opinion before and after (no change)

According to the hypothetical data from 200 audience members who participated in the study, the overall percentage reporting a favorable opinion of visiting Salt Lake City decreased from 86% (172 of 200) before the show to 79% (158 of 200) after the show, presumably reflecting a response to the show content. The null hypothesis to be tested is that the show produced no true change in audience opinion, and the following formula would be used:

$$\text{McNemar } \chi^2 = \frac{(|b-c|-1)^2}{b+c}$$

The formula uses only cells b and c in the 2 × 2 table. This is because cells a and d do not change and do not contribute to the standard error. Note also that the formula tests data with 1 degree of freedom. The subtraction of 1 in the numerator is called a "correction for continuity." (For further discussion or to calculate the McNemar chi-square, see http://www.graphpad.com/quickcalcs/McNemar1.cfm.)

The McNemar chi-square value for the data shown in Box 11-3 is 5.63. This result is statistically significant (p < 0.025), so that the null hypothesis is rejected. Care must be taken when interpreting these data, however, because the test of significance only states the following: "Among those audience members *who changed their opinion*, significantly more changed from positive to negative than vice versa." Any adequate interpretation of the data also would need to indicate the following:

1. Of the audience members, 75% had a good opinion throughout the study.
2. The percentage of the audience who changed their opinion was relatively small (15%).

2. McNemar Test of Matched Data

In medical research, the McNemar chi-square test is used frequently in case-control studies, where the cases and controls are *matched* on the basis of characteristics such as age, gender, and residence, then *compared* for the presence or absence of a specific risk factor. Under these circumstances, the data can be set up in a 2 × 2 table similar to that shown in Box 11-4.

To illustrate the use of the McNemar test in matched data, the observations made in an actual case-control study are discussed here and reported in the second part of Box 11-4.[11] In this study the investigator wanted to examine the association between mycosis fungoides (a type of lymphoma that begins in the skin and eventually spreads to internal organs) and a history of employment in an industrial environment with exposure to cutting oils. After matching 54 participants who had the disease (the cases) with 54 participants who did not have the disease (the controls), the investigator recorded whether or not the study participants had a history of this type of industrial employment.

When the McNemar chi-square formula was used to test the null hypothesis that prior occupation was not associated with the development of mycosis fungoides (see Box 11-4), the chi-square value was 5.06. Because the result was statistically significant (p = 0.021), the null hypothesis was rejected, and the alternative hypothesis, that mycosis fungoides was associated with industrial exposure, was accepted.

A **matched odds ratio** also can be calculated (see Chapter 6). When the data are set up as in Box 11-4, the ratio

| Box II-3 | McNemar Chi-Square Analysis of Relationship between Data before and Data after an Event (Two Dichotomous Variables, Paired) in a Study of 200 Participants (Fictitious Data) |

PART I Standard 2 × 2 Table Format on which Equations Are Based

	Findings after Event		
Findings before Event	Positive	Negative	Total
Positive	a	b	$a + b$
Negative	c	d	$c + d$
Total	$a + c$	$b + d$	$a + b + c + d$

PART 2 Data for Study of Opinions of Audience Members toward Travel to Salt Lake City before and after Seeing a Particular Broadway Show

	Postshow Opinion		
Preshow Opinion	Positive	Negative	Total
Positive	150	22	172
Negative	8	20	28
Total	158	42	200

PART 3 Calculation of the McNemar Chi-Square (χ^2) Value

$$\text{McNemar } \chi^2 = \frac{(|b-c|-1)^2}{b+c}$$

$$= \frac{(|22-8|-1)^2}{22+8} = \frac{(13)^2}{30} = \frac{169}{30} = 5.63$$

PART 4 Calculation of Degrees of Freedom (df) for Contingency Table, Based on Number of Rows (R) and Columns (C)

$$df = (R-1)(C-1) = (2-1)(2-1) = 1$$

PART 5 Determination of the p Value

Value from the chi-square table for 5.63 on 1 df: $p < 0.025$ (statistically significant)

Interpretation: A statistically significant difference was noted between the audience preshow opinion and postshow opinion. Specifically, for the audience members who changed their attitude toward visiting Salt Lake City after the show, most of these changes were from a positive attitude to a negative attitude, rather than vice versa.

is calculated simply as b/c. Here, the ratio is 13/3, or 4.33, indicating that the *odds* of acquiring mycosis fungoides was more than four times as great in participants with a history of industrial exposure as in those without such a history.

D. Fisher Exact Probability Test

When one or more of the expected counts in a 2 × 2 table is small (i.e., <2), the chi-square test cannot be used. It is possible, however, to calculate the exact probability of finding the observed numbers by using the Fisher exact probability test. The formula is as follows:

$$\text{Fisher } p = \frac{(a+b)!(c+d)!(a+c)!(b+d)!}{N!a!b!c!d}$$

where p is probability; a, b, c, and d denote values in the top left, top right, bottom left, and bottom right cells in a 2 × 2 table; N is the total number of observations; and ! is the symbol for factorial. (The factorial of $4 = 4! = 4 \times 3 \times 2 \times 1$.)

The Fisher exact probability test would be extremely tedious to calculate manually; unless one of the four cells contains a 0, the sum of more than one calculation is needed. Most commercially available statistical packages now calculate the Fisher probability automatically when an appropriate situation arises in a 2 × 2 table.

E. Standard Errors for Data in 2 × 2 Tables

Standard errors for proportions, risk ratios, and odds ratios are sometimes calculated for data in 2 × 2 tables, although they are not used for data in larger $R \times C$ tables.

1. Standard Error for a Proportion

In a 2 × 2 table, the proportion of success (defined, for example, as survival) can be determined for each of the two levels (categories) of the independent variable, and the standard error can be calculated for each of these proportions. This is valuable when an objective of the study is to

Box 11-4 **McNemar Chi-Square Analysis of Relationship between Data from Cases and Data from Controls (Two Dichotomous Variables, Paired) in Case-Control Study of 54 Participants**

PART 1 **Standard 2 × 2 Table Format on which Equations Are Based**

	Controls		
Cases	Risk Factor Present	Risk Factor Absent	Total
Risk Factor Present	a	b	$a+b$
Risk Factor Absent	c	d	$c+d$
Total	$a+c$	$b+d$	$a+b+c+d$

PART 2 **Data for Case-Control Study of Relationship between Mycosis Fungoides (Disease) and History of Exposure to Industrial Environment Containing Cutting Oils (Risk Factor)**

	Controls		
Cases	History of Industrial Exposure	No History of Industrial Exposure	Total
History of Industrial Exposure	16	13	29
No History of Industrial Exposure	3	22	25
Total	19	35	54

PART 3 **Calculation of the McNemar Chi-Square (χ^2) Value**

$$\text{McNemar } \chi^2 = \frac{(|b-c|-1)^2}{b+c}$$

$$= \frac{(|13-3|-1)^2}{13+3} = \frac{(9)^2}{16} = \frac{81}{16} = \textbf{5.06}$$

PART 4 **Calculation of Degrees of Freedom (_df_) for Contingency Table, Based on Number of Rows (_R_) and Columns (_C_)**

$$df = (R-1)(C-1) = (2-1)(2-1) = \textbf{1}$$

PART 5 **Determination of the _p_ Value**

Value from the chi-square table for 5.06 on 1 _df_: $p = 0.021$ (statistically significant)

Interpretation: The data presented in this 2 × 2 table are statistically significant. The cases (participants with mycosis fungoides) were more likely than expected by chance alone to have been exposed to an industrial environment with cutting oils than were the controls (participants without mycosis fungoides).

PART 6 **Calculation of the Odds Ratio (OR)**

$$OR = b/c = 13/3 = \textbf{4.33}$$

Interpretation: When a case and a matched control differed in their history of exposure to cutting oils, the odds that the case was exposed was 4.33 times as great as the odds that the control was exposed.

Data from Cohen SR: New Haven, Conn, 1977, Yale University School of Medicine.

estimate the true proportions of success when using the new intervention.

In Box 11-2, the proportion of 28-day survivors in the propranolol-treated group was 0.84 (shown as 84% in the percentage column), and the proportion of 28-day survivors in the placebo-treated group was 0.63. Knowing this information allows the investigator to calculate the standard error and the 95% confidence interval for each survival percentage by the methods described earlier (see z-tests in Chapter 10). In Box 11-2, when the calculations are performed for the proportions surviving, the 95% confidence interval for

survival in the propranolol-treated group is expressed as (0.73, 0.95), meaning that the true proportion probably is between 0.73 and 0.95, whereas the confidence interval for the placebo-treated group is expressed as (0.49, 0.77).

2. Standard Error for a Risk Ratio

If a 2 × 2 table is used to compare the proportion of disease in two different exposure groups or is used to compare the proportion of success in two different treatment groups, the relative risk or relative success can be expressed as a risk ratio. Standard errors can be set around the risk ratio, and if the 95% confidence limits exclude the value of 1.0, there is a statistically significant difference between the risks, at an alpha level of 5%.

In Box 11-2, because the proportion of 28-day survivors in the propranolol-treated group was 0.84 and the proportion of 28-day survivors in the placebo-treated group was 0.63, the risk ratio was 0.84/0.63, or 1.34. This ratio indicates that for the patients with myocardial infarction studied, the 28-day survival probability with propranolol was 34% better than that with placebo.

There are several approaches to computing the standard error of a risk ratio. Because all the methods are complicated, they are not shown here. One or another of these methods is provided in every major statistical computer package. When the risk ratio in Box 11-2 is analyzed by the Taylor series approach used in the EPIINFO computer package, for example, the 95% confidence interval around the risk ratio of 1.34 is reported as (1.04, 1.73).[12] This means that the true risk ratio has a 95% probability of being between 1.04 and 1.73. This finding confirms the chi-square test finding of statistical significance because the 95% confidence interval does not include a risk ratio of 1.0 (which means no true difference between the groups).

3. Standard Error for an Odds Ratio

If a 2×2 table provides data from a case-control study, the odds ratio can be calculated. Although Box 11-2 is best analyzed by a risk ratio, because the study method is a cohort study (randomized control trial), rather than a case-control study, the odds ratio also can be examined. Here the odds of surviving in the propranolol-treated group are 38/7, or 5.43, and the odds of surviving in the placebo-treated group are 29/17, or 1.71. The odds ratio is 5.43/1.71, or 3.18, which is much larger than the risk ratio. As emphasized in Chapter 6, the odds ratio is a good estimate of the risk ratio only if the risk being studied by a case-control study is rare. Because the risk event (mortality) in Box 11-2 is not rare, the odds ratio is not a good estimate of the risk ratio.

Calculating the standard error for an odds ratio also is complicated and is not discussed here. When the odds ratio in Box 11-2 is analyzed by the Cornfield approach used in the EPIINFO 5.01 computer package, the 95% confidence interval around the odds ratio of 3.18 is reported as (1.06, 9.85).[12] The lower-limit estimate of 1.06 with the odds ratio is close to the lower-limit estimate of 1.04 with the risk ratio, and it confirms statistical significance. The upper-limit estimate for the odds ratio is much larger than that for the risk ratio, however, because the odds ratio itself is much larger than the risk ratio.

F. Strength of Association and Clinical Utility of Data in 2×2 Tables

Earlier in this chapter, the strength of association between two continuous variables was measured as r^2. For the data shown in 2×2 tables, an alternative method is used to estimate the strength of association. A fictitious scenario and set of data are used here to illustrate how to determine strength of association and why it is important to examine associations for strength and statistical significance.

Assume that an eager male student was pursuing a master's degree and based his thesis on a study to determine if there was a true difference between the results of a certain blood test in men and the results in women. After obtaining the data shown in the first part of Box 11-5, he calculated the chi-square value and found that the difference between findings in men and findings in women was not statistically significant ($\chi^2 = 0.32$; $p = 0.572$). His advisor pointed out that even if the difference had been statistically significant, the data would not have been clinically useful because of the small gender difference in the proportion of participants with positive findings in the blood test (52% of men vs. 48% of women).

The student decided to obtain a PhD and to base his dissertation on a continued study of the same topic. Believing that small numbers were the problem with the master's thesis, this time he decided to obtain blood test findings in a sample of 20,000 participants, half from each gender. As shown in the second part of Box 11-5, the difference in proportions was the same as before (52% of men vs. 48% of women), so the results were still clinically unimportant (i.e., trivial). Now, however, the student had obtained (perhaps felt rewarded with) a statistical association that was highly significant ($\chi^2 = 32.0$; $p < 0.0001$).

Findings can have statistical significance, especially if the study involves a large number of participants, and at the same time have little or no clinical value. This example shows an interesting point. Because the sample size in the PhD study was 100 times as large as that in the master's study, the chi-square value for the data in the PhD study (given identical proportions) also was 100 times as large. It would be helpful to measure the strength of the association in Box 11-5 to show that the magnitude of the association was not important, even though it was statistically significant.

In 2×2 tables, the strength of association is measured using the phi coefficient, which basically adjusts the chi-square value for the sample size; it can be considered as analogous to the correlation coefficient (r) for the data in a 2×2 table. The formula is as follows:

$$phi = \sqrt{\frac{\chi^2}{N}}$$

The phi value in the first part of Box 11-5 is the same as that in the second part (i.e., 0.04) because the strength of the association is the same, very small. If phi is squared (similar to r^2), the proportion of variation in chi-square that is explained by gender in this example is less than 0.2%, which is extremely small. Although phi is not accurate in larger (R $\times$ C) tables, a related test, called **Cramer's V**, can be used in these tables.[13]

Every association should be examined for strength of association, clinical utility, and statistical significance. Strength of association can be shown by a risk ratio, a risk difference, an odds ratio, an r^2 value, a phi value, or a Cramer's V value. A statistically significant association implies that the association is real (i.e., is not caused by chance alone), but not that it is important. A **strong association** is likely to be important if it is real. Looking for statistical significance *and* strength of association is as important to statistical analysis as having the right *and* left wings is to an airplane.

There is a danger of automatically rejecting as unimportant statistically significant associations that show only

Box 11-5   **Analysis of Strength of Association (phi) between Blood Test Results and Gender (Two Nonparametric Variables, Unpaired) in Initial Study of 200 Participants and Subsequent Study of 20,000 Participants (Fictitious Data)**

PART 1   **Data and Calculation of phi Coefficient for Initial Study (Master's Thesis)**

Blood Test Result	Gender Male No.	Male (%)	Female No.	Female (%)	Total No.	Total (%)
Positive	52	(52)	48	(48)	100	(50)
Negative	48	(48)	52	(52)	100	(50)
Total	100	(100)	100	(100)	200	(100)

chi-square (χ^2) value: 0.32
degrees of freedom (*df*): 1
p value: **0.572** (not statistically significant)

$$\text{phi} = \sqrt{\frac{\chi^2}{N}} = \sqrt{\frac{0.32}{200}} = \sqrt{0.0016} = \mathbf{0.04}$$

Interpretation: The association between gender and the blood test result was neither statistically significant nor clinically important.

PART 2   **Data and Calculation of phi Coefficient for Subsequent Study (PhD Dissertation)**

Blood Test Result	Gender Male No.	Male (%)	Female No.	Female (%)	Total No.	Total (%)
Positive	5,200	(52)	4,800	(48)	10,000	(50)
Negative	4,800	(48)	5,200	(52)	10,000	(50)
Total	10,000	(100)	10,000	(100)	20,000	(100)

chi-square (χ^2) value: 32.0
degrees of freedom (*df*): 1
p value: **<0.0001** (highly statistically significant)

$$\text{phi} = \sqrt{\frac{\chi^2}{N}} = \sqrt{\frac{32}{20,000}} = \sqrt{0.0016} = \mathbf{0.04}$$

Interpretation: The association between gender and the blood test result was statistically significant. It was clinically unimportant (i.e., it was trivial), however, because the phi value was 0.04, and the proportion of chi-square that was explained by the blood test result was only $(0.04)^2$, or 0.0016, much less than 1%.

limited strength of association. As discussed in Chapter 6, the risk ratio (or odds ratio if from a case-control study) and the prevalence of the risk factor determine the population attributable risk. For a prevalent disease such as myocardial infarction, a common risk factor that showed a risk ratio of only 1.3 could be responsible for a large number of preventable infarctions. In general, clinical significance depends on the magnitude of effect in an individual, and the population prevalence of the factor in question. A small change in blood pressure or LDL cholesterol that might be trivial in an individual could translate to many lives saved if a large population is affected.

G. Survival Analysis

In clinical studies of medical or surgical interventions for cancer, success usually is measured in terms of the length of time that some desirable outcome (e.g., survival or remission of disease) is maintained. An analysis of the time-related patterns of survival typically involves using variations of life table techniques that were first developed in the insurance field. Insurance companies needed to know the risk of death in their insured populations so that they knew what rates to charge for the company to make profit.

The mere reporting of the proportion of patients who are alive at the termination of a study's observation period is inadequate because it does not account for how long the individual patients were observed, and it does not consider when they died or how many were lost to follow-up. Techniques that statisticians use to control for these problems include the following:

- Person-time methods
- Survival analysis using the *actuarial life table method* or the *Kaplan-Meier method*

Survival analysis requires that the dependent (outcome) variable be dichotomous (e.g., survival/death, success/

failure) and that the time to failure or loss to observation be known.

1. Person-Time Methods

In a survival study, some participants are lost to follow-up, and others die during the observation period. To control for the fact that the length of observation varies from participant to participant, the person-time methods, introduced in an earlier discussion of incidence density (see Chapter 2), can be used to calculate the likelihood of death. Briefly, if one person is observed for 3 years, and another person is observed for 1 year, the total duration of observation would be equal to *4 person-years*. Calculations can be made on the basis of years, months, weeks, or any other unit of time. The results can be reported as the number of events (e.g., deaths or remissions) per person-time of observation.

Person-time methods are useful if the risk of death or some other outcome does not change greatly over the follow-up period. If the risk of death does change with the amount of time elapsed since baseline (e.g., amount of time since diagnosis of a disease or since entry into a study), person-time methods are not helpful. For example, certain cancers tend to kill quickly if they are going to be fatal, so the amount of risk per person-time depends on whether most of the years of observation were soon after diagnosis or much later. As mentioned in Chapter 2, person-time methods are especially useful for studies of phenomena that can occur repeatedly over time, such as otitis media, bouts of angina pectoris, and exacerbations of asthma.

2. Life Table Analysis

In follow-up studies of a single dichotomous outcome such as death, a major problem is that some participants may be lost to follow-up (unavailable for examination), and some may be censored (when a patient is terminated from a study early because the patient entered late and the study is ending). The most popular solution to this problem is to use life table analysis. The two main methods of life table analysis—the actuarial method and the Kaplan-Meier method—treat losses to follow-up and censorship in slightly different ways, but both methods make it possible to base the analysis on the findings in all the participants for whom data are available. Both methods require the following information for each patient:

1. Date of entry into the study
2. Reason for withdrawal: death, loss to follow-up, or censorship
3. Date of withdrawal: date of death for patients who died, the last time seen alive for patients who were lost to follow-up, and the date withdrawn alive for patients who were censored

If different treatment groups are being compared, the method also requires knowing in which group each study participant was enrolled.

ACTUARIAL METHOD

The actuarial method, which was developed to calculate risks and premium rates for life insurance companies and retirement plans, was the basis of the earlier methods used in life table analysis. In medical studies the actuarial method is used to calculate the survival rates of patients during fixed intervals, such as years. First, it determines the number of people surviving to the beginning of each interval. Next, it assumes that the individuals who were censored or lost to follow-up during the interval were observed for only half that interval. Finally, the method calculates the mortality rate for that interval by dividing the number of deaths in the interval by the total person-years of observation in that interval for all those who began the interval.

The survival rate for an interval (p_x) is 1.0 minus the mortality rate. The rate of survival of the study group to the end of three of the fixed intervals (p_3) is the product of the survival of each of the three component intervals. For example, assume that the intervals were years; the survival rate to the end of the first interval (p_1) was 0.75 (i.e., 75%); for participants who began the second year, the survival rate to the end of the second interval (p_2) was 0.80; and for participants who began the third year, the survival rate to the end of the third interval (p_3) was 0.85. These three numbers would be multiplied together to arrive at a 3-year survival rate of 0.51, or 51%.

An important example of a study in which the actuarial method was used is the U.S. Veterans Administration study of the long-term effects of coronary artery bypass grafts versus medical treatment of patients with stable angina.[14] Figure 11-4 shows the 11-year cumulative survival for surgically and medically treated patients who did not have left

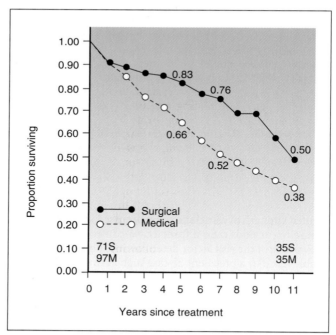

Figure 11-4 Graph showing results of survival analysis using actuarial method. From a study of long-term effects of coronary artery bypass grafts versus medical treatment of patients with stable angina. Depicted here is the 11-year cumulative survival for surgically and medically treated patients who did not have left main coronary artery disease, but were nevertheless at high risk according to angiographic analysis in the study. Numbers of patients at risk at the beginning and end of the study are given at the bottom of the figure, where *S* denotes surgical and *M*, medical. (From Veterans Administration Coronary Artery Bypass Surgery Cooperative Study Group: *N Engl J Med* 311:1333–1339, 1984.)

main coronary artery disease, but were nevertheless at high risk according to angiographic analysis in the study.

The actuarial method also can be used in studies of outcomes other than death or survival. Investigators used this method in a study of subsequent pregnancies among two groups of teenage mothers.[15] The teenage mothers in one group were enrolled in special programs to help them complete their education and delay subsequent pregnancies, whereas the girls in the other group had access to the services that are usually available. The actuarial method was used to analyze data concerning the number and timing of subsequent pregnancies in each group. When tests of significance were performed, the observed differences between the groups were found to be statistically significant.

The actuarial method is still used at times in the medical literature if there are large numbers of study participants, but the Kaplan-Meier method has many advantages, particularly if the sample size is small.

KAPLAN-MEIER METHOD

The Kaplan-Meier method has become the most commonly used approach to survival analysis in medicine.[16] In the medical literature, it is usually referred to as the **Kaplan-Meier life table method.** It also is sometimes referred to as the **product-limit method** because it takes advantage of the N year survival rate (P_N) being equal to the product of all the survival rates of the individual intervals (e.g., p_1, p_2) leading up to time N.

The Kaplan-Meier method is different from the actuarial method in that it calculates a new line of the life table every time a new death occurs. Because deaths occur unevenly over time, the intervals are uneven, and there are many intervals. For this reason, the graph of a Kaplan-Meier life table analysis often looks like uneven stair steps.

In a Kaplan-Meier analysis, the deaths are not viewed as occurring during an interval. Rather, they are seen as instantaneously terminating one interval and beginning a new interval at a lower survival rate. The periods of time between when deaths occur are *death-free intervals,* and the proportion surviving between deaths does not change, although losses to follow-up and censorship are applied during this interval. During the death-free intervals, the curve of the proportion surviving is horizontal rather than sloping downward. A death produces an instantaneous drop in the proportion surviving, and another death-free period begins.

To illustrate the method, the following example was taken from Kaplan and Meier's original article[16](Box 11-6). The article assumed eight fictitious patients, four of whom died and the remaining four of whom were losses (i.e., either lost to follow-up or censored). The four deaths occurred at 0.8, 3.1, 5.4, and 9.2 months. The four losses occurred at 1.0, 2.7, 7.0, and 12.1 months. Because losses to follow-up and censored patients are removed from the study group during the between-death interval in which they occur, they do not appear in the denominator when the next death occurs.

In Box 11-6, p_x is the proportion surviving interval x (i.e., from the time of the previous death to just before the next death), and P_x is the proportion surviving from the beginning of the study to the end of that interval. (P_x is obtained by multiplying together the p_x values of all the intervals up to and including the row of interest.) The p_x of the first

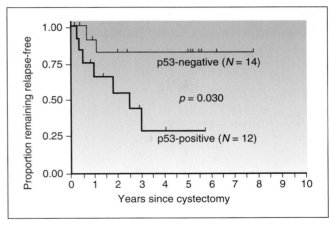

Figure 11-5 **Graph showing life table analysis using Kaplan-Meier method.** From a study of the probability of remaining relapse free over time for two groups of patients who had organ-confined transitional cell cancer of the bladder with deep invasion into the muscularis propria (stage 3a disease), but without regional lymph node metastases. One group consisted of 14 patients with negative results in a test for p53 protein in the nuclei of tumor cells, and the other group consisted of 12 patients with positive results in the same test. (From Esrig D, Elmajian D, Groshen S, et al: *N Engl J Med* 331:1259–1264, 1994.)

interval is always 1 because the first death ends the first study interval, and all the patients not lost to follow-up survive until the first death.

To illustrate the use of Kaplan-Meier analysis in practice, Figure 11-5 shows a Kaplan-Meier life table of the probability of remaining relapse free over time for two groups of patients who had cancer of the bladder.[17] All the patients had organ-confined transitional cell cancer of the bladder with deep invasion into the muscularis propria (stage 3a disease), but without regional lymph node metastases. One group consisted of 14 patients with negative results in a test for p53 protein in the nuclei of tumor cells, and the other group consisted of 12 patients with positive results in the same test. Despite small numbers, the difference in the survival curves for the p53-positive group and the p53-negative group is visually obvious, and it was found to be statistically significant ($p = 0.030$).

Life table methods do not eliminate the bias that occurs if the losses to follow-up occur more frequently in one group than in another, particularly if the characteristics of the patients lost from one group differ greatly from those of the patients lost from the other group. (For example, in a clinical trial comparing the effects of an experimental antihypertensive drug with the effects of an established antihypertensive drug, the occurrence of side effects in the group treated with the experimental drug might cause many in this group to drop out of the study and no longer maintain contact with the investigators.) The life table method is a powerful tool, however, if the losses are few, if the losses represent a similar percentage of the starting numbers in the groups to be compared, and if the characteristics of those who are lost to follow-up are similar. One of these survival methods is usually considered the method of choice for describing dichotomous outcomes in longitudinal studies, such as randomized clinical trials.

Box 11-6   Survival Analysis by Kaplan-Meier Method in Eight Study Participants

PART 1 Beginning Data

Timing of deaths in four participants: 0.8, 3.1, 5.4, and 9.2 months
Timing of loss to follow-up or censorship in four participants: 1.0, 2.7, 7.0, and 12.1 months

PART 2 Tabular Representation of Data

No. Months at Time of Subject's Death	No. Living Just before Subject's Death	No. Living Just after Subject's Death	No. Lost to Follow-up between This and Next Subject's Death	Fraction Surviving after This Death	p_x	Survival Interval (for p_x)	P_x Surviving to End of Interval
—	—	—	—	—	1.000	0 < 0.8	1.000
0.8	8	7	2	7/8	0.875	0.8 < 3.1	0.875
3.1	5	4	0	4/5	0.800	3.1 < 5.4	0.700
5.4	4	3	1	3/4	0.750	5.4 < 9.2	0.525
9.2	2	1	0	1/2	0.500	9.2 <12.1	0.263
No deaths	1	1	1	1/1	1.000	>12.1	0.263

Note: p_x is the proportion surviving interval x (i.e., from time of previous death to just before next death), and P_x is the proportion surviving from the beginning of the study to the end of that interval.

PART 3 Graphic Representation of Data

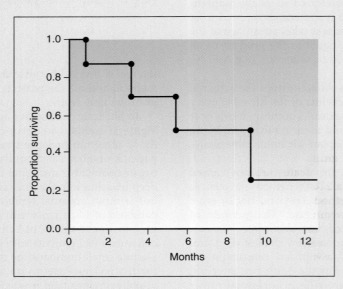

Data from Kaplan EL, Meier P: *J Am Stat Assoc* 53:457–481, 1958.

In statistics, it is always crucial to look at the raw data, and nowhere is this more important than in survival analysis, where examining the pattern of survival differences may be more important for making a clinical decision than examining whether the difference is statistically significant. For example, a surgical therapy for cancer might result in a greater initial mortality, but a higher 5-year survival (i.e., the therapy is a "kill or cure" method), whereas a medical therapy may result in a lower initial mortality, but also a lower 5-year survival. It might be important for patients to know this difference when choosing between these therapies. Patients who preferred to be free of cancer quickly and at all costs might choose the surgical treatment. In contrast, patients who wanted to live for at least a few months to finish writing a book or to see the birth of a first grandchild might choose the medical treatment.

3. Tests of Significance for Differences in Survival

Two or more life table curves can be tested to see if they are significantly different from each other. Statistical computer packages do this by using complicated tests, such as the Breslow test and the Cox test. There are reasonably good simple tests of significance, however, for differences between actuarial survival curves (z-test for proportions) and between Kaplan-Meier curves; for example, the logrank test can be done by hand.

SIGNIFICANCE TESTS FOR PROPORTIONS

See Chapter 10 for a discussion of t-tests and z-tests. The t-test for a difference between actuarial curves depends on the Greenwood formula for the standard error of a proportion and is not described here.[1,18]

LOGRANK TEST

Despite its name, the logrank test does not deal with logarithms or with ranked data. The test is often used to compare data in studies involving treatment and control groups and to test the null hypothesis that each group has the same death rate over time.

In the logrank test, each time a death occurs, the investigator calculates the probability that the observed death would have occurred in the treatment group and the probability that it would have occurred in the control group, if the null hypothesis were true. These probabilities are proportional to the number of survivors to that point in time in each group. Suppose the study started with 100 patients in each group, but at a certain point there were 60 left in the treatment group and 40 in the control group. Under the null hypothesis, the probability that the next death would occur in the treatment group is 0.6, and the probability that the next death would occur in the control group is 0.4.

Within each study group, the expected probabilities for each death are summed to form the total expected number of deaths (E) for that group. The actual deaths in each group also are summed to form the observed number of deaths (O). Then the observed deaths are compared with the expected deaths using the following chi-square test on 1 degree of freedom:

$$\text{logrank } \chi^2 = \sum \frac{(O_T - E_T)^2}{E_T} + \frac{(O_C - E_C)^2}{E_C}$$

where O_T and E_T are the observed and expected deaths in the treatment group, and where O_C and E_C are the observed and expected deaths in the control group. Only two terms are needed because the expected counts are not determined from row and column totals in a 2×2 table, but instead are obtained by an independent method. There is only 1 degree of freedom here because the total number of deaths is already known, and when the number of deaths in one of the two groups is known, the number of deaths in the other group is fixed and is no longer free to vary.

PROPORTIONAL HAZARDS MODELS (COX MODELS)

The Kaplan-Meier approach has been made even more powerful by the development of statistical models that enable dichotomous outcomes to be used as dependent variables in multiple logistic regression analyses, despite losses to follow-up and censorship of patients. Although a detailed discussion of these models is beyond the scope of this book, students should be aware that they are called **proportional hazards models** or, in some studies, **Cox models,** and that their application in clinical trials is common.[19-22]

V. SUMMARY

Bivariate analysis studies the relationship between one independent variable and one dependent variable. The relationships between two variables that are both continuous should first be examined graphically. Then the data can be analyzed statistically to determine whether there is a real relationship between the variables, whether the relationship is linear or nonlinear, whether the correlation (r) is positive or negative, and whether the association is sufficiently strong that it is not likely to have occurred by chance alone. The strength of an association between two continuous variables can be determined by calculating the value of r^2, and the impact that variable x has on variable y can be determined by calculating the slope of the regression.

Correlation and regression analyses indicate whether there is an association between two continuous variables, such as weight (y) and height (x). Correlation tells what proportion of the variation in y is explained by the variation in x. Linear regression estimates the value of y when the value of x is 0, and it predicts the degree of expected change in y when x changes by one unit of measure.

The relationship between an ordinal variable and dichotomous variable can be determined by the Mann-Whitney U test (which is used to compare two groups and is similar to the Student's t-test). The Wilcoxon matched-pairs signed-ranks test is similar to the paired t-test. The relationship between an ordinal variable and a nominal variable can be determined by the Kruskal-Wallis test (which is similar to the F-test). The most important tests measuring the correlation between two ordinal variables are the Spearman and the Kendall correlation coefficients (rho and tau).

The bivariate analysis of dichotomous or nominal data may begin by placing the data for the two variables in a contingency table. The null hypothesis of independence between the two variables usually is then tested by using the chi-square test for unpaired data. Sometimes the Fisher exact probability test must be used in the analysis of dichotomous unpaired data, when the expected numbers are small in one or more cells. For paired or matched dichotomous data, the McNemar chi-square test for paired data may be used. For data in 2×2 tables, the phi coefficient can be used to test the strength of association, and methods are available to calculate standard errors and confidence intervals for proportions, risk ratios, or odds ratios.

Survival analysis employs various methods to study dichotomous outcome variables (e.g., death/survival) over time. Although the actuarial method of analysis is sometimes still used, the Kaplan-Meier (product-limit) method has become the most frequently used approach. Life table curves are constructed from the data, and two or more curves can be tested to see if they are significantly different. For actuarial curves, significance tests for proportions can be used. For Kaplan-Meier curves, the logrank test is the most straightforward test of statistical significance. Proportional hazards (Cox) models are used to perform a survival analysis while controlling for many variables.

References

1. Dawson B, Trapp RG: *Basic and clinical biostatistics*, ed 4, New York, 2004, Lange Medical Books/McGraw-Hill.
2. Holford TR: *Multivariate methods in epidemiology*, New York, 2002, Oxford University Press.
3. Siegel S: *Nonparametric statistics*, New York, 1956, McGraw-Hill.
4. Koo V, Young M, Thompson T, et al: Cost-effectiveness and efficiency of shockwave lithotripsy vs. flexible ureteroscopic holmium:yttrium-aluminium-garnet laser lithotripsy in the treatment of lower pole renal calculi. *BJU Int* 108:1913–1916, 2011.
5. Vimalavathini R, Agarwal SM, Gitanjali B: Educational program for patients with type-1 diabetes mellitus receiving free monthly

supplies of insulin improves knowledge and attitude, but not adherence. *Int J Diabetes Dev Countr* 28:86–90, 2008.

6. Hahn KA, Ohman-Strickland PA, Cohen DJ, et al: Electronic medical records are not associated with improved documentation in community primary care practices. *Am J Med Qual* 26:272–277, 2011.

7. Periyakoil VS, Noda AM, Kraemer HC: Assessment of factors influencing preservation of dignity at life's end: creation and the cross-cultural validation of the preservation of dignity card-sort tool. *J Palliat Med* 13:495–500, 2010.

8. Stoddard HA, Piquette CA: A controlled study of improvements in student exam performance with the use of an audience response system during medical school lectures. *Acad Med* 85:S37–S40, 2010.

9. Snow PJ: Effect of propranolol in myocardial infarction. *Lancet* 2:551–553, 1965.

10. Emerson JD, Colditz GA: Use of statistical analysis. *N Engl J Med* 309:709–713, 1983.

11. Cohen SR: Mycosis fungoides: clinicopathologic relationships, survival, and therapy in 54 patients, with observation on occupation as a new prognostic factor (master's thesis), New Haven, Conn, 1977, Yale University School of Medicine.

12. Dean J, et al: *EPIINFO, version 5.01*, Atlanta, 1991, Epidemiology Program Office, Centers for Disease Control and Prevention. http://wwwn.cdc.gov/epiinfo/

13. Feinstein A: *Principles of medical statistics*, Boca Raton, Fla, 2002, Chapman & Hall/CRC.

14. Veterans Administration Coronary Artery Bypass Surgery Cooperative Study Group: Eleven-year survival in the Veterans Administration randomized trial of coronary bypass surgery for stable angina. *N Engl J Med* 311:1333–1339, 1984.

15. Currie J, Jekel JF, Klerman LV: Subsequent pregnancies among teenage mothers enrolled in a special program. *Am J Public Health* 62:1606–1611, 1972.

16. Kaplan EL, Meier P: Nonparametric estimation from incomplete observations. *J Am Stat Assoc* 53:457–481, 1958.

17. Esrig D, Elmajian D, Groshen S, et al: Accumulation of nuclear p53 and tumor progression in bladder cancer. *N Engl J Med* 331:1259–1264, 1994.

18. Cutler SJ, Ederer F: Maximum utilization of the life table method in analyzing survival. *J Chron Dis* 8:699–713, 1958.

19. Schneider M, Zuckerman IH, Onukwugha E, et al: Chemotherapy treatment and survival in older women with estrogen receptor-negative metastatic breast cancer: a population-based analysis. *J Am Geriatr Soc* 59:637–646, 2011.

20. Thourani VH, Keeling WB, Kilgo PD, et al: The impact of body mass index on morbidity and short- and long-term mortality in cardiac valvular surgery. *J Thorac Cardiovasc Surg* 142:1052–1061, 2011.

21. Appleby PN, Allen NE, Key TJ: Diet, vegetarianism, and cataract risk. *Am J Clin Nutr* 93:1128–1135, 2011.

22. Park JY, Mitrou PN, Keogh RH, et al: Self-reported and measured anthropometric data and risk of colorectal cancer in the EPIC-Norfolk study. *Int J Obes Lond* 36:107–118, 2012.

Select Readings

Dawson B, Trapp RG: *Basic and clinical biostatistics*, ed 4, New York, 2004, Lange Medical Books/McGraw-Hill.

Lee ET: *Statistical methods for survival data analysis*, Belmont, Calif, 1980, Lifetime Learning Publications.

Siegel S: *Nonparametric statistics*, New York, 1956, McGraw-Hill. [A classic.]

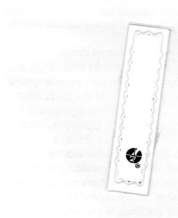

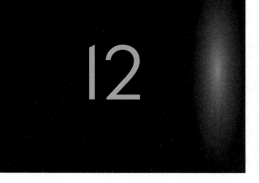

12

Applying Statistics to Trial Design: Sample Size, Randomization, and Control for Multiple Hypotheses

I. SAMPLE SIZE

The determination of sample size is critical in planning clinical research because sample size is usually the most important factor determining the time and funding necessary to perform the research. The sample size has a profound impact on the likelihood of finding statistical significance.

Members of committees responsible for evaluating and funding clinical studies look closely at the assumptions used to estimate the number of study participants needed and at the way in which calculations of sample size were performed. Part of their task when reviewing the sample size is to determine whether the proposed research is realistic (e.g., whether adequate participants are included in the intervention and control groups in a randomized clinical trial, or in the groups of cases and controls in a case-control study). In research reported in the literature, inadequate sample size may explain why apparently useful clinical results are not statistically significant.

Statisticians are probably consulted more often because an investigator wants to know the sample size needed for a study than for any other reason. Sample size calculations can be confusing, even for people who can do ordinary statistical analyses without trouble. As a test of intuition regarding sample size, try to answer the following three questions:

1. What size sample—large or small—would be needed if there was a very large variance in the outcome variable?
2. What size sample would be needed if the investigator wanted the answer to be extremely close to the true value (i.e., have narrow confidence limits or small *p* value)?
3. What size sample would be needed if the difference that the investigator wanted to be able to detect was extremely small?

If your intuition suggested that all these requirements would create the need for a large sample size, you would be correct. If intuition did not suggest the correct answers, review these questions again after reading the following information about how the basic formulas for sample size are derived.

Other factors affecting the number of participants required for a study include whether the:

1. Research design involves *paired data* (e.g., each subject has a pair of observations from two points in time—before treatment and after treatment) or *unpaired data* (e.g., observations are compared between an experimental group and a control group).
2. Investigator anticipates a large or small variance in the variable of interest.
3. Investigator wants to consider beta (β, type II or false-negative) errors in addition to alpha (α, type I or false-positive) errors.
4. Investigator chooses the usual alpha level (*p* value of 0.05 or confidence interval of 95%) or chooses a smaller level of alpha.
5. Alpha chosen is one-sided or two-sided.
6. Investigator wants to be able to detect a fairly small or extremely small difference between the means or proportions of the outcome variable.

A. Derivation of Basic Sample Size Formula

To derive the basic formula for calculating the sample size, it is easiest to start with the formula for the *paired t-test* (see Chapter 10):

$$t_\alpha = \frac{\overline{d}}{\frac{s_d}{\sqrt{N}}}$$

where t_α is the critical ratio to determine the probability of a false-positive (α) error if the null hypothesis is rejected; $\overline{d}$ is the mean difference that was observed in the outcome variable, s_d is the standard deviation of the before-after differences, and N is the sample size.

To solve for N, several rearrangements and substitutions of terms in the equation must be made. First, everything can be squared and the equation rearranged so that N is in the numerator and s^2 is the variance of the distribution of d:

$$t_\alpha{}^2 = \frac{\left(\bar{d}\right)^2}{\left(s_d / \sqrt{N}\right)^2} = \frac{\left(\bar{d}\right)^2 \cdot N}{(s)^2}$$

Next, the terms can be rearranged so that the equation for N in a paired (before and after) study becomes:

$$N = \frac{t_\alpha{}^2 \cdot (s)^2}{\left(\bar{d}\right)^2}$$

Now the t in the formula must be replaced with z. This provides a solution to a circular problem: To know the value of t, the degrees of freedom (df) must be known. The df depends on N, however, which is what the investigator is initially trying to calculate. Because the value of z is not dependent on df, and because z is close to t when the sample size is large, z can be used instead of t. The formula becomes:

$$N = \frac{z_\alpha{}^2 \cdot (s)^2}{\left(\bar{d}\right)^2}$$

In theory, using z instead of t might produce a slight underestimate of the sample size needed. In practice, however, using z seems to work well, and its use is customary. The previous formula is for a study using the *paired t-test*, in which each participant serves as his or her own control. For a study using Student's t-test, such as a randomized controlled trial (RCT) with an experimental group and a control group, it would be necessary to calculate N for each group. The previous formula considers only the problem of alpha error; to minimize the possibility of beta error, a z term for beta error must be introduced as well. Before these topics are discussed, however, the answers to the three questions posed earlier should be explored more fully in light of the information provided by the formula for the calculation of N.

1. The larger the variance (s^2), the larger the sample size must be because the variance is in the numerator of the formula for N. This makes sense intuitively because with a large variance (and large standard error), a larger N is needed to compensate for the greater uncertainty of the estimate.
2. To have considerable confidence that a mean difference shown in a study is real, the analysis must produce a small p value for the observed mean difference, which implies that the value for t_α or z_α was large. Because z_α is in the numerator of the sample size formula, the larger z_α is, the larger the N (the sample size) that is needed. For a two-tailed test, a p value of 0.05 (the alpha level chosen) would require a z_α of 1.96, which, when squared as in the formula, would equal 3.84. To be even more confident, the investigator might set alpha at 0.01. This would require a z_α of 2.58, which equals 6.66 when squared, 73% greater than when alpha is set at 0.05. To decrease the probability of being wrong from 5% to 1% would require the sample size to be almost doubled.
3. If the investigator wanted to detect with confidence a very small difference between the mean values of two study groups (i.e., a small $\bar{d}$), a very large N would be needed because the difference (squared) is in the denominator. The smaller the denominator is, the larger the ratio is, and the larger the N must be. A precise estimate and a large sample size are needed to detect a small difference.

Whether a small difference is considered clinically important often depends on the topic of research. Studies showing that a new treatment for hypertension reduces the systolic blood pressure by 2 to 3 mm Hg would be considered clinically trivial. Studies showing that a new treatment for pancreatic cancer improves the survival rate by 10% (0.1) would be considered a major advance. Clinical judgment is involved in determining the minimum difference that should be considered clinically important.

B. Beta (False-Negative) Error

If a difference is examined with a t-test, and it is statistically significant at the prestated level of alpha (e.g., 0.05), beta error is not an issue. What if a reported finding seems to be clinically important, but it is not "statistically significant" in that study? Here the question of a possible false-negative (beta) error becomes important. Beta error may have occurred because the sample size was too small. When planning a study, investigators want to avoid the likelihood of beta (false-negative) error and the likelihood of alpha (false-positive) error, and readers of the literature should be on the lookout for this problem as well. The relationship between the results of a study and the true status can be seen in a "truth table" (Table 12-1). The similarity of Table 12-1 to the relationship between a test result and the disease status is obvious (compare with Table 7-1).

A seminal article illustrated the need to be concerned about beta error: in most of 71 *negative* RCTs of new therapies published in prominent medical journals, the sample sizes were too small "to provide reasonable assurance that a clinically meaningful 'difference' (i.e., therapeutic effect) would not be missed."[1] In the study, "reasonable assurance" was 90%. In 94% of these negative studies, the sample size was too small to detect a 25% improvement in outcome with reasonable (90%) assurance. In 75% of the studies, the sample size was too small to detect a 50% improvement in outcome with the same level of assurance. Evidence indicates that this problem has persisted over time.[2]

Table 12-1 "Truth Table" Showing Relationship between Study Results and True Status

Study Result	True Status	
	True Difference	No Difference
Statistically significant difference	True-positive result	False-positive result (alpha error)
Not statistically significant	False-negative result (beta error)	True-negative result

A study with a large beta error has a low sensitivity for detecting a true difference because, as discussed in Chapter 7:

$$\text{Sensitivity} + \text{False-negative (beta) error} = 1.00$$

When investigators speak of a research study versus a clinical test, however, they usually use the term "statistical power" instead of "sensitivity." With this substitution in terms:

$$\text{Statistical power} + \text{Beta error} = 1.00$$

which means that statistical power is equal to (1 − beta error). When calculating a sample size, if the investigators accept a 20% possibility of missing a true finding (beta error = 0.2), the study should have a statistical power of 0.8, or 80%. That means the investigators are 80% confident that they would be able to detect a true mean difference of the size they specify with the sample size they determine. The best way to incorporate beta error into a study is to include it beforehand in the determination of sample size. Incorporating the statistical term for beta error (z_β) in the sample size calculation is simple but likely to increase the sample size considerably.

C. Steps in Calculation of Sample Size

The first step in calculating sample size is to choose the appropriate formula to use, based on the type of study and the type of error to be considered. Four common formulas for calculating sample size are discussed in this chapter and listed in Table 12-2, and their use is illustrated in Boxes 12-1 through 12-4.[3] The second step in calculating sample size requires that the investigators specify the following values: the variance expected (s^2); the z_α value for the level of alpha desired; the smallest clinically important difference ($\overline{d}$); and, usually, beta (measured as z_β). All values except the variance must come from clinical and research judgment, although the estimated variance should be based on knowledge of data. If the outcome variable being studied is continuous, such as blood pressure, the estimate of variance can be obtained from the literature or from a small pilot study.

If the outcome is a proportion, such as the proportion of patients who survive for 5 years, the variance is easier to estimate. The investigators need to estimate only the proportion that would survive 5 years with the new experimental treatment (which is p_1; e.g., 60%) and the proportion expected to survive with the control group's treatment (p_2; e.g., 40%). Assuming the two study groups are of approximately equal size, the investigators must determine the mean survival in the combined group ($\overline{p} = 50\%$ in this example). The formula for the variance of a proportion is simply the following:

$$\text{Variance (proportion)} = \overline{p}(1 - \overline{p})$$

When the investigators are armed with all this information, it is straightforward to compute the needed sample size, as shown in Boxes 12-1 through 12-4 and discussed subsequently. The N determined using the formulas in Boxes 12-2, 12-3, and 12-4 is only for the experimental group. If there is a control group, the study must have N experimental

Table 12-2 Formulas for Calculation of Sample Size for Common Studies in Medical Research

Type of Study and Type of Errors Considered for Use*	Appropriate Formula
Studies using paired t-test (e.g., **before-and-after studies**) and considering alpha (type I) error only	$N = \dfrac{(z_\alpha)^2 \cdot (s)^2}{(\overline{d})^2}$
Studies using Student's t-test (e.g., **RCTs with one experimental group and one control group**) and considering alpha error only	$N = \dfrac{(z_\alpha)^2 \cdot 2 \cdot (s)^2}{(\overline{d})^2}$
Studies using Student's t-test (e.g., **RCTs with one experimental group and one control group**) and considering alpha (type I) and beta (type II) errors	$N = \dfrac{(z_\alpha + z_\beta)^2 \cdot 2 \cdot (s)^2}{(\overline{d})^2}$
Studies using a test of differences in proportions (e.g., **RCTs with one experimental group and one control group**) and considering alpha and beta errors	$N = \dfrac{(z_\alpha + z_\beta)^2 \cdot 2 \cdot \overline{p}(1 - \overline{p})}{(\overline{d})^2}$

*The appropriate formula is based on the study design and type of outcome data. In these formulas, N = sample size; z_α = z value for alpha error; z_β = z value for beta error; s^2 = variance; $\overline{p}$ = mean proportion of success; and $\overline{d}$ = mean difference to be detected. See Boxes 12-1 to 12-4 for examples of calculations using these formulas. *RCTs*, Randomized controlled (clinical) trials.

participants and N control participants. For some studies, investigators may find it easier to obtain control participants than cases. When cases are scarce or costly, it is possible to increase the sample size by matching two or three controls with each case in a case-control study or by obtaining two or three control group participants for each experimental participant in a clinical trial. The incremental benefits in statistical power decline, however, as the number of cases per control increases, so it is seldom cost-effective to have more than three controls for each case. The application of the formulas described here assumes the research objective is to have *equal numbers of experimental and control participants*. If the number of controls is planned to be much greater than the number of cases, the sample size formulas discussed in this chapter would need to be modified.[4]

D. Sample Size for Studies Using t-Tests

Box 12-1 shows the formula and the calculations for a paired, before-after study of an antihypertensive drug, a study of patients whose blood pressure is checked before starting the drug and then after taking the drug. A paired t-test would be used for this type of paired data. Given the variance, alpha, and difference chosen by the investigator, only nine participants would be needed altogether. This type of study is efficient in terms of the sample size required. However, even most paired studies require considerably more than nine participants. Also, note that a very small sample tends to limit the external validity, or *generalizability,* of a trial; a few study participants are less likely than many to resemble the general population from which they are drawn.

Box 12-2 shows the formula and the calculations for an RCT of an antihypertensive drug, a study for which **Student's t-test** would be used. This formula differs from the

Box 12-1   Calculation of Sample Size for a Study Using the Paired $\pm$ t-Test and Considering Alpha Error Only

PART I   **Data on Which the Calculation is Based**

Study Characteristic	Assumptions Made by Investigator
Type of study	Before-and-after study of antihypertensive drug
Data sets	Pretreatment and posttreatment observations in the same participants
Variable	Systolic blood pressure
Losses to follow-up	None
Standard deviation (s)	15 mm Hg
Variance (s^2)	225 mm Hg
Data for alpha (z_α)	$p = 0.05$; 95% confidence desired (two-tailed test); $z_\alpha = 1.96$
Difference to be detected ($\overline{d}$)	≥10 mm Hg difference between pretreatment and posttreatment blood pressure values

PART 2   **Calculation of Sample Size (N)**

$$N = \frac{(z_\alpha)^2 \cdot (s)^2}{(\overline{d})^2} = \frac{(1.96)^2 \cdot (15)^2}{(10)^2}$$

$$= \frac{(3.84)(225)}{100} = \frac{864}{100} = 8.64 = \textbf{9 participants total}$$

Interpretation: Only nine participants are needed for this study because each paired subject serves as his or her own control in a before-and-after study, thereby greatly reducing the variance (i.e., variance between a subject and him/herself before and after a particular treatment is almost certain to be much less than the variance between one person and another). When the estimated N is a fraction, the N used should be rounded up to be safe.

Box 12-2   Calculation of Sample Size for a Study Using Student's t-Test and Considering Alpha Error Only

PART I   **Data on Which the Calculation Is Based**

Study Characteristic	Assumptions Made by Investigator
Type of study	Randomized controlled trial of antihypertensive drug
Data sets	Observations in one experimental group and one control group of the same size
Variable	Systolic blood pressure
Losses to follow-up	None
Standard deviation (s)	15 mm Hg
Variance (s^2)	225 mm Hg
Data for alpha (z_α)	$p = 0.05$; 95% confidence desired (two-tailed test); $z_\alpha = 1.96$
Difference to be detected ($\overline{d}$)	≥10 mm Hg difference between mean blood pressure values of the experimental group and control group

PART 2   **Calculation of Sample Size (N)**

$$N = \frac{(z_\alpha)^2 \cdot 2 \cdot (s)^2}{(\overline{d})^2} = \frac{(1.96)^2 \cdot 2 \cdot (15)^2}{(10)^2}$$

$$= \frac{(3.84)(2)(225)}{100} = \frac{1728}{100} = 17.28$$

$$= \textbf{18 participants per group} \times 2 \text{ groups}$$

$$= \textbf{36 participants total}$$

Interpretation: For the type of study depicted in this box, 18 participants are needed in the experimental group and 18 in the control group, for a total N of 36 study participants. The N needed to be rounded up. The total N needed in this box is four times as large as the total N needed in Box 12-1, although the values for z_α, s, and $\overline{d}$ are the same in both boxes. One reason for the larger sample size for a randomized controlled trial is that there are two groups, and the N calculated is for the intervention group only. The other reason is the fact that there are two variances to consider (i.e., the intervention and control groups contribute to the overall variance), so the estimated variance must be multiplied by 2.

formula in Box 12-1 only in that the variance estimate must be multiplied by 2. Given the same assumptions as in Box 12-1 concerning variance, alpha, and difference, it would be necessary to have a total of 36 study participants for this RCT (18 in experimental group and 18 in control group), which is four times the number of participants required for the paired, before-after study described in Box 12-1. The larger sample size is needed for two reasons. Studies using Student's *t*-test have *two sources of variance* instead of one because the study and control groups each contribute to the variance (thus the number 2 in the numerator). Second, the *N* obtained is *only for the intervention group,* and another person serves as the control for each experimental participant (so that the total sample size for equal numbers of cases and controls would be 2*N*). The only difference between the formula shown in Box 12-2 and that in Box 12-3 is the latter considers **beta error** in addition to alpha error. Although there is no complete agreement on the level of beta error acceptable for most studies, usually a beta error of 20% (one-tailed test) is used; this corresponds to a *z* value of 0.84. When this beta estimate is used in Box 12-3, with the same z_α, variance, and mean difference as in Box 12-2, the calculations show that 72 study participants are needed for the randomized controlled trial. In contrast, only 36 participants were needed if only alpha was considered, as shown in Box 12-2.

The issue of adequate versus excessive sample sizes continues to be debated. Some believe that the medical world may have overreacted to the concerns about beta error, with the result that many investigators are now using larger samples than necessary. Nevertheless, for safety, investigators may want the actual sample size to be larger than that calculated from the formulas, particularly if the investigator expects significant losses to follow-up or is uncertain of the accuracy of the variance estimate.

It is true that when z_α and z_β are added together before squaring, as shown in the formula in Box 12-3, the sample size may be excessive. Depending on the value of z_β used, this would at least double and could as much as quadruple the estimated value of *N*, which could increase the cost of a study astronomically. The large sample sizes required when beta error is included in the sample-size formulas are partly responsible for the limited number of major studies that now can be funded nationally. A needlessly large sample size introduces other problems for the investigators, who previously set the minimum difference they thought was clinically important. If the sample size is larger than necessary, they may find that differences smaller than what they publicly affirmed to be clinically important are now statistically significant. What do they do now with clinically trivial findings that are, nevertheless, statistically significant? In the research described in Boxes 12-2 and 12-3, the investigators sought to detect a difference of 10 mm Hg or more in systolic blood pressure, presumably because they believed that a smaller difference would be clinically unimportant. With a total sample size of 36 (see Box 12-2), a difference smaller than 10 mm Hg would not be statistically significant. With a total sample size of 72 (see Box 12-3), however, a difference of

Box 12-3	Calculation of Sample Size for a Study Using Student's *t*-Test and Considering Alpha and Beta Errors

PART 1 **Data on Which the Calculation Is Based**

Study Characteristic	Assumptions Made by Investigator
Type of study	Randomized controlled trial of antihypertensive drug
Data sets	Observations in one experimental group and one control group of the same size
Variable	Systolic blood pressure
Losses to follow-up	None
Standard deviation (*s*)	15 mm Hg
Variance (*s²*)	225 mm Hg
Data for alpha (z_α)	*p* = 0.05; 95% confidence desired (two-tailed test); $z_\alpha = 1.96$
Data for beta (z_β)	20% beta error; 80% power desired (one-tailed test); $z_\beta = 0.84$
Difference to be detected $(\overline{d})$	≥10 mm Hg difference between mean blood pressure values of the experimental group and control group

PART 2 **Calculation of Sample Size (*N*)**

$$N = \frac{(z_\alpha + z_\beta)^2 \cdot 2 \cdot (s)^2}{(\overline{d})^2}$$

$$= \frac{(1.96 + 0.84)^2 \cdot 2 \cdot (15)^2}{(10)^2}$$

$$= \frac{(7.84)(2)(225)}{100} = \frac{3528}{100} = 35.28$$

$$= \textbf{36 participants per group} \times 2 \text{ groups} = \textbf{72 participants total}$$

Interpretation: The total number of participants needed is 72. Including z_β (for beta error) in the calculation approximately doubled the sample size here compared with the sample size in Box 12-2. If the investigators had chosen a smaller beta error, the sample size would have increased even more.

only 8 mm Hg would be statistically significant ($t = 2.26$; p is approximately 0.03 on 70 degrees of freedom). In cases such as this, it is important to focus on the original hypotheses of the research rather than report as important every statistically significant finding.

E. Sample Size for a Test of Differences in Proportions

Often a dependent variable is measured as success/failure and is described as the proportion of outcomes that represent some form of success, such as improvement in health, remission of disease, or reduction in mortality. In this case the formula for sample size must be expressed in terms of proportions, as shown in the formula in Box 12-4.

Box 12-4 provides an example of how to calculate the sample size for an RCT of a drug to reduce the 5-year mortality in patients with a particular form of cancer. Before the calculations can be made, the investigators must decide which values they will use for z_α, z_β, variance, and the smallest difference to be detected. For alpha and beta, they decide to use a level of 95% confidence (two-tailed test, $p = 0.05$)

Box 12-4	Initial and Subsequent Calculation of Sample Size for a Study Using a Test of Differences in Proportions and Considering Alpha and Beta Errors

PART 1A   Data on Which the Initial Calculation is Based

Study Characteristic	Assumptions Made by Investigator
Type of study	Randomized controlled trial of a drug to reduce 5-year mortality in patients with a particular form of cancer
Data sets	Observations in one experimental group (**E**) and one control group (**C**) of the same size
Variable	**Success** = 5-year survival after treatment (expected to be 0.6 in experimental group and 0.5 in control group)
	Failure = death within 5 years of treatment
Losses to follow-up	None
Variance, expressed as $\bar{p}(1-\bar{p})$	$\bar{p} = 0.55$; $(1-\bar{p}) = 0.45$
Data for alpha (z_α)	$p = 0.05$; 95% confidence desired (two-tailed test); $z_\alpha = 1.96$
Data for beta (z_β)	20% beta error; 80% power desired (one-tailed test); $z_\beta = 0.84$
Difference to be detected ($\bar{d}$)	≥0.1 difference between the success (survival) of the experimental group and that of the control group (i.e., 10% difference because $p_E = 0.6$, and $p_C = 0.5$)

PART 1B   Initial Calculation of Sample Size (N)

$$N = \frac{(z_\alpha + z_\beta)^2 \cdot 2 \cdot \bar{p}(1-\bar{p})}{(\bar{d})^2} = \frac{(1.96+0.84)^2 \cdot 2 \cdot (0.55)(0.45)}{(0.1)^2}$$

$$= \frac{(7.84)(2)(0.2475)}{0.01} = \frac{3.88}{0.01} = 388$$

$$= \textbf{388 participants per group} \times 2 \text{ groups} = \textbf{776 participants total}$$

Interpretation: A total of 776 participants would be needed, 388 in each group.

PART 2A   Changes in Data on Which Initial Calculation Was Based (Because First N Was Too Large for Study to Be Feasible; See Text)

Study Characteristic	Assumptions Made by Investigator
Difference to be detected ($\bar{d}$)	≥0.2 difference between the success (survival) of the experimental group and that of the control group (i.e., 20% difference because $p_E = 0.7$, and $p_C = 0.5$)
Variance, expressed as $\bar{p}(1-\bar{p})$	$\bar{p} = 0.60$; $(1-\bar{p}) = 0.40$

PART 2B   Subsequent (Revised) Calculation of Sample Size (N)

$$N = \frac{(z_\alpha + z_\beta)^2 \cdot 2 \cdot \bar{p}(1-\bar{p})}{(\bar{d})^2} = \frac{(1.96+0.84)^2 \cdot 2 \cdot (0.60)(0.40)}{(0.2)^2}$$

$$= \frac{(7.84)(2)(0.2400)}{0.04} = \frac{3.76}{0.04} = 94$$

$$= \textbf{94 participants per group} \times 2 \text{ groups} = \textbf{188 participants total}$$

Interpretation: Now a total of 188 participants would be needed, 94 in each group. As a result of changes in the data on which the initial calculation was based, the number of participants needed would be reduced from 776 to 188.

and 80% power (one-tailed test), so that z_α equals 1.96 and z_β equals 0.84.

Initially, as shown in the first part of Box 12-4, the investigators decide they want to detect a 10% improvement in survival (i.e., difference of 0.1 between 5-year mortality of experimental group and that of control group). They also assume that the survival rate will be 50% (0.5) in the control group and 10% better (0.6) in the experimental group. They assume the mean proportion of success $(\bar{p})$ for all participants enrolled in the study will be 0.55. Based on these assumptions, the calculations show that they would need 388 participants in the experimental group and 388 in the control group, for a total of 776 participants. If it is difficult to find that many participants or to fund a study this large, what can be done?

Theoretically, any of the estimated values in the formula might be altered. The alpha and beta values used in these boxes (alpha = 0.05 two-sided, and beta = 0.20 one-sided) are the ones customarily used, however, and the best estimate of variance should always be used. The best place to rethink the sample size calculation is the requirement for the minimum clinically important difference. Perhaps a 10% improvement is not large enough to be meaningful. What if it were changed to 20% (a difference of 0.2, based on a survival rate of 70% in the experimental group and 50% in the control group)? As shown in the second part of Box 12-4, changing the improvement requirement to 20% changes the variance estimate, so that $\bar{p}$ is now equal to 0.6. Based on these revised assumptions, the calculations show that the investigators would need only 94 participants in the experimental group and 94 in the control group, for a total of 188 participants. A study with this smaller sample size seems much more reasonable to perform and less costly. Changing the difference the investigators want to detect after an initial sample size calculation is performed, however, may seem to be trying to adjust truth to what is convenient. If the investigators really believe the difference they chose a priori is clinically important, they should try to obtain funding for the large sample required.

When choosing the 10% difference initially, the investigators may have intuitively assumed (incorrectly) that it is easier to detect a small difference than a large one. Alternately, they may have had an interest in detecting a small difference, even though it would not be clinically important. In either case, the penalty in sample size may alert the investigators to the statistical realities of the situation and force them to think seriously about the smallest difference that would be clinically important.

II. RANDOMIZING STUDY PARTICIPANTS

Randomized clinical trials and randomized field trials require that the allocation of study participants to an intervention or a control status be done by randomization. There is a distinction between **randomization,** which entails allocating the available participants to one or another study group, and **random sampling,** which entails selecting a small group for study from a much larger group of potential study participants. Randomization is usually used in clinical trials. It is an important technique for achieving *internal validity* in a study because it reduces the possibility of bias, whereas random sampling helps to ensure *external validity* because it seeks to ensure a representative sample of people (see Chapter 4).

A. Goals of Randomization

An experimental design, of which the randomized controlled clinical trial (RCCT, or RCT) is the standard in clinical research, depends on an **unbiased allocation of study participants** to the experimental and control groups. For most purposes, the only evidence of an unbiased allocation that would be accepted is randomization. Contrary to popular opinion, randomization does not guarantee that the two (or more) groups created by random allocation are identical in either size or subject characteristics (although block randomization can guarantee identical group sizes). What randomization does guarantee, if properly done, is that the different groups will be free of selection bias and problems resulting from regression toward the mean.

Selection bias can occur if participants are allowed to choose whether they will be in an intervention group or a control group, as occurred in the 1954 polio vaccine trials (see Chapter 4). Another form of selection bias, *allocation bias,* can occur if investigators influence the assignment of participants to one group or another. There may be considerable pressure from a patient and the family members or other caregivers to alter the randomization process and allow the patient to enroll in the intervention group, especially in studies involving a community intervention, but this pressure must be resisted.[5]

Regression toward the mean, also known as the **statistical regression effect,** affects patients who were chosen to participate in a study precisely because they had an extreme measurement on some variable (e.g., high number of ear infections during the past year). They are likely to have a measurement that is closer to average at a later time (e.g., during the subsequent year) for reasons unrelated to the type or efficacy of the treatment they receive. In a study comparing treatment methods in two groups of patients, both of which had extreme measurements at the beginning of the study, randomization cannot eliminate the tendency to regress toward the mean. Randomization may *equalize* this tendency between the study groups, however, preventing bias in the comparison. When one group undertook an RCT of surgical treatment (tonsillectomy and adenoidectomy) versus medical treatment (antibiotics) of children with recurrent throat infections, they found that the children in both groups had fewer episodes of throat infection in the year after treatment than in the year before treatment (an effect attributed to regression toward the mean), but that the surgically treated patients showed more improvement than the medically treated patients (an effect attributed to the intervention).[6]

B. Methods of Randomization

Before-and-after studies sometimes randomize the study participants into two groups, with one group given the experimental intervention first and the other group given the placebo first. Then, after a **washout period,** when no intervention is given and physiologic values are expected to return to baseline, the group previously given the experimental intervention "crosses over" to receiving the placebo, and vice versa; thus such studies are referred to as *crossover trials.* By careful analysis, it is possible to determine whether being randomized to receive the experimental intervention first or second made any difference.

When a study involving an experimental group and a control group is planned, the investigators must decide what method of randomization will be used to ensure that each subject has an equal (or at least a known) probability of being assigned to each group. As described subsequently, some methods incorporate the use of a random-number table such as that shown in Table A in the Appendix, although computer-generated random numbers are routinely used. Regardless of the method chosen, the best way to keep human preferences from influencing the randomization process is to hide the results of randomization until they are needed for the analysis. If possible, the study participants should not know the group to which they are assigned. This often can be accomplished by "blinding" the study participants (e.g., giving control group a placebo that looks, tastes, and smells the same as treatment for experimental group) and blinding the individuals who dispense the treatment, and the individuals who record the findings from the study participants. If both these blinding efforts are made, it is a called a **double-blind** study. Blinding protects against bias in any of the study procedures that might favor one group or another if either the participants or the investigators knew who was receiving the treatment and who was not. Examples of this would occur if such knowledge influenced the way the patients experienced the treatment or illness, or the way investigators treated study participants or measured their progress.

The methods described subsequently all assume that an equal number of participants is desired in the experimental and control groups. The methods can be modified easily, however, to provide two or more control participants for each experimental subject.

1. Simple Random Allocation

Simple random allocation uses a random-number table or a computerized random-number generator to allocate potential participants to a treatment or control status. The simplest approach is to create a stack of sequentially numbered envelopes (e.g., numbered from 1 to 100 in a study with 100 participants). The investigators blindly put a pencil on a number in the random-number table and proceed from that number in a predetermined direction (e.g., up the columns of the table). If the first number is even, they write "experimental group" on a slip of paper and put it in the first envelope. If the next number is odd, they write "control group" on a slip of paper and insert it in the second envelope. They continue until all of the envelopes contain a random group assignment. The first patient enrolled in the study is assigned to whatever group is indicated in the first envelope. As each new eligible patient is enrolled, the investigators open the next sequentially numbered envelope to find out the patient's group assignment.

2. Randomization into Groups of Two

If it is important to have equally sized groups, study participants can be randomized two at a time (i.e., block randomization). Envelopes are numbered (or a comparable strategy is applied electronically) sequentially (e.g., from 1 to 100) and separated into groups of two. As in the previous method, the investigators could begin by blindly putting down a pencil on a number in the random-number table

and proceeding in a predetermined direction, or having a computerized random-number generator do this. If the first number is even, they write "experimental group" on a slip of paper and put it in the first envelope. For the paired envelope, they automatically write the alternative group, in this case, "control group." They use the random-number table to determine the assignment of the first envelope in the second pair and continue in this manner for each pair of envelopes. Any time an even number of patients have been admitted into the study, exactly half would be in the experimental group and half in the control group.

3. Systematic Allocation

Systematic allocation in research studies is equivalent to the military call, "Sound off!" The first patient is randomly assigned to a group, and the next patient is automatically assigned to the alternate group. Subsequent patients are given group assignments on an alternating basis. This method also ensures that the experimental and control groups are of equal size if there is an even number of patients entered in the study.

There are advantages to this method beyond simplicity. Usually, the variance of the data from a systematic allocation is smaller than that from a simple random allocation, so the statistical power is improved. If there is any form of periodicity in the way patients enter, however, there may be a bias. For example, suppose systematic sampling is used to allocate patients into two groups, and only two patients are admitted each day to the study (e.g., first two new patients who enter the clinic each morning). If each intake day started so that the first patient was assigned to the experimental group and the second was assigned to the control group, all the experimental group participants would be the first patients to arrive at the clinic, perhaps early in the morning. They might be systematically different (e.g., employed, eager, early risers) compared with patients who come later in the day, in which case bias might be introduced into the study. This danger is easy to avoid, however, if the investigator reverses the sequence frequently, sometimes taking the first person each day into the control group. The convenience and statistical advantages of systematic sampling make it desirable to use whenever possible. The systematic allocation method also can be used for allocating study participants to three, four, or even more groups.

4. Stratified Allocation

In clinical research, stratified allocation is often called **prognostic stratification.** It is used when the investigators want to assign patients to different risk groups depending on such baseline variables as the severity of disease (e.g., stage of cancer) and age. When such risk groups have been created, each stratum can be allocated randomly to the experimental group or the control group. This is usually done to ensure homogeneity of the study groups by severity of disease. If the homogeneity was achieved, the analysis can be done for the entire group and within the prognostic groups.

C. Special Issues with Randomization

Randomization does not guarantee that two or more groups would be identical. Suppose an investigator, when checking how similar the experimental and control groups were after randomization, found that the two groups were of different size, and that 1 of 20 characteristics being compared showed a statistically significant difference between the groups. Occasional differences being statistically significant does not mean the randomization was biased; some differences are expected by chance. There may be a legitimate concern, however, that some of the observed differences between the randomized groups could confound the analysis. In this case the variables of concern can be controlled for in the analysis.

Although randomization is the fundamental technique of clinical trials, many other precautions still must be taken to reduce bias, such as ensuring the accuracy of all the data by blinding patients and observers and standardizing data collection instruments. A major problem with RCTs involves the generalization of study findings. Patients have the right to refuse to participate in a study before or after randomization. This means that a particular study is limited to patients who are willing to participate. Are these patients similar to patients who refused to participate, or are they an unusual subset of the entire population with the problem being studied? The results of a clinical trial can be safely generalized only to similar patients.

What happens if, after randomization, a patient is not doing well, and the patient or clinician wants to switch from the experimental treatment to another medication? Ethically, the patient cannot be forced to continue a particular treatment. When the switch occurs, how would the data for this patient be analyzed? The choice among several possible strategies represents a philosophic position. Currently, the popular approach is to analyze the data *as if the patient had remained in the original group,* so that any negative outcomes are assigned to their original treatment. This strategy, called the **"intention to treat" approach,** is based on the belief that if the patient was doing so poorly as to want to switch, the outcome should be ascribed to that treatment. Other investigators prefer to exclude this patient and analyze the data as if the patient had never participated in the study; however, this could lead to a smaller, and probably biased, sample. Still others prefer to reassign the patient to a third group and analyze the data separately from the original groups. The original groups are still changed, however, and it is unclear whom the remaining groups represent.

Another problem in randomized trials of treatment is deciding what to consider as the starting point for measuring the outcome. If surgical treatment and medical treatment are being compared, should surgical mortality (dying as a result of the surgery) be included as part of the debit side for surgical treatment? Or does measuring the outcome start with the question, "Given survival from the initial surgical procedure, do patients treated surgically or those treated medically do better?"[7] Most investigators recommend beginning the analysis at the time of randomization.

III. CONTROLLING FOR THE TESTING OF MULTIPLE HYPOTHESES

In studies with large amounts of data, there is a temptation to use modern computer techniques to see which variables are associated with which other variables and to grind out many associations. This process is sometimes referred to as *data dredging,* and it is often used in medical research, although sometimes that is not made clear in the article. There are special dangers in this activity about which the reader of medical literature should be aware (also see Chapter 5).

The search for associations can be appropriate as long as the investigator keeps two points in mind. First, the scientific process requires that hypothesis development and hypothesis testing be based on *different* data sets. One data set is used to develop the hypothesis or model, which is used to make predictions, which are then tested on a new data set. Second, a **correlational study** (e.g., using Pearson correlation coefficient or chi-square test) is useful only for developing hypotheses, not for testing them. Stated in slightly different terms, a correlational study is only a type of screening method, to identify associations that might be real. Investigators who keep these points in mind are unlikely to make the mistake of thinking every association found in a data set represents a true association.

One notable example of the problem of data dredging was the report of an association between coffee consumption and pancreatic cancer, obtained by looking at many associations in a large data set, without repeating the analysis on another data set to determine if it was consistent.[8] This approach was severely criticized at the time, and subsequent studies failed to find a true association between coffee consumption and pancreatic cancer.[9]

How does this problem arise? Suppose there were 10 variables in a descriptive study, and the investigator wanted to try to associate each one with every other one. There would be 10×10 possible cells (see Chapter 5, Fig. 5-6). Ten of these would be each variable times itself, however, which is always a perfect correlation. That leaves 90 possible associations, but half of these would be "$x \times y$" and the other half "$y \times x$." Because the p values for bivariate tests are the same regardless of which is considered the independent variable and which is considered the dependent variable, there are only half as many truly independent associations, or 45. If the $p = 0.05$ cutoff point is used for alpha, 5 of 100 independent associations would be expected to occur by chance alone.[10] In the example, it means that slightly more than two *statistically significant* associations would be expected to occur just by chance.

The problem with multiple hypotheses is similar to the problem with multiple associations: The greater the number of hypotheses that are tested, the more likely it is that at least one of them will be found *statistically significant* by chance alone. One possible way to handle this problem is to lower the p value required before rejecting the null hypothesis (e.g., make it <0.05). This was done in a study testing the same medical educational hypothesis at five different hospitals.[11] If the alpha level in the study had been set at 0.05, there would have been almost a 25% probability of finding a statistically significant difference by chance alone in at least one of the five hospitals because each hospital had a 5% (alpha = 0.05) probability of showing a difference from chance alone. To keep the risk of a false-positive finding in the entire study to no more than 0.05, the alpha level chosen for rejecting the null hypothesis was made more stringent by dividing alpha by 5 (number of hospitals) to make it 0.01. This method of adjusting for multiple hypotheses is called the **Bonferroni adjustment to alpha,** and it is quite stringent.

Other possible adjustments are less stringent but are more complicated statistically and used in different situations. Examples include the Tukey, Scheffe, and Newman-Keuls procedures.[12]

IV. SUMMARY

Biostatisticians are most often consulted for help in calculating sample sizes needed for studies; such help is readily provided only if the investigator already has determined the numbers to be used in the calculations: level of alpha and beta, clinically important difference in outcome variables to be detected, and variance expected. Determining the needed sample size is usually straightforward if these values are known. Another essential process in clinical research is random allocation, which can be accomplished effectively if certain steps are followed carefully, especially keeping the selection process secret (e.g., using sealed envelopes). Blinding is used to help eliminate bias. Ideally, neither study participants (subjects), those providing the intervention, nor those collecting data should know group assignments. The basic methods of random allocation include simple random allocation, randomization into groups of two, systematic allocation, and stratified allocation. In the analysis of data, investigators should be alert to the problem of data dredging; testing multiple hypotheses increases the probability of false-positive statistical associations (alpha errors).

References

1. Freiman JA, Chalmers TC, Smith H, Jr, et al: The importance of beta, the type II error, and sample size in the design and interpretation of the randomized control trial: a survey of 71 "negative" trials. *N Engl J Med* 299:690–695, 1978.
2. Williams HC, Seed P: Inadequate size of negative clinical trials in dermatology. *Br J Dermatol* 128:317–326, 1993.
3. Chow SC, Wang H, Shao J: *Sample size calculation in clinical research*, ed 2, New York, 2007, Chapman & Hall/CRC.
4. Kelsey JL, Whittemore AS, Evans AS, et al: *Methods in observational epidemiology*, ed 2, New York, 1996, Oxford University Press.
5. Lam JA, et al: "I prayed real hard, so I know I'll get in": living with randomization. *New Dir Prog Eval* 63:55–66, 1994.
6. Paradise JL, Bluestone CD, Bachman RC, et al: Efficacy of tonsillectomy for recurrent throat infection in severely affected children. *N Engl J Med* 310:674–683, 1984.
7. Sackett DL, Gent M: Controversy in counting and attributing events in clinical trials. *N Engl J Med* 301:1410–1412, 1979.
8. MacMahon B, Yen S, Trichopoulos D, et al: Coffee and cancer of the pancreas. *N Engl J Med* 304:630–633, 1981.
9. Feinstein AR, Horwitz RI, Spitzer WO, et al: Coffee and pancreatic cancer: the problems of etiologic science and epidemiologic case-control research. *JAMA* 246:957–961, 1981.
10. Jekel JF: Should we stop using the *p*-value in descriptive studies? *Pediatrics* 60:124–126, 1977.
11. Jekel JF, Chauncey KJ, Moore NL, et al: The regional educational impact of a renal stone center. *Yale J Biol Med* 56:97–108, 1983.
12. Dawson B, Trapp RG: *Basic and clinical biostatistics*, ed 4, New York, 2004, Lange Medical Books/McGraw-Hill.

Select Readings

Dawson B, Trapp RG: *Basic and clinical biostatistics*, ed 4, New York, 2004, Lange Medical Books/McGraw-Hill.

13 Multivariable Analysis

I. OVERVIEW OF MULTIVARIABLE STATISTICS

Multivariable analysis helps us to understand the relative importance of different independent variables for explaining the variation in a dependent (outcome) variable (y), when they act alone and when they work together (interaction). There may be considerable overlap in the ability of different independent variables to explain a dependent variable. For example, in the first two decades of life, age and height predict body weight, but age and height are usually correlated. During the growth years, height and weight increase with age, so age can be considered the underlying explanatory variable, and height can be viewed as an *intervening variable* influencing weight. Children grow at different rates, so height would add additional explanatory power to that of age: Children who are tall for their age, on the average, also would be heavier than children of the same age who are short for their age. Each independent variable may share explanatory power with other independent variables and explain some of the variation in y beyond what any other variable explains.

All statistical equations attempt to model reality, however imperfectly. They may represent only one dimension of reality, such as the effect of one variable (e.g., a nutrient) on another variable (e.g., growth rate of an infant). For a simple model such as this to be of scientific value, the research design must try to equalize all the factors *other than* the independent and dependent variables being studied. In animal studies, this might be achieved by using genetically identical animals. Except for some observational studies of identical twins, this cannot be done for humans.

For *experimental* research involving humans, the first step is to make the experimental and control groups similar by randomizing the allocation of study participants to study groups. Sometimes randomization is impossible, however, or important factors may not be adequately controlled by this strategy. In this situation the only way to remove the effects of these unwanted factors is to control for them by using **multivariable statistical analysis** as follows:

1. To equalize research groups (i.e., make them as comparable as possible) when studying the effects of medical or public health interventions.
2. To build causal models from *observational studies* that help investigators understand which factors affect the risk of different diseases in populations (assisting clinical and public health efforts to promote health and prevent disease and injury).
3. To create *clinical indices* that can suggest the risk of disease in well people or a certain diagnosis, complications, or death in ill people.

Statistical models that have one outcome variable but more than one independent variable are generally called **multivariable models** (or *multivariate models*, but many statisticians reserve this term for models with multiple *dependent* variables).[1] Multivariable models are intuitively attractive to investigators because they seem more "true to life" than models with only one independent variable. A bivariate (two-variable) analysis simply indicates whether there is significant movement in Y in tandem with movement in X. Multivariable analysis allows for an assessment of the influence of change in X and change in Y once the effects of other factors (e.g., A, B, and C) are considered.

Multivariable analysis does not enable an investigator to ignore the basic principles of good research design, however, because multivariable analysis also has many limitations. Although the statistical methodology and interpretation of findings from multivariable analysis are difficult for most clinicians, the methods and results are reported routinely in the medical literature.[2,3] To be intelligent consumers of the medical literature, health care professionals should at least understand the use and interpretation of the findings of multivariable analysis as usually presented.

II. ASSUMPTIONS UNDERLYING MULTIVARIABLE METHODS

Several important assumptions underlie most multivariable methods in routine use, and those addressed in this chapter. Most methods of regression analysis require an assumption that the relationship between any of the independent variables and the dependent variable is linear (assumption of **linearity**). The effects of independent variables are assumed to be independent (assumption of **independence**), and if not, testing of interaction is warranted (entering a term in a multivariable equation that represents the interaction between two of the independent variables). The assumption of **homoscedasticity** refers to homogeneity of variance across all levels of the independent variables. In other words, it is assumed that variance and error are constant across a range of values for a given variable in the equation. Computer software packages in routine use for multivariable analysis provide means to test these assumptions. (For our purposes in this chapter, we accept that the conditions of these assumptions are satisfied.)

A. Conceptual Understanding of Equations for Multivariable Analysis

One reason many people are put off by statistics is that the equations look like a jumble of meaningless symbols. That is especially true of multivariable techniques, but it is possible to understand the equations conceptually. Suppose a study is done to predict the prognosis (in terms of survival months) of patients at the time of diagnosis for a certain cancer. Clinicians might surmise that to predict the length of survival for a patient, they would need to know at least four factors: the patient's *age;* anatomic *stage* of the disease at diagnosis; degree of systemic *symptoms* from the cancer, such as weight loss; and presence or absence of other diseases, such as renal failure or diabetes *(comorbidity).* That prediction equation could be written conceptually as follows:

$$\text{Cancer prognosis varies with Age and Stage and Symptoms and Comorbidity} \tag{13-1}$$

This statement could be made to look more mathematical simply by making a few slight changes:

$$\text{Cancer prognosis} \approx \text{Age} + \text{Stage} + \text{Symptoms} + \text{Comorbidity} \tag{13-2}$$

The four independent variables on the right side of the equation are almost certainly not of exactly equal importance. Equation 13-2 can be improved by giving each independent variable a **coefficient,** which is a **weighting factor** measuring its *relative importance* in predicting prognosis. The equation becomes:

$$\text{Cancer prognosis} \approx (\text{Weight}_1)\,\text{Age} + (\text{Weight}_2)\,\text{Stage} + (\text{Weight}_3)\,\text{Symptoms} + (\text{Weight}_4)\,\text{Comorbidity} \tag{13-3}$$

Before equation 13-3 can become useful for estimating survival for an individual patient, two other factors are required: (1) a measure to quantify the *starting point* for the calculation and (2) a measure of the *error* in the predicted value of *y* for each observation (because statistical prediction is almost never perfect for a single individual). By inserting a *starting point* and an *error term*, the $\approx$ symbol (meaning "varies with") can be replaced by an equal sign. Abbreviating the weights with a *W*, the equation now becomes:

$$\text{Cancer prognosis} = \text{Starting point} + W_1\text{Age} + W_2\text{Stage} + W_3\text{Symptoms} + W_4\text{Comorbidity} + \text{Error term} \tag{13-4}$$

This equation now can be rewritten in common statistical symbols: *y* is the dependent (outcome) variable (cancer prognosis) and is customarily placed on the left. Then x_1 (age) through x_4 (comorbidity) are the independent variables, and they are lined up on the right side of the equation; b_i is the statistical symbol for the weight of the *i*th independent variable; *a* is the *starting point,* usually called the **regression constant;** and *e* is the *error term.* Purely in statistical symbols, the equation can be expressed as follows:

$$y = a + b_1x_1 + b_2x_2 + b_3x_3 + b_4x_4 + e \tag{13-5}$$

Although equation 13-5 looks complex, it really means the same thing as equations 13-1 through 13-4.

What is this equation really saying? It states that the dependent variable (*y*) can be *predicted* for each person at diagnosis by beginning with a standard *starting point* (*a*), then making an *adjustment* for the new information supplied by the first variable (age), plus a further adjustment for the information provided by the second variable (anatomic stage), and so on, until an adjustment is made for the last independent variable (comordity) and for the almost inevitable error in the resulting prediction of the prognosis for any given study participant.

B. Best Estimates

In the example of cancer prognosis, to calculate a general prediction equation (the index we want for this type of patient), the investigator would need to know values for the regression constant (*a*) and the slopes (b_i) of the independent variables that would provide the best prediction of the value of *y*. These values would have to be obtained by a research study, preferably on two sets of data, one to provide the estimates of these parameters and a second (validation set) to determine the reliability of these estimates. The investigator would assemble a large group of newly diagnosed patients with the cancer of interest, record the values of the independent variables (x_i) for each patient at diagnosis, and follow the patients for a long time to determine the length of survival (y_i). The goal of the statistical analysis would be to solve for the best estimates of the regression constant (*a*) and the coefficients (b_i). When the statistical analysis has provided these estimates, the formula can take the values of the independent variables for new patients to predict the prognosis. The statistical research on a sample of patients would provide estimates for *a* and *b*, and then the equation could be used clinically.

How does the statistical equation know when it has found the best estimates for the regression constant and the coefficients of the independent variables? A little statistical theory is needed. The investigator would already have the observed y value and all the x values for each patient in the study and would be looking for the best values for the starting point and the coefficients. Because the error term is unknown at the beginning, the statistical analysis uses various values for the coefficients, regression constant, and observed x values to *predict* the value of y, which is called "y-hat" ($\hat{y}$). If the values of all the observed ys and xs are inserted, the following equation can be solved:

$$\hat{y} = a + b_1 x_1 + b_2 x_2 + b_3 x_3 + b_4 x_4 \qquad (13\text{-}6)$$

This equation is true because $\hat{y}$ is only an estimate, which can have error. When equation 13-6 is subtracted from equation 13-5, the following equation for the error term emerges:

$$(y - \hat{y}) = e \qquad (13\text{-}7)$$

This equation states that the error term (e) is the difference between the *observed* value of the outcome variable y for a given patient and the *predicted* value of y for the same patient. How does the computer program know when the best estimates for the values of a and b_i have been obtained? They have been achieved in this equation *when the sum of the squared error terms has been minimized*. That sum is expressed as:

$$\sum (y_i - \hat{y})^2 = \sum (y_O - y_E)^2 = \sum e^2 \qquad (13\text{-}8)$$

This idea is not new because, as noted in previous chapters, variation in statistics is measured as the sum of the squares of the observed value (O) minus the expected value (E). In multivariable analysis, the error term e is often called a **residual.**

In straightforward language, the best estimates for the values of a and b_1 through b_i are found when the total quantity of error (measured as the sum of squares of the error term, or most simply e^2) has been *minimized*. The values of a and the several bs that, taken together, give the smallest value for the squared error term (squared for reasons discussed in Chapter 9) are the best estimates that can be obtained from the set of data. Appropriately enough, this approach is called the **least-squares solution** because the process is stopped when the sum of squares of the error term is the least.

C. General Linear Model

The multivariable equation shown in equation 13-6 is usually called the *general linear model.* The model is general because there are many variations regarding the types of variables for y and x_i and the number of x variables that can be used. The model is linear because it is a linear combination of the x_i terms. For the x_i variables, a variety of transformations might be used to improve the model's "fit" (e.g., square of x_i, square root of x_i, or logarithm of x_i). The combination of terms would still be linear, however, if all the coefficients (the b_i terms) were to the first power. The model does not remain linear if any of the coefficients is taken to any power other than 1 (e.g., b^2). Such equations are much more complex and are beyond the scope of this discussion.

Numerous procedures for multivariable analysis are based on the general linear model. These include methods with such imposing designations as analysis of variance (ANOVA), analysis of covariance (ANCOVA), multiple linear regression, multiple logistic regression, the log-linear model, and discriminant function analysis. As discussed subsequently and outlined in Table 13-1, the choice of which procedure to use depends primarily on whether the dependent and independent variables are continuous, dichotomous, nominal, or ordinal. Knowing that the procedures listed in Table 13-1 are all variations of the same theme (the general linear model) helps to make them less confusing. Detailing these methods is beyond the scope of this text but readily available both online* and in print.[4]

---

*For example, http://www.icpsr.umich.edu/icpsrweb/sumprog/courses/0009.

Table 13-1 Choice of Appropriate Procedure to Be Used in Multivariable Analysis (Analysis of One Dependent Variable and More than One Independent Variable)

Characterization of Variables to Be Analyzed		
Dependent Variable	Independent Variables*	Appropriate Procedure or Procedures
Continuous	All are categorical.	Analysis of variance (ANOVA)
Continuous	Some are categorical and some are continuous.	Analysis of covariance (ANCOVA)
Continuous	All are continuous.	Multiple linear regression
Ordinal	—	There is no formal multivariable procedure for ordinal dependent variables; treat the variables as if continuous (see above procedures), or perform log-linear analysis.
Dichotomous	All are categorical.	Logistic regression; log-linear analysis
Dichotomous	Some are categorical and some are continuous.	Logistic regression†
Dichotomous	All are continuous.	Logistic regression or discriminant function analysis
Nominal	All are categorical.	Log-linear analysis
Nominal	Some are categorical and some are continuous.	Group the continuous variables and perform log-linear analysis.
Nominal	All are continuous.	Discriminant function analysis; or group the continuous variables and perform log-linear analysis.

*Categorical variables include ordinal, dichotomous, and nominal variables.
†If the outcome is a time-related dichotomous variable (e.g., live/die), proportional hazards (Cox) models are best.

D. Uses of Multivariable Statistics

Straightforward bivariate findings and relationships should be presented by a contingency table or a graph (see Chapter 11). Subtle findings and interactions among multiple independent variables are difficult to find using tables, however, and thus multivariable analysis is usually required. Multivariable analysis can often tease out how variables work *synergistically* (with each other to strengthen an effect), *antagonistically* (against each other to weaken an effect), or with *mixed effects.*

Multivariable techniques enable investigators to determine whether there is an interaction between variables. **Interaction** is present when the value of one independent variable influences the way another independent variable explains *y*. For example, a large blood pressure survey in Connecticut found that in African Americans younger than 50, hypertension was more likely to occur in men than in women.[5] In people older than 50, however, that trend was reversed, and hypertension was more likely to occur in women than in men. There was an interaction between age and gender when explaining the prevalence rate of hypertension.

The net effect of the complex calculations of multivariable analysis is to help the investigators determine which of the independent variables are the strongest predictors of *y*, and which of the independent variables overlap with one another in their ability to predict *y*, or oppose each other, or interact.

In a clinical setting, such as an emergency department, it is helpful to have a scale or index that predicts whether or not a patient with chest pain is likely to have a myocardial infarction. Several multivariable techniques might be used to develop such a **prediction model**, complete with coefficients for use in prediction. Logistic regression was used to develop a prognostic index for 4-year mortality in older adults, for example.[6] Using various combinations of symptoms, signs, laboratory values, and electrocardiographic findings, investigators developed estimates for the probability of myocardial infarction and other diseases.[7-10] More recently, multiple logistic regression has become a common technique for developing clinical prediction models (see next section). Although such clinical prediction models usually work well on average, their predictions for an individual patient may be less satisfactory. Clinical prediction models are applied increasingly to chronic disease as well as in acute disease[11] (see Websites list at end of chapter).

Multivariable analysis also can be used to develop clinical prediction models for the risk of disease or death among the general population, based on their known risk factors. Investigators in the Framingham Heart Study used multivariable analysis to develop prediction equations for the 8-year risk of developing cardiovascular disease in people with various combinations of risk factors: smoking, elevated cholesterol levels, hypertension, glucose intolerance, and left ventricular hypertrophy (see Table 5-2 and reference/website listed). These prediction equations, or updated versions, are being used in various health risk assessment programs, as well as by health insurers interested in the costs and likely benefits associated with interventions directed toward the modification of specific chronic disease risk factors.

As stated earlier, an increasingly important role for multivariable analysis in clinical research is to adjust for intergroup differences that remain after randomization, matching, or other attempts to equalize comparison groups. The relation between blood pressure and mortality from coronary heart disease in men from different parts of the world was studied, for example, after using multivariable statistical methods to adjust for age, total cholesterol level, and cigarette smoking.[12] A relatively new strategy for this purpose is called **propensity matching.** This is typically used in observational cohort studies, where preexisting demographic and clinical differences exist between people who received some type of treatment and people who did not receive the treatment because the allocation to treatment was not randomized. Study participants who did receive treatment are matched with participants who did not receive treatment who have a similar **propensity score** (based on multivariable analysis). The objective is to make the matched groups who did and did not receive the treatment similar on all relevant variables except the treatment.[12,13] It is hoped that this will accomplish approximately the same goal as randomization and allow meaningful conclusions about the effects of treatment, even from nonrandomized studies.

III. PROCEDURES FOR MULTIVARIABLE ANALYSIS

As shown in Table 13-1, the choice of an appropriate statistical method for multivariable analysis depends on whether the dependent and independent variables are continuous, ordinal, dichotomous, or nominal. In cases in which more than one method could be used, the final choice depends on the investigator's experience, personal preference, and comfort with methods that are appropriate. Because there are many potential pitfalls in the use of multivariable techniques in medical research, these techniques should not be used without experience or expert advice, and as a general rule, there should be at least 10 observations for each independent variable in the multivariable equation.[2]

A. Analysis of Variance (ANOVA)

If the dependent variable is continuous, and if all the independent variables are categorical (i.e., nominal, dichotomous, or ordinal), the correct multivariable technique is analysis of variance. One-way ANOVA and *N*-way ANOVA are discussed briefly next. This technique is based on the general linear model and can be used to analyze the results of an experimental study. If the design includes only one independent variable (e.g., treatment group), the technique is called **one-way** ANOVA, regardless of how many different treatment groups are compared. If it includes more than one independent variable (e.g., treatment group, age group, and gender), the technique is called *N*-**way** ANOVA (the *N* standing for the number of different independent variables).

B. One-Way ANOVA (*F*-Test)

Suppose a team of investigators wanted to study the effects of drugs A and B on blood pressure. They might randomly allocate hypertensive patients into four treatment groups: patients taking drug A alone, patients taking drug B alone, patients taking drugs A and B in combination, and patients taking a placebo. Alternatively, they might choose to compare three different dosage patterns of the same drug against a placebo. The investigators could measure systolic blood pressure (SBP) before and after treatment in each patient and calculate a *difference score* (posttreatment SBP − pretreatment SBP) for each study participant. This difference score would become the dependent (outcome) variable. A mean difference score would be calculated for each of the four treatment groups (three drug groups and one placebo group) so that these mean scores could be compared by using ANOVA.

The investigators would want to determine whether the differences (presumably declines) in SBP found in one or more of the drug groups were large enough to be clinically important. A decrease in mean SBP from 150 to 148 mm Hg would be too small to be clinically useful. If the results were not clinically useful, there would be little point in doing a test of significance. If one or more of the groups showed a clinically important decrease in SBP compared with the placebo, however, the investigators would want to determine whether the difference was likely to have occurred by chance alone. To do this, an appropriate statistical test of significance is needed.

Student's *t*-test could be used to compare each pair of groups, but this would require six different *t*-tests: each of the three drug groups (A, B, and AB) versus the placebo group; drug A versus drug B; drug A versus drug combination AB; and drug B versus drug combination AB. Testing these six hypotheses raises the problem of multiple comparisons (see Chapter 12). Even if the investigators decided that the primary comparison should be each drug or the drug combination with the placebo, this still would leave three hypotheses to test instead of just one. If two or three treatment groups performed significantly better than the placebo group, it would be necessary to determine if one of the treatment groups was significantly superior to the others.

The best approach when analyzing such a study would be first to perform an *F*-test (i.e., one-way ANOVA). The *F*-test is a type of *super t-test* that allows the investigator to compare more than two means simultaneously. In the antihypertensive drug study, the *null hypothesis* for the *F*-test is that the mean change in blood pressure ($\bar{d}$) will be the *same* for all four groups ($\bar{d}_A = \bar{d}_B = \bar{d}_{AB} = \bar{d}_P$). This would indicate that all samples were taken from the same underlying population (called a *universe*), and that any observed differences between the means are caused by chance variation.

When creating the *F*-test, Fisher reasoned that there were two different ways to estimate the variance. One estimate is called **between-groups** variance and is based on the variation between (or among) the means. The other is called **within-groups** variance and is based on the variation within the groups (i.e., variation around the group means). Assuming the null hypothesis that all the study groups were sampled from the same population (i.e., the treatments made no difference), these two estimates of variance should be similar. The ratio of the between-groups variance to the within-groups variance is called *F* (in honor of Fisher). It is another form of *critical ratio* because it enables a decision to be made either to reject or not to reject the null hypothesis. The *F*-test has the same general form as other critical ratios: the ratio of a measure of the effect (the differences between means)

divided by a measure of the variability of the estimates. As proof that Student's *t*-test and the *F*-test have the same underlying method, when an ANOVA is used instead of a *t*-test to compare *two* means, the *p* values are identical, and the value of $F = t^2$.

In ANOVA the two measures of variance are called the **between-groups *mean square*** and the **within-groups *mean square*. (Mean square** is simply the ANOVA name for variance, which is defined as a sum of squares, or SS, divided by the appropriate number of degrees of freedom [*df*]). The ratio of the two measures of variance can be expressed as follows:

$$F \text{ ratio} = \frac{\text{Between-groups variance}}{\text{Within-groups variance}}$$
$$= \frac{\text{Between-groups mean square}}{\text{Within-groups mean square}}$$

If the *F* ratio is close to 1.0, the two estimates of variance are similar, and the null hypothesis—that all the means came from the same underlying population—is not rejected. This occurs when the treatment has too small an effect to *push apart* the observed means of the different groups. If the *F* ratio is much larger than 1.0, however, some force, presumably the treatment, caused the means to differ, so the null hypothesis of no difference is rejected. The assumptions for the *F*-test are similar to those for the *t*-test. First, the dependent variable (in this case, blood pressure difference scores) should be normally distributed, although with large samples this assumption can be relaxed because of the central limit theorem. Second, the several samples of the dependent variable should be independent random samples from populations with approximately equal variances. This need for equal variances is more acute in the *F*-test than it is in the *t*-test, where an adjustment is available to correct for a large difference between the two variances. As with the *t*-test, the *F*-test requires that an alpha level be specified in advance. After the *F* statistic has been calculated, its *p* value can be looked up in a table of the *F* distribution to determine whether the results are statistically significant. With the *F*-test, this task is more complicated than with the *t*-test, however, because ANOVA has two different degrees of freedom to deal with: one for the numerator (the model mean square) and one for the denominator (the error mean square), as explained in Box 13-1.

If the results of the *F*-test are *not* statistically significant, either the null hypothesis must be accepted, or the study must be repeated using a larger sample (but only if the observed decrease in blood pressure was impressive but still not statistically significant). If the results *are* statistically significant, however, the investigators must take additional steps to determine which of the differences between means are greater than would be expected by chance alone. In the case of the example introduced earlier involving four treatment groups (drug A alone, drug B alone, drugs A and B combined, and placebo), statistical significance could be found if any of the following were true:

1. The mean difference of one group differed greatly from that of the other three groups.
2. The means of two groups differed greatly from those of the remaining two groups.
3. The means of the four groups were strung along a line (e.g., if drugs A and B combined showed the best results,

| Box 13-1 | Analysis of Variance (ANOVA) Table |

The goal of ANOVA, stated in the simplest terms, is to explain (i.e., to model) the total variation found in one analysis. Because the total variation is equal to the sum of squares (SS) of the dependent variable, the process of explaining that variation entails partitioning the SS into component parts. The logic behind this process was introduced in Chapter 10 (see the section on variation between groups versus variation within groups). That discussion focused on the example of explaining the difference between the heights of men and women (fictitious data). The heights of 100 female and 100 male university students were measured, the total variation (SS from the grand mean) was found to be 10,000 cm^2, and 4000 cm^2 of the variation was attributed to gender. Because that example is uncomplicated and involves round numbers, it is used here to illustrate the format for an ANOVA table.

Source of Variation	Sum of Squares (SS)	Degrees of Freedom (df)	Mean Square (MS)	F Ratio
Total	10,000	199		
Model (gender)	4,000	1	4000.0	132.0
Error	6,000	198	30.3	

The model in this example has only one independent variable—gender, a dichotomous variable. In the SS column the figure of 4000 represents the amount of variation explained by gender (i.e., the between-groups SS noted in the ANOVA), and 6000 represents the amount of SS not explained by gender (i.e., the within-groups variation). In the df column the total df is listed as 199, reflecting there were 200 participants and that 1 df was lost in calculating the grand mean for all observations. The df for the model is calculated as the number of categories (groups) minus 1. Gender has only two categories (men and women), so 1 df is assigned to it. The df for error is calculated as the total df minus the number of df assigned to the model: $199 - 1 = 198$.

The mean square is simply another name for variance and is equal to the SS divided by the appropriate df: $4000/1 = 4000.0$ for the model mean square, and $6000/198 = 30.3$ for the error mean square.

The F ratio is a ratio of variances, or in ANOVA-speak, a ratio of mean squares. Specifically, the F ratio here is calculated by dividing the model mean square by the error mean square: $4000/30.3 = 132.0$. To look up the p value that corresponds to this F ratio in the table of F distributions, it is necessary to know the df for the denominator and the df for the numerator. In this case, as described previously, the df for the numerator would be 1, and the df for the denominator would be 198. Because the F ratio is so large, 132.0, the p value would be extremely small ($p < 0.00001$), and the null hypothesis that there is no true (average) difference between the mean heights of men and women would be rejected.

If there were more than one independent variable in the model being analyzed, there would be more entries under the column showing the source of variation: total, model, *interaction*, and error. The model also would contain separate lines for the other independent variable(s), such as height of the participant's mother. The *interaction* term refers to the portion of the variation caused by interactions between the independent variables in the model (here that might be written as *gender* × *motherheight*). The error SS would be the variation not explained by *either* of the independent variables *or* their interaction.

When performed using standard software packages, the full results automatically include the critical ratio and the p value, along with other details.

drug A second-best results, drug B third-best results, and placebo least impressive results).

Most advanced statistical computer packages include options in the ANOVA program that allow investigators to determine which of the differences are "true" differences; this involves making adjustments for more than one hypothesis being tested simultaneously.[14] Although a detailed discussion of the various adjustment methods is beyond the scope of this book, it is important for readers to understand the logic behind this form of analysis and to recognize the circumstances under which one-way ANOVA is appropriate. As an example of the use of ANOVA, a clinical trial was performed in which asthma patients were randomized into three treatment groups: one who received 42 μg of salmeterol two times daily, one who received 180 μg of albuterol four times daily, and one who received a placebo.[15] At the beginning and end of the study, the investigators measured the asthma patients' forced expiratory volume in 1 second (FEV_1), and they used F-tests to compare the changes in FEV_1 values seen in the three different treatment groups. Based on the results of one-way ANOVA, they concluded that salmeterol was more effective than albuterol or placebo in increasing the morning peak expiratory flow rate.

C. N-Way ANOVA

The goal of ANOVA is to explain (to model) as much variation in a continuous variable as possible, by using one or more categorical variables to predict the variation. If only one independent variable is tested in a model, it is called an F-test, or a one-way ANOVA. If two or more independent variables are tested, it is called a two-way ANOVA, or an N-way ANOVA (the N specifying how many independent variables are used). If one variable for an F-test is gender (see Box 13-1), the total sum of squares (SS) in the dependent variable is explained in terms of how much is caused by gender and how much is not caused by gender. Any variation not caused by the model (gender) is considered to be error (residual) variation.

If two independent variables are tested in a model, and those variables are treatment and gender, the total amount of variation is divided into how much variation is caused by each of the following: independent effect of treatment, independent effect of gender, interaction between (i.e., joint effect of) treatment and gender, and error. If more than two independent variables are tested, the analysis becomes increasingly complicated, but the underlying logic remains the same. As long as the research design is "balanced" (i.e., there are equal numbers of observations in each of the study groups), N-way ANOVA can be used to analyze the individual and joint effects of categorical independent variables and to partition the total variation into the various component parts. If the design is not balanced, most computer programs provide an alternative method to do an *approximate* ANOVA; for example, in SAS, the PROC GLM procedure can be used. The details of such analyses are beyond the scope of this book.

As an example, N-way ANOVA procedures were used in a study to determine whether supplementing gonadotropin-releasing hormone with parathyroid hormone would reduce the osteoporosis-causing effect of gonadotropin-releasing hormone.[16] The investigators used ANOVA to examine the effects of treatment and other independent variables on the bone loss induced by estrogen deficiency.

D. Analysis of Covariance (ANCOVA)

Analysis of variance and analysis of covariance are methods for evaluating studies in which the dependent variable is continuous (see Table 13-1). If the independent variables are all of the categorical type (nominal, dichotomous, or ordinal), ANOVA is used. If some of the independent variables are categorical and some are continuous, however, ANCOVA is appropriate. ANCOVA could be used, for example, in a study to test the effects of antihypertensive drugs on SBP in participants of varying age. The change in SBP after treatment (a continuous variable) is the dependent variable, and the independent variables might be age (a continuous variable) and treatment (a categorical variable). One study used ANCOVA to evaluate the results of a controlled clinical trial of dichloroacetate to treat lactic acidosis in adult patients.[17] ANCOVA adjusted the dependent variable for the pretreatment concentrations of arterial blood lactate in the study participants and tested the difference between the adjusted means of the treatment groups.

E. Multiple Linear Regression

If the dependent variable and all the independent variables are continuous, the correct type of multivariable analysis is multiple linear regression. The formula looks like the general linear model formula shown in equation 13-6. Of the several computerized methods for analyzing data in a multiple linear regression, the most common is probably **stepwise linear regression.** The investigator chooses which variable to begin with (i.e., to enter first in the analysis) or instructs the computer to start by entering the independent variable that has the strongest association with the dependent variable. In either case, when only the first variable has been entered, the result is a simple regression analysis. Next, the second variable is entered according to the investigator's instructions. The explanatory strength of all the variables entered (i.e., their r^2; see Chapter 11) changes as each new variable is entered. The "stepping" continues until all the remaining independent variables have been entered, or until the remaining ones meet the predetermined criterion for being dropped (e.g., $p > 0.1$ or increase in $r^2 < 0.01$).

In addition to the statistical significance of the overall equation and each variable entered, the investigator closely watches the increase in the overall r^2, which is the proportion of variation the model has explained so far. The increase in the total r^2 after each step indicates how much additional variation is explained by the variable just entered.

Multiple linear regression is no longer used frequently in clinical medicine because many clinical variables are nominal, dichotomous, or ordinal. It is used frequently, however, in economics, health economics, and health services research. The dependent variable in such research may be the amount of profit (or loss) in dollars for a hospital over a time period. The independent variables may be the average length of stay, bed occupancy rate, and proportion of patients who require surgical care.

F. Other Procedures for Multivariable Analysis

Other major multivariable procedures include **logistic regression, log-linear analysis,** and **discriminant function analysis.** Similar to the procedures discussed previously, these also are forms of the general linear model and function in an analogous manner (see Table 13-1).

Multiple logistic regression is a procedure that is appropriate to use when the outcome variable in a clinical prediction model is dichotomous (e.g., improved/unimproved or survived/died). This procedure was used to test a model that was developed to predict on admission to the hospital whether patients with bacterial meningitis would experience a good outcome (complete recovery) or a poor outcome (residual neurologic sequelae or death).[18]

In recent years a commonly used form of logistic regression has been the *proportional hazards* (Cox) model. It enables logistic regression to be done on a *time-related,* dichotomous dependent variable, such as survival/death, even when there are losses to follow-up and censored cases. The Cox model is used to test for differences between Kaplan-Meier survival curves while controlling for other variables. It also is used to determine which variables are associated with better survival. Logistic regression was used, for example, to compare the relapse-free survival of two groups of patients with rectal cancer: patients treated with radiation plus a protracted infusion of fluorouracil and patients given a bolus injection of fluorouracil.[19] The mechanics of such methods are beyond the scope of this text, but knowing when they are warranted is important in interpreting the medical literature.

IV. SUMMARY

Multivariable analysis comprises statistical methods for determining how well several independent (possibly causal) variables, separately and together, explain the variation in a single, dependent (outcome) variable. In medical research, there are three common uses for multivariable analysis: (1) to improve the testing of an intervention in a clinical trial by controlling for the effects of other variables on the outcome variable; (2) to shed light on the etiology or prognosis of a disease in observational studies by estimating the relative impact of one or more independent variables on the risk of disease or death; and (3) to develop weights for the different variables used in a diagnostic or prognostic scoring system. As shown in Table 13-1, the choice of an appropriate procedure to be used for multivariable analysis depends on whether the dependent and independent variables are continuous, dichotomous, nominal, ordinal, or a combination of these. Because the use of multivariable techniques has many potential problems and pitfalls in clinical research, these procedures should be used and interpreted with understanding and care. A more extensive and detailed table of multivariable methods is accessible at http://www.ats.ucla.edu/stat/stata/whatstat/default.htm.

References

1. Kleinbaum DG, Kupper LL: *Applied regression analysis and other multivariable models*, North Scituate, Mass, 1978, Duxbury Press.
2. Horton NJ, Switzer SS: Statistical methods in the *Journal*. *N Engl J Med* 353:1977–1979, 2005.
3. Arbogast PG, Ray WA: Performance of disease risk scores, propensity scores, and traditional multivariable outcome regression in the presence of multiple confounders. *Am J Epidemiol* 174:613–620, 2011.
4. Holford TR: *Multivariate methods in epidemiology*, New York, 2002, Oxford University Press.
5. Freeman DH, Jr, D'Atri DA, Hellenbrand K, et al: The prevalence distribution of hypertension: Connecticut adults, 1978-1979. *J Chron Dis* 36:171–181, 1983.
6. Lee SJ, Lindquist K, Segal MR, et al: Development and validation of a prognostic index for 4-year mortality in older adults. *JAMA* 295:801–808, 2006.
7. http://cancernet.nci.nih.gov/bcra_tool.html
8. http://hp2010.nhlbihin.net/atpiii/calculator.asp
9. Yoo HH, De Paiva SA, Silveira LV, et al: Logistic regression analysis of potential prognostic factors for pulmonary thromboembolism. *Chest* 123:813–821, 2003.
10. Ayanian JZ, Landrum MB, Guadagnoli E, et al: Specialty of ambulatory care physicians and mortality among elderly patients after myocardial infarction. *N Engl J Med* 347:1678–1686, 2002.
11. D'Agostino RB, Jr: Propensity score methods for bias reduction in the comparison of a treatment to a non-randomized control group. *Stat Med* 17:2265–2281, 1998.
12. Nakayama M, Osaki S, Shimokawa H: Validation of mortality risk stratification models for cardiovascular disease. *Am J Cardiol* 108:391–396, 2011.
13. Van den Hoogen PCW, Feskens EJ, Nagelkerke NJ, et al: The relation between blood pressure and mortality due to coronary heart disease among men in different parts of the world. *N Engl J Med* 342:1–8, 2000.
14. Dawson B, Trapp RG: *Basic and clinical biostatistics*, ed 4, New York, 2004, Lange Medical Books/McGraw-Hill.
15. Pearlman DS, Chervinsky P, LaForce C, et al: A comparison of salmeterol with albuterol in the treatment of mild-to-moderate asthma. *N Engl J Med* 327:1420–1425, 1992.
16. Finkelstein JS, Klibanski A, Schaefer EH, et al: Parathyroid hormone for the prevention of bone loss induced by estrogen deficiency. *N Engl J Med* 331:1618–1623, 1994.
17. Stacpoole PW, Wright EC, Baumgartner TG, et al: A controlled clinical trial of dichloroacetate for treatment of lactic acidosis in adults. *N Engl J Med* 327:1564–1569, 1992.
18. Aronin SI, Peduzzi P, Quagliarello VJ: Community-acquired bacterial meningitis: risk stratification for adverse clinical outcome and effect of antibiotic timing. *Ann Intern Med* 129:862–870, 1998.
19. O'Connell MJ, Martenson JA, Wieand HS, et al: Improving adjuvant therapy for rectal cancer by combining protracted-infusion fluorouracil with radiation therapy after curative surgery. *N Engl J Med* 331:502–507, 1994.

Select Readings

Dawson-Saunders B, Trapp RG: *Basic and clinical biostatistics*, ed 4, New York, 2004, Lange Medical Books/McGraw-Hill. (Tests for multiple comparisons.)
Feinstein AR: *Multivariable analysis: an introduction*, New Haven, Conn, 1996, Yale University Press.

Websites

http://www.ncbi.nlm.nih.gov/pubmed/20466793
http://www.ncbi.nlm.nih.gov/pubmed/21480970
http://www.ncbi.nlm.nih.gov/pubmed/21697214

3

Preventive Medicine and Public Health

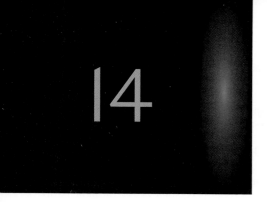

14 Introduction to Preventive Medicine

Sections 1 and 2 of this text focus on epidemiology and biostatistics, two basic sciences for preventive medicine and public health. This section (3) focuses on the theory and practice of preventive medicine. Preventive medicine and public health share common goals, such as promoting general health, preventing specific diseases, and applying epidemiologic concepts and biostatistical techniques toward these goals. However, preventive medicine seeks to enhance the lives of **individuals** by helping them improve their own health, whereas public health attempts to promote health in **populations** through the application of organized community efforts. Although this section (Chapters 14-23) emphasizes preventive medicine and Section 4 (Chapters 24-30) focuses on public health issues, a seamless continuum binds the practice of preventive medicine by clinicians, the attempts of individuals and families to promote their own and their neighbors' health, and the efforts of governments and voluntary agencies to achieve analogous health goals for populations.

I. BASIC CONCEPTS

Western medical education and practice have traditionally focused on the diagnosis and treatment of disease. Diagnosing and treating disease will always be important, but equal importance should be placed on the preservation and enhancement of health. Although specialists undertake research, teaching, and clinical practice in the field of preventive medicine, prevention is no longer the exclusive province of preventive medicine specialists, just as the care of elderly persons is not limited to geriatricians. *All* clinicians should incorporate prevention into their practice.

A. Health Defined

Health is more difficult to define than disease. Perhaps the best known definition of health comes from the preamble to the constitution of the World Health Organization: "Health is a state of complete physical, mental, and social well-being and not merely the absence of disease or infirmity." This definition is strengthened by recognizing that any meaningful concept of health must include all dimensions of human life, and that a definition must be positive, not only the absence of disease. Nevertheless, the definition has been criticized for two weaknesses: (1) its overly idealistic expectation of complete well-being and (2) its view of health as static, rather than as a dynamic process that requires constant effort to maintain.

B. Health as Successful Adaptation

In the 1960s, Dubos[1] noted that "the states of health or disease are the expressions of the success or failure experienced by the organism in its efforts to respond adaptively to environmental challenges." Environmental challenges have also been called "stress." Stress denotes any response of an organism to *demands,* whether biologic, psychological, or mental.[2] Researchers who developed the concept of **stress** correctly understood that different **stressors** could induce stress that is either helpful (**eustress**) or harmful (**distress**). Good health requires the presence of eustress in such forms as exercise (for the heart, muscles, and bones) or infant stimulation. An individual in good health also may experience some distress, but in the interest of maintaining good health, this must be limited to a level to which the organism can adapt.[3] An individual may adapt successfully to environmental stressors in the short term, but a requirement for constant, major adaptation may exact a serious toll on the body, particularly on the lungs and the neural, neuroendocrine, and immune systems. The ongoing level of demand for adaptation to stressors in an individual is called the **allostatic load** on an individual, and it may be an important contributor to many chronic diseases.[4]

C. Health as Satisfactory Functioning

Often what matters most to people about their health is how they function in their own environment. The inability to function at a satisfactory level brings many people to a physician more quickly than does the presence of discomfort. Functional problems might impinge on a person's ability to see, to hear, or to be mobile. As Dubos[5] states, "Clearly, health and disease cannot be defined merely in terms of anatomical, physiological, or mental attributes. Their real measure is the ability of the individual to function in a manner acceptable to himself and to the group of which he is a part." Breslow[6] describes health as "both (1) the current state of a human organism's equilibrium with the environment, often called health status, and (2) the potential to maintain that balance."

However health is defined, it derives principally from forces other than medical care. Appropriate nutrition, adequate shelter, a nonthreatening environment, supportive relationships, and a prudent lifestyle contribute far more to health and well-being than does the medical care system. Nevertheless, medicine contributes to health not only through patient care, but also indirectly by developing and disseminating knowledge about health promotion, disease prevention, and treatment.

II. MEASURES OF HEALTH STATUS

Measures of health status can be based on mortality, on the impact of a particular disease on quality of life, and on the ability to function. Historically, measures of health status have been based primarily on **mortality data** (see Chapter 2). Researchers assumed that a low age-adjusted death rate and a high life expectancy reflected good health in a population. Another way to account for premature mortality in different age groups is the measure of **years of potential life lost** (YPLL). This measure is used mainly in the field of injury prevention. In YPLL, deaths will be weighted depending on how many years a person might have lived if he or she had not died prematurely. This measure gives more weight to deaths occurring in young people.

Using measures of mortality alone has seemed inadequate as an increasing proportion of the population in developed countries lives to old age and accumulates various chronic and disabling illnesses. An appropriate societal goal is for people to age in a healthy manner, with minimal disability until shortly before death.[7] Therefore, health care investigators and practitioners now show increased emphasis on improving and measuring the **health-related quality of life.** Measures of the quality of life are *subjective* and thus more challenging to develop than measures of mortality. However, efforts to improve the methods for measuring quality of life are ongoing.[8]

An example of such a measure is a **health status index.** A **health index** summarizes a person's health as a single score, whereas a **health profile** seeks to rate a person's health on several separate dimensions.[9] Most health indices and profiles require that each subject complete some form of questionnaire. Many health status indices seek to adjust life expectancy on the basis of morbidity, the perceived quality of life, or both. Such indices also can be used to help guide clinical practice and research. For example, they might show that a country's emphasis on reducing mortality may not be producing equal results in improving the function or self-perceived health of the country's population. When clinicians consider which treatments to recommend to patients with a chronic disease, such as prostate cancer, this approach allows them to consider not only the treatment's impact on mortality but also its side effects, such as incontinence and impotence. Describing survival estimates in terms of the quality of life communicates a fuller picture than survival rates alone.

Life expectancy traditionally is defined as the average number of years of life remaining at a given age. The metric of **quality-adjusted life years** (QALY) incorporates both life expectancy and "quality of life," the perceived impact of illness, pain, and disability on the patient's quality of life.[10] For example, a patient with hemiparesis from a stroke might be asked to estimate how many years of life with this disability would have a value that equals to 1 year of life with good health (healthy years). If the answer were that 2 limited years is equivalent to 1 healthy year, 1 year of life after a stroke might be given a quality weight of 0.5. If 3 limited years were equivalent to 1 healthy year, each limited year would contribute 0.33 year to the QALY. Someone who must live in a nursing home and is unable to speak might consider life under those conditions to be as bad as, or worse than, no life at all. In this case the weighting factor would be 0.0 for such years.

Healthy life expectancy is a less subjective measure that attempts to combine mortality and morbidity into one index.[11] The index reflects the number of years of life remaining that are expected to be free of serious disease. The onset of a serious disease with permanent sequelae (e.g., peripheral vascular disease leading to amputation of a leg) reduces the healthy life expectancy index as much as if the person who has the sequela had died from the disease.

Other indices combine several measures of health status. The **general well-being adjustment scale** is an index that measures "anxiety, depression, general health, positive well-being, self-control, and vitality."[12] Another index is called the **life expectancy free of disability**, which defines itself. The U.S. Centers for Disease Control and Prevention (CDC) developed an index called the **health-related quality of life** based on data from the Behavioral Risk Factor Surveillance System (BRFSS).[13] Using the BRFSS data, CDC investigators found that 87% of U.S. adults considered their health to be "good to excellent." Also, the average number of good health days (the number of days free of physical and mental health problems during the 30-day period preceding the interview) was 25 days in the adults surveyed.[14]

Several scales measure the ability of patients to perform their daily activities. These functional indices measure activities that directly contribute to most people's quality of life, without asking patients to estimate the quality of life compared to how they would feel if they were in perfect health. Such functional indices include Katz's **activity of daily living** (ADL) **index** and Lawton-Brody's **instrumental activities of daily living** (IADL) **scale.** These scales have been used extensively in the geriatric population and for developmentally challenged adults. The ADL index measures a person's ability independently to bathe, dress, toilet, transfer, feed, and control their bladder and bowels. Items in the IADL scale include shopping, housekeeping, handling finances, and taking responsibility in administering medications. Other scales are used for particular diseases, such as the **Karnofsky index** for cancer patients, and the **Barthel index** for stroke patients.

III. NATURAL HISTORY OF DISEASE

The natural history of disease can be seen as having three stages: the predisease stage, the latent (asymptomatic) disease stage, and the symptomatic disease stage. Before a disease process begins in an individual—that is, during the **predisease stage**—the individual can be seen as possessing various factors that promote or resist disease. These factors include genetic makeup, demographic characteristics (especially age), environmental exposures, nutritional history, social environment, immunologic capability, and behavioral patterns.

Over time, these and other factors may cause a disease process to begin, either slowly (as with most noninfectious diseases) or quickly (as with most infectious diseases). If the disease-producing process is underway, but no symptoms of disease have become apparent, the disease is said to be in the **latent (hidden) stage.** If the underlying disease is detectable by a reasonably safe and cost-effective means during this stage, screening may be feasible. In this sense, the latent stage may represent a **window of opportunity** during which detection followed by treatment provides a better chance of cure or at least effective treatment, to prevent or forestall symptomatic disease. For some diseases, such as pancreatic cancer, there is no window of opportunity because safe and effective screening methods are unavailable. For other diseases, such as rapidly progressive conditions, the window of opportunity may be too short to be useful for screening programs. Screening programs are detailed in Chapter 16 (see Table 16-2 for screening program criteria).

When the disease is advanced enough to produce clinical manifestations, it is in the **symptomatic stage.** Even in this stage, the earlier the condition is diagnosed and treated, the more likely the treatment will delay death or serious complications, or at least provide the opportunity for effective rehabilitation.

The **natural history of a disease** is its normal course in the absence of intervention. The central question for studies of prevention (field trials) and studies of treatment (clinical trials) is whether the use of a particular preventive or treatment measure would change the natural history of disease in a favorable direction, by delaying or preventing clinical manifestations, complications, or deaths. Many interventions do not prevent the progression of disease, but instead slow the progression so that the disease occurs later in life than it would have occurred if there had been no intervention.

In the case of myocardial infarction, risk factors include male gender, a family history of myocardial infarction, elevated serum lipid levels, a high-fat diet, cigarette smoking, sedentary lifestyle, other illnesses (e.g., diabetes mellitus, hypertension), and advancing age. The speed with which coronary atherosclerosis develops in an individual would be modified not only by the diet, but also by the pattern of physical activity over the course of a lifetime. Hypertension may accelerate the development of atherosclerosis, and it may lead to increased myocardial oxygen demand, precipitating infarction earlier than it otherwise might have occurred and making recovery more difficult. In some cultures, coronary artery disease is all but unknown, despite considerable genetic overlap with cultures in which it is hyperendemic, showing that genotype is only one of many factors influencing the development of atherosclerosis.

After a myocardial infarction occurs, some patients die, some recover completely, and others recover but have serious sequelae that limit their function. Treatment may improve the outcome so that death or serious sequelae are avoided. Intensive changes in diet, exercise, and behavior (e.g., cessation of smoking) may stop the progression of atheromas or even partially reverse them.

IV. LEVELS OF PREVENTION

A useful concept of prevention that was developed or at least popularized in the classic account by Leavell and Clark[15] has come to be known as **Leavell's levels.** Based on this concept, all the activities of clinicians and other health professionals have the goal of prevention. There are three levels of prevention (Table 14-1). The factor to be prevented depends on the stage of health or disease in the individual receiving preventive care.

Primary prevention keeps the disease process from becoming established by eliminating causes of disease or by increasing resistance to disease (see Chapter 15). **Secondary prevention** interrupts the disease process before it becomes symptomatic (Chapter 16). **Tertiary prevention** limits the physical and social consequences of symptomatic disease (Chapter 17). Which prevention level is applicable also depends on which disease is the focus or what conditions are considered diseases. For example, controlling cholesterol levels in an otherwise healthy person can be primary prevention for coronary artery disease (e.g., if the physician treats incidental high cholesterol before the patient has any signs or symptoms of coronary artery disease). However, if the physician considers hypercholesterolemia itself to be a disease, treating cholesterol levels could be considered secondary prevention (i.e., treating cholesterol level before fatty atheromatous deposits form). For hypertension, efforts to lower blood pressure can be considered primary, secondary, or tertiary prevention; primary prevention might be measures to treat prehypertension, secondary prevention if the physician is treating a hypertensive patient, or tertiary prevention for a patient with symptoms from a hypertensive crisis.

A. Primary Prevention and Predisease Stage

Most noninfectious diseases can be seen as having an early stage, during which the causal factors start to produce physiologic abnormalities. During the predisease stage, atherosclerosis may begin with elevated blood levels of the "bad" low-density lipoprotein (LDL) cholesterol and may be accompanied by low levels of the "good" or *scavenger* high-density lipoprotein (HDL) cholesterol. The goal of a health intervention at this time is to modify risk factors in a favorable direction. Lifestyle-modifying activities, such as changing to a diet low in saturated and *trans* fats, pursuing a consistent program of aerobic exercise, and ceasing to smoke

Table 14-1 Modified Version of Leavell's Levels of Prevention

Stage of Disease and Care	Level of Prevention	Appropriate Response
Predisease Stage		
No known risk factors	Primary prevention	**Health promotion** (e.g., encourage healthy changes in lifestyle, nutrition, and environment)
Disease susceptibility	Primary prevention	**Specific protection** (e.g., recommend nutritional supplements, immunizations, and occupational and automobile safety measures)
Latent Disease		
"Hidden" stage; asymptomatic disease	Secondary prevention	**Screening** (for populations) or **case finding** (for individuals in medical care) and treatment if disease is found
Symptomatic Disease		
Initial care	Tertiary prevention	**Disability limitation*** (i.e., institute medical or surgical treatment to limit damage from the disease and institute primary prevention measures)
Subsequent care	Tertiary prevention	**Rehabilitation** (i.e., identify and teach methods to reduce physical and social disability)

Modified from Leavell HR, Clark EG: *Preventive medicine for the doctor in his community,* ed 3, New York, 1965, McGraw-Hill.
*Although Leavell originally categorized disability limitation under secondary prevention, it has become customary in Europe and the United States to classify disability limitation as tertiary prevention because it involves the management of symptomatic disease.

cigarettes, are considered to be methods of primary prevention because they are aimed at keeping the pathologic process and disease from occurring.

1. Health Promotion

Health-promoting activities usually contribute to the primary (and often secondary and tertiary) prevention of a variety of diseases and enhance a positive feeling of health and vigor. These activities consist of nonmedical efforts, such as changes in lifestyle, nutrition, and the environment. Such activities may require structural improvements in society to enable more people to participate in them. These improvements require societal changes that make healthy choices easier. Dietary modification may be difficult unless a variety of healthy foods are available in local stores at a reasonable cost. Exercise is more difficult if bicycling or jogging is a risky activity because of automobile traffic or social violence. Even more basic to health promotion is the assurance of the basic necessities of life, including freedom from poverty, environmental pollution, and violence.

Health promotion applies to noninfectious diseases and to infectious diseases. Infectious diseases are reduced in frequency and seriousness where the water is clean, where liquid and solid wastes are disposed of in a sanitary manner, and where animal vectors of disease are controlled. Crowding promotes the spread of infectious diseases, whereas adequate housing and working environments tend to minimize the spread of disease. In the barracks of soldiers, for example, even a technique as simple as requiring soldiers in adjacent cots to sleep with their pillows alternating between the head and the foot of the bed can reduce the spread of respiratory diseases, because it doubles the distance between the soldiers' upper respiratory tracts during sleeping time.

2. Specific Protection

Usually, general health-promoting changes in environment, nutrition, and behavior are not fully effective. Therefore, it becomes necessary to employ specific protection (see Table 14-1). This form of primary prevention is targeted at a specific disease or type of injury. Examples include immunization against poliomyelitis; pharmacologic treatment of hypertension to prevent subsequent end-organ damage; use of ear-protecting devices in loud working environments, such as around jet airplanes; and use of seat belts, air bags, and helmets to prevent bodily injuries in automobile and motorcycle crashes. Some measures provide specific protection while contributing to the more general goal of health promotion. Fluoridation of water supplies not only helps to prevent dental caries but also is a nutritional intervention that promotes stronger bones.

B. Secondary Prevention and Latent Disease

Sooner or later, depending on the individual, a disease process such as coronary artery atherosclerosis progresses sufficiently to become detectable by medical tests, such as cardiac stress test, although the individual is still asymptomatic. This may be thought of as the latent (hidden) stage of disease.

For many infectious and noninfectious diseases, *screening tests* allow the detection of latent disease in individuals considered to be at high risk. Presymptomatic diagnosis through screening programs, along with subsequent treatment when needed, is referred to as *secondary prevention* because it is the secondary line of defense against disease. Although screening programs do not prevent the causes from initiating the disease process, they may allow diagnosis at an earlier stage of disease, when treatment is more effective.

C. Tertiary Prevention and Symptomatic Disease

When disease has become symptomatic and medical assistance is sought, the goal of the clinician is to provide tertiary prevention in the form of disability limitation for patients with early symptomatic disease, or rehabilitation for patients with late symptomatic disease (see Table 14-1).

1. Disability Limitation

Disability limitation describes medical and surgical measures aimed at correcting the anatomic and physiologic components of disease in symptomatic patients. Most care provided by clinicians meets this description. Disability limitation can be considered prevention because its goal is to halt or slow the disease process and prevent or limit complications, impairment, and disability. An example is the surgical removal of a tumor, which may prevent the spread of disease locally or by metastasis to other sites. Discussions about a patient's disease also may provide an opportunity ("teachable moment") to convince the patient to begin health promotion techniques designed to delay disease progression (e.g., to begin exercising and improving the diet and to stop smoking after a myocardial infarction).

2. Rehabilitation

Although many are surprised to see rehabilitation designated a form of prevention, the label is correctly applied. Rehabilitation may mitigate the effects of disease and prevent some of the social and functional disability that would otherwise occur. For example, a person who has been injured or had a stroke may be taught self-care in activities of daily living (ADLs; e.g., feeding, bathing). Rehabilitation may enable the person to avoid the adverse sequelae associated with prolonged inactivity, such as increasing muscle weakness that might develop without therapy. Rehabilitation of a stroke patient begins with early and frequent mobilization of all joints during the period of maximum paralysis. This permits easier recovery of limb use by preventing the development of stiff joints and flexion contractures. Next, physical therapy helps stroke patients to strengthen remaining muscle function and to use this remaining function to maximum effect in performing ADLs. Occupational and speech therapy may enable such patients to gain skills and perform some type of gainful employment, preventing complete economic dependence on others. It is legitimate, therefore, to view rehabilitation as a form of prevention.

V. ECONOMICS OF PREVENTION

In an era of "cost consciousness," there are increasing demands that health promotion and disease prevention be proven economically worthwhile. Furthermore, many people in the political arena promote prevention as a means of controlling rising health care costs. This argument is based on the belief that prevention is always cost-saving. One way to examine that claim is to look at the cost-effectiveness of various preventive measures and compare them to the cost-effectiveness of treatment for existing conditions.

As outlined in Chapter 6, **cost-benefit analysis** compares the costs of an intervention to its health benefits. In order to compare different interventions, it becomes necessary to express the health benefits of different interventions with the same metric, called **cost-effectiveness analysis** (Box 14-1). Examples for such metrics are mortality, disease, and costs, or their inverse: longevity, disease-free time, and savings. A subtype of cost-effectiveness analysis is **cost-utility analysis,** which has the outcome of the cost/quality-adjusted life year, also called the **cost-effectiveness ratio** (CER). A recent comparison of the CER of various preventive measures with treatments for existing conditions found that both preventive and curative measures span the cost-effectiveness spectrum; both can be cost-saving, favorable, or unfavorable.[16]

Much depends on the frequency of the disease in the population and the characteristics of the preventive measures. Tables of the most valuable clinical services are available.[17] The Partnership for Prevention has been founded as a national not-for-profit health organization dedicated to evidence-based prevention grounded in "value."[18]

There are particular challenges to demonstrating benefits for preventive measures and achieving meaningful adoption.

A. Demonstration of Benefits

Scientific proof of benefits may be difficult because it is often impractical or unethical to undertake randomized trials of harm using people as subjects. For example, it is impossible to assign people randomly to smoking and nonsmoking groups. Apart from some research done on animal models, investigators are limited to observational studies, which usually are not as convincing as experiments. Life is filled with risks for one disease or another, and many of these operate together to produce the levels of health observed in a population. These risks may be changing in frequency in different subpopulations, making it impossible to infer what proportion of the improvement observed over time is caused by a particular preventive measure. If there is a reduction in the incidence of lung cancer, it is difficult to infer what proportion is caused by smoking reduction programs and what proportion by the elimination of smoking in workplaces and public areas, the increase in public awareness of (and action against) the presence of radon in homes, and other factors as yet poorly understood. Lastly, clinical research is expensive. A majority of research on treatment and diagnosis modalities is sponsored by pharmaceutical companies. The money spent by them to support clinical research is vastly greater than the research dollars spent on prevention. Therefore, some of the lack of data might result from the lack of large-scale, well-funded studies.

B. Delay of Benefits

With most preventive programs, there is a long delay between the time the preventive measures are instituted and the time that positive health changes become discernible. Because the latent period (incubation period) for lung cancer caused by cigarette smoking is 20 years or more, benefits resulting from investments made now in smoking reduction programs may not be identified until many years have passed. There are similar delays between the time of smoking cessation and the demonstration of effect for other smoking-related pulmonary problems, such as obstructive pulmonary disease. Most chronic diseases can be shown to have long latent periods between when the causes start and the disease appears.

C. Accrual of Benefits

Even if a given program could be shown to produce meaningful economic benefit, it is necessary to know to whom the benefits would accrue. For example, a financially stressed health insurance plan or health maintenance organization might cover a preventive measure if the financial benefit were fairly certain to be as great as or greater than the cost of providing that benefit, but only if most or all of the

Box 14-1	Cost-Benefit and Cost-Effectiveness Analysis

Cost-benefit analysis measures the costs and the benefits of a proposed course of action in terms of the same units, usually monetary units such as dollars. For example, a cost-benefit analysis of a poliomyelitis immunization program would determine the number of dollars to be spent toward vaccines, equipment, and personnel to immunize a particular population. It would determine the number of dollars that would be saved by not having to pay for the hospitalizations, medical visits, and lost productivity that would occur if poliomyelitis were not prevented in that population.

Incorporating concepts such as the dollar value of life, suffering, and the quality of life into such an analysis is difficult. Cost-benefit analysis is useful, however, if a particular budgetary entity (e.g., government or business) is trying to determine whether the investment of resources in health would save money in the long run. It also is useful if a particular entity with a fixed budget is trying to make informed judgments about allocations between various sectors (e.g., health, transportation, education) and to determine the sector in which an investment would produce the greatest economic benefit.

Cost-effectiveness analysis provides a way of comparing different proposed solutions in terms of the most appropriate measurement units. For example, by measuring hepatitis B cases prevented, deaths prevented, and life-years saved per 10,000 population, Bloom and colleagues were able to compare the effectiveness of four different strategies of dealing with the hepatitis B virus:

1. No vaccination
2. Universal vaccination
3. Screening followed by vaccination of unprotected individuals
4. A combination of the screening of pregnant women at delivery, the vaccination of the newborns of women found to be antibody positive during screening, and the routine vaccination of all 10-year-old children

After estimating the numbers of persons involved in each step of each method and determining the costs of screening, purchasing, and administering the vaccine, and delivering medical care for various forms and complications of hepatitis, Bloom et al. calculated that the fourth strategy would have an undiscounted cost of about $367 (or a discounted cost of $1205) per case of hepatitis B prevented and concluded this was the strategy with the lowest cost. (The CDC now recommends immunizing all infants against hepatitis B.)

The chaotic situation in the United States regarding costs and charges under different health insurance plans and in different hospitals makes it difficult to estimate medical care costs. The situation can be dealt with partly by performing a **sensitivity analysis** with spreadsheets in which different costs per item are substituted to see how they affect the total cost.

In addition, the concept of **discounting,** which is important in business and finance, must be used in medical cost-benefit and cost-effectiveness analysis when the costs are incurred in the present but the benefits will occur in the future. Discounting is a reduction in the **present value** of delayed benefits (or increase in present costs) to account for the **time value of money.** If the administrators of a prevention program spend $1000 now to save $1000 of expenses in the future, they will take a net loss. This is because they will lose the use of $1000 in the interim, and because with inflation the $1000 eventually saved will not be worth as much as the $1000 initially spent. The use of discounting is an attempt to adjust for these forces.

To discount a cost-benefit or cost-effectiveness analysis, the easiest way is to increase the present costs by a yearly factor, which can be thought of as the interest that would have to be paid to borrow the prevention money until the benefits occurred. For example, if it costs $1000 today to prevent a disease that would have occurred 20 years in the future, the present cost can be multiplied by $(1 + r)^n$, where r is the yearly interest rate for borrowing and n is the number of years until the benefit is realized. If the average yearly interest rate is 5% over 20 years, the formula becomes: $(1 + 0.05)^{20} = (1.05)^{20} = 2.653$. When this is multiplied by the present cost of $1000, the result is $2653. The expected savings 20 years in the future from a $1000 investment today would have to be greater than $2653 for the initial investment to be a net (true) financial gain.

From Bloom BS, Hillman AL, Fendrick AM, et al: A reappraisal of hepatitis B virus vaccination strategies using cost-effectiveness analysis. *Ann Intern Med* 118:298–306, 1993.

financial benefit would accrue to the insurance plan in the near future. If plan members switch insurance plans frequently, or if most of the financial benefit would go to the enrollees or a government rather than to the insurance plan, the prevention program would be seen as only a financial cost by the insurance plan.

The same principle is true for the even more financially strapped budgets of local, state, and federal governments. If the savings from prevention efforts would go directly to individuals, rather than to a government budget, the elected representatives might not support the prevention effort, even if the benefits clearly outweighed the costs. Elected representatives may want to show results before the next election campaign. Disease prevention may show results only over an extended time and may not lend itself to political popularity. Even so, there seems to be growing political support for at least the concept of prevention as a medical priority.

D. Discounting

If a preventive effort is made now by a government body, the costs are present-day costs, but any financial savings may not be evident until many years from now. Even if the savings are expected to accrue to the same budgetary unit that provided the money for the preventive program, the delay in economic return means that the benefits are worth less to that unit now. In the jargon of economists, the present value of the benefits must be discounted (see Box 14-1), making it more difficult to show cost-effectiveness or a positive benefit-cost ratio.

E. Priorities

As the saying goes, "the squeaky wheel gets the grease." Current, urgent problems usually attract much more attention and concern than future, subtle problems. Emergency care for victims of motor vehicle crashes is easy to justify, regardless of costs. Although prevention may be cost-effective, it may be difficult to justify using money to prevent crises that have not yet occurred. The same dilemma applies to essentially every phase of life. It is difficult to obtain money for programs to prevent the loss of topsoil, prevent illiteracy, and prevent the decay of roads and bridges. Even on an individual level, many patients do not want to make changes in their lives, such as eating a healthier diet, exercising, and stopping smoking, because the risk of future problems does not speak to them urgently in the present. As a broader example, although the level-five hurricane Katrina was expected for the U.S. Gulf Coast, inadequate preparations were made by the individuals, cities, and states involved and by the federal government.

VI. PREVENTIVE MEDICINE TRAINING

Physicians desiring to become board-certified as specialists in preventive medicine may seek postgraduate residency training in a program approved for preventive medicine training by the **Accreditation Council for Graduate Medical Education**.[19] Certification in preventive medicine must be in one of the following three **subspecialty areas:**

- General preventive medicine and public health
- Occupational medicine
- Aerospace medicine

Occasionally, a physician becomes certified in two subspecialties (most often the first and second areas listed). A few medical residency programs offer a combined residency in a clinical specialty (e.g., internal medicine) and preventive medicine. A residency program in medical toxicology is governed by a tripartite board, with representatives from the American boards of preventive medicine, pediatrics, and emergency medicine.

Certification in preventive medicine requires 3 years of residency. The first postgraduate year is called the *clinical year*. It consists of an internship with substantial patient care responsibility, usually in internal medicine, family practice, or pediatrics, although other areas are acceptable if they provide sufficient patient responsibility. The internship may be done in any accredited, first-postgraduate-year residency program. A few preventive medicine residency programs offer the first postgraduate year, but most do not. The second postgraduate year is called the *academic year* and consists of course work to obtain the master of public health (MPH) degree or its equivalent. The course work may be pursued in any accredited MPH program and need not be done in a formal preventive medicine residency program, although there are some advantages in doing so. The third postgraduate year is called the *practicum year*, and it must be completed in an accredited preventive medicine residency program. It consists of a year of supervised practice of the subspecialty in varied rotation sites, and it is tailored to fit an individual resident's needs. It typically includes clinical practice of the subspecialty; experience in program planning, development, administration, and evaluation; analysis and solution of problems (e.g., problems related to epidemics); research; and teaching. Some residency programs offer preventive medicine training combined with other specialties, such as internal medicine, pediatrics, or family

medicine. Typically, in these cases, the training time is shorter in a combined program than if residents did both programs sequentially.[20]

The certification examination has two parts: a core examination and a subspecialty examination. The core examination is the same for all three subspecialties and covers topics such as epidemiology, biostatistics, environmental health, health policy and financing, social science as applied to public health, and general clinical preventive medicine. Further information for specialty training and board examination is available on the Internet (see Websites).

VII. SUMMARY

Preventive medicine seeks to enhance the lives of patients by helping them promote their health and prevent specific diseases or diagnose them early. Preventive medicine also tries to apply the concepts and techniques of health promotion and disease prevention to the organization and practice of medicine (clinical preventive services). Health is an elusive concept but means more than the absence of disease; it is a positive concept that includes the ability to adapt to stress and the ability to function in society. The three levels of prevention define the various strategies available to practitioners to promote health and prevent disease, impairment, and disability at various stages of the natural history of disease. Primary prevention keeps a disease from becoming established by eliminating the causes of disease or increasing resistance to disease. Secondary prevention interrupts the disease process by detecting and treating it in the presymptomatic stage. Tertiary prevention limits the physical impairment and social consequences from symptomatic disease. It is not easy for prevention programs to compete for funds in a tight fiscal climate because of long delays before the benefits of such investments are noted. Specialty training in preventive medicine prepares investigators to demonstrate the cost-effectiveness and cost benefits of prevention.

References

1. Dubos R: *Man adapting*, New Haven, Conn, 1965, Yale University Press.
2. Selye H: Confusion and controversy in the stress field. *J Hum Stress* 1:37–44, 1975.
3. Selye H: The evolution of the stress concept. *Am Sci* 61:692–699, 1973.
4. McEwen BS, Stellar E: Stress and the individual. *Arch Intern Med* 153:2093–2101, 1993.
5. Dubos R: *Mirage of health*, New York, 1961, Doubleday.
6. Breslow L: From disease prevention to health promotion. *JAMA* 281:1030–1033, 1999.
7. Fries JF, Crapo LM: *Vitality and aging*, San Francisco, 1981, WH Freeman.
8. Haywood KL, Garratt AM, Fitzpatrick R: Quality of life in older people: a structured review of generic self-assessed health instruments. *Qual Life Res* 14:1651–1668, 2005.
9. McDowell I, Newell C: *Measuring health: a guide to rating scales and questionnaires*, ed 2, New York, 1996, Oxford University Press.
10. Last JM: *A dictionary of epidemiology*, ed 4, New York, 2001, Oxford University Press.
11. Barendregt JJ, Bonneux L, Van der Maas PJ: Health expectancy: an indicator for change? *J Epidemiol Community Health* 48:482–487, 1994.

12. Revicki DA, Allen H, Bungay K, et al: Responsiveness and calibration of the General Well Being Adjustment Scale in patients with hypertension, *J Clin Epidemiol* 47:1333–1342, 1994.

13. US Centers for Disease Control and Prevention: Quality of life as a new public health measure: Behavioral Risk Factor Surveillance System. *MMWR* 43:375–380, 1994.

14. US Centers for Disease Control and Prevention: Health-related quality of life measures: United States, 1993. *MMWR* 44:195–200, 1995.

15. Leavell HR, Clark EG: *Preventive medicine for the doctor in his community*, ed 3, New York, 1965, McGraw-Hill.

16. Cohen JT, Neumann PJ, Weinstein MD: Does preventive care save money? Health economics and the presidential candidates. *N Engl J Med* 358:661–663, 2008.

17. Maciosek MV, Coffield AB, Edwards NM, et al: Priorities among effective clinical preventive services: results of a systematic review and analysis. *Am J Prev Med* 31:52–61, 2006.

18. Partnership for Prevention. http:www.prevent.org, accessed under http://www.prevent.org/About-Us.aspx

19. http://www.acpm.org/?GME_MedStudents.

20. Wild DMG, Tessier-Sherman B, D'Souza S, et al: Experiences with a combined residency in internal and preventive medicine. *Am J Prev Med* 33:393–397, 2008.

Select Readings

Dubos R: *Mirage of health*, New York, 1961, Doubleday. [The concept of prevention.]

Fries JF, Crapo LM: *Vitality and aging*, San Francisco, 1981, WH Freeman. [The concept of prevention.]

Muir Gray JA: *Evidence-based healthcare: how to make health policy and management decisions*, ed 2, Edinburgh, 2001, Churchill Livingstone.

Task Force on Principles for Economic Analysis of Health Care Technology: Economic analysis of health care technology: a report on principles. *Ann Intern Med* 123:61–70, 1995. [Cost-effectiveness and cost-benefit analysis.]

Websites

http://www.acpm.org/?GME_MedStudents [American College of Preventive Medicine]

http://www.acpm.org/?page=GME_Home [American College of Preventive Medicine: Graduate Training and Careers in Preventive Medicine]

http://www.amsa.org/AMSA/Homepage/About/Committees/PreventiveMedicine.aspx [American Medical Student Association; Information on Preventive Medicine]

https://research.tufts-nemc.org/cear4/default.aspx [Cost-Effectiveness Analysis Registry]

http://www.prevent.org [Partnership for Prevention]

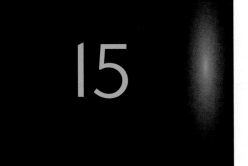

15 Methods of Primary Prevention: Health Promotion

The most fundamental sources of health are food, the environment, and behavior. Whereas public health managers are concerned with the availability of healthy food and the safety of the environment for the population (see Section 4), this chapter and Chapter 16 explore how preventive medicine clinicians can intervene *with individual patients* for better health. Here we discuss primary prevention of disease through general health promotion and specific protection. General health promotion by preventive medicine practitioners requires effective counseling driven by theories of behavior change. Chapters 16 and 17 discuss secondary and tertiary prevention for the general population. Chapters 18 to 23 discuss clinical prevention specific diseases for particular populations.

I. SOCIETY'S CONTRIBUTION TO HEALTH

In addition to the sometimes profound effects of genetics, the most fundamental sources of health do not come from access to the health care system, but rather from the following[1,2]:

1. Adequate healthy food
2. A clean and safe environment
3. Prudent behavior

The health care system is of vital importance when it comes to treating disease (and injury), but all of society, and personal actions, provide the basic structure for these three sources of health. Examples for societal sources of health include socioeconomic conditions, opportunities for safe employment, environmental systems (e.g., water supply, sewage disposal), and the regulation of the environment, commerce, and public safety. Society also helps to sustain social support systems (e.g., families, neighborhoods) that are fundamental to health and facilitate healthful behaviors.[3]

Because socioeconomic and other conditions vary greatly from country to country and over time, health problems and the success of health promotion efforts also vary. For example, wartime conditions in Sudan (1998) precluded adequate nutrition and medical assistance, and even international relief efforts were hindered. Immediately after the chemical disaster in Bhopal, India (1984), or the radiation disaster in Chernobyl, Ukraine (1986), it was impossible for people in the immediate area to find an environment safe from these toxic exposures. In both cases the toxic effects were spread rapidly by wind, and there were no effective evacuation plans. Natural disasters, such as tsunamis (Indian Ocean, 2004), earthquakes (Haiti, 2010), or both (Japan, 2011), may create conditions such as damaged roads and transportation systems that hinder quick and effective responses.

Even in reasonably ordered societies, income must be sufficient to allow for adequate nutrition and a safe environment for individuals and families. Education enhances employment opportunities and helps people understand the forces that promote good health. Coordinated systems of resource distribution are needed to avoid disparities and deprivation that compromise health. A landmark study among British civil servants showed that lower socioeconomic status correlates with poorer health, regardless of the country studied.[4] This trend applies not only to direct measures of health or lack of health (e.g., death rates), but also to nutrition, health behaviors, fertility, and mental health.[5] Debate continues about what factors to consider in defining socioeconomic groups. In the 1990s, using educational background as a measure of socioeconomic status, investigators showed that disparities between socioeconomic groups in the United States persisted.[6] Currently, U.S. statistics are stratified by educational attainment and sometimes by income level or poverty status, but not by a comprehensive measure of socioeconomic status. It is becoming increasingly clear that unhealthy lifestyles and access to medical care explain only some of the socioeconomic differences observed in the United Kingdom and the United States.[7]

Once people have access to adequate nutrition, clean water, and a safe environment, *behavior* becomes the major determining factor for health (see Chapters 20 and 21). Genetic makeup and behavior also interact; people's genes may increase their risk of developing certain diseases. However, it is their behavior that can hasten, prevent, or delay the onset of such diseases.

II. GENERAL HEALTH PROMOTION

The World Health Organization (WHO) defines health promotion as "the process of enabling people to increase control over their health and its determinants, and thereby improve their health."[8] It is customary to distinguish general health promotion from specific health protection. *General* health promotion addresses the underpinnings of general health, especially the following six suggested health behaviors[9]:

- Monitoring and limiting dietary fat intake.
- Consuming at least 5 servings of fruits and vegetables per day.
- Performing regular physical activity and exercise.
- Abstaining from tobacco.
- Adhering to medication regimen.
- Practicing stress management and weight loss as needed.

Specific health protection activities such as vaccines, antimicrobial drugs, and nutritional interventions are aimed at preventing specific diseases.

III. BEHAVIORAL FACTORS IN HEALTH PROMOTION

Human behavior is fundamental to health. The actual, primary causes of death in the United States and most other countries involve modifiable lifestyle behaviors: cigarette smoking, poor diet, and lack of exercise.[2] Therefore, efforts to change patients' behavior can have a powerful impact on their short-term and long-term health. Clinicians may not be aware of individual behavioral choices made by their patients, and if they are aware, they may not feel comfortable in trying to influence patient choices. Clinicians may also be more likely to counsel patients regarding topics with clear scientific support, such as nutrition and exercise, or that require medical techniques, such as screening or family planning. They are more likely to counsel patients when they discover

definite risk factors for disease, such as obesity, hypertension, elevated cholesterol levels, or unprotected sexual activity.

An important window of opportunity for counseling occurs after the development of symptomatic disease, such as an acute myocardial infarction, when a patient's motivation to modify diet, begin exercising regularly, and quit smoking may be at its peak ("teachable moment"). Another situation in which many patients are open to behavior change is pregnancy.

Boxes 15-1 and 15-2 provide specific recommendations for promoting a healthy diet and for smoking cessation. The most recent U.S. Preventive Services Task Force report offers recommendations for clinician counseling on a variety of additional topics, including motor vehicle, household, and recreational injury prevention; youth violence; sexually transmitted diseases; unintended pregnancy; gynecologic cancer; low back pain; and dental/periodontal disease.[10]

A. Theories of Behavior Change

In order to impact behavior, it is helpful to understand how health behavior is shaped and how people change. Behavior change is always difficult. The advantage of intervening in accordance with a valid theory of behavior change is that the intervention has a higher chance of success. Most health behavior models have been adapted from the social and behavioral sciences. Theories also help in targeting interventions, choosing appropriate techniques, and selecting appropriate outcomes to measure.[11] We can only sketch out the basics of the most common health theories here. For further details, readers should consult monographs on the topic.[11] Other theories support the approach to changing group norms and helping communities identify and address health problems (see Chapter 25).

Most health behavior theories have been adapted from the social and behavioral sciences. Therefore, they share common assumptions, as follows:

- Knowledge is necessary, but not sufficient, for behavior change.
- Behavior is affected by what people know and how they think.
- Behavior is influenced by people's perception of a behavior and its risks, their own motivation and skills, and the social environment.

An important part of motivation is also their self-perceived ability to influence their life. The degree to which people believe this is most often called *self-efficacy*.

The most common theories for health behavior counseling are the health belief model, transtheoretical model (stages of change), theory of planned behavior, and precaution adoption process model (Table 15-1).

1. Health Belief Model

The health belief model holds that, before seeking preventive measures, people generally must believe the following[12]:

- The disease at issue is serious, if acquired.
- They or their children are personally at risk for the disease.
- The preventive measure is effective in preventing the disease.
- There are no serious risks or barriers involved in obtaining the preventive measure.

Box 15-1   Health-Promoting Dietary Guidelines

In the past, various expert panels and organizations have recommended different types of diets for the prevention of particular diseases. These individual disease-preventing diets have largely been supplanted by one health-promoting diet designed to prevent multiple diseases by enhancing health. Dietary guidelines generated by the U.S. Department of Agriculture, American Heart Association, American Cancer Society, National Cancer Institute, and Institute of Medicine differ only in minor points, whereas all support the goal of maintaining and promoting health by engaging in regular physical activity; eating appropriately sized portions of food; limiting the intake of saturated and *trans* fats; and eating relatively generous amounts of whole grains, vegetables, and fruits. Also encouraged is the inclusion of healthful polyunsaturated and monounsaturated fats from such sources as nuts, seeds, olives, avocado, and olive and canola oils. Recommended intake ranges for the major nutrient classes—carbohydrate, fat, and protein—are provided by the Food and Nutrition Board of the Institute of Medicine at the National Academy of Sciences.

With regard to macronutrient distribution, the Institute of Medicine guidelines call for 20% to 35% of total calories from total fat, 45% to 65% from carbohydrates, and 10% to 35% from proteins. The guidelines further emphasize the restriction of saturated and *trans* fat and their replacement with monounsaturated and polyunsaturated fat. Processed foods should be eaten sparingly. Alcohol consumption should be modest, with ethanol levels not exceeding 15 g/day for women or 30 g/day for men (one drink for women or two drinks for men).*

From Otten JJ, Hellwig JP, Meyers LD, editors: Dietary reference intakes: the essential guide to nutrient requirements, Institute of Medicine of the National Academies, Washington, DC, 2006, National Academies Press.
*Katz DL: *Nutrition in clinical practice,* Philadelphia, 2008, Lippincott, Williams & Wilkins.
See these websites:
http://www.iom.edu/About-IOM/Leadership-Staff/Boards/Food-and-Nutrition-Board.aspx
http://www.cnpp.usda.gov/Publications/DietaryGuidelines/2010/PolicyDoc/ExecSumm.pdf
http://www.choosemyplate.gov/
http://fnic.nal.usda.gov/nal_display/index.php?info_center=4&tax_level=3&tax_subject=256&topic_id=1342&level3_id=5140

1. *Ask* **about tobacco use during every office visit.**
   Include questions about tobacco use when assessing the patient's vital signs. Placing tobacco-use status stickers on patient charts, noting tobacco use in electronic medical records, or using computer reminder systems also may be helpful.

2. *Advise* **all smokers to quit.**
   Advice should be:
   Clear: "I think it is important for you to quit smoking now. Cutting down or changing to light cigarettes is not enough."
   Strong: "As your physician, I need to tell you that smoking cessation is one of the most important decisions you can make for your health."
   Personalized: Physicians should talk with patients about how smoking has affected their health, children, or other family members; the social and economic costs of smoking; and the patient's readiness to quit.

3. *Assess* **the patient's willingness to quit.**
   Assess the patient's willingness to quit by asking, "On a scale from 0 to 10, with 0 being 'not at all motivated' and 10 being 'extremely motivated,' how motivated are you to quit smoking?" Use the patient's level of motivation to determine the next step:
   If the patient is willing to make a quit attempt, offer medication, brief counseling, and self-help resources and schedule a follow-up visit.
   If the patient is unwilling to quit, identify why the patient is not motivated. Explore what he or she likes and does not like about smoking and the potential advantages and disadvantages of quitting. Identify the patient's core values (e.g., health, being a role model for children) and how smoking affects these values.

4. *Assist* **the patient in his or her attempt to quit.**
   Help the patient make a quit plan:
   Set a quit date, ideally within 2 weeks of the office visit.
   Request encouragement and support from family and friends.
   Anticipate triggers and cues to smoking, and identify alternative coping strategies.
   Help the patient change his or her environment:
   Throw away cigarettes, matches, lighters, and ashtrays; launder clothing; and vacuum home and car.
   Avoid smoking in places where the patient spends a lot of time (e.g., home, work, car).
   Avoid other smokers and drinking alcohol.
   Provide basic information about smoking and cessation (e.g., addictive nature of smoking, importance of complete abstinence, possible withdrawal symptoms).
   Recommend pharmacotherapy, unless contraindications exist, and behavior therapy for smoking cessation.
   Provide supplementary self-help materials.

5. *Arrange* **follow-up contact.**
   Follow-up should occur within the first week after the quit date. A second follow-up contact is recommended within the first month. Further follow-up visits should be scheduled as needed.
   During a follow-up visit, success should be congratulated. If the patient has relapsed, review the circumstances and elicit a new commitment to quit. Consider referral for more intensive treatment.
   Follow-up contact can be by telephone, e-mail, or in person.

Modified from National Heart, Lung, and Blood Institute and American Lung Association recommendations.
http://www.ncbi.nlm.nih.gov/books/bv.fcgi?rid=hstat2.section.7741, cited from http://www.aafp.org/afp/2006/0715/p262.html#afp20060715p262-b2.
*The five "A"s from Fiore MC: *Treating tobacco use and dependence,* Rockville, Md, 2000, US Department of Health and Human Services, Public Health Service.

Table 15-1 **Overview of Common Theories of Behavior Change**

Theory	Focus	Key Concepts
Individual Level		
Health belief model	Individuals' perceptions of the threat posed by a health problem, the benefit of avoiding the threat, and factors influencing the decision to act	Perceived susceptibility Perceived severity Perceived benefits Perceived barriers Cues to action Self-efficacy
Stages of change model	Individuals' motivation and readiness to change a problem behavior	Precontemplation Contemplation Preparation Action Maintenance
Theory of planned behavior	Individuals' attitudes toward a behavior, perceptions of norms, and beliefs about the ease or difficulty of changing	Behavioral intention Attitude Subjective norm Perceived behavioral control
Precaution adoption process model	Individuals' journey from lack of awareness to action and maintenance	Unaware of issue Unengaged by issue Deciding about acting Deciding not to act Deciding to act Acting Maintenance
Interpersonal Level		
Social cognitive theory	Personal factors, environmental factors, and human behavior exert influence on each other	Reciprocal determinism Behavioral capability Expectations Self-efficacy Observational learning Reinforcements

Modified from Rimer BP, Glanz K: Theory at a glance: a guide for health promotion practice. http://www.cancer.gov/cancertopics/cancerlibrary/theory.pdf.

In addition, cues to action are needed, consisting of information regarding how and when to obtain the preventive measure and the encouragement or support of other people. This theory has been used to promote screening.

2. Stages of Change (Transtheoretical Model)

The transtheoretical model was developed first by Prochaska and DiClemente to explain how patients quit smoking. The underlying insight was that people do not change their behavior dramatically in one moment. Change is a *process,* and patients have different counseling and informational needs depending on where they are in this process. This model addressed both the stages of change and the process of changing. The stages of change are called precontemplation, contemplation, preparation, action, and maintenance.

In **precontemplation** the patient is not convinced there is a problem and is unwilling to consider change. In **contemplation** the patient has some ambivalence about the behavior but is not ready to take direct action. Acceptance of the need to act and **preparation** for action follow. In the **action** stage the patient is planning for change. Action is when people actually quit or make changes. This phase is followed by **maintenance** (and often, **relapse**). Many people cycle through the process many times before they make sustained changes. This theory has informed many efforts to change addictive behaviors.

3. Theory of Planned Behavior and Theory of Reasoned Action

Both the theory of planned behavior (TPB) and the associated theory of reasoned action (TRA) explore how people form intentions for behavior change and how beliefs and attitudes play a role in those intentions. **Behavioral intentions** are the most important factor in predicting behavior. In turn, behavioral intentions are influenced by a person's attitude and the presumed attitudes of other important individuals (subjective norms). In addition to this construct, TPB includes perceived behavioral control. This concept is similar to self-efficacy and describes how much people believe they can control their behavior. TPB/TRA has been used to target a wide range of behaviors, such as dieting, questioning genetically engineered food, and limiting sun exposure.

4. Precaution Adoption Process Model

The precaution adoption process model distinguishes seven steps, from unawareness of a problem to behavior change. People progress from ignorance or unawareness (stage 1) through un-engagement (stage 2) through a decision to act (stages 3 and 4). If a decision to act has been made (stage 5), the next steps involve acting (stage 6) and maintenance (stage 7) of behavior change. Although it has some similarities to the stages of change model, this model assumes that the development is *linear* (people cannot go back to stage 1 and become unaware of an issue). The precaution adoption process model is particularly suited for newly recognized hazards, such as radon or osteoporosis, and provides guidance on how to impact people in stages before they make decisions.

5. Social Learning Theory and Social Cognitive Theory

Behavior and behavior change do not occur in a vacuum. For most people, their social environment is a strong influence to change or maintain behaviors. **Social learning theory** asserts that people learn not only from their own experiences but also from observing others. **Social cognitive theory** builds on this concept and describes **reciprocal determinism;** the person, the behavior, and the environment all influence each other. Therefore, recruiting credible role models who perform the intended behavior may be a powerful influence. This theory has been successfully used to influence condom use.[13]

B. Behavioral Counseling

Patients often want and need counseling, particularly those with risk factors for significant diseases. If medications can be prescribed, it is tempting for the physician to provide these as the first line of treatment for obesity, smoking, hypertension, and elevated cholesterol levels. Nevertheless, unless the problem is severe when the patient is first seen, generally the best approach is to try first to modify diet, exercise, or other aspects of lifestyle. If these approaches to reducing risk factors are refused or are unsuccessful within a reasonable time, or if the risk to the patient is high, medications can be considered. However, medications should not replace counseling, only supplement it.

Many clinicians are uncomfortable with risk factor counseling, thinking they lack counseling skills or time. However, good data show that even brief interventions can have a profound impact on patients. Each year, millions of smokers quit smoking because they want to, because they are concerned about their health, and because their providers tell them to quit. At the same time, even more individuals begin smoking worldwide. Box 15-2 summarizes the approach that the National Heart, Lung, and Blood Institute and the American Lung Association recommend for use by clinicians in counseling their patients. Many online training programs are available to assist clinicians in counseling.[14]

Across a broad area of behavior, patient adherence is based on a functioning physician-patient relationship and skilled physician communication.[15] Beyond a good relationship, it matters *how* clinicians counsel. Despite its venerable tradition, simply giving advice is rarely effective.[16] Given the importance of social determinants of health, physician counseling is only one, often minor influence. Even though insufficient to cause change, however, counseling can provide motivation and support behavior change.

1. Motivational Interviewing

Motivational interviewing is a counseling technique aimed at increasing patients' motivation and readiness to change. It has been shown to be effective across a broad range of addictive and other health behaviors[17] and outperforms traditional advice giving.[16] Motivational interviewing fits well with the transtheoretical model of change and provides concrete strategies on how to increase people's motivation toward change. The model rests on three main concepts, as follows:

1. Patients with problem behaviors are ambivalent about their behavior.
2. "I learn what I believe as I hear myself talk." If the clinician presents one side of the argument and argues for change, it causes the patient to take up the opposite position. It is important to let the patient explore the advantages of changing, and allow the patient to do most of the talking.[18]
3. Change is motivated by a perceived disconnect between present behavior and important personal goals and values (cognitive dissonance).

Therefore, successful counseling involves increasing patients' cognitive dissonance and directing the dissonance toward behavior change. These steps are achieved by the following four strategies:

1. Expressing empathy.
2. Developing cognitive dissonance.
3. Rolling with resistance (resistance is a signal for the counselor to respond differently).
4. Supporting self-efficacy.

Table 15-2 gives some examples of how a skilled counselor might encourage a patient to "talk change."

Regardless of the extent of the clinician's activity in behavior change, the clinician is responsible for monitoring the progress of the patient on a regular basis and for changing the approach if sufficient progress is not being made. If necessary, the clinician can assist the process of risk factor modification by recommending appropriate medications, such as nicotine patches or nicotine inhalers for cessation of smoking or statins for reduction or modification of blood lipid levels.

2. Shared Decision Making

Shared decision making is a relatively new concept. It is a process by which patients and providers consider outcome probabilities and patient preferences and reach a mutual decision. This method is best used for areas of true uncertainty,[19] such as prostate cancer screening, treatment of early breast cancer, or abnormal uterine bleed. For these problems, which treatment or screening option is preferable depends on how patients view risks and benefits. During shared decision making, provider and patient explore together treatment options, consequences, expected benefits and consequences, and patient preferences. Many computerized decision aids have been developed to help this process. Examples include aids regarding prostatectomy for benign prostatic hyperplasia, hysterectomy for uterine bleed, and back surgery for chronic pain.[20]

Table 15-2 **Specific Motivational Interviewing Techniques for Early Stages of Change**

Stage	Technique	Example
Precontemplation	Eliciting self-motivational statements	What concerns do you have about your drinking?
	Provide only objective assessment	Your liver function indicates some damage, likely from your drinking. I don't know whether this is of any concern to you or not. …
	Reflective listening and affirmation	You have expressed a lot of concerns to me, and I respect you for that. Let me try to put all of these together. …
Contemplation	Increasing cognitive dissonance	I can see how this might be confusing to you. On the one hand, you see there are serious problems around your alcohol use. And on the other hand, it seems like the label "alcoholic" doesn't quite fit.
	Paradoxical interventions	There are many advantages you see from drinking. It is possible that you will never be able to change.
	Education	
Action	Providing information on treatment options	You have taken a big step today, and I respect you for it.
	Continued affirmation	
Maintenance	Providing information and support	What do you remember as the most important reason to quit drinking?
	Continued affirmation	
Relapse	Increasing self-efficacy	You've been through a lot, and I admire you for the commitment you've shown to stay sober for so long.

Modified from Miller WR: *Behav Psychother* II:147–172, 1983 and Miller WR et al: *Motivational enhancement therapy manual*, 1995.

IV. PREVENTION OF DISEASE THROUGH SPECIFIC PROTECTION

The major goals of primary prevention by specific protection involve prevention in the following three areas:

- **Specific diseases** (e.g., by using vaccines and antimicrobial prophylaxis)
- **Specific deficiency states** (e.g., by using iodized salt to prevent iodine deficiency goiter; by using fluoride to prevent dental caries)
- **Specific injuries and toxic exposures** (e.g., by using helmets to prevent head injuries in construction workers, goggles to prevent eye injuries in machine tool operators, or filters and ventilation systems to control dust)

This section discusses vaccinations, prevention of deficiency, and microbial prophylaxis. Chapter 22 discusses injury prevention in detail.

A. Prevention of Disease by Use of Vaccines

An intact immune system in a well-nourished and otherwise healthy individual provides basic protection against infectious diseases. **Intact immunity** implies that the immune system was normal at birth and has not been damaged by a disease, such as infection with human immunodeficiency virus (HIV) or side effects from medications (e.g., anticancer drugs, long-term steroid use). Some evidence suggests that depression and loneliness may suppress normal functioning of the immune system. Similarly, experimental animals are more resistant to infections when in the presence of other animals of the same species.[21]

I. Types of Immunity

Passive immunity is protection against an infectious disease provided by circulating antibodies made in another organism. Newborn infants are protected by **maternal antibodies** transferred through the placenta before birth and through breast milk after birth. If recently exposed to hepatitis B virus (HBV) and not immunized with HBV vaccine, a person can be given **human immune globulin,** which confers passive immunity and protects against HBV infection. In an emergency a specific type of **antitoxin**, if available, can be used to confer passive immunity against bacterial toxins, such as diphtheria antitoxin in the patient with clinical diphtheria or trivalent botulinum antitoxin for botulism. Passive immunity provides incomplete protection and usually is of short duration.

Vaccines confer **active immunity.** Some types of vaccines, such as the inactivated polio vaccine, do this by stimulating the production of **humoral** (blood) **antibody** to the antigen in the vaccine (see Chapter 1). Other types, such as the live attenuated polio vaccine, not only elicit this humoral antibody response but also stimulate the body to develop **cell-mediated immunity.** This tissue-based cellular response to foreign antigens involves mobilization of killer T cells. Active immunity is much superior to passive immunity because active immunity lasts longer (a lifetime in some cases) and is rapidly stimulated to high levels by a reexposure to the same or closely related antigens. All approved vaccines provide most immunized persons with some level of **individual immunity** to a specific disease (i.e., they themselves are protected).

Some vaccines also reduce or prevent the shedding (spread) of infectious organisms from an immunized person to others, and this contributes to **herd immunity** (see Fig. 1-2).

2. Types of Vaccines

Some vaccines are **inactivated** (killed), some are **live attenuated** (altered), and others are referred to as **toxoids** (inactivated or altered bacterial exotoxins). To reduce the likelihood of negative side effects, the antigens are increasingly being prepared in a cell-free (acellular) manner. Other vaccines consist of only antigenic fragments from the organisms of concern (e.g., polysaccharides), usually conjugated to a harmless biologic moiety. Newer, genomic methods increasingly permit the identification and replication of antigenic sequences of base pairs (epitopes) that are recognized by T or B lymphocytes, which then produce antibodies.

The older pertussis and typhoid vaccines are examples of **inactivated bacterial vaccines,** and injected influenza vaccine and the inactivated polio vaccine are examples of **inactivated viral vaccines.** The bacille Calmette-Guérin (BCG) vaccine against tuberculosis is an example of a **live attenuated bacterial vaccine,** and the measles and oral polio vaccines are examples of **live attenuated viral vaccines.** Live attenuated vaccines are created by altering the organisms so that they are no longer pathogenic, but still have antigenicity.

Diphtheria and tetanus vaccines are the primary examples of **toxoids** (vaccines against biologic toxins). *Corynebacterium diphtheriae,* the organism that causes diphtheria, produces a potent toxin when it is in the lysogenic state with corynebacteriophage. *Clostridium tetani,* an organism that is part of the normal flora of many animals and is found frequently in the soil, can cause tetanus in unimmunized individuals with infected wounds. This is because *C. tetani* produces a potent toxin when it grows under anaerobic conditions, such as are often found in wounds with necrotic tissue. Tetanus is almost nonexistent in populations with high immunization levels.

3. Immunization Recommendations and Schedules

ACTIVE IMMUNIZATION OF ADULTS

The need for adequate immunization levels in adults was shown by the dramatic epidemic of diphtheria that occurred in the independent states of the former Soviet Union, where more than 50,000 cases, with almost 2000 deaths, were reported between 1990 and 1994. In 70% of the cases, diphtheria occurred in persons 15 years or older.[22] Most of these individuals had been immunized against diphtheria as children, but the immunity had waned.

The immunization schedule for adults as of 2012 is shown in Figure 15-1. The immunization of adults builds on the foundation of vaccines given during childhood. If an adult is missing diphtheria and tetanus vaccines, these should be started immediately. Many adults need boosters because they were immunized as children, and their immunity levels have declined since they were immunized. For protection against tetanus, several combination preparations are available; however, adults usually are given the combined tetanus and diphtheria (Td) vaccine, which contains a reduced amount of diphtheria antigen to decrease the number of reactions. For adults who have a high risk of exposure to pertussis, some experts recommend that adults be immunized with the acellular pertussis (aP) vaccine because it may provide some herd immunity against pertussis to children.

The measles, mumps, and rubella (MMR) vaccine should be administered to adults who were born after 1957 and lack evidence of immunity to measles (a definite history of measles or measles immunization after age 12 months). Exceptions are pregnant women and immunocompromised patients.

Pneumococcal polysaccharide vaccine should be given at least once to persons 65 years and older, to persons age 2 to 64 with chronic diseases that increase their risk of mortality or serious morbidity from pneumococcal infection (chronic pulmonary or cardiac disease, cancer, renal or hepatic disease, asplenia, immunosuppression), to smokers, and to residents of long-term care facilities. Experts recommend that influenza vaccine be given annually in the late autumn to everybody over age 6 months, regardless of risk level. Hepatitis A is a disease acquired by eating or drinking contaminated substances. Vaccination against it is recommended for persons living in or traveling to areas of high or moderate risk. It also is recommended for persons who have significant occupational exposure, engage in homosexual activities, or use illegal drugs. Immunization against hepatitis B, a disease acquired through contact with blood and other body fluids, is recommended for persons who are at high risk because of their professions (e.g., health care workers), jobs in certain countries overseas, homosexual activities, intravenous drug use, or frequent exposure to blood or blood products.

International travelers should ensure that all their basic immunizations are up-to-date (e.g., poliomyelitis, tetanus, diphtheria, measles). Before traveling to less developed countries, it may be necessary or desirable to receive immunizations against hepatitis A, hepatitis B, typhoid, cholera, yellow fever, polio, and other diseases. For recommendations and help in determining requirements, individuals planning to travel abroad should consult a local clinician who specializes in international travel, their local or state health department, or the Centers for Disease Control and Prevention (CDC). The Internet has country-specific information regarding preventive measures needed for travel there, such as vaccines, immune globulins, and chemoprophylaxis.[23]

4. Passive Immunization

The medical indications for passive immunization are much more limited than the indications for active immunization. Table 15-3 provides information about biologic agents available in the United States and the indications for their use in immunocompetent persons (those with normal immune systems) and immunocompromised persons (those with impaired immune systems).

For immunocompetent individuals who are at high risk for exposure to hepatitis A, usually because of travel to a country where it is common, hepatitis A vaccine can be administered if there is time, or immune globulin can be administered before travel as a method of **preexposure prophylaxis.** For individuals recently exposed to hepatitis B or rabies and not known to have a protective antibody titer, a specific immune globulin can be used as a method of **postexposure prophylaxis** (see also Chapter 20). For individuals who lack active immunity to exotoxin-producing bacteria already causing symptoms, such as *Clostridium botulinum,* the organism responsible for botulism, the injection of a specific antitoxin is recommended after tests are performed to rule out hypersensitivity to the antitoxin.[24] For immunocompromised persons who have been exposed to a common but potentially life-threatening infection, such as chickenpox, immune globulin can be lifesaving if given intravenously soon after exposure.

B. Vaccine Surveillance and Testing

As discussed in Chapter 3, the rates and patterns of reportable diseases are monitored, and any cases thought to be vaccine associated are investigated. The goals are to monitor

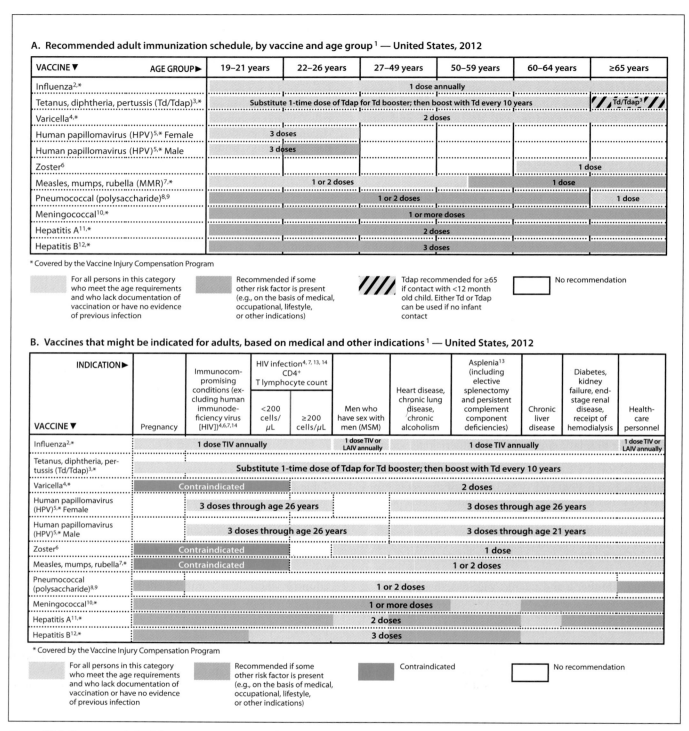

Figure 15-1 Recommended adult vaccination schedule. (From http://www.cdc.gov/vaccines/recs/schedules/downloads/adult/mmwr-adult-schedule.pdf. For footnotes, see http://www.cdc.gov/vaccines/recs/schedules/downloads/adult/mmwr-adult-schedule.pdf.)

the effectiveness of vaccines and to detect vaccine failures or adverse effects.

I. Randomized Field Trials

The standard way to measure the effectiveness of a new vaccine is through a randomized field trial, the public health equivalent of a randomized controlled trial. In this type of trial, susceptible persons are randomized into two groups and are given the vaccine or a placebo, usually at the beginning of the high-risk season of the year. The vaccinated subjects and unvaccinated controls are followed through the high-risk season to determine the **attack rate** (AR) in each group.

$$AR = \text{Number of persons ill}/$$
$$\text{Number of persons exposed to the disease}$$

Table 15-3 **Indications for Use of Immune Globulins and Antitoxins Available in the United States***

Immunobiologic Agent	Type	Indications
Botulinum antitoxin	Specific equine antibodies	Treatment of botulism
Botulinum antitoxin (BIG)	Specific human antibodies	Treatment of botulism in infants
Cytomegalovirus immune globulin, intravenous (CMV-IGIV)	Specific human antibodies	Prophylaxis in hematopoietic stem cell and kidney transplant recipients
Diphtheria antitoxin Some, but no U.S, trade names; click for drug monograph	Specific equine antibodies	Treatment of respiratory diphtheria

Hepatitis B immune globulin (HBIG)
Some trade names
  HepaGam B
  HyperHep B S/D
  NABI-HB
	Specific human antibodies	Prophylaxis for hepatitis B postexposure

Immune globulin (IG)	Pooled human antibodies	Prophylaxis for hepatitis A preexposure and postexposure, measles postexposure, immunoglobulin deficiency, rubella during 1st trimester of pregnancy, varicella (if varicella-zoster immune globulin unavailable)
Intravenous immune globulin (IVIG)	Pooled human antibodies	Prophylaxis for and treatment of severe bacterial and viral infections (e.g., HIV infection in children), primary immunodeficiency disorders, autoimmune thrombocytopenic purpura, chronic B-cell lymphocytic leukemia, Kawasaki disease, autoimmune disorders (myasthenia gravis, Guillain-Barré syndrome, poly/dermatomyositis) Prophylaxis for graft-versus-host disease
Subcutaneous immune globulin (SCIG)	Pooled human antibodies	Treatment of primary immunodeficiency disorders
Rabies immune globulin (HRIG)†	Specific human antibodies	Management of rabies postexposure in people not previously immunized with rabies vaccine
Respiratory syncytial virus immune globulin, intravenous (RSV-IGIV)	Specific human antibodies	Prevention of RSV in infants with a history of premature birth (<35 wks gestation) or children with a chronic lung disorder (e.g., bronchopulmonary dysplasia)
Respiratory syncytial virus murine monoclonal antibody (RSV-mAb) Some trade names (Synagis); click for drug monograph	Murine monoclonal antibody (palivizumab)	Prevention of RSV in infants with history of premature birth (<35 wks gestation) or children with chronic lung disorder (e.g., bronchopulmonary dysplasia)
Tetanus immune globulin (TIG)	Specific human antibodies	Treatment of tetanus Postexposure prophylaxis in patients not adequately immunized with tetanus toxoid
Vaccinia immune globulin (VIG)	Specific human antibodies	Treatment of eczema vaccinatum, vaccinia necrosum, and ocular vaccinia
Varicella-zoster immune globulin (VZIG)	Specific human antibodies	Postexposure prophylaxis in susceptible immunocompromised people, certain susceptible pregnant women, and perinatally exposed neonates

From General Recommendations on immunization. Recommendations of the Advisory Committee on Immunization Practices (ACIP), *MMWR* 43:1, 1994. Updated through the Center for Biologics Evaluation and Research, US Food and Drug Administration, 2008.
*Immune globulin preparations and antitoxins are given intramuscularly (IM) unless otherwise indicated.
†HRIG is administered topically around wounds as well as IM.

Here, AR among the vaccinated is the number of vaccinated persons ill with the disease divided by the total number vaccinated. For the unvaccinated, AR is the number of unvaccinated persons in the study group who are ill divided by the total number of unvaccinated persons in the study group.

Next, the **vaccine effectiveness** (VE) (sometimes called *protective efficacy*), when calculated as a percentage, is:

$$VE = AR_{(unvaccinated)} - AR_{(vaccinated)} \times 100 / AR_{(unvaccinated)}$$

In the VE equation, the numerator is the observed reduction in AR as a result of the vaccination, and the denominator represents the total amount of risk that could be reduced by the vaccine. The VE formula is a specific example of the general formula for **relative risk reduction.**

Testing the efficacy of vaccines by randomized field trials is costly, but it may be required the first time a new vaccine is introduced. Field trials were used to evaluate inactivated polio vaccine, oral polio vaccine, measles vaccine, influenza vaccine, and varicella vaccine. An example of such a trial of a new vaccine is a recent study of an HIV vaccine, showing a vaccine efficacy of about 26%.[25]

2. Retrospective Cohort Studies

The antigenic variability of influenza virus necessitates frequent (often yearly) changes in the constituents of influenza vaccines to keep them up-to-date with new strains of the virus (see Chapter 1). This requires constant surveillance of the disease and the protective efficacy of the vaccine. Because there are insufficient resources and time to perform a randomized controlled trial of each new influenza vaccine, retrospective cohort studies are done sometimes during the influenza season to evaluate the protective efficacy of the vaccines.

In these studies, because there is no randomization, investigators cannot ensure that no selection bias occurred on the part of the clinicians who recommended the vaccine or the individuals who agreed to be immunized. If selection bias were present, the participants who were immunized might be either sicker or more interested in their health than those who were not immunized. Studies of influenza vaccine protective effectiveness in nursing homes have suggested that rates vary from almost 0% to about 40%.[26] The relatively low vaccine effectiveness may be caused by inadequate antibody production by older people and the delay from vaccine administration until an outbreak appears. However, evidence shows that the vaccination reduces influenza mortality rates in community-dwelling elderly people, and this reduction is greater among persons who are revaccinated each year.[27]

3. Case-Control Studies

Because randomized field trials require large sample sizes, they are usually impossible to perform for relatively uncommon diseases, such as *Haemophilus influenzae* infections or pneumococcal pneumonia. To overcome this problem, some investigators have recommended using case-control studies.[28] This is based on the fact that when the risk of disease in the population is low, the vaccine effectiveness formula, expressed as a percentage, may be rewritten as follows:

$$VE = 1 - [AR_{(vaccinated)} / AR_{(unvaccinated)}] = (1 - RR) \approx (1 - OR)$$

The risk ratio (RR) is closely approximated by the odds ratio (OR) when the disease is uncommon, as in the cases of *H. influenzae* infections in children and pneumococcal infections in adults.

When one group of investigators performed a case-control study of pneumococcal vaccine, which was a polyvalent vaccine containing capsular polysaccharide antigens of 23 strains of *Streptococcus pneumoniae,* they found that the vaccine showed fairly good efficacy against the strains contained in the vaccine and no efficacy against other *S. pneumoniae* strains.[29] That the risks from strains not in the vaccine were comparable in the case and control groups suggests that the differences in protective efficacy for strains that were in the vaccine were not caused by selection bias.

4. Incidence Density Measures

The questions that vaccine research and surveillance are designed to answer include the following:

- When should a new vaccine be given?
- What is the duration of the immunity produced?

In the case of measles vaccine, initial surveillance studies suggested that when the vaccine was given to infants before 12 months of age, often it was ineffective, presumably because the vaccine antigen was neutralized by residual maternal antibody.

To determine answers to both these questions, one group of investigators performed a study in which they monitored the incidence density of measles cases in Ohio over a full winter and spring season.[30] To adjust for the duration of exposure to measles, which varied between individuals, they used the incidence density as their measure of measles incidence (see results in Box 15-3 and description in Chapter 2). The formula for **incidence density** (ID) is as follows:

$$ID = \text{Number of new cases of a disease/Person-time of exposure}$$

The denominator (person-time) can be expressed in terms of the number of person-days, person-weeks, person-months, or person-years of exposure to the risk.

Box 15-3	Data Showing Why Measles Vaccine Is Now Postponed until Children Are 15 Years Old

PART 1 Relationship between the age at measles vaccination and (1) measles incidence density (incidence of disease per 1000 person-weeks) and (2) relative risk of measles per 1000 person-weeks of exposure at different ages of vaccination compared with children vaccinated at 15 months old

Age at Vaccination	Measles Incidence per 1000 Person-Weeks	Relative Risk Compared with Risk in Children Vaccinated at 15 Months Old
Never	155.3	33
<11 months	39.6	8.5
11 months	15	3.2
12 months	7.1	1.5
13 months	5.2	1.1
14 months	4.7	1

PART 2 Relationship of time elapsed since measles vaccination and (1) measles incidence density (incidence of measles per 1000 person-weeks) and (2) relative risk of measles compared with children vaccinated recently (0-3 years)

Time Since Vaccination	Measles Incidence per 1000 Person-Weeks	Relative Risk
0-3 years	4	1
4-6 years	4.2	1.1
7-9 years	5.4	1.4
10-12 years	11.7	2.9

Data from Marks J, Halpin TJ, Orenstein WA: *Pediatrics* 62:955–960, 1978.

The results shown in Box 15-3, along with other studies, suggested that measles vaccine should be postponed until children are approximately 15 months old. One concern in delaying the vaccine is that measles is more severe in newborns than in older infants. Partly to reduce the risk that new schoolchildren will be exposed to measles and bring the disease home to younger siblings, experts recommend that all children be revaccinated with measles vaccine before they enter school, at age 5 or 6 years. This also serves as a booster dose to protect the children as they enter school.

Another concern has been the duration of immunity. As shown in the second part of Box 15-3, the measles vaccine lost its protective ability slowly during the first 6 years, but the relative risk of acquiring measles had almost tripled by 10 to 12 years after immunization. This was another line of evidence that led to the recommendation that children be revaccinated before entering school, at age 5 or 6 years.

C. Immunization Goals

The strategy of developing disease control programs through the use of vaccines depends on the objectives of the vaccine campaign. The goal may be **eradication of disease** (as has been achieved for smallpox), **regional elimination of disease** (as has been achieved for poliomyelitis in the Western Hemisphere), or **control of disease** to reduce morbidity and mortality (as in chickenpox). Global efforts to eradicate poliomyelitis have been underway for several decades. Total eradication has seemed close several times, yet achieving it has remained—so far—elusive.[31] Disease eradication by immunization is feasible only for diseases in which humans are the sole reservoir of the infectious organism. Although vaccines are available to prevent some diseases with reservoirs in other animals (e.g., rabies, plague, encephalitis) and some diseases with reservoirs in the environment (e.g., typhoid fever), these infections are not candidates for eradication programs. The surveillance systems to achieve eradication or regional elimination must be excellent, and any eradication or elimination program requires considerably more resources and time and general political and popular support than a disease control program. For these reasons, immunization strategies are frequently the subject of much scrutiny and debate.

1. Vaccine-Related Supplies and Lawsuits

Recent shortages of some vaccines have caused concern about vaccine supplies. Far fewer companies now make vaccines for the United States,[32] citing the cost and risk of developing and making vaccines, tighter regulation of production, and the risk of liability for the companies. As a consequence of being named in lawsuits, many vaccine manufacturers ceased to make vaccines.

In response to the problem, the U.S. Federal Government instituted the National Vaccine Injury Compensation Program, which covers diphtheria, tetanus, pertussis, measles, mumps, rubella, and oral and inactivated polio vaccines. It is limited to claims for injuries or deaths attributable to vaccines given after October 1, 1988. Claims concerning injury must be filed within 3 years of the first symptoms (e.g., anaphylactic shock, paralytic poliomyelitis, seizure disorders, encephalopathy). Claims of death must be filed within 4 years of the first symptoms and 2 years of death. The program essentially protects vaccine manufacturers from liability lawsuits, unless it can be shown that their vaccines differed from the federal requirements. It also simplifies the legal process and reduces the costs for people making a claim, and almost all the costs of the program and payouts to patients are borne by the federal government (and by taxpayers).

Even though this program has significantly reduced the liability costs to for-profit vaccine producers, the vaccine market remains fragile and prone to mismatches between demand and supply.[33] Another problem caused by few companies being willing to make vaccines is the reduction of worldwide capacity to produce large amounts of vaccines in a short time if required by an emergency. Specifically, it would take at least 6 months from the time an influenza H5N1 pandemic strain of virus is isolated until significant amounts of the vaccine can be produced.[34] This difficulty was brought into stark relief in 2009, when a novel H1N1 strain with characteristics of an epidemic strain appeared, and there were substantial difficulties in distributing vaccines to high-risk groups.[35]

The number and type of missed opportunities for immunization have been studied in the context of medical care, especially during sick-child visits.[36] Often, clinicians do not vaccinate children who have mild upper respiratory tract infections, even though the office visit included a vaccination. More recent guidelines emphasize that children should receive the appropriate vaccines despite having mild infections. Also, the parent often brings the child's siblings, who should receive vaccinations if their immunization records are not up-to-date; however, this is seldom done. These two scenarios are common in outpatient clinics and especially emergency departments, where opportunities may be missed because providers lack records, time, and a relationship with patients.

Hospitalized children and adults whose immunization records are not up-to-date should be given the appropriate vaccines unless contraindications exist. Clinicians are often poorly informed about contraindications. *The following factors are* **not** *considered contraindications to immunizing children or adults:*

1. Mild reaction to a previous DTP or DTaP dose, consisting of redness and swelling at the injection site or a temperature less than 40.5° C (<105° F) or both
2. Presence of nonspecific allergies
3. Presence of a mild illness or diarrhea with low-grade fever in an otherwise healthy patient scheduled for vaccination
3. Current therapy with an antimicrobial drug in a patient who is convalescing well
4. Breastfeeding of an infant scheduled for immunization
5. Pregnancy of another woman in the household

Updated vaccination recommendations and contraindications to vaccinations can be found online.[23]

D. Prevention of Disease by Use of Antimicrobial Drugs

Another form of specific protection, which can be used for varying lengths of time, is **antimicrobial prophylaxis.**

For travelers to countries where malaria is endemic, antimicrobial protection against the causative organism, *Plasmodium*, is desirable. Oral chemoprophylaxis for adults may consist of the use of chloroquine phosphate before and during travel, followed by primaquine for a few weeks after

Table 15-4 Criteria for Tuberculin Positivity, Millimeters of Induration (mm), by Risk Group

Reaction	Groups at Risk
≥5 mm	Human immunodeficiency virus (HIV)–positive patients
	Recent contacts of tuberculosis (TB) case patients
	Fibrotic changes on chest radiograph consistent with prior TB
	Patients with organ transplants and other immunosuppressed patients (receiving equivalent of ≥15 mg/day of prednisone for ≥1 month)*
≥10 mm	Recent immigrants (within last 5 years) from high-prevalence countries
	Injection drug users
	Residents and employees† of high-risk congregate settings: prisons/jails, nursing homes/other long-term facilities for elderly persons, hospitals, other health care facilities, residential facilities for AIDS patients, homeless shelters
	Mycobacteriology laboratory personnel
	Patients with clinical conditions that place them at high risk: silicosis, diabetes mellitus, chronic renal failure, some hematologic disorders (e.g., carcinoma of head/neck or lung), weight loss ≥10% of ideal body weight, gastrectomy, jejunoileal bypass
	Children <4 years of age or infants, children, and adolescents exposed to adults at high risk
≥15 mm	Persons with no risk factors for TB

Modified from US Centers for Disease Control and Prevention (CDC): Screening for tuberculosis and tuberculosis infection in high-risk populations: recommendations of the Advisory Council for the Elimination of Tuberculosis, *MMWR* 44(RR-11):19–34, 1995; and CDC: *MMWR* 49(RR-6):1–71, 2000.
*Risk of TB in patients treated with corticosteroids increases with higher dose and longer duration.
†For persons who are otherwise at low risk and are tested at the start of employment, a reaction of ≥15 mm of induration is considered positive.
AIDS, Acquired immunodeficiency syndrome.

returning home. However, plasmodia are resistant to chloroquine in many areas. In those cases, atorvaquone/proguanil can be used, or an alternative drug, such as mefloquine, may be given instead. Because resistance rates change rapidly and new regimens become available, travelers should consult CDC websites[37] or travel medicine clinics.

The natural history of tuberculosis (TB) is discussed in Chapter 20. Patients with latent TB should be treated to prevent active TB. Latent TB is diagnosed through a positive purified protein derivative (PPD) test. The cutoff of the PPD test depends on the risk to the patient[38] (Table 15-4). The different cutoff points reflect different relative risks of developing disease. The usual prophylactic regimen is isoniazid (INH, isonicotine hydrazine) daily for 6 to 9 months, beginning from the recognition of a recent exposure or the diagnosis of skin test conversion. Shorter regimens have been associated with higher risks of liver toxicity in trials.

In some patients with severe structural heart disease, a short-term course of bactericidal antibiotics is recommended before dental or other manipulative medical procedures are performed. Individuals who have been exposed to a virulent meningococcal disease (either meningitis or meningococcal sepsis) should receive prophylactic treatment with an antibiotic, such as rifampin, ciprofloxacin, or ceftriaxone. The tetravalent meningococcal vaccine is recommended to control outbreaks of serogroup C meningococcal disease and possibly of particular serogroups against which vaccines are ineffective.[39] A large dose of ceftriaxone may be given to prevent syphilis or gonorrhea in patients who had sexual contact with an infected person when the disease was communicable.

After needlesticks from high-risk patients, health care workers can be treated with a 4-week prophylactic anti-HIV regimen.[40]

E. Prevention of Deficiency States

When specific vitamin and mineral deficiencies were identified in the past, food or water was fortified to ensure that most people would obtain sufficient amounts of nutrients of a specific type. Iodine in salt has essentially eliminated goiter;

vitamin D in milk has largely eliminated rickets; and fluoridated water has greatly reduced dental caries in children. A more recent example is the enrichment of cereal grain products with folic acid so that newly pregnant women are not deficient in folic acid. This practice was initiated in January 1998 to prevent neural tube defects. By 2001, there had been a 23% decrease in neural tube defect–affected births.[41]

The frequent use of vitamin and mineral supplements and the fortification of most breakfast cereals with numerous vitamins and minerals have largely eliminated vitamin B deficiencies in U.S. populations with reasonably normal nutrition. Nevertheless, vitamin B deficiencies are still found in some elderly persons.

V. EFFECTING BEHAVIOR CHANGE IN UNDERSERVED POPULATIONS

Ample data sources show that important health care disparities exist and persist in the United States. Racial minorities receive lower-quality care and have less access to interventions.[42] Such disparities result from different underlying rates of illness because of genetic predisposition, local environmental conditions, poorer care, poor lifestyle choices, different care-seeking behaviors, linguistic barriers, and lack of trust in health care providers.[43] The impact of these disparities on health, life, and well-being are profound. For example, black and low-income children are less likely to receive all recommended vaccines. Black children are hospitalized 3.6 times more often than white children for asthma and are more likely to die as a result of asthma.[44] One strategy to decrease such disparities is to provide *culturally and linguistically appropriate services* (CLAS), which encompass cultural competency and health literacy.

A. Cultural Competency

Cultural competency is defined as health care services delivered in a way that is respectful of and responsive to the health beliefs, practices, and needs of diverse patients.[43] This concept posits that cultural issues and communication about culture underlie all clinical and preventive services. Cultural competency usually includes language-access services and translated patient education materials, but also requires providers to be familiar with the cultural perspectives and beliefs more prevalent in certain groups. For example, some American Indian cultures believe that the mention of an illness will cause the illness; Haitians may think that losing blood through a blood test might weaken them; and many African groups expect family members to have an important role in treatment decisions and believe telling terminally ill patients about their condition is uncaring.[45] Such facts may or may not be true for the individual whom the provider is treating. Beyond memorizing such facts, true cultural competency requires providers to reflect on their own attitudes, beliefs, biases, and behaviors that may influence care, and to explore with their patients how they see their illness.

Suggested questions to explore the cultural context of a disease include the following[46]:

What do your call your problem? What name does it have?

What do you think caused your problem?

What do you fear most about your disorder?

What kind of treatment do you think you should receive?

What are the most important results you hope to receive from the treatment?

What do friends, family, or others say about these symptoms?

What kind of medicines, home remedies, or other treatments have you tried for this illness?

Is there anything you eat, drink, or do/avoid on a regular basis to stay healthy?

Have you sought any advice from alternative/folk healer, friend, or other people (nondoctors) for help with your problem?

B. Health Literacy

Health literacy, a relatively new concept in medicine, refers to "an individual's ability to read, understand, and use healthcare information to make effective healthcare decisions and follow instructions for treatment."[47] Low health literacy is common,[48] with up to 50% of the U.S. population unable to comprehend and act on basic medical information. For example, many individuals do not understand the terms *polyp, tumor,* or *screening test.* Providers must realize that native speakers of English may not understand the information presented and may be ashamed to speak up about problems or lack of understanding.[49] Differences in health literacy level were consistently associated with increased hospitalizations and emergency department visits, lower use of preventive services, poorer ability to interpret labels and health messages, and among seniors, poorer overall health status and higher mortality. Health literacy level potentially mediates health care disparities between blacks and whites.[49] Improving consumer health literacy is one of the U.S. *Healthy People* goals.

Several factors account for low health literacy, but it is probably best to assume that no patient will understand information presented at a reading level higher than 6th grade ("universal health literacy precautions"). Recommended interventions to improve information uptake for patients with low health literacy include the following[50]:

- Redesigning patient information at lower reading levels and simplifying the content and design.
- *Teach-back:* Asking the patient to teach the information back to the provider to confirm understanding.
- *Ask me 3:* This model promotes three simple but essential questions that patients should ask their providers in every health care interaction:
  1. What is my main problem?
  2. What do I need to do?
  3. Why is it important for me to do this?

VI. SUMMARY

Primary prevention begins with health promotion, which is working to improve the nutritional, environmental, social, and behavioral conditions in which people are conceived, born, and raised and live. The clinician's role in counseling patients regarding personal habits is underused. In particular, many clinicians do not counsel patients until after a health problem is detected or an adverse event occurs. Theories of behavior change are important to design and evaluate health promotion efforts and include the health belief model, stages of change model, theory of reasoned action, and precaution adoption process model. Motivational interviewing is a counseling method that encourages the patient to "talk change" and outperforms traditional advice giving for many addiction and health behavior problems. Many primary prevention strategies focus on the use of specific biologic, nutritional, or environmental interventions to protect individuals against certain diseases, deficiency states, injuries, or toxic exposures. The prototype of specific protection is the vaccine, which is directed against one disease and prevents the disease by increasing host resistance. Host resistance can be temporarily increased by passive immunization or sometimes by prophylactic antibiotic therapy. Nutritional deficiencies can be eliminated by adding nutrients (e.g., iodine) to common foods (salt) to prevent a particular disease (goiter). To decrease health care disparities among their patients, providers need to provide culturally and linguistically appropriate services. Cultivation of widespread healthy literacy is a social and public health priority as well.

References

1. McGinnis MJ, Foege WH: Actual causes of death in the United States. *JAMA* 270:2207–2212, 1993.
2. Mokdad AH, Marks JS, Stroup DF, et al: Actual causes of death in the United States, 2000. *JAMA* 291:1238–1245, 2004.
3. Pratt L: *Changes in health care ideology in relation to self-care by families,* Miami, 1976, Annual Meeting of American Public Health Association.
4. Marmot MG, Shipley MJ, Rose G: Inequalities in death: specific explanations of a general pattern? *Lancet* 1:1003–1006, 1984.
5. Hollingshead AB, Redlich FC: *Social class and mental illness,* New York, 1958, Wiley & Sons.
6. Pappas G, Queen S, Hadden W, et al: The increasing disparity in mortality between socioeconomic groups in the United States, 1960 and 1986. *N Engl J Med* 329:103–109, 1993.
7. Marmot MG: Status syndrome: a challenge to medicine. *JAMA* 295:1304–1307, 2007.
8. World Health Organization: Bangkok Charter, 2005. http://www.who.int/healthpromotion/conferences/HPJA_2005-3Tang.pdf.

9. Ory MG, Jordan PJ, Bazarre T: The Behavior Change Consortium: setting the stage for a new century of health behavior–change research. *Health Educ Res* 17:500–511, 2002.

10. http://www.uspreventiveservicestaskforce.org/recommendations.htm.

11. Rimer BP, Glanz K: Theory at a glance: a guide for health promotion practice. http://www.cancer.gov/cancertopics/cancerlibrary/theory.pdf.

12. Rosenstock IM: Historical origins of the health belief model. *Health Educ Monogr* 2:328–335, 1974.

13. Carlos JA, Bingham TA, Stueve A, et al: The role of peer support on condom use among black and Latino MSM in three urban areas. *AIDS Educ Prev* 22:430–444, 2010.

14. Free OWCH program. www.turnthetidefoundation.org.

15. Zolnierek KB, DiMatteo MR: Physician communication and patient adherence to treatment: a meta-analysis. *Med Care* 47:826–834, 2009.

16. Rubak S, Lauritzen T, Christensen B: Motivational interviewing: a systematic review and meta-analysis. *Br J Gen Pract* 55:305–312, 2005.

17. Hettema J, Steele J, Miller WR: Motivational interviewing. *Ann Rev Clin Psychol* 1:91–111, 2005.

18. Miller WR: Motivational interviewing with problem drinkers. *Behav Psychother* II:147–172, 1983.

19. Frosch DL, Kaplan RM: Shared decision making in clinical medicine. *Am J Prev Med* 17:285–294, 1999.

20. O'Connor AM, Llewellyn-Thomas HA, Flood AB: Modifying unwarranted variations in health care: shared decision making using patient decision aids. *Health Affairs* 2004; Suppl Variation:VAR63-72.

21. Cassel J: Psychosocial processes and stress: theoretical formulation. *Int J Health Serv* 4:471–482, 1974.

22. US Centers for Disease Control and Prevention (CDC): Diphtheria epidemic: new independent states of the former Soviet Union, 1990-1994. *MMWR* 44:177–181, 1995.

23. CDC: Traveler's health: vaccines. http://wwwnc.cdc.gov/travel/page/vaccinations.htm.

24. CDC: National Center for Emerging and Zoonotic Infectious Diseases. http://www.cdc.gov/nczved/divisions/dfbmd/diseases/botulism/#treat.

25. Rerks-Ngarm S, Pitisuttithum P, Nitayaphan S, et al: Vaccination with ALVAC and AIDSVAX to prevent HIV-1 infection in Thailand. *N Engl J Med* 361:2209–2220, 2009.

26. Cartter ML, Renzullo PO, Helgerson SD, et al: Influenza outbreaks in nursing homes: how effective is influenza vaccine in the institutionalized elderly? *Infect Control Hosp Epidemiol* 11:473–478, 1990.

27. Voordouw ACG, Sturkenboom MC, Dieleman JP, et al: Annual revaccination against influenza and mortality risks in community-dwelling elderly persons. *JAMA* 292:2089–2095, 2004.

28. Clemens JD, Shapiro ED: Resolving the pneumococcal vaccinate controversy: are there alternatives to randomized clinical trials? *Rev Infect Dis* 6:589–600, 1984.

29. Shapiro ED, Berg AT, Austrian R, et al: The protective efficacy of polyvalent pneumococcal polysaccharide vaccine. *N Engl J Med* 325:1453–1460, 1991.

30. Marks J, Halpin TJ, Orenstein WA: Measles vaccine efficacy in children previously vaccinated at 12 months of age. *Pediatrics* 62:955–960, 1978.

31. Cochi SL, Kew O: Polio today: are we on the verge of global eradication? *JAMA* 300:839–841, 2008.

32. Sloan FA, Berman S, Rosenbaum S, et al: The fragility of the U.S. vaccine supply. *N Engl J Med* 351:2443–2447, 2004.

33. Parmet WE: Pandemic vaccines—the legal landscape. *N Engl J Med* 362:1949–1952, 2010.

34. Shute N: *US News & World Report* 64–66, 2006.

35. SteelFisher GK, Blendon RJ, Bekheit MM: The public's response to the 2009 H1N1 influenza pandemic. *N Engl J Med* 362:e65, 2010.

36. CDC: Vaccines for Children Program, 1994. *MMWR* 43:705, 1994.

37. CDC: Malaria: choosing a drug to prevent malaria. http://www.cdc.gov/malaria/travelers/drugs.html.

38. CDC: Targeted tuberculin testing and treatment of latent tuberculosis infection. *MMWR* 49(RR-6):1–71, 2000.

39. Advisory Committee on Immunization Practices: Prevention and control of meningococcal disease. *MMWR* 54(RR-07):1–21, 2005.

40. CDC: Updated U.S. Public Health Service guidelines for the management of occupational exposures to HIV and recommendations for postexposure prophylaxis. *MMWR* 54(RR-09):1–17, 2005.

41. CDC: Folic acid and prevention of spina bifida and anencephaly. *MMWR* 51(RR-13):1–19, 2002.

42. US Institute of Medicine: *Unequal treatment*, Washington, DC, 2002, National Academies Press.

43. Office of Minority Health: Think cultural health. http://cccm.thinkculturalhealth.hhs.gov.

44. Agency for Healthcare Research and Quality: National Healthcare Disparities Report, 2003. http://www.ahrq.gov/qual/nhdr03/nhdr03.htm.

45. A provider's handbook on culturally competent care, 1999, Kaiser Permanente San Francisco Medical Center.

46. Office of Minority Health: A physician's practical guide to culturally competent care. http://cccm.thinkculturalhealth.hhs.gov.

47. Weiss BD: Health literacy and patient safety. In *AMA manual*. http://www.ama-assn.org/ama1/pub/upload/mm/367/healthlitclinicians.pdf.

48. Berkman ND, DeWalt DA, Pignone MP, et al: Health literacy and outcomes: an updated systematic review, *AHRQ Evid Rep/Technol Assess* 199. http://archive.ahrq.gov/downloads/pub/evidence/pdf/literacy/literacy.pdf.

49. Institute of Medicine: *Health literacy: a prescription to end confusion*, Washington, DC, 2004, National Academies Press.

50. National Patient Safety Foundation: Ask me 3. http://www.npsf.org/for-healthcare-professionals/programs/ask-me-3.

Select Readings

Berkman ND, DeWalt DA, Pignone MP, et al: Health literacy and outcomes: an updated systematic review, *AHRQ Evid Rep/Technol Assess* 199. http://archive.ahrq.gov/downloads/pub/evidence/pdf/literacy/literacy.pdf.

Glanz K, Rimer BK: *Theory at a glance: a guide for health promotion practice*, National Cancer Institute, National Institutes of Health, US Department of Health and Human Services, NIH Pub Jp 97-3896, Washington, DC, 1997 (revised), NIH.

Katz DL: *Nutrition in clinical practice*, Philadelphia, 2008, Lippincott, Williams & Wilkins.

Smedley BD, Syme SL, editors: *Promoting health: strategies from social and behavioral research*, Institute of Medicine, Washington, DC, 2000, National Academies Press.

US Centers for Disease Control and Prevention: Epidemiology and prevention of vaccine-preventable diseases. In *The pink book: course textbook*, ed 12, Atlanta, 2011, CDC. http://www.cdc.gov/vaccines/pubs/pinkbook.

US Institute of Medicine: *Speaking of health; assessing health communication strategies for diverse populations*, Washington, DC, 2002, National Academies Press.

US Institute of Medicine: *Unequal treatment*, Washington, DC, 2002, National Academies Press.

Websites

http://cccm.thinkculturalhealth.hhs.gov/ [Health care disparities and culturally and linguistically appropriate services (CLAS).].

www.idsociety.org [Infectious Disease Society.]

http://fnic.nal.usda.gov/nal_display/index.php?info_center=4&tax_level=3&tax_subject=256&topic_id=1342&level3_id=5140 [Nutritional intake.]

http://www.ahrq.gov/clinic/cpgsix.htm [Resources to treat tobacco use and dependence.]

http://www.cdc.gov/vaccines/ [Vaccinations and antimicrobial prophylaxis.]

Principles and Practice of Secondary Prevention

Secondary prevention is based on early detection of disease, through either screening or case finding, followed by treatment. **Screening** is the process of evaluating a group of people for asymptomatic disease or a risk factor for developing a disease or becoming injured. In contrast to case finding (defined later), screening usually occurs in a **community setting** and is applied to a population, such as residents of a county, students in a school, or workers in an industry. Because a positive screening test result usually is not diagnostic of a disease, it must be followed by a *diagnostic* test. For example, a positive finding on a screening mammogram examination must be followed by additional diagnostic imaging or a biopsy to rule out breast cancer.

As shown in Figure 16-1, the process of screening is complex and involves a cascade of actions that should follow if each step yields positive results. In this regard, initiating a screening program is similar to boarding a roller coaster; participants must continue until the end of the process is reached. Many members of the public assume that any screening program will automatically be valuable or cost-effective; this explains the popularity of mobile imaging vans that offer full-body computed tomography (CT) and the direct-to-consumer marketing of genomic analysis. In contrast, many preventive medicine specialists demand the same standards of evidence and cost-effectiveness as for therapeutic interventions in patients with known disease. A case may be made for even higher standards. Screening means looking for trouble. It involves, by definition, people with no perception of disease, most of whom are well; therefore great potential exists to do net harm if screening is performed haphazardly.

Screening usually is distinguished from **case finding,** which is the process of searching for asymptomatic diseases and risk factors among people in a **clinical setting** (i.e., among people who are under medical care). If a patient is being seen for the first time in a medical care setting, clinicians and other health care workers usually take a thorough medical history and perform a careful physical examination and, if indicated, obtain laboratory tests. Establishing baseline findings and laboratory values in this way may produce case finding, if problems are discovered, and is considered "good medicine" but is not referred to as "screening."

A program to take annual blood pressure of employees of a business or industry would be considered screening, whereas performing chest radiography for a patient who was just admitted to a hospital for elective surgery would be called "case finding." The distinction between screening and case finding is frequently ignored in the literature and in practice. Most professional societies do not distinguish between the two in their recommendations regarding screening. We use the two terms interchangeably in this chapter. Chapter 7 discusses some of the quantitative issues involved in assessing the accuracy and performance of screening, including sensitivity, specificity, and predictive value of tests. In this chapter we assume the reader is comfortable with these concepts. The purpose here is to discuss broader public health issues concerning screening and case finding. Chapter 18 provides an extensive discussion of the U.S. Preventive Services Task Force in the clinical encounter.

I. COMMUNITY SCREENING

A. Objectives of Screening

Community screening programs seek to test large numbers of individuals for one or more diseases or risk factors in a community setting (e.g., educational, work, recreational) on a voluntary basis, often with little or no direct financial outlay by the individuals being screened (Table 16-1).

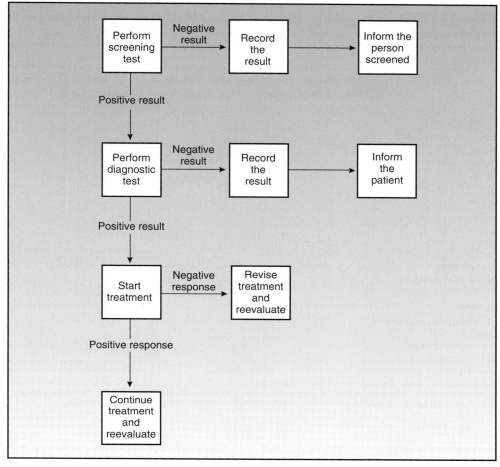

Figure 16-1 **The process of screening.**

Table 16-1 **Objectives of Screening Programs**

Target	Objective	Examples
Disease	Treatment to reduce mortality	Cancer
	Treatment to prevent complications	Hypertension
	Treatment to eradicate infection and prevent its spread	Gonorrhea, syphilis, tuberculosis
	Change in diet and lifestyle	Coronary artery disease, type 2 diabetes mellitus
Risk Factors		
Behavioral	Change in lifestyle	Cigarette smoking, unsafe sexual practices
Environmental	Change in occupation	Chronic obstructive pulmonary disease from work in a dusty trade
Metabolic	Treatment or change in diet and lifestyle	Elevated serum cholesterol levels

B. Minimum Requirements for Community Screening Programs

The minimum requirements for establishing a safe, ethical, and cost-effective screening program fall into the following three areas:

- Disease requirements
- Screening test requirements
- Health care system requirements

If any of the requirements is not at least partially met, an extensive population-wide screening program may be inappropriate. Table 16-2 outlines these requirements in four common screening programs, for hypertension, high cholesterol, cervical cancer, and ovarian cancer, as further discussed in Application of Minimum Screening Requirements to Specific Programs.

1. Disease Requirements

1. The disease must be *serious* (i.e., produce significant morbidity or mortality), or there is no reason to screen in the first place.
2. Even if a disease is serious, there must be an *effective therapy* for the disease if it is detected. Screening is of no value unless there is a good chance that detecting the

Table 16-2　Requirements for Screening Programs and Ratings of Example Methods to Detect Hypertension, Elevated Cholesterol Levels, Cervical Cancer, and Ovarian Cancer

Requirements	Screening Method and Rating*			
	Sphygmomanometer Reading (Hypertension)	Serum Cholesterol Test (Dyslipidemia)	Pap Smear (Cervical Cancer)	Computed Tomography (Ovarian Cancer)
Disease Requirements				
Disease is serious.	++	++	++	++
Effective treatment exists.	++	+	+	+/−
Natural history of disease is understood.	++	+	++	+
Disease occurs frequently.	++	++	++	++
Other diseases or conditions may be detected.	−	−	−	+
Screening Test Requirements				
Test is quick to perform.	++	+	+	++
Test is easy to administer.	++	+	+	+
Test is inexpensive.	++	+	+	+
Test is safe.	++	++	+	+
Test is acceptable to participants.	++	+	+	++
Sensitivity, specificity, and other operating characteristics are acceptable.	++	+	+	−
Health Care System Requirements				
Method meets the requirements for screening in a community setting.	++	++	+	−
Method meets the requirements for case finding in a medical care setting.	++	++	++	+

*Ratings are applied to four conditions for which community screening has often been undertaken: hypertension, tested by a sphygmomanometer reading of blood pressure; elevated cholesterol levels, with total cholesterol measurement based on a rapid screening of blood; cervical cancer, tested by Papanicolaou (Pap) smear; and ovarian cancer, tested by computed tomography (CT) scanning. Ratings are as follows: ++, good; +, satisfactory; −, unsatisfactory; +/−, depends on disease stage.

disease in the *presymptomatic stage* would be followed by effective therapy. Furthermore, the benefits of detecting the condition in a few people should outweigh the harms that occur (and accrue) to people with a false-positive test, including unnecessary, invasive workups and treatment. For example, at present, there is no value in screening for pancreatic cancer because the chance of cure by standard medical and surgical methods is extremely small. The controversy around prostate cancer screening is largely about the benefits of treatment versus the possible harm of unnecessary treatment.

3. The natural history of a disease must be understood clearly enough to know that there is a significant window of time during which the disease is detectable, and a cure or at least effective treatment would occur. For example, colon cancer follows an established disease mechanism from small polyps in the colon to colon cancer. Early detection and surgical removal of a polyp in the colon could prevent intestinal obstruction and morbidity, and likely is curative.

4. The disease or condition must not be too rare or too common. Screening for a rare disease usually means that many false-positive test results would be expected for each true finding (see Chapter 7). This increases the cost and difficulties of discovering persons who truly are ill or at high risk, and it causes anxiety and inconvenience for individuals who must undergo more testing because of false-positive results. Unless the benefits from discovering one case are very high, as in treating a newborn who has phenylketonuria or congenital hypothyroidism, it is seldom cost-effective to screen general populations for a rare disease.

Screening for common conditions may produce such a large proportion of positive results that it would not be cost-effective; common conditions are best sought in the context of care. It is possible, however, that screening for some common risk factors, such as elevated cholesterol levels, may provide opportunities for education and motivation to seek care and behavior change.

2. Screening Test Requirements

1. The screening test must be reasonably quick, easy, and inexpensive, or the costs of large-scale screening in terms of time, effort, and money would be prohibitive.
2. The screening test must be safe and acceptable to the persons being screened and to their clinicians. If the individuals to be screened object to a procedure (as frequently occurs with colonoscopy), they are unlikely to participate.
3. The sensitivity, specificity, positive predictive value, and other operating characteristics of a screening test must be known and acceptable. False-positive and false-negative test results must be considered. An additional difficulty in using screening tests in the general population is that the characteristics of the screening test may be different in the population screened from the population for whom the screening was developed.

3. Health Care System Requirements

1. People with positive test results must have access to follow-up. Because screening only sets apart a high-risk group, persons who have positive results must receive

further diagnostic testing to rule in or rule out actual disease. Follow-up testing may be expensive, time-consuming, or painful, with some risk. With many screening programs, most of the efforts and costs are in the follow-up phase, not in the initial screening.

2. Before a screening program for a particular disease is undertaken, treatment already should be available for people known to have that disease. If there are limited resources, it is not ethical or cost-effective to allow persons with symptoms of the disease to go untreated and yet screen for the same disease in apparently well persons.

3. Individuals who are screened and diagnosed as having the disease in question must have access to treatment, or the process is ethically flawed. In addition to being unethical, it makes no medical sense to bring the persons screened to the point of informing them of a positive test result and then abandon them. This is a major problem for community screening efforts because many people who come for screening have little or no medical care coverage. Therefore, the cost for the evaluation of the positive screening tests and the subsequent treatment (if disease is detected) are often borne by a local hospital or other institution.

4. The treatment should be acceptable to the people being screened. Otherwise, individuals who require treatment would not undertake it, and the screening would have accomplished nothing. For example, some men may not want treatment for prostate cancer because of possible incontinence and impotence.

5. The population to be screened should be clearly defined so that the resulting data are epidemiologically useful. Although screening at "health fairs" and in shopping centers provides the opportunity to educate the public about health topics, the data obtained are seldom useful because the population screened is not well defined and tends to be self-selected and highly biased in favor of those concerned about their health.[1]

6. It should be clear who is responsible for the screening, which cutoff points are to be used for considering a test result "positive," and how the findings will become part of participants' medical record at their usual place of care.

4. Application of Minimum Screening Requirements to Specific Programs

Table 16-2 applies the previously described criteria to the following four conditions for which community screening has been undertaken:

- Hypertension, tested by a sphygmomanometer reading of blood pressure
- Elevated cholesterol levels, based on a screening of blood
- Cervical cancer, with Papanicolaou smear
- Ovarian cancer, for which CT scan screening was considered but rejected

As shown in Table 16-2, screening for hypertension, hypercholesterolemia, and cervical cancer generally fulfill the minimum requirements for a community screening program. Investigators have agreed that a screening program using CT scans to detect ovarian cancer in the general population fails at two critical points. First, the yield of detection is low. Second, as numerous studies have shown, only a small proportion of cancers can be cured by the time they are detected.[2] Because of these problems, community screening for ovarian cancer is not recommended.

For many screening programs, debate surrounds general screening issues such as what age to start the screening, when to stop, how often to repeat the screening, and whether the methods yield accurate results. Screening for breast cancer is an example of a controversial screening program because the benefits seem to be less than originally hoped and risks are associated with screening mammography.[3] The age at which to begin screening women for breast cancer is particularly controversial because breast cancer is less common in younger women, but often more aggressive than later in life, and the risks of screening (e.g., false positives) are higher (Box 16-1).

C. Ethical Concerns about Community Screening

The ethical standards are important to consider when an apparently well population of individuals who have *not* sought medical care is screened. In this case the professionals involved have an important obligation to show that the benefits of being screened outweigh the costs and potential risks. The methods used in performing any public screening program should be safe, with minimal side effects.

D. Potential Benefits and Harms of Screening Programs

The potential benefits of screening include reduced mortality, reduced morbidity, and reassurance. With the goal of screening programs to identify disease in the early, presymptomatic stage so that treatment can be initiated, the potential benefits are reduced mortality for many programs. However, some screening programs have a goal of early detection using less invasive treatment (e.g., taking a small piece of breast tissue rather than removing the entire breast). Another potential benefit of screening is the reassurance to both individuals and providers.

The potential adverse effects (harms) of all screening programs need to be considered. Some screening procedures may be uncomfortable, such as mammography, or require preparation, such as colonoscopy (colon cleansing). Colonoscopy also carries procedural risks (bleeding, perforation). Other harms of screening include anxiety from false-positive results, false reassurance for patients with false-negative tests, and costs to individuals and society from lost work.

Test errors are a major concern in screening (see Chapter 7). **False-positive test results** lead to extra time and costs and can cause anxiety and discomfort to individuals whose results were in error. In the case of screening for breast cancer, one study showed that the more screening mammograms or clinical breast examinations given, the more likely one or more false-positive results occurred.[4] An estimated 49% of women who had undergone 10 mammograms had at least one false-positive reading, equal to a false-positive error rate of 6% to 7% on each mammogram.

False-negative test results can be even worse. One implied promise made to people is that if they are screened for a particular disease and found to have negative results, they need not worry about that disease. False-negative results may lead people with early symptoms to be less concerned.

Breast cancer and prostate cancer in particular illustrate the challenge in weighing evidence of small changes in mortality against side effects of screening and treatment. Because of the impact of screening biases, only a change in overall mortality in the screened population is considered evidence of an effective screening program. The debate about changes in the U.S. Preventive Services Task Force (USPSTF) recommendations on breast cancer also demonstrate that few issues in preventive medicine have more power to polarize the public, politicians, and health care professionals than screening.[30]

Breast Cancer

Many women die prematurely of breast cancer. Unfortunately, only a fraction of breast abnormalities detected on a mammogram truly lead to a saved life; the majority are false-positive findings or lead to unnecessary diagnosis and treatment of lesions such as ductal carcinoma in situ (DCIS), which is not harmful to the majority of women. Most women would not have known they had these DCIS lesions had it not been for the screening mammography. Women with DCIS are at increased risk for a subsequent diagnosis of invasive breast cancer. Unfortunately, we cannot predict which women with DCIS will ultimately go on to have invasive breast cancer. Thus, women who are diagnosed with DCIS after a screening mammography often undergo breast surgery, chemotherapy, and radiation treatment that can be costly and traumatic. Similarly, many women whose cancers are detected by mammography still die of their disease. If mammograms saved lives, both breast cancer–associated mortality and total mortality in populations screened should decrease. This hypothesis has been tested in multiple trials.

As of 2011, the strongest evidence shows that any difference in **overall** mortality between populations exposed to screenings and those not screened is small: for every 2000 women invited for screening throughout 10 years, one will have her life prolonged; 10 healthy women who would not have been diagnosed if there had not been screening will be treated unnecessarily, and more than 200 women will experience important psychological distress for many months because of false-positive findings.[30]

In 2009, USPSTF changed its screening recommendations regarding breast cancer for women age 40 to 49. Previously recommending routine screening in this population, the Task Force now argued that the improvement in mortality in women between age 40 and 49 was small and that possible harms needed to be considered. Instead, USPSTF recommended that physicians discuss the risks and benefits of screening with the women and to proceed according to their risk/benefit preferences. This change led to a significant media backlash. Many people claimed the decision amounted to "care rationing," and that the USPSTF had overstepped its mandate by weighing mortality benefits against anxiety.[31] The Task Force argued that the evidence did not support a "one size fits all" recommendation and that their guidelines empowered patients and their physicians to make rational decisions based on evidence and more respectful of individual values.[32] As of 2012, the rating is a "B" for women age 50 to 74 (recommended) and a "C" for women 40 to 49, indicating that USPSTF believes the decision to screen should be individualized, and the net benefit is likely small.

Prostate Cancer

Prostate cancer affects men in a broad age range and has a wide variability in its impact on mortality; some are rapidly fatal, whereas others are slow-growing and indolent. False-positive results of prostate-specific antigen (PSA) testing are common and often lead to other unnecessary invasive testing (e.g., biopsy). This testing can then lead to diagnosis (often without a reliable way to distinguish between indolent and aggressive disease), treatment (e.g., surgery, radiation, and/or chemotherapy), and serious harm, including erectile dysfunction, bladder and bowel incontinence, and death, to manage a disease that might otherwise have never been problematic (most men die *with* prostate cancer, not *of* prostate cancer). To date, there is no compelling evidence that prostate cancer screening decreases all-cause or prostate cancer–specific mortality.[33] If there is any benefit, it likely accrues over more than 10 years. Therefore, USPSTF advised in 2012 against routine screening with PSA (D-rating).

Both these controversies illustrate the need of **personalizing** screening decisions. The decision to be screened for breast cancer or prostate cancer should be based on the patient's risk preferences and willingness to have false-positive test results and invasive follow-up testing. Many decision aids have been developed to help individuals make informed decisions.

They may delay medical visits that they might otherwise have made promptly. False-negative results also may falsely reassure clinicians. False-negative results can be detrimental to the health of the people whose results were in error, and if test results delay the diagnosis in people who have an infectious disease, such as tuberculosis, the screening tests can be dangerous to the health of others as well.

Overdiagnosis is another potential harm of screening programs. For example, screening mammography may lead to a diagnosis of a preinvasive lesion that is not invasive breast cancer (see Box 16-1). Actions taken in response to such findings, including surgery, may result in a scenario where the ostensible "cure" is in fact worse than the disease.

E. Bias in Screening Programs

It is not easy to establish the value of a community screening effort, unless a randomized controlled trial (RCT) is conducted. An RCT is needed to reduce the potential for bias. In cancer an association between screening and longer survival does not prove a cause-and-effect relationship because of possible problems such as selection bias, lead-time bias, and length bias.[5]

Selection bias may affect a screening program in different directions, all of which may make it difficult to generalize findings to the general population. On one hand, individuals may want to participate because they have a family history of the disease or are otherwise aware that they are at higher risk of contracting the disease. In this case the screening program would find more cases than expected in the general population, exaggerating the apparent utility of screening. On the other hand, individuals who are more "health conscious" may *preferentially* seek out screening programs or may be less likely to drop out.

Lead-time bias occurs when screening detects disease earlier in its natural history than would otherwise have

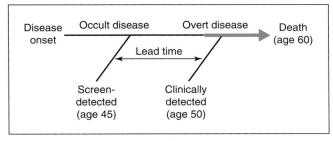

Figure 16-2 **Lead-time bias.** Overestimation of survival duration among screen-detected cases (relative to those detected by signs and symptoms) when survival is measured from diagnosis. This one patient survives for 10 years after clinical diagnosis and survives for 15 years after the screening-detected diagnosis. However, this simply reflects earlier diagnosis, because the overall survival time of the patient is unchanged. (From Black WC, Welch HG: Advances in diagnostic imaging and overestimates of disease prevalence and the benefits of therapy, N Engl J Med 328:1237–1243, 1993.)

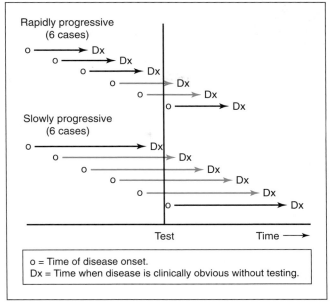

Figure 16-3 **Overestimation of survival duration among screening-detected cases.** This is caused by the relative excess of slowly progressing cases, which are disproportionately identified by screening because the probability of detection is directly proportional to the length of time during which they are detectable (and thereby inversely proportional to the rate of progression.) In these 12 patients, 2 of 6 rapidly progressive cases are detected, whereas 4 of 6 slowly progressive cases are detected. (From Black WC, Welch HG: Advances in diagnostic imaging and overestimates of disease prevalence and the benefits of therapy, N Engl J Med 328: 1237–1243, 1993.)

occurred, so that the period from diagnosis to death is increased. However, the additional *lead time* (increased time during which diagnosis is known) may not have changed the natural history of the disease or extended the longevity of life. This lead-time bias tends to operate in screening for cancers, no matter how aggressive the tumors (Fig. 16-2).

Length bias occurs when the full spectrum of a particular tumor, such as prostate cancer, includes cancers that range from very aggressive to very slow-growing. Individuals with slow-growing tumors live longer than individuals with the aggressive tumors, so they are more likely to be discovered by screening. Screening programs often select for the less aggressive, slower-growing tumors, and these patients are likely to survive longer after detection, regardless of the treatment given (Fig. 16-3).

Selection, lead-time, and length biases apply to both case finding and to community screening. Given the potential problems in showing the true effectiveness of screening, great care must be exercised to ensure a community screening program is worthwhile.

F. Repetition of Screening Programs

There are pitfalls in not carefully considering the details of repeat screening efforts. This is particularly true if an initial major screening effort is considered a great success, and enthusiasm may lead the organizers to repeat the screening too soon (e.g., 1 year later). Unless the population screened the second time is very different from the one screened the first time, a screening effort repeated after a short interval is likely to be disappointing. This is because the initial screening would have detected **prevalent cases** (cases accumulated over many years), whereas the repeated screening would detect only **incident cases** (new cases since the last screening), making the number of cases detected in the second screening effort smaller.[6]

Again, the more screening tests done on an individual, the more likely positive findings will occur, both true positive and false positive. If a woman begins annual breast cancer screening at age 40, she would undergo 30 screening mammograms by age 70. One study followed 2400 women age 40 to 69 for a 10-year period to determine the number of mammograms and clinical breast examinations done.[7] The

women had an average of four mammograms and five clinical breast examinations during this decade, and almost one third had at least one false-positive examination. Recommending frequent repeat examinations carries a significant burden of cost and anxiety to rule out disease in individuals with false-positive examinations.

G. Simultaneous Screening for Multiple Diseases (Multiphasic Screening)

Multiphasic screening programs involve screening for a variety of diseases in the same individual at one point in time. Some investigators have argued that multiphasic screening makes community efforts more efficient. When a sample of blood is drawn, for example, it is easy to perform a variety of tests, using modern, automated laboratory equipment.

However, the yield of multiphasic screening is doubtful.[8] One problem is that multiphasic screening in an elderly population detects many diseases or abnormal conditions that have been found earlier and are already being treated, in which case funds are being used for unnecessary testing. Another problem is that multiphasic screening results in a relatively high frequency of false-positive results, which requires many participants to return for more expensive follow-up tests.

For each disease-free person screened with a battery of **independent tests** (tests that measure different values), the

Table 16-3 **Correlation between Number of Screening Tests and Persons with False-Positive Result**

No. of Screening Tests Performed*	Percentage of Persons with at Least One False-Positive Test Result†
1	5%
2	9.8%
4	18.5%
5	22.6%
10	40.1%
20	64.2%
25	72.3%

Data from Schoenberg BS: The "abnormal" laboratory result, *Postgrad Med* 47:151–155, 1970.
*It is assumed that the tests measure different values (i.e., the tests are independent).
†Percentages are based on tests that each has a 5% false-positive error rate.

probability that at least one of the screening tests would yield a false-positive finding can be expressed as $[1 - (1 - \text{alpha})^n]$, where alpha is the false-positive error rate (see Chapter 7) and *n* is the number of screening tests done. If two screening tests are performed and alpha is 5% (making the test specificity 95%), the probability of a disease-free person's being recalled for further testing is $[1 - (0.95)^2] = [1 - (0.9025)]$ = almost 10%. If four tests are performed, the probability is $[1 - (0.95)^4] = [1 - (0.8145)] = 18.5\%$. As Table 16-3 shows, if 25 tests are performed, more than 70% of disease-free individuals would return for unnecessary but often costly follow-up testing.

One study described a controlled trial of multiphasic screening in which one group of individuals received a battery of special screening tests that included hearing and vision tests, glaucoma screening, blood pressure measurements, spirometry, electrocardiography, mammography and breast examination, Papanicolaou smear, chest x-ray film, urinalysis, complete blood count, and 12 blood chemistry tests. Comparison of the findings in this group with the findings in a similar control group not subjected to the battery of tests (but receiving their regular care) found *no major differences* in the health knowledge, mortality rates, or morbidity rates of the two groups. The group who underwent multiphasic screening, however, spent more nights in the hospital.[9]

It is very difficult at present to integrate all recommended screening tests into a clinical encounter.[10]

H. Genetic Screening

Recent advances in genetic testing have made it more and more feasible to screen individual patients and populations for many different diseases. Indications for genetic testing may include **presymptomatic testing,** such as a patient tested for Huntington's disease. If the test is positive, patients are virtually certain of developing the disease over their lifetime. Alternatively, testing might be done to establish the predisposition for a disease, called **susceptibility testing.** This is the dominant form of testing for many common diseases, such as coronary artery disease (CAD). Most CAD cases follow a multifactorial pattern, with many different genes interacting with environmental factors to produce similar disease. For these diseases, the presence or absence of particular genetic traits can neither rule in nor rule out that the patient will develop the disease.[11]

However, the psychological impact of genetic test results on patients is often counterintuitive and poorly understood. So far, there is little evidence for significant adverse psychological impact, significant lifestyle changes, or screening adherence from consumer genetic testing.[12,13]

In contrast, **prenatal screening** has made a significant impact on population health for certain groups. This is particularly well established for individuals of Jewish Ashkenazi heritage, who have a significant carrier rate of "Jewish genetic disorders" (e.g., Tay-Sachs disease, familial dysautonomia) For this group, genetic testing combined with careful pretest and posttest counseling, has helped couples make informed decisions regarding their family planning. Such testing has also led to a decrease in the incidence of certain diseases.[14]

Several quality requirements beyond the accuracy of the test are specific to genetic screening tests. The genetic abnormality found must also correspond to a specific disease or increased risk for disease (**clinical validity**). Even if the test detects a genetic abnormality that meaningfully predicts disease, the information may not be useful to the patient (**clinical utility**).[15] For most genetic tests, there is little evidence of clinical utility, and the standards for analytic and clinical validity are much lower than for any other diagnostic test. Lastly, genomic screening seems to be predicated on the idea that the only way to change genetic vulnerability is through changing genes. In fact, gene expression is influenced by environmental stimuli, and lifestyle interventions may change gene expression.[16]

II. INDIVIDUAL CASE FINDING

A. Periodic Health Examination

Historically, the most common method of prevention in clinical medicine, especially for adults, was the annual physical examination (checkup), now known as the *periodic health examination.* After World War II the number of available treatments for chronic illnesses increased greatly, and more people began to have an annual checkup, usually consisting of a medical history, physical examination, complete blood count, urinalysis, chest x-ray film, and electrocardiogram. Despite the popularity of these checkups, the number of recipients was limited because many insurance plans would not cover their costs, although some corporations provided them as a benefit for high-level managers ("executive physicals"). Most research on the periodic health examination before the 1960s concerned examinations that were sponsored by businesses or industries or were conducted by the few large health plans existing at the time.

An annotated bibliography of 152 early studies of periodic health examinations showed that reports published before 1940 were mostly anecdotal and were enthusiastic about the examinations.[17] Reports between 1940 and 1962 were more likely to include quantitative data and, although still supportive, increasingly raised serious questions about routine use of examinations. The subsequent increase in the number of health maintenance organizations (HMOs) in turn increased the use of periodic examinations in larger populations. Although most investigators agreed that examinations in children were beneficial, increasingly the studies began to cast doubts about the cost-effectiveness of periodic health examinations in adults.[18-20]

During the 1970s, investigators began moving toward the idea of modifying the periodic examination to focus only on the conditions and diseases that would be most likely to be found in a person of a given age, gender, and family history. This approach was termed "lifetime health monitoring."[21] The greatest support for a new approach came in 1979, when the Canadian Task Force on the Periodic Physical Examination recommended that the traditional form of periodic checkup be replaced by the use of **health protection packages** that included gender-appropriate and age-appropriate immunizations, screening, and counseling of patients on a periodic basis.[22] Specifically, the Task Force recommended that "with certain exceptions, the procedures be carried out as case finding rather than screening techniques; that is, they should be performed when the patient is attending for unrelated symptoms rather than for a specific preventive purpose." Among the certain exceptions noted by the task force were pregnant women, the very young, and the very old, for whom they recommended regular visits specifically for *preventive purposes.*

B. Health Risk Assessments

Health risk assessments (HRAs) use questionnaires or computer programs to elicit and evaluate information concerning individuals in a clinical or industrial medical practice. Each assessed person receives information concerning his or her estimated life expectancy and the types of interventions that are likely to have a positive impact on health and longevity.

For many years, the idea of HRAs has been promoted by clinicians enthusiastic about detecting disease and risk factors in individuals. Based on the founders' original work, the Society for Prospective Medicine was formed,[23] to improve the construction and use of HRAs and the practice of preventive (*prospective*) medicine in a clinical or industrial medical practice.[24] Toward this end, the Society promotes the use of HRAs for the following:

- Assessing the needs of individual patients as they enter a medical care system or of employees in an industrial setting.
- Developing health education information tailored to the needs of the individuals who complete the assessment.
- Developing cost-containment strategies based on better acquisition of health risk information from individuals.

Most HRAs use questionnaires or interactive computer programs to gather data concerning each person being assessed. In addition to data such as height, weight, blood pressure, cholesterol level, and previous and present diseases, the information usually includes details concerning the person's lifestyle and family history. Using an algorithm, a computer calculates the person's "risk age" on the basis of the data. Most HRAs use an algorithm based on findings of the Framingham Heart Study. The **risk age** is defined as the age at which the average individual would have the same risk of dying as the person being assessed. If the assessed person's risk age is older than his or her chronologic age, that means he or she has a higher risk of dying than the average individual of the same chronologic age. Likewise, if the assessed person's risk age is younger than the chronologic age, the person has a lower risk of dying than the average individual of the same chronologic age.

The HRAs usually provide a printed report about the assessed person's relative risk of dying or risk age, combined with some sort of educational message regarding the types of interventions that would have the most positive effect on the person's life expectancy, if instituted. The printed HRA reports have become more sophisticated in recent years and are sometimes supplemented with individualized educational messages.

Studies have extensively evaluated HRAs, with mixed results.[25-27] Criticisms focus on errors or lack of information by the persons entering the data, difficulties in validating the predictions, uncertainties about the correct reference population for baseline risks, and limitations related to the instruments focusing mainly or exclusively on mortality and not on morbidity or the quality of life. The greatest strength of HRAs may be the ability to estimate disease levels at the population level, clarify how nutritional and lifestyle factors affect an assessed person's risk of death, and motivate the person to make changes in a positive direction. HRAs principally serve to *raise awareness,* which is just one of several domains, and generally not the most important, related to behavior change.[28]

III. SCREENING GUIDELINES AND RECOMMENDATIONS

The many organizations that issue screening guidelines and recommendations include the following:

- Specialty organizations (e.g., American Urological Association)
- Organizations representing primary care specialties (e.g., American College of Physicians, American Academy of Family Physicians)
- Foundations for the treatment and prevention of particular diseases (e.g., American Cancer Society)
- Organizations dedicated to evaluating screening recommendations (e.g., U.S. Preventive Services Task Force [USPSTF], American College of Preventive Medicine [ACPM], Canadian Task Force on the Periodic Health Examination)

In many cases, these organizations agree on their screening recommendations. However, certain diseases and screening methods have led to major controversy, such as breast cancer screening and prostate cancer screening. In general, the specialty organizations tend toward recommending screening methods related to their field, unless there is evidence of harm. In contrast, the ACPM and USPSTF tend to only recommend screening programs for which there is unequivocal evidence of benefits in patient outcomes. (See Box 16-2 and Chapter 18.)

In an effort to clarify many of the issues concerning screening and case finding and to make evidence-based recommendations, the U.S. Department of Health and Human Services created the **U.S. Preventive Services Task Force.** In its investigations, USPSTF reviews data concerning the efficacy of three broad categories of interventions:

- **Screening** for disease in asymptomatic clinical populations and in certain high-risk groups (secondary prevention)

| Box 16-2 | Lung Cancer Screening: Simulation Models, Stage Differences, and RCTs |

The development of new diagnostic methods offers new screening possibilities. Conducting a randomized controlled trial (RCT) of a new screening intervention is arduous and time-consuming. In the absence of RCTs, preventive medicine practitioners sometimes rely on single-arm studies or mathematical modeling of screening interventions through cost-utility analysis (see Chapter 6). The history of lung cancer screening illustrates the pitfalls of such sources of evidence.

Lung cancer remains the number-one cause of cancer mortality in the United States. For a long time, there was no viable way to screen for lung cancer. Chest x-ray and sputum examination had been tested but only led to more invasive testing, with no difference in mortality. Then, helical computed tomography (CT) imaging became available and seemed to offer the capacity to find small lung cancer nodules early.[34] Several uncontrolled trials were performed and showed higher cancer detection rate.[35] Several authorities advocated to start screening immediately based on the difference in the distribution of cancer stages found in the screened group from that usually found in clinical practice; patients in the screened group were much more likely to be diagnosed with early and small, potentially curable cancers.[36] Several modeling studies of screening with helical CT were then published, with conflicting results.[37,38]

In 2002 the National Lung Screening Trial was launched. More than 53,000 participants were randomized to either three annual helical CT scans or chest x-ray films. In 2011 the results were published: There were 247 deaths from lung cancer per 100,000 person-years in the low-dose CT group and 309 deaths per 100,000 person-years in the radiography group, representing a relative reduction in mortality from lung cancer with low-dose CT screening of 20.0%.[39] Although less than expected by proponents, this mortality reduction was still clinically significant. However, the trial also likely showed evidence of overdiagnosis; even after the gap in detection time between the two screening modalities closed, the screened group had more cancer than the control arm.[40]

This example shows that modeling can inform decisions when no evidence is available. However, given the significant biases at work to have uncontrolled studies overestimate screening benefits, there is no alternative to rigorous RCTs.

■ **Counseling** to promote good health habits and prevent disease (health promotion)
■ **Immunizations** and **chemoprophylaxis** to prevent specific diseases (primary prevention)

The first report of the USPSTF was issued in 1989. Since then, there have been regular literature reviews and updated screening recommendations for the entire spectrum of diseases amenable to screening, counseling, and prophylaxis. Recommendations are upgraded regularly and are available online.[29]

IV. SUMMARY

The goal of secondary prevention is the detection of disease or risk factors in the presymptomatic stage, when medical, environmental, nutritional, and lifestyle interventions can be most effective. Screening is done in a community setting, whereas case finding is done in a clinical setting. To be beneficial and cost-effective, community screening programs must fulfill various requirements on the health problem to be detected, the screening test used, and the system available to provide health care for people with positive screening results. Selection, lead-time, and length biases can lead to overestimates of benefit from screening, particularly the program detecting cancer. Although multiphasic screening seeks to make the process efficient by searching for many conditions at the same time, the high incidence of false-positive results and associated problems have made this technique less successful than was originally anticipated. Genetic screening introduces a new subset of requirements for screening tests, including clinical validity and clinical utility.

Historically, the periodic health examination has been the most common method of case finding. Because of disappointing benefits, however, it is now being replaced by lifetime health monitoring. This approach focuses on monitoring individuals for the specific set of conditions and diseases most likely to be found in persons of a certain age and gender, and its use has been advocated by experts on preventive medicine in Canada and the United States. Many practitioners who emphasize preventive medicine prefer to see their patients for checkups more often than may be recommended, such as 1 or 2 years, to maintain a relationship of trust and to repeat health promotion messages that are important for efforts to change behavior.

References

1. Berwick DM: Screening in health fairs: a critical review of benefits, risks, and costs. *JAMA* 254:1492–1498, 1985.
2. Nelson HD et al: Screening for ovarian cancer: a brief update. http://www.uspreventiveservicestaskforce.org/3rduspstf/ovariancan/ovcanup.htm.
3. Nelson HD, Tyne K, Naik A, et al: Screening for breast cancer: an update for the U.S. Preventive Services Task Force. *Ann Intern Med* 151:727–737, 2009.
4. Elmore JG, Armstrong K, Lehman CD, et al: Screening for breast cancer. *JAMA* 293:1245–1256, 2005.
5. Bailar JD III: Mammography: a contrary view. *Ann Intern Med* 84:77–84, 1976.
6. Christopherson WM, Parker JE, Drye JC: Control of cervical cancer: preliminary report on a community program. *JAMA* 182:179–182, 1962.
7. Elmore JG, Barton MB, Moceri VM, et al: Ten-year risk of false-positive screening mammograms and clinical breast examinations. *N Engl J Med* 338:1089–1096, 1998.
8. Bates B, Yellin JA: The yield of multiphasic screening. *JAMA* 222:74–78, 1972.
9. Olsen DM, Kane RL, Proctor PH: A controlled trial of multiphasic screening. *N Engl J Med* 294:925–930, 1976.
10. Yarnall KS, Pollak KI, Østbye T, et al: Primary care: is there enough time for prevention? *Am J Public Health* 93:635–641, 2003.
11. Robin NH, Tabereaux PB, Benza R, et al: Genetic testing in cardiovascular disease. *J Am Coll Cardiol* 50:727–737, 2007.

12. Heshka JT, Palleschi C, Howley H, et al: A systematic review of perceived risks, psychological and behavioural impacts of genetic testing. *Genet Med* 10:19–32, 2008.

13. Bloss CS, Schork NJ, Topol EJ: Effect of direct-to-consumer genome-wide profiling to assess disease risk. *N Engl J Med* 364:524–534, 2011.

14. Gross SJ: Carrier screening in individuals of Ashkenazi Jewish descent. *Genet Med* 10:54–56, 2008.

15. Hogarth S, Javitt G, Melzer D: The current landscape for direct-to-consumer genetic testing: legal, ethical, and policy issues. *Annu Rev Genomics Hum Genet* 9:161–182, 2008.

16. Ornish D, Magbanua MJ, Weidner G, et al: Changes in prostate gene expression in men undergoing an intensive nutrition and lifestyle intervention. *Proc Natl Acad Sci USA* 105:8369–8374, 2008.

17. Siegel GS: *Periodic health examinations: abstracts from the literature*, Washington, DC, 1963, US Department of Health, Education, and Welfare.

18. Schor SS, Clark TW, Parkhurst LW, et al: An evaluation of the periodic health examination: the findings in 350 examinees who died. *Ann Intern Med* 61:999–1005, 1964.

19. Roberts NJ, Ipsen J, Elsom KO, et al: Mortality among males in periodic health examination programs. *N Engl J Med* 281:20–24, 1969.

20. Spitzer WO, Brown BP: Unanswered questions about the periodic health examination. *Ann Intern Med* 83:257–263, 1975.

21. Breslow L, Somers AR: The lifetime health monitoring program: a practical approach to preventive medicine. *N Engl J Med* 296:601–608, 1977.

22. Canadian Task Force on the Periodic Physical Examination: The periodic health examination. *Can Med Assoc J* 121:1193–1254, 1979.

23. Robbins LC, Hall J: *How to practice prospective medicine*, Indianapolis, 1970, Methodist Hospital of Indiana.

24. Society for Prospective Medicine: Managing health care, measuring lives: expanding the definition and scope of health risk appraisal. Thirty-First Annual Meeting of the Society for Prospective Medicine, New Orleans, 1995.

25. Foxman B, Edington DW: The accuracy of health risk appraisal in predicting mortality. *Am J Public Health* 77:971–974, 1987.

26. Schoenbach VJ: Appraising health risk appraisal (editorial). *Am J Public Health* 77:409–411, 1987.

27. Smith KW, McKinlay SM, McKinlay JB: The reliability of health risk appraisals: a field trial of four instruments. *Am J Public Health* 79:1603–1607, 1989.

28. O'Donnell MP: A simple framework to describe what works best: improving awareness, enhancing motivation, building skills, and providing opportunity. *Am J Health Promot* 20(1 suppl):1–7 (following 84, iii), 2005.

29. US Preventive Services Task Force. http://www.uspreventiveservicestaskforce.org/.

30. US Preventive Services Task Force: *Guide to clinical preventive services*, ed 2, Baltimore, 1996, Williams & Wilkins.

31. When evidence collides with anecdote, politics, and emotions: breast cancer screening. *Ann Intern Med* 152:531–532, 2010.

32. Gøtzsche PC, Nielsen M: Screening for breast cancer with mammography. *Cochrane Database Syst Rev* (1):CD001877, 2011.

33. Chou R, Croswell JM, Dana T, et al: Screening for prostate cancer: a review of the evidence for the U.S. Preventive Services Task Force. *Ann Intern Med* 155:762–771, 2011.

34. Kramer BS, Berg CD, Aberle DR, et al: Lung cancer screening with low-dose helical CT: results from the National Lung Screening Trial. *J Med Screen* 18:109–111, 2011.

35. The National Lung Screening Trial: overview and study design. NLST Research Team. *Radiology* 258:243–253, 2011.

36. Henschke CI: CT screening for lung cancer is justified. *Nat Clin Pract Oncol* 4:440–441, 2007.

37. Mahadevia PJ, Fleisher LA, Frick KD, et al: Lung cancer screening with helical computed tomography in older adult smokers: a decision and cost-effectiveness analysis. *JAMA* 289:313–322, 2003.

38. Bach PB, Jett JR, Pastorino U, et al: Impact of computed tomography screening on lung cancer outcomes. *JAMA* 297:1–9, 2007.

39. National Lung Screening Trial Research Team: Reduced lung-cancer mortality with low-dose computed tomographic screening. *N Engl J Med* 365:395–409, 2011.

40. Sox HC: Better evidence about screening for lung cancer. *N Engl J Med* 365:455–457, 2011.

Select Readings

Fletcher RH, Fletcher SW: *Clinical epidemiology: the essentials*, ed 4, Philadelphia, 2005, Lippincott, Williams & Wilkins.

Katz DL, Nawaz H, Greci L: *Clinical epidemiology and evidence-based medicine: fundamental principles of clinical reasoning and research*. Thousand Oaks, Calif, 2001, Sage.

Welch HG: *Should I be tested for cancer? Maybe not and here's why*, Berkeley, Calif, 2004, University of California Press.

Woolf SH, Jonas S, Kaplan-Liss E, editors: *Health promotion and disease prevention in clinical practice*, ed 2, Philadelphia, 2007, Lippincott, Williams & Wilkins.

Website

http://www.uspreventiveservicestaskforce.org/   [U.S. Preventive Services Task Force]

Methods of Tertiary Prevention

In practice, tertiary prevention resembles treatment of established disease. The difference is in perspective. Whereas treatment is expressly about "fixing what is wrong," tertiary prevention looks ahead to potential progression and complications of disease and aims to forestall them. Thus, although treatment and tertiary prevention often share methods, their motives and goals diverge.

Methods of tertiary prevention are designed to limit the physical and social consequences of disease or injury after it has occurred or become symptomatic. There are two basic categories of tertiary prevention. The first category, **disability limitation,** has the goal of halting the progress of the disease or limiting the damage caused by an injury. This category of tertiary prevention can be described as the "prevention of further impairment." The second category, called **rehabilitation,** focuses on reducing the social disability produced by a given level of impairment. It aims to strengthen the patient's remaining functions and to help the patient learn to function in alternative ways. Disability limitation and rehabilitation usually should be initiated at the same time (i.e., when the disease is detected or the injury occurs), but the emphasis on one or the other depends on factors

such as the type and stage of disease, the type of injury, and available methods of treatment. This chapter discusses opportunities for tertiary prevention and provides specific clinical examples of disability limitation and rehabilitation.

I. DISEASE, ILLNESS, DISABILITY, AND DISEASE PERCEPTIONS

Although sometimes used interchangeably, there are important distinctions among disease, disability, and illness. Typically, *disease* is defined as the medical condition or diagnosis itself (e.g., diabetes, heart disease, chronic obstructive lung disease). *Disability* is the adverse impact of the disease on objective physical, psychological, and social functioning. For example, although stroke and paralytic polio are different diseases, both can result in the same disability: weakness of one leg and inability to walk. *Illness* is the adverse impact of a disease or disability on how the patient feels. One way to distinguish these terms is to specify that disease refers to the medical diagnosis, disability to the objective impact on the patient, and illness to the subjective impact.

Disability and illness obviously derive from the medical disease. However, illness is also powerfully influenced by patients' perceptions of their disease, its duration and severity, and their expectations for a recovery; together, these beliefs are called **illness perceptions.** Disease and illness interact; a patient's illness perceptions strongly predict recovery, loss of work days, adherence, and health care utilization.[1,2] To be successful, tertiary prevention and rehabilitation must not only improve patients' physical functioning, but also influence their illness perceptions. Although there is some evidence of effective psychological interventions on illness perceptions,[3] a recent systematic review of interventions of illness perceptions in cardiovascular health found too much heterogeneity among studies to allow for general conclusions.[4] Despite the mixed quality of the data, the practicing clinician should consider the patients' illness perceptions, if only to understand which patients are at high risk of poor outcomes.

II. OPPORTUNITIES FOR TERTIARY PREVENTION

The first sign of an illness provides an excellent opportunity to initiate methods of tertiary prevention. The sooner disability limitation and rehabilitation are begun, the greater the chance of preventing significant impairment. In the case of infectious diseases, such as tuberculosis and sexually transmitted diseases, early treatment of a disease in one person may prevent its transmission to others, making treatment of one person the primary prevention of that disease in others. Similarly, early treatment of alcoholism or drug addiction in one family member may prevent social and emotional problems, including codependency, from developing in other family members.

Symptomatic illness can identify individuals most in need of preventive efforts. In this sense, the symptoms function similar to screening, by defining individuals especially in need. When they feel well, people may not be convinced by health promotion and disease prevention messages. When they become ill, however, they may understand for the first time the value of changing their diet, behavior, or environment. For example, a person at risk for coronary artery disease who has experienced no symptoms will generally be less open to changes in diet and exercise than someone who has experienced chest pain. The onset of symptoms may provide a window of opportunity for health promotion aimed at preventing progression of the disease (**"teachable moment"**). Cardiovascular disease is used here to illustrate the approach to prevention after the disease has made its presence known. However, almost any hospitalization or major life event (e.g., pregnancy, birth of a grandchild) can be a teachable moment for patients, and the prognosis for most diseases improves with better diet, exercise, and adherence.

III. DISABILITY LIMITATION

Disability limitation includes therapy as well as attempts to halt or limit future progression of the disease, called **symptomatic stage prevention.** Most medical or surgical therapy of symptomatic disease is directed at preventing or minimizing impairment over the short-term and long-term. For example, both coronary angioplasty and coronary artery bypass are aimed at both improving function and extending life. These are attempts to undo the threat or damage from an existing disease, in this case, coronary artery disease (CAD). The strategies of symptomatic stage prevention include the following:

1. Modifying diet, behavior, and environment
2. Screening frequently for incipient complications
3. Treating any complication that is discovered

In this section, CAD, hyperlipidemia, hypertension, and diabetes mellitus are used to illustrate how methods of disability limitation can be applied to patients with chronic diseases. The emphasis is on symptomatic stage prevention.

A. Cardiovascular Disease

Cardiovascular disease encompasses coronary artery disease, cerebrovascular accident (CVA, stroke), heart failure, and peripheral artery disease (PAD). If cardiovascular disease has already occurred, the clinician's immediate goal is to prevent death and permanent damage. Beyond that, the clinician's goal is to slow, stop, or even reverse the progression of the disease process.

1. Risk Factor Modification

When cardiovascular disease becomes symptomatic (e.g., with a heart attack), the acute disease needs to be addressed with interventions, such as thrombolysis, rhythm stabilization, and perhaps stents or surgical bypass. When a patient is stabilized, the risk factors to be addressed to slow or reverse disease progression are generally similar to those for primary prevention, but the urgency for action is increased. The following *modifiable* risk factors are important to address when cardiovascular disease has already occurred: hypertension, smoking, dyslipidemia, diabetes, diet, and exercise.

In practice, which risk factor to address first should be negotiated between clinician and patient. The most important risk factor to modify should be the one the patient is actually motivated and able to change. Any change there will improve risk, and successful behavior change in one area can provide motivation for further change later.

CIGARETTE SMOKING

Smoking accelerates blood clotting, increases blood carbon monoxide levels, and causes a reduction in the delivery of oxygen. In addition, nicotine is *vasoconstrictive* (causes blood vessels to tighten). The age-related risk of myocardial infarction (MI) in smokers is approximately twice that in nonsmokers. For individuals who stop smoking, the excess risk declines fairly quickly and seems to be minimal after 1 year of nonsmoking. Smoking cessation is probably the most effective behavioral change a patient can make when cardiovascular disease is present. Smoking cessation also helps to slow related smoking-induced problems most likely to complicate the cardiovascular disease, such as chronic obstructive pulmonary disease (COPD).

DIABETES MELLITUS

Type 2 diabetes mellitus increases the risk of repeat MI or restenosis (reblockage) of coronary arteries. Keeping the level of glycosylated hemoglobin (a measure of blood sugar control; e.g., Hb A_{1c}) at less than 7% significantly reduces the effect of diabetes on the heart, kidneys, and eyes. Many authorities advocate treating diabetes as a **coronary heart disease equivalent,** based on a Finnish study that showed that patients with diabetes (who had not had a heart attack) had a similar risk of MI as patients with established CAD.[5] Even though this study's methods and results are in dispute, the management of diabetes mellitus has shifted. The approach no longer focuses only on sugar control, but instead aims for multifactorial strategy to identify and target patients' broader cardiovascular risk factors.[6] This approach includes treating lipids and controlling blood pressure (BP).

HYPERTENSION

Any hypertension increases the risk of cardiovascular disease, and severe hypertension (systolic BP ≥195 mm Hg) approximately quadruples the risk of cardiovascular disease in middle-aged men.[7,8] Effects of hypertension are direct (damage to blood vessels) and indirect (increasing demand on heart). Control of hypertension is crucial at this stage to prevent progression of cardiovascular disease.

SEDENTARY LIFESTYLE

It seems that at least 30 minutes of moderate exercise (e.g., fast walking) at least three times per week reduces the risk of cardiovascular disease. There is increasing evidence that sitting itself, independent of the amount of exercise, increases the risk of MI.[9] The uncertainty occurs partly because it is difficult to design observational studies that completely avoid the potential bias of self-selection (e.g., people with incipient heart disease may have cues that tell them to avoid exercise). Nevertheless, there is increasing emphasis on the potential benefits of even modest physical activity, which has direct effects on lipids and also helps to keep weight down, which itself improves the blood lipid profile. Conversely, there is a growing appreciation for adverse health effects of "sedentariness."[9]

EXCESS WEIGHT

In people who are overweight, the risk for cardiovascular disease partly depends on how the body fat is distributed. Fat can be distributed in the hips and legs (*peripheral adiposity,* giving the body a pear shape) or predominantly in the abdominal cavity (*central adiposity,* giving the body an apple shape, more common in men than women.) Fat in the hips and legs does not seem to increase the risk of cardiovascular disease. In contrast, fat in the abdominal cavity seems to be more metabolically active, and the risk of cardiovascular disease is increased. This is not surprising, because fat mobilized from the omentum goes directly to the liver, which is the center of the body's lipid metabolism. Centrally located body fat is implicated in the *insulin resistance syndrome* and is associated with increased sympathetic tone and hypertension.

Weight loss ameliorates some important cardiac risk factors, such as hypertension and insulin resistance. Some studies suggest that alternating dieting and nondieting, called *weight cycling,* is a risk factor in itself,[10] but other studies question this conclusion.[11] The most recent findings in this area suggest that weight gain and loss may result in lasting hormonal and cytokine alterations that facilitate regaining weight.[12] Although weight cycling may have specific associated risks, whether any such risks are truly independent of obesity itself remains unclear.[13-16] At present, expert opinion generally supports a benefit from weight loss, with greater benefit clearly attached to sustainable weight loss[17] (http://www.nwcr.ws/). Achieving sustained weight loss remains a considerable challenge (see Chapter 19).

DYSLIPIDEMIA

The risk of progression of cardiovascular disease is increased in patients with dyslipidemia (abnormal levels of lipids and the particles that carry them), which can act synergistically with other risk factors (see later and also Chapter 5, especially Table 5-2, and Chapter 19). Disease progression can be slowed by improving blood lipid levels or by addressing other modifiable risk factors (e.g., hypertension, diabetes) that benefit from diet and exercise.

2. Therapy

The immediate care and long-term care of patients with symptomatic CAD depend on the extent to which the disease has progressed when the patient comes under medical care. Even in the presence of severe CAD, there may be little or no warning before MI occurs. After acute medical and surgical therapy (tertiary prevention) is provided, the provider should initiate efforts directed at symptomatic stage prevention (also tertiary prevention in this case).

3. Symptomatic Stage Prevention

Every patient with symptomatic cardiac disease needs evaluation for risk factors and a plan to reduce the risk of adverse cardiac events. If the patient already has had an MI or undergone revascularization (opening up blocked arteries) through percutaneous transluminal coronary angioplasty (cardiac catheterization) or coronary artery bypass surgery, the goals include preventing restenosis and slowing the progression of atherosclerosis elsewhere.

BEHAVIOR MODIFICATION

Patients should be questioned about smoking, exercise, and eating habits, all of which affect the risks of cardiovascular disease. Smokers should be encouraged to stop smoking (see Chapter 15 and Box 15-2), and all patients should receive nutrition counseling and information about the types and appropriate levels of exercise to pursue. Hospitalized patients with elevated blood lipids should be placed on a "heart healthy" diet (see Chapter 19) and encouraged to continue this type of diet when they return home. This change in diet requires considerable coaching, often provided by a specialized cardiac rehabilitation nurse, dietitian, or both.

OTHER MEASURES

The assessment and appropriate management of known risk factors, such as dyslipidemia, hypertension, and diabetes mellitus, are essential for reducing the risk of adverse cardiac events in patients with symptomatic CAD.

B. Dyslipidemia

Dyslipidemia, sometimes imprecisely called "hyperlipidemia," is a general term used to describe an abnormal elevation in one or more of the lipids or lipid particles found in the blood. The **complete lipid profile** provides information on the following:

- Total cholesterol (TC)
- High-density lipoprotein (HDL) cholesterol
- Low-density lipoprotein (LDL) cholesterol
- Very-low-density lipoprotein (VLDL) cholesterol, which is associated with triglycerides (TGs)

The **TC** level is equal to the sum of the HDL, LDL, and VLDL levels:

$$TC = HDL + LDL + VLDL$$
$$= (HDL) + (LDL) + (TGs/5)$$

The "good cholesterol," **HDL,** is actually not only cholesterol but rather a particle (known as *apoprotein*) that contains cholesterol and acts as a scavenger to remove excess cholesterol in the body (also known as *reverse cholesterol transport*). HDL is predominantly protein, and elevated HDL levels have been associated with decreased cardiovascular risk. **LDL**, the "bad cholesterol," is likewise not just cholesterol but a particle that contains it. Elevated LDL levels have been associated with increased cardiovascular risk. A high level of certain LDL particles may be a necessary precursor for *atherogenesis* (development of fatty arterial plaques). Much of the damage may be caused by oxidative modification of the LDL, making it more atherogenic.[12] **VLDL**, another "bad cholesterol," is actually a precursor of LDL. The particle is predominantly **triglyceride.**

The previous formulas clarify why total cholesterol alone is not the best measure for cardiovascular risk. Cholesterol is cholesterol, but the risk for heart disease comes from how it is *packaged* in different VLDL, LDL, and HDL particles. Additional measures of potential interest in risk stratification are related to lipids not routinely included in the lipid panel. These include HDL subfractions, the size and density of LDL particles, and lipoprotein (a), or Lp(a) lipoprotein.

I. Assessment

A variety of index measures have been proposed to assess the need for intervention and to monitor the success of preventive measures. The most frequently used guidelines are those of the Third National Cholesterol Education Program (NCEP),[18] as modified based on more recent research.[19] This discussion and Table 17-1 indicate the levels of blood lipids suggested by the widely accepted NCEP recommendations for deciding on treatment and follow-up. New NCEP recommendations are expected in 2012.

TOTAL CHOLESTEROL LEVEL

Some screening programs measure only the total cholesterol (TC) level. In adults without known atherosclerotic disease, a TC level less than 200 mg/dL does not require the need for action, although the level should be checked every 5 years. A level between 200 and 239 mg/dL is considered borderline high, and a fasting lipid profile is recommended, with action determined on the basis of the findings. If TC level is 240 mg/dL or greater, diagnosis based on a fasting lipid profile is needed, and dietary and lifestyle changes should be initiated; in addition, lipid-lowering drugs should be considered.

The TC level may be misleading and is a poor summary measure of the complicated lipoprotein-particle distributions that more accurately define risk. In insulin resistance,

for example, TC tends to be normal, but there is an adverse pattern of lipoproteins—high triglycerides and low HDL. This pattern originally was discerned in the Framingham Heart Study and is sometimes referred to as *syndrome X*. In the Helsinki Heart Study, primary dyslipidemia was defined as the presence of a non-HDL cholesterol level 200 mg/dL or greater on two successive measurements.[20] Many clinicians find this index useful because it uses the total contribution of cholesterol fractions currently considered harmful. Some specialists pay attention to the ratio of the TC level to the HDL level, as discussed later.

HIGH-DENSITY LIPOPROTEIN LEVEL

In general, the higher the HDL level is, the better. The minimum recommended HDL level is 50 mg/dL in women and 40 mg/dL in men. An HDL level less than 40 mg/dL is of special concern if the LDL level or the triglyceride level is high (see later). An HDL level greater than 60 mg/dL is considered a **negative risk factor**, or a **protective factor**, reducing an individual's risk of cardiovascular disease.

LOW-DENSITY LIPOPROTEIN LEVEL

In an adult without known atherosclerotic disease or major risk factors for cardiovascular disease, an LDL level of less than 130 mg/dL is considered acceptable, and another lipid profile is recommended within 5 years. If the LDL is borderline elevated (130-159 mg/dL), and the patient has no more than one cardiovascular risk factor, the lipid profile should be repeated within 1 year. If two or more risk factors are present, however, dietary and lifestyle changes should be recommended. If the LDL level is 160 mg/dL or greater, dietary and lifestyle changes should be recommended, and lipid-lowering therapy should be considered. A LDL greater than 190 mg/dL usually calls for pharmacotherapy.

In the presence of demonstrated atherosclerotic disease or multiple major risk factors, the criteria have been tightened. LDL was the primary focus of the revisions to the NCEP-III recommendations.[18] For high-risk patients, an LDL level of 100 mg/dL or more should lead to the institution of dietary and lifestyle changes and to treatment with lipid-lowering medications. The NCEP-III recommendations state that the LDL target should be less than 70 mg/dL in very-high-risk patients, such as patients with CAD or CAD equivalents, such as peripheral vascular disease, carotid

Table 17-1 **Evaluation of Blood Lipid Levels in Persons without and with Coronary Risk Factors or Coronary Artery Disease (CAD)**

Lipid Fraction	Optimal mg/dL	Acceptable mg/dL	Borderline mg/dL	Abnormal mg/dL
For Persons with No CAD and No More than One Risk Factor*				
Total cholesterol	—	<200	200-239	≥240
LDL	<100	100-129	130-159	≥160
HDL	≥60	40-59	—	<40
Triglycerides	<150	—	150-199	200
For Persons with Major CHD Risk Factors or Existing CHD				
LDL	<70	—	<100	≥100

*Risk factors are cigarette smoking, diabetes, hypertension, and family history of early CAD.
CHD, Coronary heart disease; *HDL,* high-density lipoprotein; *LDL,* low-density lipoprotein; *mg/dL,* milligrams per deciliter.

artery disease, or diabetes mellitus. Achieving this target usually requires aggressive statin therapy along with good diet and exercise (see Table 17-1).

TRIGLYCERIDE AND VERY-LOW-DENSITY LIPOPROTEIN LEVELS

The VLDL level can be determined for most patients by dividing the triglyceride (TG) level by 5. The desired TG level is less than 150 mg/dL. Although levels greater than 200 mg/dL were previously considered reasons for concern and treatment, the clinical perspective on TG levels is evolving. Some experts believe that treating high TG levels may not be helpful in mitigating the risk of cardiovascular disease, and that treatment is only indicated at very high TG levels (e.g., >500 mg/dL) to reduce the risk of pancreatitis.

TOTAL CHOLESTEROL–TO–HIGH-DENSITY LIPOPROTEIN RATIO

Some investigators monitor the TC/HDL ratio. Using this approach, one group reported that angiograms in patients with a TC/HDL ratio greater than 6.9 showed progression of coronary atherosclerosis during the study, whereas those in patients with a lower TC/HDL ratio did not show progression.[21] Currently, a TC/HDL ratio of less than 4.5 is recommended if atherosclerotic disease is absent, and a ratio of less than 3.5 is recommended if atherosclerotic disease is present.

TRIGLYCERIDE–HIGH-DENSITY LIPOPROTEIN RELATIONSHIP

Research suggests that the combination of an HDL level less than 30 mg/dL and a TG level greater than 200 mg/dL places an individual at high risk for CAD, and the possibility of genetic hyperlipidemia should be considered. This pattern is often associated with insulin resistance and hypertension, sometimes referred to as the **metabolic syndrome.** This adverse pattern, as noted earlier, may be concealed by a "normal" total cholesterol level. This is one reason why lipid screening should generally include the standard panel rather than total cholesterol alone.

HOMOCYSTEINE LEVEL

Elevated homocysteine levels are associated with an increased risk of atherogenesis.[22] Thus far, however, interventions through dietary supplements of folic acid, pyridoxine, or vitamin B_{12} have not shown improved outcomes.[23] Some believe that homocysteine is merely a marker for the "true" culprit. Likewise, all the lipid fractions, lipoprotein particles, and indices previously discussed may actually be markers of the true culprits; none is consistently explanatory, and improving the patient's *numbers,* even for the most explanatory components, does not consistently lead to improved patient outcomes.

2. Therapy and Symptomatic Stage Prevention

Any primary care clinician should be able to treat patients with a moderately elevated total cholesterol level or abnormal lipid levels and should be aware of the therapeutic options. Patients with severe or esoteric lipid abnormalities probably should be treated by specialists, however. In the primary prevention of CAD, clinicians should recommend a trial of lifestyle modifications (dietary changes, increased

exercise, and smoking cessation) before prescribing a lipid-lowering medication, such as an **HMG-CoA reductase inhibitor** (**statin** drug). When CAD becomes symptomatic, lifestyle modifications *and* drug treatment (usually statins) should be started as soon as possible. When statins are not well tolerated or do not achieve targeted lipid reductions on their own, newer drugs, such as ezetimibe, are available. Although newer drugs may improve lipid numbers, however, as yet there is no good evidence that these improve patient outcomes, such as preventing heart attacks and strokes or delaying death.

C. Hypertension

In the United States, 43 million to 50 million people are estimated to have hypertension, and approximately half have not yet been diagnosed. Groups at increased risk include pregnant women, women taking estrogens or oral contraceptives, elderly persons, and African Americans. Children also are at risk for hypertension.

The Joint National Committee on Prevention, Detection, Evaluation, and Treatment of High Blood Pressure (JNC) is convened by the National Heart, Lung, and Blood Institute. It publishes period reports addressing the diagnosis, treatment, and prevention of hypertension.[24] According to the Seventh Joint National Committee Report (JNC 7), *hypertension* is defined as an average systolic BP of 140 mm Hg or greater, or an average diastolic BP of 90 mm Hg or greater, when blood pressure is properly measured on two or more occasions in a person who is not acutely ill and not taking antihypertensive medications. These levels are high enough for treatment to bring proven benefits. New recommendations from JNC 8 are expected in 2012.

1. Assessment

Hypertension may be detected by community or occupational screening, by individual case finding (e.g., when a person seeks care for dental problems or for medical problems unrelated to hypertension), or when a person develops one or more common complications of hypertension, such as visual problems, early renal failure, congestive heart failure, stroke, or MI. Over the last 20 years, the risk of mortality from CAD and stroke in hypertensive individuals has decreased, in part because of the early detection and improved management of high blood pressure. However, much still remains to be done. Only slightly more than one third of patients with hypertension are "well controlled" (up from 29% in 2000).[25] This fact underscores how many lives could be saved and how much disability could be prevented if we were better at delivering consistent care (see Chapter 28).

Table 17-2 provides information regarding the evaluation and staging of hypertension, based on average systolic BP and diastolic BP. In addition to listing the ranges for normal BP and prehypertension, Table 17-2 shows the ranges for two stages of hypertension.

2. Therapy and Symptomatic Stage Prevention

After the stage of hypertension has been determined, JNC 7 recommends the following actions (see also Table 17-2). Individuals with **normal blood pressure** should be

Table 17-2 Evaluation of Blood Pressure (BP) and Staging of Hypertension, Based on Average Systolic BP and Diastolic BP in Persons Not Acutely Ill and Not Taking Antihypertensive Medications*

Systolic BP (mm Hg)	Diastolic BP (mm Hg)	Interpretation	Initiate Drug Treatment?
<120	<80	Normal BP	No
120-139	80-89	Prehypertension	In some cases
140-159	90-99	Stage 1 hypertension	Yes; thiazides for most
≥160	≥100	Stage 2 hypertension	Yes; two-drug combination

Data from National Institutes of Health: The seventh report of the Joint National Committee on Prevention, Detection, Evaluation, and Treatment of High Blood Pressure (JNC-7), 2003. www.nhlbi.nih.gov/guidelines/hypertension.
*The highest stage for which either systolic BP or diastolic BP qualifies is taken as the stage of hypertension. For example, if systolic is 165 and diastolic 95 mm Hg, this is stage 2 hypertension. *Note:* For patients with diabetes or chronic kidney disease, the BP goal should be less than 130/80 mm Hg.

monitored at 2-year intervals. Individuals with **prehypertension** should be counseled about lifestyle changes and monitored at 1-year intervals. Patients with **stage 1 hypertension** should begin diet and lifestyle changes and should receive one antihypertensive medication, usually a thiazide diuretic. Patients with **stage 2 hypertension** should begin diet and lifestyle changes and should be treated with two antihypertensive medications. During evaluation the clinician should check for any evidence of target organ damage, because any stage of hypertension is more severe if there is evidence of such damage.

Most hypertension is classified as **essential hypertension,** meaning that the specific underlying cause is unknown. Depending on the patient, however, hardening of the arteries, fluid retention, or changes in the renin-angiotensin-aldosterone system may be involved. **Nonessential (secondary) hypertension** is caused by other, often treatable causes, such as renal artery disease, chronic kidney disease, or obstructive sleep apnea.

Symptomatic stage prevention and therapy are aimed at reducing systolic BP to less than 140 mm Hg, reducing diastolic BP to less than 90 mm Hg, and monitoring patients to ensure that these levels are maintained. The goal is to prevent damage to the organs at risk from hypertension to prevent disability, organ failure, and death. For patients with any stage of hypertension, the following lifestyle modifications are indicated: weight reduction, increased physical activity, and institution of a healthy diet. In the Dietary Approaches to Stop Hypertension (DASH) trials, investigators found that instituting a diet that was rich in fruits, vegetables, grains, and nonfat dairy products was associated with a reduction in systolic BP, and even greater BP reductions were seen if sodium intake was restricted to no more than 1200 mg/day.[26] Other dietary measures to reduce BP include the moderation of alcohol intake and an increase in the intake of potassium, calcium, and magnesium. Smokers should be encouraged to stop smoking, because smoking cessation reduces the risk of damage to many of the same organs that hypertension damages.

For patients whose BP levels remain elevated despite these lifestyle modifications, use of one or more antihypertensive medications is indicated. Because most hypertension is asymptomatic, providers must counsel patients about the importance of taking medications and the risks of stopping treatment. The major classes of effective antihypertensive agents include diuretics, beta blockers, angiotensin-converting enzyme (ACE) inhibitors, angiotensin receptor blockers (ARBs), calcium channel blockers, alpha blockers, and vasodilators. Although many antihypertensive medications cause significant side effects, the wide range of choices should be used to develop a treatment plan that is satisfactory to the patient.

In controlled clinical trials, *thiazide-type diuretics* have been shown to reduce cardiovascular disease and are a good first choice in asymptomatic patients either alone or with other drugs. Thiazide diuretics should be used with caution in elderly patients because of possible orthostatic hypotension (lightheadedness or fainting), acute renal failure, and electrolyte imbalances (particularly low potassium). *Beta blockers* are a good choice for patients who have CAD, heart failure, or diabetes. Beta blockers are contraindicated, however, in patients with conduction abnormalities, and cardioselective beta blockers are often used in patients with asthma or COPD. Beta blockers seem to be less effective as first-time treatment of high BP in patients without heart disease; meta-analyses suggest an association with increased risk of cardiovascular events and death.[27,28]

In the Heart Outcomes Prevention Evaluation (HOPE) trials, investigators found clear evidence that ACE inhibitors can prevent deaths caused by MI and stroke and can reduce the mortality in many groups of high-risk cardiac patients.[29] However, ACE inhibitors should not be used in patients who might become pregnant (due to the risk of birth defects) or in patients who have bilateral renal artery stenosis.

D. Diabetes Mellitus

More than 26 million people in the United States have diabetes, and this number is rising. If current trends continue, one in three adults will have diabetes by 2050.[30] About 5% of diabetic patients have **type 1 diabetes mellitus,** a disease that requires lifelong treatment with insulin and places them at higher risk for a variety of cardiovascular, renal, and other serious complications. The remaining 95% of patients have **type 2 diabetes mellitus,** usually associated with obesity and **insulin resistance.**

Much can be done to prevent target organ damage from diabetes, as shown in the landmark Diabetes Control and Complications Trial (DCCT) and the United Kingdom Prospective Diabetes Study (UKPDS). In patients with type 1 diabetes, DCCT showed that improved control of blood glucose levels significantly reduced the incidence of **microvascular disease** (retinopathy, nephropathy, neuropathy) and reduced the incidence of **macrovascular disease** (atherosclerosis of large blood vessels, MI, angina pectoris, stroke, aneurysm, amputations of distal lower extremity).[31,32]

Similarly, in patients with type 2 diabetes, UKPDS found that in general the lower the average glycemic level in patients, the fewer the complications.[33]

Patients in the DCCT intervention group had to self-monitor their blood glucose level, keep detailed records of insulin dosage and glucose level, regulate dietary intake and level of insulin based on self-monitoring results, and be actively involved in other aspects of their care. Although the risk of hypoglycemic episodes was three times as high in the intervention group as in the control group, no serious sequelae of hypoglycemia occurred in the intervention group. One death from hypoglycemia occurred in the control group. Weight gain was a common side effect of tight diabetic control.

Based on the results of DCCT, "tight control" (defined as control as good as that obtained in DCCT) may benefit patients who are willing to participate actively in their own care. Currently, the most used definition of tight control is hemoglobin A_{1c} (glycohemoglobin, or sugar linked to Hb) values less than 7% of total hemoglobin. Many U.S. patients with diabetes may have glycohemoglobins above the recommended level (57% with Hb A_{1c} <7% in 2004).[34] Tight control should be supplemented with frequent examination of the retina and with laser treatment of microvascular lesions when indicated. The use of ACE inhibitors has proved valuable not only in controlling hypertension but also in reducing the incidence of microalbuminuria (albumin protein in the urine) a sign of diabetic kidney damage, and delaying the onset of diabetes-induced renal failure.

All patients with type 1 or type 2 diabetes should be advised of the need for moderate to high levels of physical activity and should receive individual counseling about nutrition. They should be informed of the common complications of diabetes and the importance of contacting their clinician if they note early symptoms of any of these complications.

Many other hypoglycemic agents are being used to reduce insulin resistance before it develops into frank type 2 diabetes. Current interest centers particularly on biguanides (metformin) and thiazolidinediones (glitazones), which are more effective when used in combination than used alone. Oral hypoglycemic agents that act by stimulating the pancreas to produce more insulin (sulfonylureas, short-acting secretagogues) also are being used, but over time these may exhaust the beta cells' ability to make insulin. Oral hypoglycemics also tend to foster weight gain, which compounds the problem of insulin resistance. The role, safety, and impact on outcomes of newer agents such as glucagon-like peptide-1 analogs, incretins, amylin analogs, and dipeptidyl peptidase-4 (DPP-4) inhibitors are not yet fully established. For most patients, metformin should be the first-line agent.[35]

IV. REHABILITATION

Occurring after disease already has caused damage, rehabilitation may seem to take place when there is nothing left to prevent. However, the goal of rehabilitation is to *reduce the social disability produced by a given level of impairment,* both by strengthening the patient's remaining functions and by helping the patient learn to function in alternative ways. Often, rehabilitation specialists can contribute to a patient's

progress back from an illness, but the initiation of rehabilitation should be incorporated into the patient's care from the beginning.

A. General Approach

Rehabilitation must begin in the early phases of treatment if it is to be maximally effective. In patients who have had a stroke, head injury, hip fracture, or other problem that temporarily immobilizes them, it is important to keep joints flexible from the beginning of the illness or injury, so that weakened but recovering muscles do not have to overcome stiffened joints. Beginning rehabilitation efforts early also tends to increase the cooperation of patients and family members by conveying to them that improvement is expected.

The most effective rehabilitation program is tailored to meet the physical, emotional, psychological, and occupational needs of the individual. As stated earlier, these programs also need to address patients' illness perceptions.

Often, a *rehabilitation counselor* coordinates the efforts of a team of specialists. *Physical therapists* work to strengthen weakened muscles, increase joint movement and flexibility, and teach patients ways of accomplishing routine tasks despite their disabilities. These tasks, or activities of daily living (see Chapter 14), include feeding oneself, transferring from bed to chair and back, grooming, controlling the bladder and bowels, bathing, dressing, walking on a level surface, and going up and down stairs. *Speech therapists* seek to improve the ability of patients to articulate their thoughts after a stroke or head injury that produces aphasia, and they may help to evaluate whether or not stroke patients can swallow food safely. *Occupational therapists* evaluate the occupational abilities of patients, counsel them regarding suitable types of work, provide them with job training or retraining, and help them find a suitable job. Usually, the most cost-effective efforts are those designed to help a patient return to the previous place of employment. Some patients may be able to resume their job, whereas others may obtain a new or modified job there. *Psychiatric or emotional counseling* may be important, as may be spiritual counseling by a member of the clergy. There also are specialists in cardiac and pulmonary rehabilitation.

B. Coronary Heart Disease

Coronary heart disease (or CAD) was the first disease for which rehabilitation programs were developed, and these programs still provide the template for most rehabilitation. Most cardiac rehabilitation programs follow defined components and stages[36] (Table 17-3). Core components of rehabilitation for all cardiac conditions include a comprehensive assessment of the patient's clinical and functional status. This information provides the basis for a rigorous program aimed at gradually improving physical functioning, risk factor profile, and psychosocial status.

BLOOD PRESSURE MONITORING

- If resting systolic BP is 130 to 139 mm Hg or diastolic BP is 85 to 89 mm Hg, recommend lifestyle modifications, exercise, weight management, sodium restriction, and moderation of alcohol intake (<30 g/day in men; <15 g/day in women), according to DASH diet.

Table 17-3 **Core Components of Cardiac Rehabilitation (post-ACS and post-PCI)**

Component	Established/Agreed Issues	Class (Level)	Issues?*
Patient assessment	Clinical history: review clinical courses of ACS.	I (A)	
	Physical examination: inspect puncture site of PCI and extremities for presence of arterial pulses.		
	Exercise capacity and ischemic threshold: Submaximal exercise stress testing by bicycle ergometry or treadmill maximal stress test (cardiopulmonary exercise test if available) within 4 weeks after acute events, with maximal testing at 4-7 weeks.	IIa (C)	
Physical activity counseling	*Exercise stress test guide:* With exercise capacity more than 5 METs without symptoms, patients can resume routine physical activity; otherwise, patients should resume physical activity at 50% of maximal exercise capacity and gradually increase.	I (B)	Should resistance physical activity 2 days per week be encouraged? (current evidence class IIb [C]) (21)
	Physical activity: Slow, gradual, progressive increase of moderate intensity aerobic activity, such as walking, climbing stairs, and cycling, supplemented by an increase in daily activities (e.g., gardening, housework).		
Exercise training	Program should include supervised, medically prescribed, aerobic exercise training:	I (B)	When should this training program start? After exercise stress testing?
	Low risk patients: At least three sessions of 30-60 min/wk aerobic exercise at 55%-70% of maximum workload (METs) or HR at onset of symptoms; ≥1500 kcal/wk to be expended.		
	Moderate-risk to high-risk patients: Similar to low-risk group, but starting with <50% maximum workload (METs).		
	Resistance exercise: At least 1 hr/wk with intensity of 10-15 repetitions per set to moderate fatigue.		
Diet/nutritional counseling	Caloric intake should be balanced by energy expenditure (physical activity) to avoid weight gain	I (C)	
Weight control management	Mediterranean diet with low levels of cholesterol and saturated fat	I (B)	
Lipid management	Foods rich in omega-3 fatty acids	I (B)	
	Statins for all patients, intensified to a lipid profile of cholesterol: <175 mg/dL, or <155 mg/dL in high-risk patients		
	LDL-C: <100 mg/dL, or <80 mg/dL in high-risk patients		
	Triglycerides: <150 mg/dL		
Blood pressure monitoring	Assess BP frequently at rest and as indicated during exercise. Use lifestyle modification and drugs if necessary to treat to optimal BP	I (B)	
Smoking cessation	Ask about tobacco and intervene according to stage of change	I (B)	
Psychosocial management	Screen for distress and intervene if necessary	I (B)	

Modified from Piepoli MF et al: *Eur J Cardiovasc Prev Rehabil* 17:1–17, 2010.
*Requiring further evidence.
ACS, Acute coronary syndrome; *HR,* heart rate; *LDL-C,* low-density lipoprotein cholesterol; *METs,* metabolic equivalent tasks; *PCI,* primary percutaneous coronary intervention.

■ If resting systolic BP is 140 mm Hg or greater or if diastolic BP is 90 mm Hg or greater, initiate drug therapy. Expected outcomes are BP less than 140/90 mm Hg (or <130/80 mm Hg if patient has diabetes or heart or renal failure) and BP less than 120/80 mm Hg in patients with left ventricular dysfunction.

SMOKING CESSATION

All smokers should be professionally encouraged to stop using all forms of tobacco permanently. Follow-up, referral to special programs, and pharmacotherapy (including nicotine replacement) are recommended, as a stepwise strategy for smoking cessation. Structured approaches are to be used (e.g., five "A"s: ask, advise, assess, assist, arrange; see Box 15-2).

■ Ask the patient about his/her smoking status and use of other tobacco products. Specify both amount of smoking (cigarettes per day) and duration of smoking (number of years).

■ Determine readiness to change; if ready, choose a date for quitting.

■ Assess for psychosocial factors that may impede success. Intervention: provide structured follow-up. Offer behavioral advice and group or individual counseling.

■ Offer nicotine replacement therapy, bupropion, varenicline, or both. The expected outcome is long-term abstinence from smoking.

■ Manage psychosocial issues.

■ Screen for psychological distress, as indicated by clinically significant levels of depression, anxiety, anger or hostility, social isolation, marital/family distress, sexual dysfunction/adjustment, and substance abuse of alcohol and/or other psychotropic agents.

■ Use interview and/or other standardized measurement tools.

■ Offer individual and/or small group education and counseling on adjustment to heart disease, stress management, and health-related lifestyle change (profession, motor vehicle operation, sexual activity resumption).

■ Whenever possible, include spouses and other family members, domestic partners, and/or significant others in such sessions.

■ Teach and support self-help strategies and ability to obtain effective social support.
■ Provide vocational counseling in case of work-related stress. *Expected outcome:* Absence of clinically significant psychosocial problems and acquisition of stress management skills.

Cardiac rehabilitation has been shown to be one of the most cost-effective interventions in preventing progression of heart disease. It may be particularly powerful in improving self-management by disadvantaged patients.[37] Rehabilitation usually involves the following four stages:

1. Enrollment of patients while they are in the hospital
2. Reconvalescence at home
3. Supervised group programs
4. Lifelong maintenance

C. Rehabilitation for Other Diseases

PULMONARY REHABILITATION

Evidence of the positive impact of pulmonary rehabilitation first came from a landmark study on lung reduction surgery[38] and was later confirmed in systematic reviews.[39] Since then, the indications for pulmonary rehabilitation have been broadened beyond COPD, and rehabilitation programs are now used for many chronic respiratory diseases.

CANCER REHABILITATION

More and more patients experience cancer not as an acute lethal illness but rather as a chronic disease. This trend has engendered an increased interest in the role of cancer rehabilitation. In contrast to patients with most other diseases, cancer patients often suffer as much from complications of therapy as from the disease itself.[40]

D. Categories of Disability

Disability is a socially defined concept but has practical implications for financial support. Most states delineate several categories for reimbursement of workers who have job-related injuries or illnesses covered under a workers' compensation program, as follows:

■ **Permanent total disability** (e.g., loss of two limbs or loss of vision in both eyes)
■ **Permanent partial disability** (e.g., loss of one limb or loss of vision in one eye)
■ **Temporary total disability** (e.g., fractured arm in truck driver)
■ **Temporary partial disability** (e.g., fractured arm in elementary school teacher)
■ **Death**

In these categories, state statutes stipulate benefits for disabled persons (or for their surviving family in the case of death) according to a fixed schedule. Less well-defined illnesses and injuries, such as repetitive motion or back injuries, are usually compensated by a mixture of financial and vocational rehabilitation benefits, including counseling, retraining, and even job placement.[41]

A disability is considered "temporary" if it is expected that a person will return to his or her job within a time defined by statute. If the disability is job-related, the person is partially reimbursed for lost wages and fully reimbursed for the costs of medical care from the state workers' compensation fund (see Chapters 18 and 24).

In the United States a person with a permanent disability may be reimbursed at a fixed rate for the rest of life or for a defined period. The rate varies from state to state (as stipulated by law), but it is based on the type of disability and degree of function lost (as determined by a clinician).

V. SUMMARY

The goal of tertiary prevention is to limit the physical and social consequences of an injury or disease after it has occurred or become symptomatic. The two major categories of tertiary prevention are disability limitation and rehabilitation. Whereas disease and disability describe objective diagnoses and impairments, illness also encompasses patients' perceptions, assumptions, and expectations about their disease. These illness perceptions strongly predict disease outcomes and patient recovery.

Methods of disability limitation include therapy, which seeks to undo or reduce the threat or damage from an existing disease, and symptomatic stage prevention, which attempts to halt or limit progression of disease. The strategies of symptomatic stage prevention are taken from primary prevention (modification of diet, behavior, and environment) and secondary prevention (frequent screening for complications, treatment for complications). The effective management of chronic diseases, such as coronary artery disease, dyslipidemia, hypertension, and diabetes mellitus, requires a combination of therapy and symptomatic stage prevention. This approach also can be used in the management of many other diseases, including stroke, chronic obstructive pulmonary disease, arthritis, and some cancers and infectious diseases.

Rehabilitation should begin in the early stages of treatment. Depending on the needs of the patient, the rehabilitation team may include a rehabilitation counselor; physical therapist; speech therapist; occupational therapist; and psychiatric, emotional, or spiritual counselor. Under most state laws governing workers' compensation, several categories of job-related illnesses or injuries are recognized: permanent total disability, permanent partial disability, temporary total disability, temporary partial disability, and death. The goal of rehabilitation for workers, whether their impairment is temporary or permanent, is to minimize the social and occupational consequences of the impairment.

Although it might seem that the opportunity for prevention is lost when a disease appears or an injury occurs, this is often not the case. The appearance of symptoms or the threat of severe complications may lead patients to take an active interest in their health status, seek the health care that they need, and make positive changes in their environment, diet, and lifestyle.

References

1. Petrie KJ, Jago LA, Devcich DA: The role of illness perceptions in patients with medical conditions. *Curr Opin Psychiatry* 20:163–167, 2007.
2. Giri P, Poole J, Nightingale P, et al: Perceptions of illness and their impact on sickness absence. *Occup Med* 59:550–555, 2009.

3. Keogh KM, Smith SM, White P, et al: Psychological family intervention for poorly controlled type 2 diabetes. *Am J Managed Care* 17:105–113, 2011.

4. Goulding L, Furze G, Birks Y: Randomized controlled trials of interventions to change maladaptive illness beliefs in people with coronary heart disease: systematic review. *J Adv Nurs* 66:946–961, 2010.

5. Haffner SM, Lehto S, Ronnemaa T, et al: Mortality from coronary heart disease in subjects with type 2 diabetes and in non-diabetic subjects with and without prior myocardial infarction *N Engl J Med* 339:229–234, 1998.

6. Bulugahapitiya U, Siyambalapitiya S, Sithole J, et al: Is diabetes a coronary risk equivalent? Systematic review and meta-analysis, *Diabet Med* 26:142–148, 2009.

7. Breslow L: Risk factor intervention for health maintenance. *Science* 200:908–912, 1978.

8. Dawber TR, Meadors GF, Moore FE Jr: Epidemiologic approaches to heart disease: the Framingham Study. *Am J Public Health* 41:279–286, 1951.

9. Healy GN, Matthews CE, Dunstan DW, et al: Sedentary time and cardio-metabolic biomarkers in U.S. adults: NHANES 2003–06. *Eur Heart J* 32:590–597, 2011.

10. Lissner L, Odell PM, D'Agostino RB, et al: Variability of body weight and health outcomes in the Framingham population. *N Engl J Med* 324:1839–1844, 1991.

11. Wing RR, Jeffery RW, Hellerstedt WL: A prospective study of effects of weight cycling on cardiovascular risk factors. *Arch Intern Med* 155:1416–1422, 1995.

12. Gotto AM, Pownall HJ: *Manual of lipid disorders*, ed 3, Baltimore, 2002, Williams & Wilkins.

13. Sumithran P, Prendergast LA, Delbridge E, et al: Long-term persistence of hormonal adaptations to weight loss. *N Engl J Med* 365:1597–1604, 2011.

14. Cereda E, Malavazos AE, Caccialanza R, et al: Weight cycling is associated with body weight excess and abdominal fat accumulation: a cross-sectional study. *Clin Nutr* 30:718–723, 2011.

15. Taing KY, Ardern CI, Kuk JL: Effect of the timing of weight cycling during adulthood on mortality risk in overweight and obese postmenopausal women. *Obesity* (Silver Spring) 20:407–413, 2012.

16. Strohacker K, McFarlin BK: Influence of obesity, physical inactivity, and weight cycling on chronic inflammation. *Front Biosci* (elite ed) 2:98–104, 2010.

17. Field AE, Malspeis S, Willett WC: Weight cycling and mortality among middle-aged or older women. *Arch Intern Med* 169:881–886, 2009.

18. National Cholesterol Education Program: Executive summary of the third report of the NCEP Expert Panel on Detection, Evaluation, and Treatment of High Blood Cholesterol in Adults (Adult Treatment Panel III). *JAMA* 285:2486–2497, 2001.

19. http://www.nhlbi.nih.gov/guidelines/cvd_adult/background.htm.

20. Frick MH, Elo O, Haapa K, et al: Helsinki Heart Study: primary prevention trial with gemfibrozil in middle-aged men with dyslipidemia. *N Engl J Med* 317:1237–1245, 1987.

21. Arntzenius AC, Kromhout D, Barth JD, et al: Diet, lipoproteins, and the progression of coronary atherosclerosis: the Leiden Intervention Trial. *N Engl J Med* 312:805–811, 1985.

22. Smulders YV, Blom HJ: The homocysteine controversy. *J Inherit Metab Dis* 34:93–99, 2011.

23. Mei W, Rong Y, Jinming L, et al: Effect of homocysteine interventions on the risk of cardiocerebrovascular events: a meta-analysis of randomised controlled trials. *Int J Clin Pract* 64:208–215, 2010.

24. National Institutes of Health, National Heart, Lung, and Blood Institute: The Seventh Report of the Joint National Committee on Prevention, Detection, Evaluation, and Treatment of High Blood Pressure 2003; http://www.nhlbi.nih.gov/guidelines/hypertension.

25. Ong KL, Cheung BMY, Man YB, et al: Prevalence, awareness, treatment, and control of hypertension among United States adults, 1999–2004. *Hypertension* 49:69–75, 2007.

26. Svetkey LP, Sacks FM, Obarzanek E, et al: The DASH diet, sodium intake, and blood pressure trial (DASH-sodium): rationale and design. *J Am Diet Assoc* 99(suppl 8):96–104, 1999.

27. Yusuf S, Sleight P, Pogue J, et al: Effects of an angiotensin-converting enzyme inhibitor, ramipril, on cardiovascular events in high-risk patients. *N Engl J Med* 342:145–153, 2000.

28. Bangalore S, Sawhney S, Messerli FH: Relation of beta-blocker-induced heart rate lowering and cardioprotection in hypertension. *J Am Coll Cardiol* 52:1482–1489, 2008.

29. Carlberg B, Samuelsson O, Lindholm LH: Atenolol in hypertension: is it a wise choice? *Lancet* 364(9446):1684–1689, 2004.

30. US Centers for Disease Control and Prevention: Chronic disease prevention and health prevention: diabetes successes and opportunities for population-based prevention and control at a glance, 2011. http://www.cdc.gov/chronicdisease/resources/publications/AAG/ddt.htm.

31. Diabetes Control and Complications Trial. DCCT Research Group. *N Engl J Med* 329:683–689, 1993.

32. Santiago JV: Lessons from the Diabetes Control and Complications Trial. *Diabetes* 42:1549–1554, 1993.

33. Stratton IM, Adler AL, Neil HA, et al: Association of glycaemia with macrovascular and microvascular complications of type II diabetes: prospective observational study. *BMJ* 321:405–412, 2000.

34. Hoerger TJ, Segel JE, Gregg EW, et al: Is glycemic control improving in U.S. adults? *Diabetes Care* 31:81–86, 2007.

35. Bennett WL, Maruthur NM, Singh S, et al: Comparative effectiveness and safety of medications for type 2 diabetes: an update including new drugs and 2-drug combinations. *Ann Intern Med* 154:602–613, 2011.

36. Piepoli MF, Corrà U, Benzer W, et al: Secondary prevention through cardiac rehabilitation: from knowledge to implementation. Cardiac Rehabilitation section of European Association for Cardiovascular Prevention and Rehabilitation. *Eur J Cardiovasc Prev Rehabil* 17:1–17, 2010.

37. Mead H, Andres E, Ramos C, et al: Barriers to effective self-management in cardiac patients: the patients' experience. *Patient Educ Counsel* 79:69–76, 2010.

38. Fishman A, Martinez F, Naunheim K, et al: A randomized trial comparing lung-volume-reduction surgery with medical therapy for severe emphysema. *N Engl J Med* 348:2059–2073, 2003.

39. Puhan MA, Gimeno-Santos E, Scharplatz M, et al: Pulmonary rehabilitation following exacerbations of chronic obstructive pulmonary disease. *Cochrane Database Syst Rev* (10):CD005305, 2011.

40. Spence RR, Heesch KC, Brown WJ: Exercise and cancer rehabilitation: a systematic review. *Cancer Treat Rev* 36:185–194, 2010.

41. LaDou J: *Occupational and environmental medicine*, ed 3, Stamford, Conn, 2004, Appleton & Lange.

Select Readings

Diabetes Control and Complications Trial. DCCT Research Group. *N Engl J Med* 329:683–689, 1993.

Franklin DJ: Cancer rehabilitation: challenges, approaches, and new directions. *Phys Med Rehabil Clin North Am* 18:899–924, 2007.

Gordon DL, Katz DL: Stealth health: how to sneak age-defying, disease-fighting habits into your life without really trying. Pleasantville, NY, Readers' Digest 2005. [Information for patients.]

Gotto AM, Pownall HJ: *Manual of lipid disorders*, ed 3, Baltimore, 2002, Williams & Wilkins.

Hypertension treatment guidelines: www.nhlbi.nih.gov/guidelines/hypertension.

Krumholz HM: *The expert guide to beating heart disease: what you absolutely must know*, New York, 2005, HarperCollins. [Information for patients.]

LaDou J: *Occupational and environmental medicine*, ed 3, Stamford, Conn, 2004, Appleton & Lange.

National Cholesterol Education Program: Executive summary of the third report of the NCEP Expert Panel on Detection, Evaluation, and Treatment of High Blood Cholesterol in Adults (Adult Treatment Panel III). *JAMA* 285:2486–2497, 2001.

National Institutes of Health, National Heart, Lung, and Blood Institute. The Seventh Report of the Joint National Committee on Prevention, Detection, Evaluation, and Treatment of High Blood Pressure, 2003.

Petrie KJ, Cameron LD, Ellis CJ, et al: Changing illness perceptions following myocardial infarction: an early intervention randomized controlled trial. *Psychosom Med* 20:580–586, 2002.

Petrie KJ, Jago LA, Devcich DA: The role of illness perceptions in patients with medical conditions. *Curr Opin Psychiatry* 20:163–167, 2007.

Websites

http://www.nhlbi.nih.gov/guidelines/hypertension [Joint National Committee on Prevention, Detection, Evaluation, and Treatment of High Blood Pressure (JNC 7).]

http://www.nhlbi.nih.gov/guidelines/cholesterol/index.htm [National Cholesterol Education Program.]

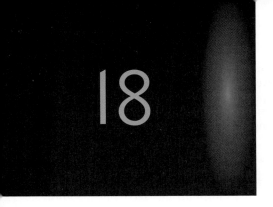

18

Clinical Preventive Services (United States Preventive Services Task Force)

In Chapter 16, we explored how screening is, in the most literal sense, "looking for trouble." Looking for trouble makes sense if, by finding it early, it can be fixed. But if you don't know what to do with the trouble you find, you are no longer just looking for trouble, you are *asking* for it.[1] The credibility of preventive medicine depends on the following two goals:

■ Screening is only done if it meets rigorous standards.
■ The screening test can realistically be integrated in the busy practice of *all* clinicians.

I. UNITED STATES PREVENTIVE SERVICES TASK FORCE

The U.S. Preventive Services Task Force (USPSTF) was founded in 1984 to address these goals. This chapter focuses on why its work is important and how busy clinicians can keep up-to-date with and incorporate the Task Force's recommendations. Recommendations for clinical preventive services change frequently with emerging evidence. For more details and updated recommendations, readers should consult USPSTF online (see Website list at end of chapter).

A. Mission and History

When the USPSTF was first convened by the U.S. Public Health Service in 1984, it was modeled on an earlier Canadian task force to serve as an independent panel of experts on prevention and evidence-based medicine (EBM). Since 1995, the Task Force has worked under the **Agency of Healthcare Research and Quality** (AHRQ). It covers all primary and secondary preventive services, including screening, counseling, and specific chemoprophylaxis.[2] The Task Force aims to provide accurate and balanced recommendations across a spectrum of populations, types of services, and disease types. Its mission is to:

1. Assess the benefits and harm of delivering preventive services to asymptomatic individuals (based on age, gender, and risk factors).
2. Recommend which services should be incorporated into primary care.

This mission is very circumscribed. The USPSTF only considers screening of **asymptomatic** patients, and it only deals with preventive services within **primary care.** Often, however, USPSTF recommendations are criticized by specialist organizations. Specialists may primarily see preselected patients with subtler symptoms that were missed earlier or may see high-risk groups. Screening decisions for such patients may be different from those for the general population, because the pretest probability of disease is much higher. On the other hand, recommendations of USPSTF are sometimes used for insurance decisions about which screening tests to cover. In these cases, recommendations may be more broadly applied than intended. In contrast to the Community Preventive Services Guide (see Chapter 26), the USPSTF does not take cost-effectiveness or financial concerns into consideration.

When the USPSTF was founded, its principles were revolutionary: that preventive care should be rigorously evaluated, and that not every screening test was worth doing. In its history, USPSTF has often recommended against or failed to endorse screening tests that were recommended by other organizations. The reason for this reluctance to endorse some interventions may be based on several assumptions of the Task Force.

B. Underlying Assumptions

As outlined in Chapter 16, screening studies are subject to many biases that lead researchers to **overestimate benefits.** Therefore the Task Force places a higher burden of evidence for benefits than for evidence of harm. For benefits, USPSTF will only accept evidence from randomized controlled trials (RCTs), community trials, meta-analyses, or systematic reviews. However, it will take into account evidence of cohort studies and case-control studies in calculations of harm.

Prevention studies describe the **upper bounds of efficacy.** In other words, controlled trials describe a best-case scenario with well-trained and highly motivated providers and patients. The Task Force assumes that in the real world, with unselected providers and in the general population, the effectiveness of a screening program will be lower.

Delivery of a screening service is not an outcome. Diagnosis of a disease also is not an outcome. Therefore the benefit of a screening program lies not in the number of patients screened or the number of patients diagnosed with disease, but only in the health outcomes. **Health outcomes** are changes in a patient's health or health perception, such as pain, shortness of breath, or death. In contrast to health outcomes, **intermediate outcomes** are measurements of pathology or physiology that can lead to health outcomes (e.g., high blood pressure). USPSTF will give no weight to evidence of number of screening events or cases found, and it gives greater weight to studies of health outcomes than to those of intermediate outcomes.

Because the standard for evidence is so high, USPSTF may wait longer than other organizations before endorsing screening modalities, as with lung cancer screening using helical computed tomography (CT). The number of patient lives potentially saved must be weighed against the risk of subjecting healthy patients to potentially harmful screening tests. With this tension and when in doubt, the Task Force seems to prefer being late to being wrong.

C. Evidence Review and Recommendations

Developing a recommendation is a two-part process: reviewing the evidence and formulating recommendations. Although the Task Force itself makes the recommendations, independent centers review the evidence. USPSTF has established 12 such **evidence-based practice centers** (EPCs).[3] The literature review and recommendation process is highly structured and includes various steps to safeguard the Task Force's integrity and to help it pursue its goals of transparency, accountability, consistency, and independence[4] (Table 18-1). Safeguards include stringent criteria for selection of members, stringent policies regarding conflict of interest, dual review of each abstract, and a comment period for community partners and the public.

CRITICAL APPRAISAL QUESTIONS

- Do the studies have the appropriate research design to answer the key questions?
- What is the internal validity?
- What is the external validity?

Table 18-1 Procedures for Developing a Recommendation Statement

Activity*	Responsible Parties	Timeline
Topic selection	Topic Prioritization Workgroup, a subset of Task Force members and AHRQ and EPC staff	The Workgroup meets periodically throughout the year.
Work plan development	The EPC writes work plans with guidance from a topic team consisting of 3 or 4 USPSTF members and a medical officer from AHRQ.	From start to finish, these activities—development, peer review, and approval—take 3-6 months.
External work plan peer review	Work plans are reviewed by experts in the field.	
Approval of peer-reviewed work plan†	All members of USPSTF	
Draft evidence report	Evidence reports are written by EPC or by AHRQ medical officers, depending on topic.	Typically completed within 6-24 months, depending on the scope of the topic.
Peer review of draft evidence report by experts and partners	All draft evidence reports are sent to limited number of experts in the field and 6 federal partners‡ for review, and Task Force leaders are asked to comment on draft evidence report.	
Draft recommendation statement	Task Force members draft recommendation statement with AHRQ medical officer.	Completed within 2-4 weeks.
USPSTF review of evidence and vote on draft recommendation statement	All members of USPSTF	
Final evidence report	EPC and AHRQ medical officer incorporate reviewer comments and finalize evidence report.	Submitted to AHRQ within 3-6 months after USPSTF vote.
Peer review of draft recommendation statement by partners	22 partners of USPSTF	Partners typically have 2-3 weeks to review draft recommendation statement.
Approval of final recommendation statement	Task Force members	USPSTF members typically approve recommendation statement as final within 1-2 months.
Release of recommendation statement and evidence report	AHRQ staff	Time from vote to release (publication in journal and posting on website) of the recommendation varies.

Modified from Guirguis-Blake J: *Ann Intern Med* 147:117–121, 2007.
*Listed in order starting with the initial step.
†This step usually occurs at a Task Force meeting, although in the case of topic updates, work plan peer review and Task Force approval are exceptional rather than usual.
‡Centers for Disease Control and Prevention, Centers for Medicare and Medicaid Services, Food and Drug Administration, Indian Health Service, National Institutes of Health, and Veterans Administration.
AHRQ, Agency for Healthcare Research and Quality; *EPC,* evidence-based practice center; *USPSTF,* U.S. Preventive Services Task Force.

- How many studies have been conducted that address the key question, and how large are the studies?
- How consistent are the results?
- Are there additional factors that raise confidence in the results (e.g., dose-response effects, consistency with biologic models)?

TASK FORCE MEMBERS

Sixteen members serve on the Task Force at any given time. About 25% of USPSTF members are replaced each year. Members are nominated in a public process and are chosen based on their expertise in the subject matter, research methods, disease prevention, application of synthesized evidence to clinical decision making, and clinical expertise in primary health care. They are chosen through a rigorous process and serve staggered 4-year terms on the committee.

KEY QUESTIONS

Once an evidence review is complete, USPSTF members vote on the eight key questions that determine if screening for a condition X is recommended:

1. Does screening for X reduce morbidity and/or mortality?
2. Can a group at high risk for X be identified on clinical grounds?
3. Are accurate screening tests available?
4. Are treatments available that make a difference in intermediate outcomes when the disease is caught early?
5. Are treatments available that make a difference in morbidity and mortality (patient outcomes) when the disease is caught early?
6. How strong is the association between the intermediate outcomes and patient outcomes?
7. What are the harms of the screening test?
8. What are the harms of treatment?

GRADING SERVICES

Once Task Force members have answered these questions, the group assigns a grade for the service of A, B, C, D, or I[5] (Table 18-2). After assigning a tentative grade, the Task Force discusses these recommendations with federal and primary care partners. Federal partners include the Centers for Disease Control and Prevention (CDC), Center for Medicare and Medicaid Services (CMS), Health Resource and Services Administration (HRSA), National Institutes of Health (NIH), and Food and Drug Administration (FDA). Examples of primary care partners include the American Medical Association, American College of Physicians, and American College of Preventive Medicine.

The results of the evidence review and the Task Force recommendations are posted for comments by the partners and public, published in reputable journals, and disseminated on the Internet.

In clinical practice there is little difference between grade **A** and **B** recommendations; in both cases the service should be strongly encouraged. Services with grades of C, D, and I should not be routinely used. However, it is important to understand the difference between these grades. For grades A through D, USPSTF is reasonably certain it understands the balance of benefits and harm. For services graded **C,** there is a net benefit, but it is likely small. A service with a C recommendation is breast cancer screening for women younger than 50 (see Chapter 16). Decisions about these C services should be individualized. In contrast, for services graded **D,** there is clear evidence that there is *no* net benefit, or that there is net harm; an example is screening for ovarian cancer. These D services should be avoided.

For services with an **I** grade, evidence is lacking or conflicting, and the Task Force has determined that they can neither recommend for nor recommend against the service. As of 2012, services with an I grade include skin cancer screening, colorectal cancer screening with CT colonography,

Table 18-2 Grades Assigned to Screening Recommendation and Suggestions for Practice

Grade	Definition	Net Benefit?	Suggestions for Practice
A	USPSTF recommends the service.	High certainty for net benefit	Offer/provide this service.
B	USPSTF recommends the service.	At least moderate certainty for net benefit	Offer/provide this service.
C	USPSTF does not recommend routinely providing this service. Clinicians may choose to provide this service to select patients depending on individual circumstances. However, for most individuals without signs or symptoms, there is likely to be only a small benefit from this service.	At least moderate certainty that the net benefit is small	Offer/provide this service *only* if other considerations support the offering or providing the service in an individual patient.
D	USPSTF recommends against the service.	Moderate or high certainty of no benefit or net harm	Discourage the use of this service.
I	USPSTF concludes that the current evidence is insufficient to assess the balance of benefits and harms of the service. Evidence is lacking, of poor quality, or conflicting.	No certainty on balance of benefits/harms	Read Clinical Considerations section of USPSTF Recommendation Statement. If the service is offered, patients should understand the uncertainty about the balance of benefits and harms.

Modified from http://www.uspreventiveservicestaskforce.org/uspstf07/ratingsv2.htm.
USPSTF, U.S. Preventive Services Task Force.

and screening for lung cancer using helical CT.[6] These services require the most time to discuss, and patients and clinicians should engage in shared decision making to understand consequences of testing and of not testing, as well as the patient's risk preferences. Such shared decision making is not only time-consuming but also requires some sophisticated evaluation of trade-offs on both sides.

II. ECONOMICS OF PREVENTION

Attitudes towards preventive services vary. Some people believe that prevention must be a good in itself. Intuition suggests that finding problems early will make them easier to treat. Many political campaigns address the rising costs of health care by promising to spend more on prevention. On the other end of the spectrum are health economists, who argue that prevention rarely reduces costs and that preventive services should be used very selectively.[7]

A more balanced approach focuses on **value.** Health is a **public good.** We do not expect other public goods (e.g., clean water, national security) to save money. However, money spent on public goods should be spent wisely; we should try to obtain as much health as we can with every dollar spent.[8] In a setting of limited health care resources, monies for disease care *and* prevention should go toward those services that deliver the most health. Fortunately, the following core set of preventive services has proved highly effective[9]:

■ Screening for hypertension, dyslipidemia, obesity, colorectal and cervical cancer, and breast cancer in women over 50
■ Childhood and adult immunizations

■ Smoking cessation counseling
■ Use of aspirin in persons at high risk for cardiovascular disease

According to the National Commission on Prevention Priorities, 100,000 deaths could be averted each year by increasing delivery of five high-value clinical preventive services.[10] Increasing use of these services might be cost-neutral or even cost-saving.[11]

Table 18-3 provides one ranking of preventive services by considerations of cost-effectiveness. **Clinically preventable burden** (CPB) is the disease, injury, and premature death that would be prevented if the service were delivered to all people in the target population. **Cost effectiveness** (**CE**) is a standard measure for comparing services' return on investment. Services with the same total score tied in the rankings: 10 = highest impact, most cost-effective, and 2 = lowest impact, least cost-effective, among these evidence-based preventive services.

A. Overuse, Underuse, and Misuse of Screening

In clinical practice, it is difficult (1) to deliver all highly effective preventive services consistently, (2) to avoid the less effective ones, and (3) to deliver services only to patients who will derive benefit. This may be even more difficult with the ascendancy of "patient-centered care"; patients may have priorities driven by passions, convictions, anxieties, and marketing that conflict with evidence-based guidelines.

Strong evidence exists for underuse of highly effective services. In the landmark Community Quality Index study published in 2003, only 54.9% of patients received all recommended preventive services.[12] This is partially driven by

Table 18-3 Ranking of Preventive Services for U.S. Population

Clinical Preventive Services	CPB	CE	Total
Discuss daily aspirin use—men 40+, women 50+	5	5	
Childhood immunizations	5	5	10
Smoking cessation advice and help to quit—adults	5	5	
Alcohol screening and brief counseling—adults	4	5	9
Colorectal cancer screening—adults 50+	4	4	
Hypertension screening and treatment—adults 18+	5	3	
Influenza immunization—adults 50+	4	4	8
Vision screening—adults 65+	3	5	
Cervical cancer screening—women	4	3	7
Cholesterol screening and treatment—men 35+, women 45+	5	2	
Pneumococcal immunizations—adults 65+	3	4	
Breast cancer screening—women 40+	4	2	
Chlamydia screening—sexually active women under 25	2	4	
Discuss calcium supplementation—women	3	3	6
Vision screening—preschool children	2	4	
Discuss folic acid use—women of childbearing age	2	3	5
Obesity screening—adults	3	2	
Depression screening—adults	3	1	
Hearing screening—adults 65+	2	2	
Injury prevention counseling—parents of children ages 0-4	1	3	4
Osteoporosis screening—women 65+	2	2	
Cholesterol screening—men < 35, women < 45 at high risk	1	1	
Diabetes screening—adults at risk	1	1	2
Diet counseling—adults at risk	1	1	
Tetanus-diphtheria booster—adults	1	1	

Modified from http://www.prevent.org/National-Commission-on-Prevention-Priorities/Rankings-of-Preventive-Services-for-the-US-Population.aspx.
CPB, Clinically preventable burden; *CE,* cost-effectiveness.

reimbursement; Medicare pays for 93% of recommended preventive services for adults, but the required counseling and coordination are mostly unreimbursed.[13] In a typical clinical practice, urgent problems and symptomatic conditions can easily supersede conversations about health maintenance.[14]

The Task Force recommends that clinicians track delivery of all services with an A or a B grade for every patient to ensure that all patients receive these services. Many electronic health records feature reminders at the point of care to help providers integrate preventive services. Alternatively, and for paper charts, an assistant can check if the patient is due for recommended services and can prepare screening test requisitions in advance. In either case, the time required is considerable. Some authors estimate it would take 7.4 hours per workday just to incorporate all recommended services into primary care.[15] This problem might prove intractable until the implementation of more innovative care models that link payments to long-term outcomes and thereby make prevention an efficient use of practice time (see Chapter 29, Cost Containment Strategies).

However, the problem is not only lack of time and reimbursement. Strong evidence also exists for overuse and misuse of screening services. Medicare reimburses physicians for 44% of services that have a D rating from the Task Force.[13] A large proportion of Medicare patients undergo screening colonoscopies more frequently than recommended.[16] Screening is overused in elderly patients and patients in poor health and at the end of life,[17,18] who are unlikely to benefit from screening. The challenge for clinicians is therefore twofold: (1) find more efficient ways to deliver preventive services to patients who need them and (2) discuss goals of care and expected benefits of screening with patients who are unlikely to benefit. This will probably require rethinking the delivery of care. No one provider can provide the array of preventive services and counseling necessary in a series of brief, one-on-one encounters. The solution may lie in a team-based model, such as the chronic care model[19] (see Chapter 28).

It is even more difficult to have a meaningful conversation about services that depend on patient preferences for risk, such as those graded C (and some graded B, such as chemoprevention of breast cancer), or services with conflicting evidence (graded I). Many patients strongly demand services based on anecdotal evidence from friends, family members, or the media. For these services, the Task Force recommends community education, use of shared decision-making aids, and trained assistants.[20] However, such a sophisticated and personnel-intensive approach is probably not feasible for many primary care providers.

III. MAJOR RECOMMENDATIONS

A. Highly Recommended Services

Table 18-4 lists preventive services that have a rating of A or B from USPSTF. Recommended services are skewed toward screening: About 25 screening services are recommended, versus seven counseling services and seven chemoprevention

Table 18-4 Recommended Preventive Health Care Screening Services

Topic	Recommendation	Grade	Date in Effect
Abdominal aortic aneurysm screening: men	One-time screening for abdominal aortic aneurysm by ultrasonography in men age 65-75 who have ever smoked.	B	February 2005
Alcohol misuse counseling	Screening and behavioral counseling interventions to reduce alcohol misuse by adults, including pregnant women, in primary care settings.	B	April 2004
Anemia screening: pregnant women	Routine screening for iron deficiency anemia in asymptomatic pregnant women.	B	May 2006
Aspirin to prevent cardiovascular disease: men	Use of aspirin in men age 45-79 when potential benefit of reduction in myocardial infarctions outweighs potential harm of increase in gastrointestinal hemorrhage.	A	March 2009
Aspirin to prevent cardiovascular disease: women	Use of aspirin in women age 55-79 when potential benefit of reduction in ischemic strokes outweighs potential harm of increase in gastrointestinal hemorrhage.	A	March 2009
Bacteriuria screening: pregnant women	Screening for asymptomatic bacteriuria with urine culture for pregnant women at 12-16 weeks' gestation or at first prenatal visit, if later.	A	July 2008
Blood pressure screening: adults	Screening for high blood pressure in adults age 18 or older.	A	December 2007
BRCA screening, counseling about	Refer women whose family history is associated with increased risk for deleterious mutations in *BRCA1* or *BRCA2* genes for genetic counseling and evaluation for *BRCA* testing.	B	September 2005
Breast cancer–preventive medication	Discuss chemoprevention with women at high risk for breast cancer and at low risk for adverse effects of chemoprevention. Clinicians should inform patients of potential benefits and harms of chemoprevention.	B	July 2002
Breast cancer screening	Screening mammography for women, with or without clinical breast examination, every 1-2 years for women age 50-75 or older.	B	December 2009*
	Individualize decision to start mammography earlier than age 50.	C	December 2009
Breastfeeding counseling	Use interventions during pregnancy and after birth to promote and support breastfeeding.	B	October 2008

Continued

Table 18-4 **Recommended Preventive Health Care Screening Services—cont'd**

Topic	Recommendation	Grade	Date in Effect
Cervical cancer screening	Screening for cervical cancer in women who have been sexually active and have a cervix age 21-64.	A	March 2012
Chlamydial infection screening: nonpregnant women	Screening for chlamydial infection for all sexually active nonpregnant young women age 24 or younger and for older nonpregnant women at increased risk.	A	June 2007
Chlamydial infection screening: pregnant women	Screening for chlamydial infection for all pregnant women age 24 or younger and for older pregnant women at increased risk.	B	June 2007
Cholesterol abnormalities screening: men ≥35	Screening men age 35 or older for lipid disorders.	A	June 2008
Cholesterol abnormalities screening: men <35	Screening men age 20-35 for lipid disorders if at increased risk for coronary heart disease.	B	June 2008
Cholesterol abnormalities screening: women ≥45	Screening women age 45 or older for lipid disorders if at increased risk for coronary heart disease.	A	June 2008
Cholesterol abnormalities screening: women <45	Screening women age 20-45 for lipid disorders if at increased risk for coronary heart disease.	B	June 2008
Colorectal cancer screening	Screening for colorectal cancer using fecal occult blood testing, sigmoidoscopy, or colonoscopy, in adults, beginning at age 50 and continuing until age 75. Risks and benefits of these screening methods vary.	A	October 2008
Dental caries chemoprevention: preschool children	Prescribe oral fluoride supplementation at currently recommended doses to preschool children older than 6 months whose primary water source is deficient in fluoride.	B	April 2004
Depression screening: adolescents	Screening of adolescents (age 12-18) for major depressive disorder when systems are in place to ensure accurate diagnosis, psychotherapy (cognitive-behavioral or interpersonal), and follow-up.	B	March 2009
Depression screening: adults	Screening adults for depression when staff-assisted depression care supports are in place to ensure accurate diagnosis, effective treatment, and follow-up.	B	December 2009
Diabetes screening	Screening for type 2 diabetes in asymptomatic adults with sustained blood pressure (either treated or untreated) >135/80 mm Hg.	B	June 2008
Fall prevention in adults at risk for falls	Exercise, physical therapy, and Vitamin D supplementation	B	May 2012
Folic acid supplementation	Recommend daily supplement containing 0.4-0.8 mg (400-800 μg) of folic acid to all women planning or capable of pregnancy.	A	May 2009
Gonorrhea prophylactic medication: newborns	Prophylactic ocular topical medication for all newborns against gonococcal ophthalmia neonatorum.	A	July 2011
Gonorrhea screening: women	Screen all sexually active women, including those who are pregnant, for gonorrhea infection if at increased risk for infection (i.e., if young or with other individual or population risk factors).	B	May 2005
Healthy-diet counseling	Intensive behavioral dietary counseling for adult patients with hyperlipidemia and other known risk factors for cardiovascular and diet-related chronic disease. Intensive counseling can be delivered by primary care clinicians or by referral to other specialists, such as nutritionists or dietitians.	B	January 2003
Hearing loss screening: newborns	Screening for hearing loss in all newborn infants.	B	July 2008
HBV screening: pregnant women	Screening for hepatitis B virus infection in pregnant women at first prenatal visit.	A	June 2009
Hemoglobinopathies screening: newborns	Screening for sickle cell disease in newborns.	A	September 2007
HIV screening	Screen for human immunodeficiency virus in all adolescents and adults at increased risk for HIV infection.	A	July 2005
Hypothyroidism screening: newborns	Screening for congenital hypothyroidism in newborns.	A	March 2008
Iron supplementation: children	Routine iron supplementation for asymptomatic children age 6-12 months at increased risk for iron deficiency anemia.	B	May 2006
Obesity screening and counseling: adults	Screen all adult patients for obesity and offer intensive counseling and behavioral interventions to promote sustained weight loss for adults with BMI >30.	B	September 2012
Obesity screening and counseling: children	Screen children age 6 years or older for obesity and offer (or refer for) comprehensive, intensive behavioral interventions to improve weight status.	B	January 2010
Osteoporosis screening: women	Screening for osteoporosis in women age 65 years or older and in younger women whose fracture risk equals or exceeds that of 65-year-old white woman who has no additional risk factors.	B	September 2011
PKU screening: newborns	Screening for phenylketonuria in newborns.	A	March 2008

Table 18-4 **Recommended Preventive Health Care Screening Services—cont'd**

Topic	Recommendation	Grade	Date in Effect
Rh incompatibility screening: first pregnancy visit	Rh (D) blood typing and antibody testing for all pregnant women during first visit for pregnancy-related care.	A	February 2004
Rh incompatibility screening: 24-28 weeks' gestation	Repeated Rh (D) antibody testing for all unsensitized Rh (D)-negative women at 24-28 weeks' gestation, unless biologic father known to be Rh (D)–negative.	B	February 2004
Sexually transmitted infections (STIs) counseling	High-intensity behavioral counseling to prevent STIs in all sexually active adolescents and in adults at increased risk for STIs.	B	October 2008
Syphilis screening: nonpregnant women	Screen nonpregnant women/persons at increased risk for syphilis infection.	A	July 2004
Syphilis screening: pregnant women	Screen all pregnant women for syphilis infection.	A	May 2009
Tobacco use counseling and interventions: nonpregnant women	Ask all nonpregnant women/adults about tobacco use, and provide tobacco cessation interventions for those who use tobacco products.	A	April 2009
Tobacco use counseling: pregnant women	Ask all pregnant women about tobacco use, and provide augmented, pregnancy-tailored counseling to those who smoke.	A	April 2009
Visual acuity screening: children	Screening to detect amblyopia, strabismus, and defects in visual acuity in children age 3-5 years.	B	January 2011

Modified from U.S. Preventive Services Task Force A and B Recommendations, March 2012. http://www.uspreventiveservicestaskforce.org/uspstf/uspsabrecs.
*In 2009 the recommendations on screening have substantially changed, particularly in regard to women ages 40 to 50 and over 75 (see Chapter 16).

Table 18-5 **Recommended Screening Tests for Women**

Screening	Ages 18-39	Ages 40-49	Ages 50-64	Age 65 and older
Blood pressure (BP) test	At least every 2 years if normal BP (<120/80 mm Hg) Once a year if BP between 120/80 and 139/89 Discuss treatment with physician or nurse if BP 140/90 or higher.	At least every 2 years if normal BP (<120/80 mm Hg) Once a year if BP between 120/80 and 139/89 Discuss treatment with physician or nurse if BP 140/90 or higher.	At least every 2 years if normal BP (<120/80 mm Hg) Once a year if BP between 120/80 and 139/89 Discuss treatment with physician or nurse if BP 140/90 or higher. Discuss with physician or nurse if you think you are at risk of osteoporosis.	At least every 2 years if normal BP (<120/80 mm Hg) Once a year if BP between 120/80 and 139/89 Discuss treatment with physician or nurse if BP 140/90 or higher.
Bone mineral density test (osteoporosis screening)				At least once at age 65 or older Talk to physician or nurse about repeat testing.
Breast cancer screening (mammogram)		Discuss with physician or nurse.	Starting at age 50, every 2 years	Every 2 years through age 74. Age 75 and older, ask physician or nurse if needed.
Cervical cancer screening: Pap test	At least every 3 years if ≥21, or <21 and sexually active for at least 3 years	At least every 3 years	At least every 3 years	Ask physician or nurse if you need Pap test.
Chlamydia test	Yearly through age 24 if sexually active or pregnant Age ≥25 if at increased risk, pregnant, or not pregnant	If sexually active and at increased risk, pregnant, or not pregnant	If sexually active and at increased risk	If sexually active and at increased risk
Cholesterol test	Starting at age 20, regularly if at increased risk for heart disease Ask physician or nurse how often you need testing.	Regularly if at increased risk for heart disease Ask physician or nurse how often you need testing.	Regularly if at increased risk for heart disease Ask physician or nurse how often you need testing.	Regularly if at increased risk for heart disease Ask physician or nurse how often you need testing.

Data from http://www.womenshealth.gov/publications/our-publications/screening-tests-for-women.pdf.

interventions. Some counseling topics that may have a bearing on health, such as firearm safety and partner violence, are missing because of lack of evidence; other issues, such as healthy-diet counseling, are restricted to high-risk groups. This imbalance of recommended services may reflect that a few healthy lifestyle choices (diet, exercise, not smoking) have an impact on many different diseases. It might also reflect which prevention research is funded or the difficulties involved with effective counseling.

In practice, it might be easier to follow a listing of services by age and gender (Tables 18-5 and 18-6). For screening of children, see Websites list at end of chapter.

Table 18-6 Recommended Screening Tests for Men

Screening	Ages 18-39	Ages 40-49	Ages 50-64	Age 65 and Older
Abdominal aortic aneurysm screening				Have this one-time screening if age 65-75 and ever smoked.
Blood pressure (BP) test	At least every 2 years if normal BP (<120/80 mm Hg) Once a year if BP between 120/80 and 139/89 Discuss treatment with physician or nurse if BP 140/90 or higher.	At least every 2 years if normal BP (<120/80 mm Hg) Once a year if BP between 120/80 and 139/89 Discuss treatment with physician or nurse if BP 140/90 or higher.	At least every 2 years if normal BP (<120/80 mm Hg) Once a year if BP between 120/80 and 139/89 Discuss treatment with physician or nurse if BP 140/90 or higher.	At least every 2 years if normal BP (<120/80 mm Hg) Once a year if BP between 120/80 and 139/89 Discuss treatment with physician or nurse if BP 140/90 or higher.
Cholesterol test	Starting at age 20 until age 35, if at increased risk for heart disease At age 35 and older, regularly Ask physician or nurse how often you need testing.	Regularly Ask physician or nurse how often you need testing.	Regularly Ask physician or nurse how often you need testing.	Regularly Ask physician or nurse how often you need testing.
Colorectal cancer screening (fecal occult blood testing, sigmoidoscopy, or colonoscopy)			Starting at age 50 Talk to physician or nurse about which screening test is best for you and how often you need it.	Through age 75 Talk to physician or nurse about which screening test is best for you and how often you need it.
Diabetes screening	If BP higher than 135/80 mm Hg or if taking medicine for high BP	If BP higher than 135/80 mm Hg or if taking medicine for high BP	If BP higher than 135/80 mm Hg or if taking medicine for high BP	If BP is higher than 135/80 mm Hg or if taking medicine for high BP
Human immunodeficiency virus (HIV) test	If at increased risk for HIV infection Discuss your risk with physician or nurse.	If at increased risk for HIV infection Discuss your risk with physician or nurse.	If at increased risk for HIV infection Discuss your risk with physician or nurse.	If at increased risk for HIV infection Discuss your risk with physician or nurse.
Syphilis screening	If at increased risk	If at increased risk	If at increased risk	If at increased risk

Data from http://www.womenshealth.gov/screening-tests-and-vaccines/screening-tests-for-men/.

B. Limits of Evidence

One important aspect of Task Force recommendations is that they can be, and often are, *noncommittal*. When evidence is lacking or inconsistent, the Task Force may conclude that neither a recommendation for nor a recommendation against a practice is justified. This has two important implications. First, judgment remains a vital element in clinical practice even in the EBM era. Although it may be reasonable to recommend neither for nor against a practice in general, a given patient will either receive or not receive a service. At the individual level, even the failure to make a decision proves to be a decision. Consequently, many topics addressed by the Task Force revert to a process of dialogue and shared decision making between clinician and patient. Such decisions are influenced by individual priorities, preferences, and at times economics; practices not formally recommended may not be routinely covered by third-party payers.

The second implication of USPSTF's noncommittal approach is that "no evidence of benefit" is not the same as "evidence of no benefit." A practice that may ultimately prove to be of decisive benefit may not be recommended because the relevant evidence has not yet accrued (see Box 16-2). The same is true of a practice that may ultimately prove to confer net harm. Practice must evolve in tandem with an evolving base of evidence.

C. Clinical Preventive Service Compliance

One of the important themes to develop recently in the field of clinical preventive service delivery is that compliance should not be measured for a given service, but rather for the "bundle of services" recommended for an individual based on age and gender. Several such "bundled metrics" have been proposed, based on Behavioral Risk Factor Surveillance System (BRFSS) data[21] or computerized records.[22] Such packaging of metrics (1) improves accountability, raising the bar for performance, and (2) directs the focus to underserved patients, because the metric only improves if most patients receive all services. For this reason, a packaged measure of up-to-date preventive services has recently been added to the *Healthy People 2020* indicators.[21]

STAYING CURRENT

The USPSTF offers many ways in which providers can stay current and access recommendations at the point of care. These include a pocket guide to the preventive services, an

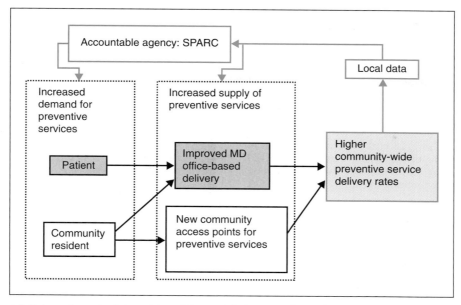

Figure 18-1 SPARC model. Sickness Prevention Achieved through Regional Collaboration (SPARC) for delivery of preventive services. (From Shenson D, Benson W, Harris AC: *Prev Chronic Dis* l5:1–8, 2008.)

electronic preventive services selector based on age and gender of patients, and a subscription to e-mail updates from the Task Force.[23]

IV. COMMUNITY-BASED PREVENTION

Despite many efforts among primary care providers, preventive services continue to be underused, and disparities in access to screening persist. Since many preventive services are *portable*, they can be delivered in a community setting as well as in a physician's office.[24] The CDC recommends linking community and clinical strategies, particularly those that focus on underserved populations.[25,26] Some states have experimented with combining linkage to community services, with enhanced reimbursement for preventive services and use of intensively trained clinical and process coaches.[27]

One way to expand prevention outside the physician's office is **community collaboration**. Historically, preventive medicine has focused on the physician as the main point of delivering preventive services.[27] However, other models are possible. For example, in the Sickness Prevention Achieved through Regional Collaboration (SPARC) model, public health agencies, hospitals, and social service organizations collaborate to integrate preventive services into other community events, such as polling stations on election day or the delivery of meals on wheels (Fig. 18-1). This approach has been used successfully to increase rates of vaccination for influenza, pneumococcus, hepatitis B, and tetanus, as well as to increase screening for colorectal cancer and mammography.[28] This model encourages accountability at the community level for delivery of preventive services. Although there is little downside to increasing the use of vaccinations, community collaboration also is not without challenges: The increase of screening rates through such programs likely carries the same problems of overuse and misuse as can occur through a physician's office (see Chapter 16).

V. SUMMARY

The U.S. Preventive Services Task Force follows a rigorous process to assess the benefits and harm of delivering preventive services to asymptomatic individuals. Five letter grades summarize the evidence for net benefits or harm for services, including chemoprevention, counseling, and screening:

A—High certainty the service is beneficial.
B—Moderate certainty service is beneficial.
C—At least moderate certainty that net benefit is small.
D—At least moderate certainty of no net benefit or net harm.
I—Evidence is lacking or conflicting.

In clinical practice, screening tests are underused, overused, and misused. Considerable clinical judgment is required in the delivery of many clinical preventive services for which evidence remains equivocal. Providers need to deliver all recommended services consistently. For services with lower grades, clinicians should engage patients in meaningful conversations about the evidence and their risk preferences. This will likely require major restructuring of care delivery and innovative models of community-based prevention.

References

1. Katz DL: PSA: please stop asking (for trouble), Huffington Post, 2011. http://www.huffingtonpost.com/david-katz-md/psa-testing_b_1000852.html.
2. US Preventive Services Task Force: *Procedure manual*, AHRQ Pub No 08-05118-EF, 2008, Agency for Healthcare Research and Quality.
3. US Preventive Services Task Force: Methods and process. http://www.uspreventiveservicestaskforce.org/methods.htm on 1/2/2011.
4. Guirguis-Blake J: Current processes of the U.S. Preventive Services Task Force: refining evidence-based recommendation development. *Ann Intern Med* 147:117–121, 2007.

5. Barton MB, Miller T, Wolff T, et al: How to read the new recommendation statement: methods update from the U.S. Preventive Services Task Force. *Ann Intern Med* 147:123–127, 2007.

6. Petitti D, Teutsch SM, Barton MB, et al: Update on the methods of the U.S. Preventive Services Task Force: insufficient evidence. *Ann Intern Med* 150:199–205, 2009.

7. Russell LB: Preventing chronic disease: an important investment, but don't count on cost savings. *Health Affairs* 28:42–45, 2009.

8. Woolf SH, Husten CG, Lewin LS, et al: The economic argument for disease prevention: distinguishing between value and savings. Partnership for Prevention. http://www.prevent.org/data/files/initiatives/economicargumentfordiseaseprevention.pdf.

9. Maciosek MV, Coffield AB, Edwards NM, et al: Priorities among effective clinical preventive services: results of a systematic review and analysis. *Am J Prev Med* 31:52–61, 2006.

10. National Commission on Prevention Priorities. *Preventive care: a national profile on use, disparities, and health benefits*, Washington, DC, 2007, Partnership for Prevention.

11. Maciosek MV, Coffield AB, Flottemesch TJ, et al: Greater use of preventive services in U.S. health care could save lives at little or no cost. *Health Affairs* 29:1656–1660, 2010.

12. McGlynn EA, Asch SM, Adams J, et al: The quality of care delivered to adults in the United States. *N Engl J Med* 348:2635–2645, 2003.

13. Lesser LI, Krist AH, Kamerow DB, et al: Comparison between U.S. Preventive Services Task Force recommendations and Medicare coverage. *Ann Fam Med* 9:44–49, 2011.

14. Crabtree BF: Delivery of clinical preventive services in family medicine offices. *Ann Fam Med* 3:430–431, 2005.

15. Yarnall KSH: Primary care: is there enough time for prevention? *Am J Public Health* 93:635–641, 2003.

16. Goodwin JS, Singh A, Reddy N, et al: Overuse of screening colonoscopy in the Medicare population. *Arch Intern Med* 171:1335–1343, 2011.

17. Bellizzi KM, Breslau ES, Burness A, et al: Prevalence of cancer screening in older, racially diverse adults: still screening after all these years. *Arch Intern Med* 171:2031, 2011.

18. Sultan S: Colorectal cancer screening in young patients with poor health and severe comorbidity. *Arch Intern Med* 166:2209–2214, 2006.

19. Chronic care model. http://www.improvingchroniccare.org/index.php?p=the_chronic_care_model&s=2.

20. Sheridan SL, Harris RP, Woolf SH: Shared decision making about screening and chemoprevention: a suggested approach from the U.S. Preventive Services Task Force. *Am J Prev Med* 26:56–66, 2004.

21. Shenson D, Bolen J, Adams M, et al: Receipt of preventive services by elders based on composite measures, 1997–2004. *Am J Prev Med* 32:11–18, 2007.

22. Vogt TM, Aickin M, Ahned F, et al: The prevention index: using technology to improve quality assessment. *Health Serv Res* 39:511–530, 2004.

23. http://www.uspreventiveservicestaskforce.org/tfsublist.htm

24. Ogden LL, Richard CL, Shenson D: Clinical preventive services for older adults: the interface between personal health care and public health services. *Am J Public Health* 102:419–425, 2012.

25. US Centers for Disease Control and Prevention: Enhancing use of clinical preventive services among older adults: closing the gap. http://www.cdc.gov/aging/pdf/Clinical_Preventive_Services_Closing_the_Gap_Report.pdf.

26. Community and Clinical Partnerships: Promoting preventive services for adults, 50–64.

27. Department of Vermont Health Access: Vermont Blueprint for Health. 2010 Annual Report, January 2011. http://hcr.vermont.gov/sites/hcr/files/final_annual_report_01_26_11.pdf.

28. Shenson D, Benson W, Harris AC: Expanding the delivery of clinical preventive services through community collaboration: the SPARC model. *Prev Chronic Dis* 15:1–8, 2008.

Select Readings

US Preventive Services Task Force: *Procedure manual*, AHRQ Pub No 08-05118-EF, 2008.

Wallace RB: Maxcy-Rosenau-Last: Public Health and Preventive Medicine: Screening.

Websites

http://innovations.ahrq.gov/innovations_qualitytools.aspx [AHRQ Health Care: Innovations Exchange]

http://www.prevent.org/ [Partnership for Prevention]

http://www.uspreventiveservicestaskforce.org/ [USPSTF]

http://www.cdc.gov/vaccines/schedules/hcp/child-adolescent.html

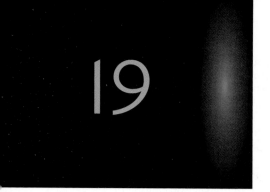

19

Chronic Disease Prevention

I. OVERVIEW OF CHRONIC DISEASE

Whereas infectious diseases were long a major determinant of both quality and length of human life, and remain so in much of the developing world, the burden of morbidity and premature mortality in developed countries shifted dramatically over the 20th century to so-called chronic diseases. The term "chronic disease" is less useful than in the past because even infectious diseases such as human immunodeficiency virus (HIV) have become "chronic" with the advent of effective treatments in the absence of cure. In essence, any disease that can be effectively managed over years or decades, but not cured, is chronic. The term *chronic disease* is applied preferentially, however, to conditions described as follows:

■ Not directly transmissible person to person
■ Routinely span years and often decades
■ Degenerative in some way, relating to aberrant or declining function of some body part or system
■ Often propagated by fundamental physiologic imbalances or disturbances, such as inflammation

The conditions of greatest concern—contributing most to years lost from life, life lost from years, and costs—are cardiovascular diseases (including stroke), cancer, pulmonary diseases, and diabetes and related metabolic derangements. These conditions now constitute the leading causes of mortality worldwide. In addition, conditions such as osteoarthritis, chronic pain syndromes, and depression exact a high toll in morbidity and cost, generally without imposing a direct mortality toll.

Of particular interest to epidemiologists is the strong body of evidence suggesting that fully 80% of chronic disease is potentially preventable by means already available, and that even genetic risk factors for chronic disease development and progression are modifiable by the effective application of lifestyle interventions.

A. The Human Toll

A short list of chronic diseases—heart disease, cancer, stroke, diabetes, and chronic lung disease—constitute the leading force of worldwide mortality. More than 60% of all deaths in the world each year are attributable to this short list of conditions.[1]

In some ways, the mortality toll of chronic diseases can exaggerate their harms. Chronic degeneration of vitality and function is, to one degree or another, the human fate until such time as the "rectangularization" of the mortality curve can be converted from an aspiration to prevailing reality[2] (Fig. 19-1). As life expectancy rises, so does the opportunity for time-dependent degeneration of organ systems. Chronic, degenerative disease is simply a point along this spectrum and thus inescapable under prevailing conditions if persons live long enough; we must eventually die of something. To the extent chronic disease merely represents this inevitable "something," the attributed death toll can make the situation seem worse than the reality. Not succumbing to infectious or traumatic causes of death early in life partly makes us vulnerable to chronic diseases later. The importance of causes of death earlier in life is best captured not by the number of deaths but by the number of *years of potential life lost* (see Chapter 24).

In another important way, however, the mortality toll of chronic diseases greatly underestimates the human cost. Long before taking years from life by causing premature death, chronic diseases take *life from years* by reducing ability, function, vitality, and quality. This is an ever more salient concern because chronic diseases, driven largely by a short list of lifestyle factors and particularly their relationship to obesity,[3] occur at ever younger ages. What was called only a generation ago "adult-onset diabetes" is now called type 2 diabetes and routinely diagnosed in children. The proliferation of cardiac risk factors in ever younger children is well

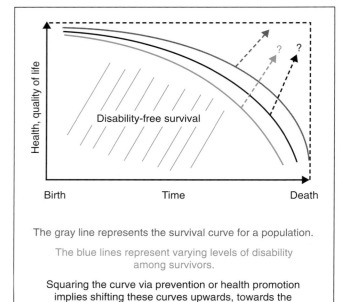

The gray line represents the survival curve for a population.

The blue lines represent varying levels of disability among survivors.

Squaring the curve via prevention or health promotion implies shifting these curves upwards, towards the hypothetical population health limit represented by the black lines.

Figure 19-1 **The concept of rectangularizing, or squaring, the survival curve.** (From *Society, the individual, and medicine*, Ottawa, Canada, 2010, University of Ottawa. www.med.uottawa.ca/sim/data/Rectangularization_of_mortality_e.htm)

documented.[4] Further, the occasional lifestyle-related cancer is diagnosed in surprisingly younger persons. A marked increase in the rate of stroke among children age 5 to 14 years also has been reported.[5]

Collectively, these trends indicate the importance of factoring the chronicity of chronic disease into any assessment of the human cost. As serious and potentially disabling disease begins at ever-younger ages, mortality becomes an increasingly less useful measure of the total impact of these conditions. A measure of attenuated quality of life, adjusted for the life span affected, is most suitable[6] (See Chapters 14 and 24 for quality-adjusted life years [QALY] and disability-adjusted life years [DALY]). By such a metric, the human cost of chronic disease is enormous, and it continues to rise.

B. The Financial Toll

There are glib expressions in the halls of medicine about the relative financial costs of life and death. Death is, in financial terms, inexpensive as expenditures related to treatment and preservation of life cease. Life, burdened by chronic disease, can be enormously expensive. As we grow ever more adept at forestalling death through the application of pharmacotherapy, procedures, and medical technology, the costs of living with chronic disease are rising. In the United States, more than 75% of Medicare expenditure (hundreds of billions of dollars annually) is for chronic disease.[7]

As with the mortality statistics, these costs represent several mixed messages. The positive message is that costs of chronic disease care rise as this care becomes more effective. When treatments are ineffective, death comes earlier. More effective treatment is unquestionably good, but means a longer treatment period before death and thus higher costs.

Advances in pharmacotherapy and technology tend to improve treatment and function (favorable) but generally involve higher costs (unfavorable). The positive message lost in gloomy statistics about cost is that we are "getting what we are paying for": longer lives despite the high and rising prevalence of chronic disease.

Other messages related to the financial costs of chronic disease are decidedly less positive. As addressed later, chronic diseases are substantially preventable by means already available. The reliance on high-cost treatment is to some degree testimony to the failure to make better use of lower-cost prevention. There is also widespread failure to treat risk factors such as high blood pressure and dyslipidemia to target levels.[8,9]

Also, the *direct* financial costs of chronic disease care do not fully capture the economic toll. Reduced productivity, absenteeism, presenteeism (attending work while sick), and related effects, known in economic terms as *externalities* or *indirect costs* (or benefits; externalities can be positive as well as negative), are high and may even exceed the direct costs.[10]

Projections about the financial costs of chronic disease are genuinely alarming and constitute nothing less than a crisis, questioning the fundamental solvency and economic viability of the U.S. health care system beyond the middle of the 21st century should current trends persist. As a result, there is increasing awareness about the importance of chronic disease prevention and the strategies that will convert what is known in this area into what is done, as well as increased attention to better management of chronic disease with patient-centered medical homes[11] and the chronic care model.[12] Professionals directly involved in public health and preventive medicine have a clear opportunity to advance the mission of prevention in responding to the dangers of the chronic disease crisis.

C. Common Elements in Pathogenesis

There is increasing appreciation for a unifying constellation of processes that underlie most if not all chronic degenerative diseases.[13,14] These pathways and their details will spawn discussion and debate for years. A case may be made, however, for a short list of common pathways, as shown in Box 19-1.

Of particular relevance in the context of epidemiology is that a common constellation of factors underlying most or all chronic diseases suggests the presence of common pathways to prevention as well. This indeed appears to be the case; the same short list of lifestyle factors appears to influence the likelihood of all major chronic diseases across the life span, other factors being equal (see Box 19-2). The notion of common pathways to diverse morbidities has been embraced by leading health agencies[15] and the National Institutes of Health (NIH).[16]

II. PREVENTABILITY OF CHRONIC DISEASE

Literature spanning at least the past two decades makes a compelling case that the leading causes of premature death—and thus the leading causes of chronic morbidity, because they are the same—are overwhelmingly preventable by means already available. A seminal 1993 paper first highlighted that chronic diseases leading to premature death were not meaningfully "causes" of death but rather "effects."[17]

| Box 19-1 | Four Pathophysiologic Pathways in Chronic Disease* |

1. Cellular Senescence

Aging, or *senescence,* at the organ system and cellular levels encompasses gradual attenuation of function (e.g., age-related decline in glomerular filtration rate) and ultimately a termination of cellular renewal and the loss of formerly functional cells through *apoptosis* (programmed cell death). Chronologic and biologic aging are related but different. *Chronologic aging* refers to a measure in units of actual time; *biologic aging* refers to function relative to age-standardized norms. By either measure, the time-dependent attenuation of functional capacity is a common element in the development and progression of chronic diseases.

2. Degeneration

Degeneration can occur as a time-dependent process but can also occur independently. Cumulative injury to the vascular lining caused by hypertension is an example of degeneration, as is the erosion of articular cartilage caused by "wear and tear" that leads to osteoarthritis.

3. Oxidation

A preoccupation with the health-promoting potential of antioxidants derives from the harmful potential of oxygen free radicals generated both in defense of the body against pathogens and as a byproduct of metabolic activity. Oxidation is implicated as a facilitator of virtually all chronic diseases.

4. Inflammation

Inflammation is a generic term referring to a range of immune system actions, both in response to and independent of infection. The action of various white blood cell lines, cytokines, immunoglobulins, and complement can defend the body against pathogens but can also cause damage to native tissue and healthy cells. Dietary imbalances, with resultant hormonal imbalances, related in particular to eicosanoids (prostaglandins), cortisol, and insulin, are implicated in chronic inflammation, which in turn is implicated in the propagation of most chronic disease.

*Common to most if not all chronic diseases. These processes provide important insights about the potential to prevent chronic disease, as well as opportunities to prevent multiple chronic diseases by addressing a common cluster of causes.

| Box 19-2 | Ten Controllable Factors in Prevention of Chronic Disease |

Tobacco	Toxic agents
Diet	Firearms
Activity patterns	Sexual behavior
Alcohol	Motor vehicles
Microbial agents	Drug use

Modified from McGinnis JM, Foege WH: *JAMA* 270:2207–2212, 1993.

These effects—the chronic diseases—were the result of 10 factors, mostly behaviors that individuals can control (Box 19-2). Using the epidemiology of 1990, this analysis found that about 80% of all premature deaths were attributable to the first three entries: tobacco, diet, and activity patterns (physical activity). Alliteratively, the leading causes of chronic disease and premature death in 1990 were "how we used our feet, our forks, and our fingers."

In 2004 the U.S. Centers for Disease Control and Prevention (CDC) updated and supported the same fundamental conclusions.[18] The same is true of subsequent related studies.[19-21] In addition, recent and accumulating evidence indicates that lifestyle interventions can modify gene expression and thus alter the risk for chronic disease development and progression at the genetic level.[22,23] In the aggregate, this literature belies the importance of the nature/nurture debate by highlighting the hegemony of "epigenetics" and the apparent human potential to "nurture nature."

The available data from diverse sources suggest that about 80% of all chronic disease could be prevented. With regard to specific conditions, 80% or more of cardiovascular disease;

90% or more of diabetes; and as much as 60% of cancer are thought to be preventable with the use of resources already available. Were this knowledge to be translated into the power of routine action, it would increase life expectancy and add much more to health expectancy, or the "health span."[24] In blunt terms, if and when we find the means to turn what we know about the prevention of chronic disease into what we routinely do, it would constitute one of the most stunning advances in the history of public health (see Chapter 28).

III. CONDITION-SPECIFIC PREVENTION

A. Obesity

There is debate about the appropriateness of classifying obesity as a chronic disease. Obesity is clearly established as a risk factor for virtually all major chronic diseases. Whether obesity itself qualifies as a disease is important in several ways. First, obesity bias is a prevalent and pernicious influence, and the establishment of obesity as a true medical condition defends against this in the form of legitimacy. The codification of obesity as a disease implies that, as with other diseases, it is (at least relatively) inappropriate to "blame the victim."

Of perhaps more direct practical importance is that the identification of obesity as a disease facilitates its inclusion among conditions with medical insurance coverage. The *International Classification of Diseases* (ICD) coding system used for billing third-party payers assigns a "diagnostic code" to any given condition. Obesity must be recognized among candidate conditions for such coverage to be processed. The U.S. Department of Health and Human Services initially designated obesity as a disease with this in mind, and relevant progress has followed. In 2011 the Centers for Medicare and Medicaid Services (CMS) authorized reimbursement for obesity counseling to physicians treating patients with a body mass index (BMI) of 30 or greater[25] (Table 19-1).

There is a potential liability, however, in cataloging obesity as a disease. Diseases are states of aberrant body function generally amenable to medical treatments (e.g., pharmacotherapy, surgery). If obesity constitutes such an aberrant state, it invites a focus on such treatments as bariatric surgery and antiobesity drugs. The effectiveness of bariatric surgery is well established and the pursuit of effective drugs for weight management well justified, but a dedicated focus on these approaches can and likely does distract attention and divert resources from policies and programs that facilitate better use of feet and forks. In other words, by *blaming* obesity on a diseased state of the body, the potential to address the *diseased* state of the **obesigenic** (obesity-causing) environment may be diminished.

An analogy well suited to clarify this perspective is drowning. Drowning is a legitimate medical condition for which medical care is warranted and for which both diagnostic codes and reimbursement are available. However, no one mistakes the propensity to drown as an "aberrant state of the body." Rather, a perfectly normal and healthy body is simply not suited to breathing under the water. Drowning (or near-drowning) is recognized universally as the inevitable outcome when a normal body spends too much time in an environment (underwater) to which it is poorly suited.

The importance of this perspective is in how it relates to prevailing societal responses. The treatment of drowning after it occurs is relatively rare and far from optimal. Many routine steps are taken—from posting lifeguards at beaches, to teaching children how to swim, to putting fences around pools—to prevent drowning from occurring. Only when the clear emphasis on environmental approaches to prevention fails does the treatment of drowning become germane, as a last resort.

Throughout most of human history, calories have been relatively scarce and often difficult to obtain, and physical activity has been an unavoidable requirement for survival. Modern society has devised an environment in which physical activity is scarce and often difficult to maintain, and calories are unavoidable. Homo sapiens are endowed with no native defenses against caloric excess and the tendency toward "sedentariness." The result is the modern obesity trends. In essence, the population is confronting an environment for which it is poorly suited and is succumbing to its toxic effects. We are *drowning* in calories. This perspective might promote an emphasis on environmentally based approaches (policies and programs that facilitate healthful eating and routine physical activity) to obesity prevention and control, even while establishing the medical legitimacy of obesity as a condition deserving treatment (Box 19-3).

Nonmodifiable risk factors for obesity include low resting energy expenditure, genetic polymorphisms that predispose to weight gain and impede weight loss, and an ethnic heritage that increases the propensity for obesity. *Modifiable* risk factors relate principally to the quality and quantity of dietary intake and energy expenditure through exercise. Lean body mass can be increased through exercise and thus also constitutes a modifiable risk factor. Insomnia increases obesity risk by several mechanisms, and thus impaired sleep is a potentially modifiable risk factor as well.

The primary and secondary prevention of obesity principally involve improvements in diet and physical activity patterns. Secondary prevention includes screening, which means clinical assessment of weight and height (BMI) as well as waist circumference, and for children the plotting of BMI on appropriate growth charts.[26]

Table 19-1 Classification of Weight Status Based on Body Mass Index (BMI)

BMI*	Classification
<18	Underweight
18-25	Normal weight
25-29.9	Overweight
30-34.9	Stage I obesity
35-39.9	Stage II obesity
>40	Stage III (severe) obesity

*Expressed as weight in kilograms divided by the square of the height in meters (weight [kg]/height^2 [m]).

Box 19-3	Summary of Obesity Risk Factors and Prevention*

Risk Factors

Nonmodifiable
Resting energy expenditure/basal metabolic rate
Genetics
Ethnicity

Modifiable
Energy consumption
Energy expenditure
Lean body mass
Sleep quality and quantity

Primary Prevention
Dietary management: improved quality, control of quantity
Physical activity

Secondary Prevention

Screening: Assessing body mass index (BMI) and waist circumference in clinical practice; plotting pediatric BMI on growth charts
Dietary management
Physical activity promotion
Possible use of pharmacotherapy

Tertiary Prevention

Bariatric surgery
Pharmacotherapy
Dietary management and physical activity promotion as important adjuncts

*Primary prevention is for nonobese individuals to prevent them from becoming obese. Secondary prevention is for asymptomatically obese individuals. Tertiary prevention is for symptomatic obesity.

Tertiary prevention, to prevent complications of established obesity, often involves pharmacotherapy for metabolic complications and bariatric surgery. The utility of bariatric surgery is well established. Pharmacotherapy for obesity is, to date, of limited utility and prone to unintended consequences. The use of medications for the metabolic complications of obesity, such as prediabetes, is more clearly supported by high-quality evidence.[27]

Figure 19-2 shows the prevalence of obesity in low-income U.S. children age 2 to 4 years.

See Figure 19-3 on studentconsult.com for obesity trends in U.S. adults. (For USPSTF recommendations on obesity, see the Websites list at end of chapter.)

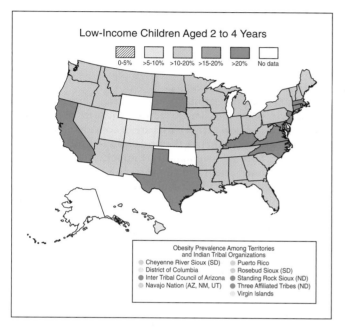

Figure 19-2 Obesity prevalence in early childhood, United States, 2009. Among low-income children age 2 to 4 years by state. *Insert,* In territories and Indian tribe organizations. (From Division of Nutrition, Physical Activity and Obesity, National Center for Chronic Disease Prevention and Health Promotion, Atlanta, 2009, US Centers for Disease Control and Prevention.)

B. Type 2 Diabetes Mellitus

In developed countries, about 95% of patients with diabetes mellitus have type 2. Whereas **type 1 diabetes** is an autoimmune disease resulting in destruction of the insulin-producing beta cells of the islets of Langerhans, type 2 diabetes is overwhelmingly a lifestyle-related disease of progressive insulin resistance mediated largely by excess body fat. Type 2 diabetes mellitus, formerly called "adult-onset diabetes," is usually preventable, both by treating the insulin resistance that often precedes it and, more fundamentally, by preventing the accumulation of excess visceral fat that is an important root cause, if not the cause, in most patients.[27]

The importance of preventing type 2 diabetes is reflected in its large contribution to current health care costs and the projections of its future prevalence. The CDC projects that as many as one in three Americans will have diabetes by the mid–21st century if current trends persist,[28] putting the fate of the U.S. health care system in doubt. Fortunately, type 2 diabetes is overwhelmingly preventable by available interventions. A fasting glucose between 100 and 125 mg/dL is indicative of **prediabetes,** whereas a level of 126 mg/dL or greater indicates diabetes.[29] The U.S. Preventive Services Task Force (USPSTF) specifically recommends diabetes screening in patients with borderline or overt hypertension.[30]

Risk factors for type 2 diabetes overlap substantially with risk factors for obesity. Rates of diabetes are considerably higher in some ethnic groups than others, and there is a known genetic predisposition. The principal driver of the epidemiology of type 2 diabetes, however, and its progression from a disease of adults into a disease of children and adults alike, is **epidemic** (or hyperendemic) **obesity.** The epidemiology of obesity has changed drastically over recent decades; genes have not. In particular, central adiposity and the accumulation of excess visceral fat in the liver are causally implicated. Diabetes can be prevented with lifestyle interventions that foster moderate weight loss; with pharmacotherapy; and with bariatric surgery. Medical management of diabetes to prevent progression and complications constitutes tertiary prevention. Box 19-4 summarizes these issues.

Box 19-4	Summary of Type 2 Diabetes Risk Factors and Prevention

Risk Factors

Nonmodifiable
Genetics
Ethnicity

Modifiable
Obesity, in particular abdominal (visceral) adiposity

Primary Prevention

Weight loss/management
Dietary management
Physical activity
Pharmacotherapy
Bariatric surgery

Secondary Prevention

Screening: Fasting glucose; glucose tolerance testing
Dietary management

Physical activity
Pharmacotherapy
Bariatric surgery

Tertiary Prevention

Pharmacotherapy
Medical assessment for potential complications (e.g., eye and foot examinations)
Bariatric surgery
Weight loss/management
Dietary management
Physical activity

C. Stroke (Cerebrovascular Accident)

Stroke, or cerebrovascular accident (CVA), is the fourth leading cause of death in the United States after heart disease, cancer, and lung disease[31] and a major cause of long-term morbidity. The incidence rate of stroke in those age 50 and older had declined in the United States, principally because of better detection and treatment of hypertension, the major risk factor.[32] The morbidity of stroke has been somewhat attenuated through the use of thrombolytic therapy that can restore blood flow and salvage brain tissue imperiled by ischemia. **Hemorrhagic stroke** is a potential side effect of such therapies and can occur independently of them. Hemorrhagic stroke is much less common than ischemic stroke, less predictable, and in general less preventable.

A marked rise in the rate of stroke in children age 5 to 14 years has been observed recently in the United States.[32] The explanation is uncertain, but childhood obesity is cited as a likely candidate.

Risk factors for stroke overlap substantially with risk factors for cardiovascular disease (see next). Medical conditions (e.g., diabetes) that increase the risk of heart disease similarly increase the risk of stroke. Atrial fibrillation is a risk factor for stroke, generally managed with anticoagulation. The main modifiable risk factor for stroke is **hypertension.** Patient adherence to management guidelines for blood pressure reliably translates into reduced stroke risk and, at the population level, reduced stroke incidence.

Revascularization, such as carotid endarterectomy after a transient ischemic attack, constitutes secondary stroke prevention. Thrombolytic and anticoagulant therapies to limit stroke-related injury to the brain and rehabilitation programs to preserve and restore function constitute the mainstays of tertiary prevention. Updated information about stroke management and prevention is available from the CDC[33] and the American Stroke Foundation.[34] As of January 2012, the USPSTF recommends against screening for carotid stenosis in asymptomatic individuals.[35]

D. Cardiovascular Disease

Cardiovascular disease has long been the leading cause of death in both men and women in the United States and remains so at this time.[36] It exerts a comparable toll in developed countries worldwide and causes a high and rising number of deaths globally.[37]

Risk factors for heart disease vary by culture and circumstance. In some parts of the world, infectious disease, such as streptococcal pharyngitis leading to rheumatic fever, or Chagas' disease resulting from infection by *Trypanosoma cruzi* in South America,[38] remains an important cause of heart disease. The focus here is preferentially on the epidemiology of heart disease, specifically **coronary artery disease** (CAD), or coronary heart disease, in the United States and comparably developed nations, in which the role of infection is minor (although not inconsequential). Chronic inflammation is now known to propagate the progression of atherosclerotic plaque, implicating such conditions as periodontal disease (see later).

The principal determinants of cardiovascular risk tend to be lifestyle behaviors. In particular, tobacco use, dietary pattern, and physical activity level are of considerable importance and greatly influence the probability of future cardiac events (e.g., unstable angina, heart attacks, sudden cardiac death). To some extent, however, such effects are indirect. Poor diet and lack of physical activity tend to contribute to dyslipidemia and hypertension, which in turn raise cardiovascular risk. It is these "downstream effects" of diet and physical activity patterns that are incorporated into quantified estimates of future risk, such as the Framingham cardiac risk score.[39]

Box 19-5 summarizes cardiovascular risk factors and prevention strategies. Many risk factors contribute to cardiovascular disease, including age, gender, hypertension, smoking, and dyslipidemia.[40] Of the modifiable risk factors, a serum cholesterol level greater than 181 mg/dL, systolic blood pressure greater than 120 mm Hg, smoking, and history of

---

Box 19-5	Summary of Cardiovascular Disease Risk Factors and Prevention

Risk Factors

Nonmodifiable
Age
Gender
Family history/genetics

Modifiable
Dyslipidemia
Hypertension
Diabetes/prediabetes (including insulin resistance)
Obesity, in particular abdominal (visceral) adiposity
Poor diet
Lack of physical activity
Smoking
Stress

Primary Prevention

Tobacco avoidance
Healthful eating

Physical activity
Stress management
Weight control
Pharmacotherapy for risk factor modification (e.g., hypertension, diabetes, dyslipidemia)
Risk factor screening (e.g., cholesterol, blood pressure)

Secondary Prevention

Risk factor management, as for primary prevention
Revascularization (angioplasty; coronary artery bypass surgery)

Tertiary Prevention

Risk factor management as for primary prevention to prevent recurrence/progression
Revascularization to preserve/restore function
Cardiac rehabilitation

diabetes together explain about 87% of coronary heart disease (CHD) risk.[41] However, the impact of changing these risk factors has variable impact on total risk. For example, for CAD, cigarette smoking increases the risk for smokers by 70% versus nonsmokers. In contrast, a long-term change of 23 mg/dL of serum cholesterol in men age 55 to 64 reduced congestive heart failure (CHF) risk by 25%. A 5–mm Hg change in diastolic blood pressure decreases CHD risk by 21%.[41] Also, risk factors have different weight on different manifestations; dyslipidemia is a stronger risk factor for CAD and peripheral artery disease (PAD) than for stroke and CHF, hypertension is more important for stroke and CHF, and smoking has the strongest impact on PAD risk.[40]

These risk factors do not act independently, and other factors, such as stress, socioeconomic status, and family history are often not captured in these studies. Also, concentrating on one risk factor at a time carries the risk of underestimating cardiovascular disease (CVD) risk in patients with multiple marginal risk factors. The best way to estimate risk is to use validated total risk score such as the Framingham risk calculator, which allows one to estimate the 10-year risk for CVD based on a combination of age, gender, and risk factors levels. In the past, there was a different risk calculator for CAD, stroke, and CHF. In 2008 a risk score for general CVD risk was published, the Framingham Heart Study general cardiovascular disease: 10-year risk,[42] which performs as well as the individual disease calculators. This score also provides a *risk age,* the biologic age that corresponds to the risk level of a patient, which is useful in communicating risk to patients. For example, if a patient is 40 years old but his risk age is 80, his cardiovascular risk is as high as if he were 80 years old. (A discussion of comprehensive cardiac risk modification is beyond the scope of this chapter.)

Epidemiologic research reports that at least 80% of all CAD is preventable by addressing a short list of lifestyle-related risk factors, notably dietary pattern, physical activity pattern, and tobacco use. Similar risk reductions are likely possible at later stages with pharmacologic management of risk factors, such as antihypertensive medications, statins (cholesterol-lowering drugs) and other drugs for dyslipidemia, and platelet inhibition with aspirin.[43] The emphasis for prevention is on lifestyle behaviors before the development and progression of risk factors, shifting toward pharmacotherapy as risk factors progress.

See Table 19-3 on studentconsult.com for a summary of lipid management recommendations of the National Heart, Lung, and Blood Institute of the NIH.

The field of cardiovascular medicine evolves rapidly, and thus readers are referred to the peer-reviewed literature and authoritative websites for up-to-date information regarding epidemiology, prevention, and treatment. Key areas at present include the detection and management of cardiac risk factors in adolescents and children; the optimal use of statins in men and women for primary prevention; the utility of diverse biomarkers of cardiac risk; and the incremental utility of various risk assessment modalities, such as coronary computed tomography (CT) imaging.

E. Chronic Lung Disease

Chronic lower respiratory tract disease, including chronic obstructive pulmonary disease (COPD), emphysema, bronchitis, and pneumoconiosis constitutes the third leading cause of death in the United States after heart disease and cancer.[44] An enormous portion of this toll is directly related to tobacco and is thus preventable with tobacco avoidance. Pneumoconioses are generally work-related diseases, and prevention is thus an occupational health issue (see Chapter 22). Asthma, an important chronic condition of the upper airway, is a relatively uncommon cause of mortality but an important cause of morbidity.

Nonmodifiable risk factors for chronic pulmonary disease include age and certain genetic disorders, such as α_1-antitrypsin deficiency[45] and cystic fibrosis.[46] Modifiable risk factors include exposure to airborne toxins caused by pollution, occupation, or tobacco smoke.

Tobacco avoidance and smoking cessation are top priorities in the prevention and treatment of chronic pulmonary diseases. There is no standard screening for pulmonary disease. The USPSTF recommends against screening for COPD[47] and currently is noncommittal about lung cancer screening,[48] a subject of ongoing study prone to change. Secondary prevention thus relates to management of early-stage disease to prevent progression. Pharmacotherapy is prominent in such efforts, notably antiinflammatory drugs (e.g., steroids) for asthma, COPD, and chronic bronchitis. Tertiary prevention may include home oxygen for patients functionally limited by hypoxemia, along with medications to manage symptoms and prevent progression, and pulmonary rehabilitation after decompensation. Both the CDC[49] and the American Lung Association[50] provide patient-friendly guidance online. The National Heart, Lung, and Blood Institute (NHLBI) provides a useful source of regularly updated information for health professionals.[51]

F. Cancer

Unlike most chronic diseases, which pertain to a particular organ system (e.g., heart disease, stroke, pulmonary disease, arthritis, diabetes), cancer—the second leading cause of death in the United States[52]—can affect any organ or tissue in the body and is relatively common and potentially lethal. Thus the topic is vast; comprehensive detail is available elsewhere, notably oncology textbooks and journals. The most important facts about cancer include the following:

- Cancer is acknowledged to be substantially (up to 60%) preventable by addressing lifestyle behaviors.
- Cancer is not the unpredictable threat that the public tends to believe it is.

Cancer development is a predictable process, analogous to the progression of atherosclerotic plaque leading to clinically significant coronary disease. The steps of that process span years to decades, with opportunity for effective prevention (Table 19-2). *Initiation* refers to the development of a potentially carcinogenic (cancer-causing) mutation. *Promotion* refers to the growth of cancer cells, before any clinical symptoms or signs develop. *Expression* refers to the first clinical evidence of the presence of cancer.

Nonmodifiable risk factors for cancer include age and predisposing genetic mutations, some of which are prevalent, important, and well known (e.g., *BRCA*).[53] Modifiable risk factors include diet, physical activity, body weight, tobacco use, exposure to infectious agents, and toxins.

Table 19-2 Steps in Development and Progression of Cancer and Opportunities for Prevention

Stage	Relevant Prevention Methods
Initiation	Toxin avoidance, particularly tobacco smoke and excess alcohol Healthful diet Weight control Physical activity Immunization, in some cases
Promotion	Early detection and treatment through screening Other methods as for initiation
Expression	Diagnosis and treatment Other methods as for initiation

The primary prevention of cancer mostly involves the avoidance of relevant pathogens, including the following:

- Human papillomavirus (HPV), implicated in cervical cancer, anal and penile cancers, and head and neck cancers
- Hepatitis B virus (HBV), implicated in hepatocellular carcinoma
- Toxins, such as tobacco and excess alcohol
- Industrial chemicals at the worksite and potentially contaminating the environment and food supply

In theory, organically grown food offers benefits in this regard, but establishing such evidence is difficult and largely nascent to date. Healthful eating, moderate physical activity, and weight control offer important defenses at all stages of cancer. As noted in the previous discussion of obesity, the link between excess body fat and cancer risk is well established and of general importance.[54] In select patients, immunization may serve as primary cancer prevention by preventing an initiating infection (e.g., against HPV and HBV).

The secondary prevention of cancer principally involves making use of effective screening protocols. The USPSTF recommends screening specific populations for cervical, breast, and colon cancers; recommends against screening for some others; and is noncommittal in certain cases, such as lung cancer, where evidence is equivocal and evolving.[55] Readers are encouraged to keep current with these often-changing topics by visiting the USPSTF website (see Chapter 18).

Tertiary cancer prevention involves effective treatment and a range of strategies aimed at preventing recurrence and progression, as well as strategies to restore function or appearance, such as rehabilitation and reconstructive cosmetic surgery. This topic potentially encompasses all aspects of cancer treatment. One example of tertiary prevention incorporated into treatment is hormonal therapy to prevent recurrence, applied notably to prostate and breast cancer. The selective estrogen receptor modulators, such as tamoxifen and raloxifene, substantially reduce breast cancer incidence. Raloxifene, approved for treating and preventing osteoporosis, may also be used for primary breast cancer prevention in high-risk women.[56]

G. Oral Health

Dental caries is one of the few conditions so common without routine care that screening is inappropriate. Instead, prophylaxis in the form of routine dental visits and cleanings, with fluoride application, is the standard of care.

In addition to caries, periodontal disease is an important form of pathology in the oral cavity. Research over recent decades has highlighted the importance of oral health to general health and the link between gingivitis and periodontitis to a variety of systemic diseases.[57] The following primary strategies help prevent chronic disease of the oral cavity:

- Good oral hygiene (routine brushing and flossing)
- Adequate intake of fluoride from water or dental treatment
- Routine dental visits
- Avoidance of excess alcohol
- Avoidance of toxins, such as tobacco

H. Dementia, Chronic Pain, and Arthritis

Other chronic conditions include dementias, back pain, recurrent headaches, neuropathies, rheumatologic disease, and atopic conditions.

Dementia is a diverse category of conditions; some are preventable by means as simple as nutrient supplementation, and others are not known to be preventable at all. Alzheimer's disease is of particular interest in this regard. Because of its rising prevalence, related in part to an aging population, and its enormous human and economic costs, Alzheimer's disease is receiving increasing attention, and resources related to prevention, early diagnosis, treatment, and cure. To the extent currently thought possible, Alzheimer's disease is preventable generally through the prevention of cardiovascular disease.[58]

Conditions of **chronic pain,** especially arthritis, are prevalent and important contributors to morbidity,[59-61] as well as indirectly to mortality. For example, the physical inactivity leading to progression of obesity and development of diabetes may be a major determinant of a fatal myocardial infarction. With the potential interplay of chronic conditions, each compounding the other, chronic pain may foster physical inactivity, which may lead to weight gain, which may exacerbate the pain. Such complexity occurs in many older patients with chronic disease, warranting meaningful applications of *holistic care.*[62]

Osteoarthritis (OA) may be the quintessential example of a degenerative disease attributable to "wear and tear." Symptoms develop and progress as friction erodes articular cartilage in the knee, hip, hand, and other joints. Some degree of secondary inflammation may occur, but inflammation is relatively unimportant in OA, in contrast to rheumatologic diseases such as rheumatoid arthritis. Strategies for the primary prevention of OA include avoiding excessive stress to joints and exercising to keep muscles well conditioned. Secondary prevention directed at symptom control and preservation of function involves analgesics, supplements, and modalities such as massage, as well as regular physical activity. Tertiary prevention—restoration of function impaired by disease progression and prevention of complications—includes physical therapy and rehabilitation, strategies to reconstitute eroded cartilage, and surgery, especially joint replacement. Relevant reviews are available for clinicians,[63] as are online sources for patients.[64]

IV. BARRIERS AND OPPORTUNITIES

A. Impediments to Chronic Disease Prevention

The toll of chronic disease and its well-established preventability by available means make a compelling case for action, especially considering the personal nature of public health statistics. Almost every family in modern society has faced some prevalent chronic disease and knows someone with heart disease, cancer, lung disease, stroke, or diabetes. If we were to find the means to turn what we know about prevention into what we practice routinely, up to 8 in 10 persons directly affected by chronic disease would not have been.[65] We as a society have the opportunity to bequeath the avoidance of that suffering and loss to our children. One barrier that might be readily overcome is the failure to part the veil of statistical anonymity and recognize the familiar faces on the other side.

1. Personal Barriers

Other barriers to fulfilling the promise of chronic disease prevention relate to lifestyle behaviors. The three leading root causes of chronic disease are tobacco use, poor diet, and lack of physical activity. Medical intervention is at best only a partial response to any of these. Patients can be supported in a smoking cessation effort, but they still must be willing to undergo the effort. Healthful diet and routine exercise may be recommended, but patients must make a longitudinal commitment to both. As the focus of prevention moves outside the clinical domain, health professionals have less direct control. Therefore an important barrier is that chronic disease prevention increasingly must be a personal endeavor, and many people lack the required skill or the will, or both.

2. Public Barriers

Many aspects of modern living conspire directly against chronic disease prevention efforts. Overconsumption of calories is routine for many reasons, including federal subsidies that foster the propagation of processed foods, the willful hyperpalatability of these foods, assertive and creative food-marketing efforts, and the ubiquity of food (especially fast food). Lack of physical activity is explained in part by an ever-expanding array of devices that perform tasks once done by muscles, at work and at play, with schedules that make the allocation of time for exercise difficult and excuses easy. In essence, almost everything about modern living that makes it modern is obesigenic, and much is **morbidigenic** (disease-causing).[66]

B. Opportunities for Chronic Disease Prevention

Opportunities, however, are as great and numerous as barriers and challenges. There is increasing attention to the importance of prevention for both the public health and the health of national economies. Federal regulations, such as reimbursement for lifestyle counseling by physicians, are evolving.[25] A medical specialty devoted to lifestyle approaches has emerged,[67] and "new age" tools provide novel means to engage health care professionals in effective behavior modification efforts.[68]

Given the traditional focus of formalized medicine on *disease care*, it is not surprising that much of the emphasis on prevention in the health care context relates to better screening, early treatment, and better management of established chronic disease. Two examples are the patient-centered medical home[11] and the chronic care model.[12] Both are designed to improve the flow of information, with the patient at the center and the goal to improve delivery of care so that outcomes are enhanced and costs reduced. Another important concept is that delivery and receipt of clinical preventive services can be enhanced by engaging nonclinical, community-based entities as partners.[69]

Although laudable and important, these models emphasize the delivery of clinical services and define the recipient as a patient. The greatest opportunities for chronic disease prevention (1) involve changing lifestyle behaviors in ways that are acceptable to most people, (2) reside largely outside the clinical setting, and (3) relate to the preservation of health in people who have no cause to be "patients."

Clinicians can learn to be more effective agents of change, but only to a certain degree. Various health-related policies could be adopted to facilitate favorable "defaults."[70] Expert guidance may be provided at decision points, such as the purchase of food.[71] Financial incentives may be used to motivate achievement of health goals[72] or to reward healthful choices.[73] The financial interest of businesses in workforce health promotion may be better leveraged to advance health promotion in other settings as well.[74]

The promise of drastic reductions in the human and financial costs of chronic disease beckons and is achievable by means already in hand. The challenge our society now confronts is to muster the resolve to traverse the miles that separate what we know about chronic disease prevention from what we do.

V. SUMMARY

The human and financial toll of chronic disease in modern society presents many opportunities for prevention, particularly in regard to the short list of factors responsible for most chronic diseases, directly or indirectly. This same list indicates the degree to which all or most chronic diseases could be prevented through one common, health-promoting approach, a promise borne out by population studies. As much as an 80% reduction in the mortality and morbidity of heart disease, cancer, pulmonary disease, stroke, and diabetes could be achieved with improvements in dietary and physical activity patterns and tobacco avoidance.

References

1. http://www.who.int/topics/chronic_diseases/en/
2. Manton KG, Tolley HD: Rectangularization of the survival curve: implications of an ill-posed question. *J Aging Health* 3:172–193, 1991.
3. Egger G: Obesity, chronic disease, and economic growth: a case for "big picture" prevention. *Adv Prev Med* 2011:149–158, 2011.
4. Nathan BM, Moran A: Metabolic complications of obesity in childhood and adolescence: more than just diabetes. *Curr Opin Endocrinol Diabetes Obes* 15:21–29, 2008.
5. http://www.bbc.co.uk/news/health-14746370

6. Prieto L, Sacristán JA: Problems and solutions in calculating quality-adjusted life years (QALYs). *Health Qual Life Outcomes* 1:80, 2003.

7. http://healthcarecostmonitor.thehastingscenter.org/kimberly swartz/projected-costs-of-chronic-diseases/

8. http://www.nhlbi.nih.gov/guidelines/hypertension/jnc8/index.htm

9. http://www.nhlbi.nih.gov/guidelines/cholesterol/

10. Thrall JH: Prevalence and costs of chronic disease in a health care system structured for treatment of acute illness. *Radiology* 235:9–12, 2005.

11. http://www.ncqa.org/tabid/631/default.aspx

12. http://www.improvingchroniccare.org/index.php?p=the_chronic_care_model&s=2

13. Probst-Hensch NM: Chronic age-related diseases share risk factors: do they share pathophysiological mechanisms, and why does that matter? *Swiss Med Wkly* 140:w13072, 2010. doi:10.4414/smw.2010.13072.

14. Diomedi M, Leone G, Renna A: The role of chronic infection and inflammation in the pathogenesis of cardiovascular and cerebrovascular disease. *Drugs Today (Barc)* 41:745–753, 2005.

15. Eyre H, Kahn R, Robertson RM, et al: Preventing cancer, cardiovascular disease, and diabetes: a common agenda for the American Cancer Society, the American Diabetes Association, and the American Heart Association. *Circulation* 109:3244–3255, 2004.

16. http://commonfund.nih.gov/about.aspx

17. McGinnis JM, Foege WH: Actual causes of death in the United States. *JAMA* 270:2207–2212, 1993.

18. Mokdad AH, Marks JS, Stroup DF, et al: Actual causes of death in the United States, 2000. *JAMA* 291:1238–1245, 2004.

19. McCullough ML, Patel AV, Kushi LH, et al: Following cancer prevention guidelines reduces risk of cancer, cardiovascular disease, and all-cause mortality. *Cancer Epidemiol Biomarkers Prev* 20:1089–1097, 2011.

20. Kvaavik E, Batty GD, Ursin G, et al: Influence of individual and combined health behaviors on total and cause-specific mortality in men and women: the United Kingdom Health and Lifestyle Survey. *Arch Intern Med* 170:711–718, 2010.

21. Ford ES, Bergmann MM, Kröger J, et al: Healthy living is the best revenge: findings from the European Prospective Investigation into Cancer and Nutrition–Potsdam study. *Arch Intern Med* 169:1355–1362, 2009.

22. Ornish D, Magbanua MJ, Weidner G, et al: Changes in prostate gene expression in men undergoing an intensive nutrition and lifestyle intervention. *Proc Natl Acad Sci USA* 105:8369–8374, 2008.

23. Ornish D, Lin J, Daubenmier J, et al: Increased telomerase activity and comprehensive lifestyle changes: a pilot study. *Lancet Oncol* 9:1048–1057, 2008.

24. Huffman DM, Barzilai N: Contribution of adipose tissue to health span and longevity. *Interdiscip Top Gerontol* 37:1–19, 2010.

25. http://www.cms.gov/medicare-coverage-database/details/nca-decision-memo.aspx?&NcaName=Intensive%20Behavioral%20Therapy%20for%20Obesity&bc=ACAAAAAAIAAA&NCAId=253&

26. http://www.cdc.gov/growthcharts/

27. Knowler WC, Barrett-Connor E, Fowler SE, et al: Reduction in the incidence of type 2 diabetes with lifestyle intervention or metformin. Diabetes Prevention Program Research Group. *N Engl J Med* 346:393–403, 2002.

28. http://www.cdc.gov/media/pressrel/2010/r101022.html

29. http://diabetes.niddk.nih.gov/dm/pubs/diagnosis/#diagnosis

30. http://www.uspreventiveservicestaskforce.org/uspstf/uspsdiab.htm

31. http://www.cdc.gov/nchs/fastats/lcod.htm

32. http://www.webmd.com/stroke/news/20110209/stroke-rates-are-rising-for-young-americans

33. http://www.cdc.gov/stroke/index.htm

34. http://www.strokeassociation.org/STROKEORG/

35. http://www.uspreventiveservicestaskforce.org/uspstf/uspsacas.htm

36. http://www.cdc.gov/nchs/fastats/lcod.htm

37. http://www.who.int/cardiovascular_diseases/resources/atlas/en/

38. http://www.ncbi.nlm.nih.gov/pubmedhealth/PMH0002348/

39. http://www.framinghamheartstudy.org/risk/hrdcoronary.html

40. D'Agostino RB, Vasan RS, Pencina MJ, et al: General cardiovascular risk profile for use in primary care. *Circulation* 117:743–753, 2008.

41. Magnus P: The real contribution of the major risk factors to the coronary epidemics. *Arch Intern Med* 161:2657–2660, 2001.

42. http://www.framinghamheartstudy.org/risk/gencardio.html

43. http://www.uspreventiveservicestaskforce.org/uspstf/uspsasmi.htm

44. http://www.cdc.gov/nchs/fastats/lcod.htm

45. http://www.alpha1.org/

46. http://www.cff.org/

47. http://www.uspreventiveservicestaskforce.org/uspstf/uspscopd.htm

48. http://www.uspreventiveservicestaskforce.org/uspstf/uspslung.htm

49. http://www.cdc.gov/copd/

50. http://www.lungusa.org/lung-disease/

51. http://www.nhlbi.nih.gov/health/indexpro.htm

52. http://www.cdc.gov/nchs/fastats/lcod.htm

53. http://www.cancer.gov/cancertopics/factsheet/Risk/BRCA

54. Calle EE, Rodriguez C, Walker-Thurmond K, et al: Overweight, obesity, and mortality from cancer in a prospectively studied cohort of U.S. adults. *N Engl J Med* 348:1625–1638, 2003.

55. http://www.uspreventiveservicestaskforce.org/uspstopics.htm#AZ

56. http://www.cancer.gov/cancertopics/druginfo/raloxifenehydrochloride

57. Teng YT, Taylor GW, Scannapieco F, et al: Periodontal health and systemic disorders. *J Can Dent Assoc* 68:188–192, 2002.

58. http://www.huffingtonpost.com/david-katz-md/alzheimers_b_1219272.html

59. Losina E, Walensky RP, Reichmann WM, et al: Impact of obesity and knee osteoarthritis on morbidity and mortality in older Americans. *Ann Intern Med* 154:217–226, 2011.

60. Johannes CB, Le TK, Zhou X, et al: The prevalence of chronic pain in United States adults: results of an Internet-based survey. *J Pain* 11:1230–1239, 2010.

61. Sacks JJ, Luo YH, Helmick CG: Prevalence of specific types of arthritis and other rheumatic conditions in the ambulatory health care system in the United States, 2001–2005. *Arthritis Care Res (Hoboken)* 62:460–464, 2010.

62. http://www.huffingtonpost.com/david-katz-md/holism-helicopters-spiral_b_828643.html

63. Sofat N, Beith I, Anilkumar PG, et al: Recent clinical evidence for the treatment of osteoarthritis: what we have learned. *Rev Recent Clin Trials* 6:114–126, 2011.

64. http://www.ncbi.nlm.nih.gov/pubmedhealth/PMH0001460/

65. Katz DL: Facing the facelessness of public health: what's the public got to do with it? *Am J Health Promot* 25:361–362, 2011.

66. Katz DL. Obesity … be dammed! What it will take to turn the tide? *Harvard Health Policy Rev* 7:135–151, 2006.

67. http://www.lifestylemedicine.org/

68. http://www.turnthetidefoundation.org/OWCH/training.htm

69. http://www.cdc.gov/aging/states/sparc.htm

70. Thaler RH, Sunstein CR: *Nudge: improving decisions about health, wealth, and happiness,* New York, 2009, Penguin.
71. www.nuval.com
72. http://www.incentahealth.com/; http://www.kardio.com/
73. http://www.huffingtonpost.com/david-katz-md/food-stamps-healthy-food_b_984684.html
74. Katz DL: Advancing the health of families: who's the BAWSS? *Childhood Obesity* 7:73–75, 2011.

Websites

http://www.cdc.gov/chronicdisease/
http://www.uspreventiveservicestaskforce.org/uspstf/uspsobes.htm *and* http://www.uspreventiveservicestaskforce.org/uspstf/uspschobes.htm [USPSTF recommendations on obesity.]
http://www.who.int/topics/chronic_diseases/en/

Prevention of Infectious Diseases

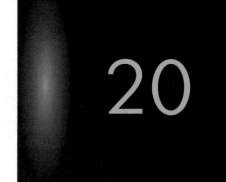

20

WITH PATRICIA E. WETHERILL

I. OVERVIEW OF INFECTIOUS DISEASE

Humans have coexisted with microbes since the beginning of the human race. One of the originators of epidemiology, John Snow, laid the foundations of the discipline by analyzing and controlling cholera, a bacterial disease caused by *Vibrio cholerae*. Immunity to infection is influenced by a person's genetic background, overall health, access to good sanitation and nutrition, and even social status. Therefore, the prevalence of infectious diseases is a good proxy for disenfranchisement and poverty in a population. Poverty plays multiple roles in the cycle of infectious diseases. Poverty can contribute to infectious diseases by making the environment more suitable for disease transmission, and poverty can also be a consequence of infectious diseases. Causal pathways include complications of pregnancy, repeated episodes of diarrheal illness in children leading to slowed mental and physical development, and the death of broad swaths of a parent generation (e.g., from AIDS).[1]

Control of infectious disease is challenging because of the adaptive capabilities of microbes. Microbes have inhabited the earth far longer than humans and have successfully adapted to all evolutionary challenges. Several recent developments fuel a global environment in which new infectious diseases emerge and become rooted in society, as summarized by the Institute of Medicine into the **convergence model**[2] (Fig. 20-1; see also Chapter 30). The convergence model is centered on the human-microbe interaction. The black box in the center of the figure indicates that these interactions can be difficult to predict in an emerging disease. More importantly, a microbe is a necessary but not sufficient cause of ill health. Humans constantly encounter millions of potentially harmful microbes without falling ill. Four domains of factors impact humans and microbes or their interactions. Each of these factors provides a starting point for thinking systematically about pathways of prevention (Box 20-1).

Understanding and controlling infectious diseases requires integrating many different preventive and public health skills. These include obtaining accurate history on sensitive topics such as sexual behaviors; geographic epidemiology; outbreak investigation; analysis of disease rates by different variables (age, gender, race, socioeconomic status) to detect high-risk groups; successful outreach to public and health professionals; screening; contact tracing; immunization; school health; counseling; sanitation; waste and wastewater management; food protection; disease registries; and prophylactic drugs. Diseases vary, but the epidemiologic skills are similar for different diseases, independent of their mode of transmission (e.g., STD vs. vector-borne disease). Public health controls disease through prevention efforts in three broad categories, as follows[2]:

- **Improving resistance of the host.** Includes such basics as hygiene and nutrition, as well as vaccination, postexposure prophylaxis, and chemoprophylaxis (see Chapter 15).
- **Improving environmental safety.** Includes sanitation, air quality control, water and food safety, and control of vectors and animal reservoirs. Public sanitation has been crucial in controlling infectious disease. Worldwide, areas without access to clean water and basic sanitation carry the highest burden of diseases that disproportionally impact children less than 5 years old.
- **Improving public health systems.** Includes improved contact tracing, education, containment, and herd immunity.

All infection control activity requires a thorough understanding of the various infectious diseases. This chapter only briefly addresses the complexity of different diseases, and important diseases are discussed elsewhere (e.g., see Chapter 3 for influenza and Select Readings for further information). On the other hand, control of an infectious disease often only requires understanding how it is transmitted. For

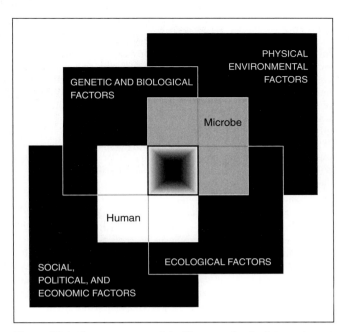

Figure 20-1 Convergence model of human-microbe interaction.
(From Smolinski MS, Hamburg MA, Lederberg J, editors: *Microbial threats to health: emergence, detection, and response*, Washington, DC, 2003, National Academies Press.)

example, John Snow determined that water from a particular company caused most of the cholera in London. Armed with this understanding and the supporting data, he was able to convince the local council to disable the well. Breaking the chain of transmission helped end the outbreak.

Diseases can be usefully grouped according to transmission[3] (Table 20-1). Often, surveys of patients and "shoe leather" epidemiology will reveal the mode of transmission, and public health officials can disrupt disease transmission before the causative agent has been identified (see Chapter 3).

A. Burden of Disease

Infectious diseases affect all countries, but the burden of disease is different in developed and developing countries. In the United States, infectious disease mortality has for the most part steadily declined since the early 1900s.[4] Most of this decline *preceded* the availability of antibiotics or vaccines and was likely the result of better hygiene, sanitation, and chlorination of drinking water.

Since the 1980s, the burden of infectious disease in the United States has again increased, largely because of emerging or reemerging infections, such as multidrug-resistant *Staphylococcus aureus*, *Clostridium difficile*, and *Mycobacterium tuberculosis*. Globally, infectious diseases account for about half the disease burden in low-income and middle-income countries. Infectious diseases especially impact children; more than half of childhood mortality is attributable to acute respiratory infections, measles, diarrheal illnesses, malaria, and human immunodeficiency virus and acquired immunodeficiency syndrome (HIV/AIDS).

To weigh the effects of disease on life span, many global health experts measure the impact of infectious disease in disability-adjusted life years (DALY). DALY take into account premature mortality and years of life lived in less than full health (see Chapter 24.) Five of the 10 leading diseases for global disease burden are infectious: HIV/AIDS, lower respiratory infections, diarrheal illnesses, malaria, and tuberculosis (TB). More importantly, many of the infectious diseases causing a large disease burden are increasing (HIV/AIDS, respiratory diseases) and are disproportionately impacting the lowest-income countries.[5]

See online Figure 20-2 on studentconsult.com for global mortality rates by cause and region.

Worldwide death rates from malaria and HIV/AIDS are increasing. These increases have negated gains derived from reduced child mortality from measles, acute respiratory infections, and diarrhea.

B. Obtaining an Accurate History

Transmission of major infectious diseases often results from a person's *behavior,* including eating and hygiene habits, pets in residence, illicit drug use, and sexual partners. Therefore, caring for a patient with an infectious disease requires taking a careful behavioral history. The behaviors resulting in transmission can be mainstream and unrelated to any social taboos, such as the restaurant visited before a diarrheal illness.

More often, patients may be embarrassed by behavior that induced the infectious disease. Examples range from people kissing their pets (leading to transmission of *Pasteurella* spp.[6]) to sexual behaviors and use of illicit drugs (leading to transmission of sexually transmitted and blood-borne diseases). Patients may not be comfortable sharing such information unless the clinician is skilled at putting people at ease and asks about intimate details in a nonjudgmental way. Taking such a history is crucial for understanding how the patient contracted the infectious disease and who else may have been infected.

Client-centered counseling means tailoring prevention messages to a patient's practices, values, and risk perceptions. For sexually transmitted diseases (STDs), or sexually transmitted infections (STIs), client-centered counseling has been shown to increase the likelihood of patients changing their behavior.[7] The same likely holds true for other behaviors. As in other areas of counseling, it is important that the clinician start with open-ended questions and reassure the patient that the information will be treated confidentially.

Counseling for STDs is discussed in detail here for several reasons. STDs play a major role in infectious disease epidemiology, have a significant impact on fertility and pregnancy outcomes, and also may cause problems in newborns (e.g., syphilis, gonorrhea). Women are often more vulnerable to STDs than men, which poses particular challenges, because many effective interventions require male condoms. Also, effective counseling for STDs has been extensively researched, but many clinicians are uncomfortable addressing this topic.

Counseling for STDs can serve as a template for other sensitive topics, such as illicit drug use, risk taking among adolescents, and addiction. For STDs and other sensitive topics, it is particularly important that the interviewing techniques be culturally appropriate and, especially with adolescents, correspond to patients' developmental levels. The interview should begin with more neutral topics in the social history (e.g., sports, activities, diet), then move to questions

I. Genetic and Biologic Factors

In human-microbe interaction, genetic and biologic factors include the makeup of the human body, with its physical, cellular, and molecular barriers to infection (**human susceptibility to infection**). Many of these factors are amenable to prevention efforts; exercise and a healthy diet contribute to intact barriers to infection. Biologic factors that **increase infectivity** of the microbe include its prevalence, stability, infectious dose, latency phase, and induction of shedding in the host. The noroviruses, the most common cause of diarrheal illness, exemplify the highly infectious microbe: viral particles are highly prevalent and can survive for a long time outside the human body; even a few viruses are enough to induce illness; and they are mainly transmitted from people who do not feel ill (viral shedding). **Microbial adaptation and change** also affects the interplay. Many microbes have successfully adapted to their environments through millions of years and continue to evolve. Their constant, rapid pace of mutation helps them develop resistance to potent antibiotics (e.g., vancomycin-intermediate staphylococcus aureus [VISA]) and complicates attempts to find vaccines (e.g., malaria, HIV).

Pathways to prevention in this domain include decreasing host susceptibility through better nutrition and vaccines, as well as constant vigilance for emerging resistance patterns.

2. Physical Environment Factors

Physical environment factors include the **climate and latitude** of an environment, which affect a location's conduciveness to microbe or vector survival. Climate can directly impact disease transmission through replication and survival of pathogens and vectors, as well as through its effects on ecology. Landslides, earthquakes, and other **natural disasters** also create conditions conducive to the spread of infectious disease, such as overcrowding, lack of sanitation, and malnutrition.

Prevention efforts in this domain include improved food safety and sanitation, as well as focused surveillance on areas conducive to emerging infections.

3. Ecological Factors

Changes in ecosystems can effect the transmission of microbes through water, soil, air, food, or vectors. Such alterations also affect microbes with animal reservoirs. Examples include the changes of malaria prevalence in response to a warming climate and the increase in prevalence of Lyme disease because of more deer in expanding New England woods. Also important are changes in land use. A growing number of emerging infectious diseases arise from increased human contact with animal reservoirs (**disruption/destabilization** of natural habitats; see Chapter 30). An example is the Nipah virus, which was endemic to Southeast Asian fruit bats. When pig farms grew in size and density and expanded into fruit orchards in the late 1990s, the virus was transmitted to the pigs and then their handlers, causing encephalitis outbreaks. Pathways to prevention in this domain can be again found mainly through surveillance.

4. Social, Political, and Economic Factors

Human demographics and behavior involve international travel and commerce that can lead to rapid dissemination of infectious diseases (e.g., SARS) or produce-borne diseases. **Advances in technology** and industry open up new transmission modes (e.g., blood transfusion, use of antibiotics in farm animals). Furthermore, **disruptions of peace** and public health services as well as **income inequality** all worsen infectious diseases transmission. For example, war and famines are closely linked to the spread of infectious diseases, and mortality from infectious diseases is closely correlated with global poverty. **Lack of political will** has also contributed to delayed control. For example, the widespread perception in the second half of the 20th century was that infectious diseases were under control and no longer posed a public health threat. This complacency probably contributed to delays in detecting and controlling multidrug-resistant TB as well as food-borne outbreaks. A relatively new factor here is also the **intent to harm** through the release of microbial agents as an act of aggression.

Pathways for prevention through social, economic, and political factors lie in taking a comprehensive view of health, advocating for improvements to the underlying determinants in populations, and helping create the political will to strengthen public health and overcome health disparities (see Chapter 26).

Table 20-1 Transmission of Infectious Diseases

Transmission Mode	Examples of Diseases	Control Measures
Close personal contact	Upper respiratory infections Meningitis EBV infection Group A streptococcal disease Tuberculosis STDs, HIV	Practice use of barriers (e.g., handwashing, masks, barrier methods [condoms]) Find and treat/isolate carriers Improve host resistance
Food/water	Typhoid Shigellosis Cholera Legionellosis Giardiasis	Improve sanitation, ensure food safety, improve water quality, improve hygiene, cook meat properly
Soil-transmitted helminths	Ascariasis Hookworm Strongyloidiasis	Improve sanitation. Ensure treatment of excreta
Arthropods	Malaria Lyme Some viral hemorrhagic fevers Dengue	Control/eliminate vectors Eliminate reservoir Use repellents/insecticides
Zoonoses	Rabies Anthrax Tularemia Toxoplasmosis	Eliminate carriers Monitor pet health Control rodents

From Wallace RB, editor: Maxcy-Rosenau-Last: *Public health and preventive medicine,* ed 15. II. Communicable diseases. New York, 2008, McGraw-Hill Medical.
EBV, Epstein-Barr virus; *HIV,* human immunodeficiency virus; *STDs,* sexually transmitted diseases (STIs).

about sexual behaviors. In broaching such topics, it is important to *frame the questions,* as in the following examples:

- For adolescents, "Now I am going to take a few minutes to ask you some sensitive questions that are important for me to help you be healthy. Anything we discuss will be completely confidential. I won't discuss this with anyone, not even your parents, without your permission."[8] After clarifying this, introduce the topic in a nonthreatening way: "Some of my patients your age have started having sex. Have you had sex?"
- For adults, "To provide the best care, I ask all my patients about their sexual activity. So, tell me about your sex life."
- Further history taking can follow the model of the "5 Ps" (partners, prevention of pregnancy, protection from STDs, practices, and past STDs).[7]
- For each of those domains, again it is important to start with open-ended questions (e.g., "Tell me about how you have sex"; "Where do you meet your partners?") before asking about specific high-risk behaviors.

Additional information on effective STD counseling and behavioral interventions can be found online.[9]

II. PUBLIC HEALTH PRIORITIES

A. HIV/AIDS, Tuberculosis, and Malaria

In some countries in sub-Saharan Africa, HIV/AIDS, tuberculosis, and malaria together account for more than 50% of deaths.[10] These illnesses decrease health and constrain growth and development of many of the poorest nations. In general, they also impact developed countries, either internally through income inequality or externally through immigration and international travel. All these diseases have important lessons to offer for successful infectious disease prevention. Prevention efforts for these three diseases are often implemented together, as through the Global Fund to Fight AIDS, Tuberculosis, and Malaria.[11] The Global Fund follows an innovative model, targeting all three diseases through partnerships among government, civil society, the private sector (including businesses and foundations), and affected communities, combined with meticulous attention to data and evaluation.

1. Human Immunodeficiency Virus/Acquired Immunodeficiency Syndrome

EPIDEMIOLOGY

No new disease in modern times has had as severe an impact worldwide as AIDS, which is caused by the human immunodeficiency virus. Although HIV transmission and management are of major concern in the United States, the situation is more serious in Southeast Asia, South America, Russia, and the Indian subcontinent. It is catastrophic in sub-Saharan Africa, where many adults are infected, death rates in the most productive age groups are extremely high, and many children have been orphaned. In 2009 an estimated 2.6 million people became newly infected with HIV, with 1.8 million deaths worldwide.[12]

The U.S. Centers for Disease Control and Prevention (CDC) estimated in 2012 that more than 1 million people are living with HIV infection in the United States, with around 18,000 deaths annually. An estimated 50,300 Americans are newly infected with HIV each year;[13] one in five people (21%) living with HIV are unaware of having the infection, presumably accounting for a large proportion of new infections.

Spread of HIV Infection Human immunodeficiency virus is spread through *horizontal transmission* (generally adult to adult) by sexual contact (both heterosexual and homosexual) and by sharing needles and other equipment for *intravenous drug use* (IDU). HIV is spread through *vertical transmission* (from parent to child) in utero or through breastfeeding. HIV can also be spread by transfusions of blood and blood products and by accidental punctures of the skin with contaminated needles or other medical equipment; these mechanisms could be either horizontal or vertical depending on the circumstances. In places where the rates of new HIV infections are approximately equal among men and women, heterosexual intercourse is the most important route of spread. Where the prevalence and new infections involve more men than women, either homosexual intercourse or IDU is likely to be the dominant route. In U.S. men the first and second most frequent routes of infection are *men who have sex with men* (MSM) and IDU. In U.S. women the most frequent route of infection is heterosexual intercourse. In central Africa and Southeast Asia, however, heterosexual intercourse is the predominant route of spread.

PREVENTION OF HIV INFECTION AND AIDS

The best ways to prevent the spread of HIV/AIDS have been known since the syndrome was discovered and before the responsible microorganism was identified. They consist of restricting sexual activity to a monogamous relationship and avoiding IDU. If a person chooses to have multiple sexual partners or to use intravenous drugs, the next best prevention is to use condoms for every sexual contact and clean needles and equipment for each IDU episode. Male circumcision, antiretroviral therapy (ART) and possibly also antiretroviral vaginal gel can also significantly decrease infection rates.[14] Treatment is prevention (see below).

Globally, an unprecedented coalition of governments, nongovernmental organizations (NGOs), pharmaceutical companies, and private foundations have worked together successfully to control the spread of the AIDS epidemic. Through these efforts, the annual number of new HIV infections has declined worldwide, and AIDS-related deaths have fallen with increased access to ART. In 33 countries (22 in sub-Saharan Africa) the HIV incidence decreased more than 25% between 2001 and 2009.[15] These successes highlight the following lessons about prevention and disease control in general:

1. Prevention and treatment exist along a continuum. HIV prevention efforts have included access for people to ART. Politically, it is difficult to generate support for case finding and prevention if diagnosed patients cannot be treated.
2. Knowledge is essential to successful prevention but not enough; motivations and behavior need to change as well. The most successful ways to impact behavior are to provide motivation and to change social norms.

3. Successful prevention targets clusters of behavioral indicators, not just one. Countries that simultaneously targeted condom use, delayed initiation of sexual activity, and reducing multiple partnerships had marked reductions in HIV prevalence.
4. Target high-risk populations. In most countries, a minority of the population has multiple sexual partners or has commercial or *transactional* sex (sex for drugs, food, or shelter). Targeting prevention efforts to these groups has a much higher impact on population health than does general prevention.
5. Empowerment is part of prevention. Many of the primary transmitters of HIV infection come from vulnerable and disempowered populations. Prevention programs combining outreach and empowerment with modification of sexual behavior have shown impressive results in South Africa and India.

Infected patients may change their behavior to protect others if they know they are infected. For this reason, anonymous HIV testing centers have been established in most U.S. areas. However, these testing centers identify less HIV infection than other health care settings, so preventive counseling and testing has shifted over the last 10 years. The changes emphasize ease of access to testing.

The CDC recommends routine, voluntary, opt-out HIV screening for all patients age 13 to 64 in health care settings, unless prevalence of undiagnosed HIV infection has been documented at less than 0.1%.[16] Box 20-2 provides additional CDC guidelines.[16,17]

Testing for HIV has developed into multiple categories, such as the following:

Screening serology: enzyme-linked immunosorbent assay (ELISA)
Confirmatory assays: Western blot
Nucleic acid testing (NAT)
Rapid HIV antibody tests
Home tests

There are multiple specimen options as well, including (but not limited to) saliva, blood, and urine. The choice of test is driven by the population served, rapidity of results, prevalence of disease in the community, and cost. In general and for most centers, testing for HIV depends on detecting antibodies in a two-step process. The standard methodology uses a third-generation, HIV antibody serum or plasma test, with confirmation of all positive results by Western blot or immunofluorescence antibody (IFA).

In two situations, however, testing for antibodies will yield incorrect results. First, patients with new HIV infection may not have yet developed antibodies. In some cases, presence of NAT or p24 antigen may represent a positive screening test. Second, newborns of HIV-positive mothers can have maternal antibodies circulating until age 18 months. For these infants, polymerase chain reaction (PCR) testing for HIV DNA is the preferred test.[18]

2. Tuberculosis

Before industrialization and urbanization transformed Western civilization, TB was a known problem, but it did not become a scourge in Europe and North America until the 19th century. Although predominantly spread within the home, TB also was frequently spread in crowded working conditions.

EPIDEMIOLOGY

Despite the lack of any specific medical prevention or therapy, TB mortality began to decline in the late 19th century and continued to decline steadily until the end of World War II. This probably resulted from improvements in socioeconomic conditions, including better nutrition, less crowding in homes and worksites, and improved sanitation. Although far advanced by the late 1940s, control of TB was improved further with the introduction of *streptomycin* as a treatment and with the subsequent discovery of additional antimicrobial drugs.

In the United States the incidence of TB continued to decline until 1985, when it resurged because of emerging resistance and HIV infection; there were 11,545 cases of TB in 2009. Since the peak of TB resurgence in the United States in 1992, the number of TB cases reported annually has decreased by approximately 57%. Most cases are among minorities; Hispanics account for 29% and Asians for 28% of all cases. California, Texas, New York, and Florida accounted for 50% of the national case total.[19]

The global burden of disease in 2010 was 8.8 million new cases and 1.45 million deaths from TB.[20] In the 21st century,

---

Box 20-2   CDC Guidelines for HIV/AIDS Screening

Screening all patients starting treatment for tuberculosis and all patients seeking treatment for sexually transmitted diseases/infections (STDs/STIs).
Repeat screening at least annually of all persons at high risk for human immunodeficiency virus (HIV) infection:
  ▪ Injection drug users and their sex partners
  ▪ Persons who exchange sex for money or drugs
  ▪ Sex partners of HIV-infected persons
Counseling of patients that they and their prospective sex partners to be tested before initiating a new sexual relationship.
Routine, voluntary, opt-out testing of all pregnant women.
Repeat testing during the third trimester:
  ▪ Women receiving health care in settings with elevated incidence of HIV or AIDS

  ▪ Women age 15 to 45 years
  ▪ Women who receive health care in facilities in which prenatal screening identifies at least one HIV-infected pregnant woman per 1000 screened
  ▪ Women at high risk for acquiring HIV
  ▪ Women with signs or symptoms consistent with acute HIV infection
Screening of women with undocumented HIV status at the time of labor with a rapid HIV test unless they decline (opt-out testing).
Rapid testing of newborns is recommended when the mother's HIV status is unknown.

treatment for TB has entered a new phase because of the emergence of widespread resistance to multiple antibiotics. Resistance to at least the two major antituberculosis drugs, *isoniazid* and *rifampicin* (rifampin) has been termed **multidrug-resistant tuberculosis** (MDR-TB). Treatment of MDR-TB requires prolonged and expensive chemotherapy using second-line drugs that have less efficacy and heightened toxicity. If resistance to these drugs also arises, the disease becomes **extensively drug-resistant tuberculosis** (XDR-TB), which is virtually untreatable. The increase of MDR-TB and XDR-TB is fueled by inadequate chemotherapy; patients stop their treatment prematurely or receive an inadequate number or choice of agents.[21]

In an era of increased mobility, problems with resistant TB can quickly spread to the United States. A substantial portion of U.S. cases are from foreign-born patients. Therefore, many experts recommend a global strategy for TB control. Control of drug-resistant TB requires a strong health care infrastructure to ensure the delivery of effective therapy, coupled with surveillance and monitoring activities to enable timely intervention to limit transmission and spread.[21]

Stages and Natural History The natural history and pathogenesis of mycobacterial infection makes the control of TB considerably more complex than the control of other bacterial diseases. Most importantly, the manifestations of TB vary greatly among patients. In about 3% of individuals who are newly infected with mycobacteria, the infection proceeds fairly rapidly either to invade lung tissue or to cause a generalized systemic disease, such as **miliary tuberculosis.** In most persons with normal immune systems, however, lesions develop in the lungs and become contained as cell-mediated immunity develops.

The initial infection is called **primary tuberculosis.** The resolution of the primary infection is only part of the interplay of the host and the disease. The disease remains in a quiet (dormant) state, but never resolves completely. This person is therefore more correctly considered to have *inactive* TB or **latent tuberculosis infection** (LTBI). The interplay of the host and the organism during the initial infection is influenced by multiple factors, including age, immune status, amount of inoculum, nutritional status, and comorbidities. The presence of cell-mediated immunity is revealed by a positive reaction in the tuberculin skin test using purified protein derivative (PPD). Recently, interferon-γ–release assays (IGRAs) have emerged as an alternative to diagnose latent TB infections.[22]

The person infected with LTBI or inactive TB, which is noninfectious, will ultimately have two possible courses, as follows:

- The TB infection will remain inactive for the rest of the infected person's life. In developed countries, this is by far the most common course.
- The infected person's own disease may reactivate later in life to become **active tuberculosis.** This occurs in 4% to 8% of infected persons (over lifetime of patient) and is called **reactivation tuberculosis.**

Conversely, TB history needs to be distinguished from patients who become exposed to a new TB infection and develop active disease from their new infection, called **reinfection tuberculosis** or *exogenous* TB.

PREVENTION

The control of TB has been assisted by the discovery of methods for primary, secondary, and tertiary prevention.

The first discovery was a vaccine derived from a live, attenuated mycobacterium called **bacille Calmette-Guérin** (BCG) vaccine. When BCG is applied to a scratch in the skin of a previously uninfected child or adult, it stimulates the production of cell-mediated immunity, which provides some protection against a first infection with *Mycobacterium tuberculosis*. Immunization with BCG is a method of primary prevention. It is the least expensive approach to TB control, and although considerable debate surrounds its efficacy,[23] BCG is widely used in developing nations that have high rates of TB. In the United States, BCG vaccine is recommended only for children who are likely to be exposed to TB in an environment where cooperation with diagnosis and treatment efforts is unlikely. Other forms of primary TB prevention include reduction of overcrowding in prisons and homeless shelters. Immunocompromised hosts are effective transmitters of TB; therefore identifying HIV coinfection, especially in patients with resistant TB, is important as a primary prevention strategy.

The U.S. Public Health Service recommends the identification of those who have positive results in the tuberculin skin test (particularly recent skin test converters) and the use of a 9-month course of isoniazid (INH) in patients at high risk of developing reactivation TB. Recently, this treatment regimen was compared to a 3-month course of rifapentine (a synthetic rifamycin antibiotic) plus INH. The shorter regimen of rifapentine and INH was as effective in preventing active TB and had a higher treatment completion rate than the 9-month regimen of INH.[24]

Subsequent discoveries have led to new strategies for secondary and tertiary TB prevention. Tuberculosis control depends on early identification and appropriate treatment to ensure complete treatment and identification of comorbidities such as HIV. The focus of global TB control is **directly observed therapy, short course** (DOTS), comprising the following five components[25]:

1. Political commitment and sustained financing
2. Case detection through quality-assured bacteriology
3. Standardized treatment with supervision and patient support
4. Effective drug supply and management system
5. Monitoring and evaluation system with impact measurement

This approach highlights the importance of patient support and monitoring systems. In addition, some hospitals have developed special negative-pressure rooms in which patients with suspected MDR-TB can be tested and treated without risking the spread of drug-resistant infection to other patients and hospital staff.[26]

3. Malaria

EPIDEMIOLOGY

Worldwide, there were 225 million cases of malaria and an estimated 781,000 deaths in 2009, a decrease from 233 million cases and 985,000 deaths in 2000. Most deaths occur among children living in Africa, where the disease accounts for approximately 20% of all childhood deaths.[27]

Malaria is caused by a parasitic protozoan called plasmodium, which is transmitted by insect vector, the female *Anopheles* species of mosquito. Of the five types of plasmodia, *Plasmodium falciparum* is the most deadly, and *P. falciparum* and *P. vivax* are most common. All plasmodia multiply inside the red blood cells, which then break open to release more parasites (hemolysis). Malaria transmission depends on a complex interplay between the parasite (e.g., resistance to antimalarials), the vector (e.g., mosquito preference for humans), the host (decreased immunity in young children and pregnant women), and the environment (e.g., increased rainfall and temperatures increasing breeding sites for mosquitoes).[28]

Malaria induces a febrile illness, with fever, chills, and anemia. In severe cases, it can lead to convulsions and widespread organ failure. Malaria is diagnosed by microscopy or rapid diagnostic tests. Patients in endemic regions gradually develop immunity to the disease. However, this immunity may wear off after a few years, and thereafter, new bouts of malaria are as severe as if the patient had never had the disease.

DISTINGUISHING MALARIA FROM SIMILAR ILLNESSES

Distinguishing malaria from other illnesses is critical. The infections with similar presentation are geographically distinct and require in-depth knowledge of regional diseases. Carefully asking patients about their type of exposure, the season involved, food and water consumed, and vaccination history all help identify the likelihood of malaria versus similar illnesses.

Geography matters alot. For example, yellow fever is endemic to sub-Saharan Africa and South America.[29] The Geosentinel database showed that for travelers returning with fever from sub-Saharan Africa, malaria was the most common diagnosis. In contrast, *dengue fever* was significantly more common than malaria in travelers returning from Southeast Asia and the Caribbean region, and of similar frequency for travelers returning from Central America, South America, and South-Central Asia.[30]

Classic nonhemorrhagic dengue fever presents similarly to malaria, is transmitted by mosquitoes, and occurs worldwide. The similarities include fever, headache, nausea, malaise, and anorexia. However, dengue has a shorter incubation period, has more pronounced and severe myalgias, and is characterized by a centrifugal rash, petechiae, lymphadenopathy, conjunctival injection, and relative bradycardia.[29]

PREVENTION

The difficulties of preventing and controlling malaria highlight the challenges inherent in controlling a disease for which the vector's animal reservoir cannot be eradicated and to which patients do not build lasting immunity. Treatment regimens were originally based on *chloroquine*. However, many regions now have chloroquine-resistant malaria. Although many antimalarial drug treatments are available, each region has specific guidelines on drug resistance patterns and potential drug options. Work on a vaccine is ongoing and appears promising, especially in children. Box 20-3 outlines primary, secondary, and tertiary prevention policies for malaria control.[27]

Box 20-3	Policies for Malaria Prevention

Primary Prevention

Providing insecticide-treated mosquito bed nets to all persons at risk for malaria
Indoor residential spraying with pesticides
Malaria vaccine once available

Secondary Prevention

Intermittent preventive treatment of vulnerable groups in areas of high transmission
Rapid parasitologic confirmation before treatment to distinguish fevers caused by malaria from nonmalarial fever

Tertiary Prevention

Treatment with combination therapy to reduce resistance

It is particularly important to sustain the malaria control effort to avoid resurgence; repeated attacks of malaria after years of no disease can be particularly severe.

B. Diseases Transmitted by Close Contact

Diseases transmitted by close contact have sometimes been called **hygiene-related diseases** or "diseases of failure to wash your hands." Although these names oversimplify the complexity of such diseases, they do highlight that many of them can be controlled with interventions as simple as handwashing, respiratory masks, and isolation of sick patients. Many contact diseases are vaccine-preventable. Most are highly infectious, so constant vigilance is necessary to maintain herd immunity.

The close-contact disease spectrum ranges from the common cold, which causes some loss of work, to diarrheal illnesses, which kill millions of children in developing countries. Many of these diseases are also seasonal: Acute respiratory infections peak in the winter, whereas most acute gastrointestinal illnesses peak in the warmer months. Many of these infectious agents also account for a large number of outbreaks to which public health officials respond (e.g., influenza, diarrheal illness, meningitis).

EPIDEMIOLOGY

By surface area, the human respiratory tract is probably the largest area of contact between humans and microbes. It is usually well protected by defense mechanisms (e.g., hairs and mucosal surfaces that prevent bacterial adhesion), as well as the normal flora of microorganisms, which compete with pathogenic bacteria for attachment sites. An important concept in acute respiratory infection epidemiology is the **reproductive number** (R_0), calculated as follows:

$$R_0 = \int_0^\infty b(a)F(a)\,da$$

where $b(a)$ is the average number of people infected by an index case per unit time, $F(a)$ is the probability that a newly infected person remains infectious for at least time a; and a is the period of infectivity.[31] R_0 indicates an agent's transmissibility and helps estimate the vaccine coverage required to induce herd immunity. For example, measles has a very high R_0 of 15 to 17. Although **severe acute respiratory syndrome** (SARS) was the first global epidemic in the 21st century, its R_0 was only 2 to 3, which has limited its spread.

Some assume that the common circulating gastrointestinal, respiratory, and skin infections are a minor concern. However, their health burden is considerable in terms of absence from work and school, together with increased pressure on health services.[32] Table 20-2 summarizes hygiene-related diseases, populations affected, and prevention measures.

Viral hepatitis is an important cause of local and sporadic outbreaks. It is associated with chronic sequelae such as chronic hepatitis, liver failure, and liver cancer. For viral hepatitis, serology is important in making the diagnosis. A complex pattern on viral surface antigen, and different antibodies indicate acute infections, chronic infection, or resolved infection. The hepatitis B virus (HBV) contains both surface antigen (HBsAg) and core protein (HBcAg). The surface antigen suggests ongoing HBV infection, either acute or chronic. People who have recovered and who are immune or have been successfully vaccinated will have HBs antibodies. However, there is a **window phase** in late convalescence when HBs antigen levels decline and HBs antibody levels slowly increase; in this window, neither may be detectable because of immune complex formation. During this period, anti-HBc immunoglobulin M (IgM) antibodies are detectable and may be the only sign of HBV infection. Because the vaccine contains only HBsAg, the presence of anti-HBc antibodies distinguishes patients who have had the disease from vaccinated patients (Table 20-3).[33]

Table 20-2 Major Diseases Transmitted by Close Contact, Populations Affected, and Prevention

Major Syndromes	Disease Burden	Significant Pathogens	Vulnerable Populations	Prevention
Respiratory infections (common cold, sore throat, otitis media, pneumonia, bronchiolitis*)	DALY: 94 million Deaths worldwide: 3.9 million (WHO, 2002)	Streptococcus pneumoniae	Adults over 65, children, patients with chronic medical conditions	Polysaccharide vaccine (e.g., Pneumovax)
		Haemophilus influenzae B (Hib) Bordetella pertussis Corynebacterium diphtheriae	Children	Vaccine combining Hib, pertussis, and diphtheria toxin
		SARS Coronavirus	Animal handlers and health care workers	Early recognition, isolation, stringent infection control
		Influenza	Adults 65 and older, pregnant women, children age 6-23 months, patients with chronic conditions	Yearly vaccinations, isolation, early antiviral treatment
		Respiratory syncytial virus*	Children, elderly, immunocompromised patients	Passive immunization in children
Viral hepatitis (acute hepatitis, chronic hepatitis, acute liver failure, liver cancer)	4.4 million living with chronic hepatitis in U.S.; 80,000 new infections/year (CDC, 2005)	Hepatitis A and E (transmitted fecal-oral, acute infections only)	Crowding, endemic in certain countries, day care centers, MSM, IDU	Personal attention to hygiene and environmental sanitation, active and passive immunization (hepatitis A)
		Hepatitis B, C, D (transmitted by parenteral exposure to blood/body fluids, can cause chronic infections)	Health care workers, IDU, MSM	Active and passive immunization (hepatitis B)
Meningitis (bacterial, viral)	Case fatality rate for meningococcal meningitis: 10%-14%	Streptococcus pneumoniae, Hib, Neisseria meningitidis	Infants, adolescents (Hib and meningococci)	Vaccines (pneumococcal, Hib, meningococcal)
		Nonpolio enteroviruses, HSV, WNV, measles, influenza	Children in day care	Isolation; hand hygiene
Acute gastrointestinal infections	7th leading cause of death worldwide; often cause large outbreaks	Norovirus Rotavirus E. coli spp. Shigella spp. Vibrio cholerae	Young children, people living in crowding, lack of clean water	Isolation, hand hygiene
Sexually transmitted diseases (STDs)†	448 million new infections globally (WHO, 2011)	HSV, lymphogranuloma venereum, syphilis Chlamydia, gonococci HPV Scabies, pediculosis pubis	Adolescents, patients engaging in unprotected sex with multiple partners	Early identification and treatment; partner management, vaccine (HPV) Antibiotics and antivirals

CDC, Centers for Disease Control and Prevention; DALY, disability-adjusted life years; HPV, human papillomavirus; HSV, herpes simplex virus; IDU, intravenous drug use; MSM, men who have sex with men; SARS, severe acute respiratory syndrome; WHO, World Health Organization; WNV, West Nile virus.
*In children.
†Sexually transmitted infections (STIs), including genital, anal, or perianal ulcers; urethritis and cervicitis; genital warts; ectoparasitic infections.

Table 20-3 **Pattern of Hepatitis Serology**

Antigens	Result	Diagnosis
HBsAg	Negative	Susceptible
Anti-HBc	Negative	
Anti-HBs	Negative	
HBsAg	Negative	Immune because of natural
Anti-HBc	Positive	infection
Anti-HBs	Positive	
HBsAg	Negative	Immune because of
Anti-HBc	Positive	hepatitis B vaccination
Anti-HBs	Positive	
HBsAg	Positive	Acutely infected
Anti-HBc	Positive	
IgM anti-HBc	Positive	
Anti-HBs	Negative	
HBsAg	Positive	Chronically infected
Anti-HBc	Positive	
IgM anti-HBc	Negative	
Anti-HBs	Negative	
HBsAg	Negative	Interpretation unclear; four
Anti-HBc	Positive	possibilities:
Anti-HBs	Negative	1. Resolved infection (most common)
		2. False-positive anti-HBc, thus susceptible
		3. "Low-level" chronic infection
		4. Resolving acute infection

Modified from CDC: *MMWR* 54(RR-16), 2005. http://www.cdc.gov/hepatitis/hbv/PDFs/SerologicChartv8.pdf

C. Foodborne and Waterborne Infections

Food-borne and waterborne infections are caused by a variety of agents and foods, but all are transmitted by oral/fecal contact. Infections are usually spread through contaminated food and water or by contact with vomit or feces. Every year, millions of cases of food-borne illness and thousands of resulting deaths occur in the United States. Therefore, this group of diseases often highlights issues in water and food safety. Meat can be contaminated during slaughter, raw produce during harvest and processing, and all food from inadequate filtering at water treatment plants. Some bacteria replicate particularly well in particular foods, for example:

Salmonella spp. (eggs)
Listeria monocytogenes (unpasteurized milk, raw cheese, cantaloupe)
Vibrio spp. (shellfish)
Cyclospora cayetanensis (fresh produce)

However, many outbreaks have been caused by raw or undercooked meat, gravies, custards, and any food in contact with contaminated drinking water. Most agents will only cause diarrhea, vomiting, cramps, and sometimes fever. However, some agents can cause other symptoms, such as the following:

- *Clostridium botulinum,* causing respiratory paralysis and death
- Enterohemorrhagic *Escherichia coli,* causing kidney failure
- Shiga toxin–producing *E. coli* (STEC), associated with hemolytic-uremic syndrome (HUS)

Box 20-4	Enteric Outbreaks—United States, 2011

Jensen Farms cantaloupes: *Listeria monocytogenes*
Ground turkey: *Salmonella heidelberg*
Whole, fresh imported papayas: *Salmonella agona*
African dwarf frogs: *Salmonella typhimurium*
Alfalfa and spicy sprouts: *Salmonella enteritidis*
Raw sprouts from a German farm: Shiga toxin–producing *Escherichia coli* O104
Chicks and ducklings: *Salmonella altona* and *S. johannesburg*
Microbiology laboratories: *Salmonella typhimurium*
Turkey burgers: *Salmonella hadar*
Lebanon bologna: *E. coli* O157:H7
Del Monte cantaloupe: *Salmonella panama*
Hazelnuts: *E. coli* O157:H7

From http://www.cdc.gov/outbreaknet/outbreaks.html.

In 2011 an outbreak of *E. coli* (O104:H4) in Germany and other European countries underscored the importance of public health in defining the outbreak, the virulence factors, the source (contaminated sprouts), surveillance, and eradication.[34] A list of the major food-borne outbreaks in the United States in 2011 shows the variety of involved foods and bacteria and emphasizes the breadth of epidemiologic detection work required in identifying outbreak sources (Box 20-4).[35]

The CDC estimates that eight known pathogens account for the vast majority of illnesses, hospitalizations, and deaths each year from food-borne illness (Table 20-4). More than half (58%) of all foodborne-disease outbreaks are caused by *Norovirus.*

In developed countries, the single most effective intervention to decrease waterborne diseases has been the widespread chlorination of water supplies and effective sewage collection and treatment. If outbreaks occur, isolation of infected patients and treatment with antibiotics for invasive diseases form effective tertiary prevention. Travelers going to developing countries with uncertain water supply should be encouraged to avoid raw fruits and vegetables, to avoid beverages with ice, and to drink only water that has been boiled or disinfected.

D. Vector-borne Diseases and Zoonoses

Mosquitoes and ticks are the most important disease vectors. Mosquitoes depend on standing water for replication, benefiting from human-made habitats (e.g., water control ditches, irrigation system runoffs), and can even breed successfully in water in discarded tires. Diseases transmitted by mosquitoes include malaria and hemorrhagic viral fevers (e.g., yellow fever, dengue) and multiple encephalitis viruses (e.g., West Nile, St. Louis encephalitis).

Ticks transmit the widest variety of pathogens of any blood-feeding arthropod. Usually, times of heavy rainfall (rainy seasons in tropics, late spring through early fall in temperate zones) coincide with seasonal variations of disease intensity. Ticks transmit many pathogens, including:

Rickettsia (Rocky Mountain spotted fever)
Spirochetes: *Borrelia burgdorferi* (Lyme disease)

Table 20-4 Clinical Presentations of Foodborne and Waterborne Infections

Pathogen	Incubation Period	Symptom Duration	Symptoms	Food	Comments
Norovirus	1-2 days	1-3 days	Voluminous D&V	Raw produce, contaminated drinking water, food handled by infected person, vomiting, contamination	Resistant to common cleaning agents
Nontyphoidal *Salmonella* spp.	24 hours	2-4 days	D&V, fever	Eggs, meat, poultry, raw milk or juice, cheese, fruits and vegetables	
Campylobacter spp.	1-7 days	1-7 days	Watery D, fever	Poultry, milk, gravy	
Staphylococcus aureus	1-6 hours	24-48 hours	Sudden onset of severe nausea, V	Improperly refrigerated meat, poultry, potato and egg salads, cream pastries	Caused by preformed toxins
Toxoplasma gondii	Variable	Variable	Enlarged lymph nodes, flulike illness	Undercooked meat, contaminated water	Causes severe disease in pregnancy and for HIV/AIDS patients; can also be transmitted by cats
E. coli (STEC)	3-4 days	5-10 days	Severe, bloody D	Undercooked beef, raw juice and milk, raw fruits and vegetables (sprouts)	Can cause kidney failure
Listeria monocytogenes	9-48 hours	Variable	Fever, muscle aches, nausea, D	Raw milk, cheese, ready-to-eat deli meat	Pregnant women at risk for premature delivery and stillbirth
Clostridium perfringens	4-24 hours	1-3 days	Intense abdominal cramps, watery D	Poultry, meat	

D&V, Diarrhea and vomiting; *STEC,* shiga-toxin producing *E. coli.*

Ehrlichia (human monocytic ehrlichiosis)
Anaplasma (human granulocytic anaplasmosis)

Other vectors include rat fleas (*Rickettsia typhi* and *Yersinia pestis*).

Globally, many other vector-borne diseases exist, mostly neglected tropical and zoonotic infections. These disproportionately impact the poorest populations.

PREVENTION

Primary prevention includes using insect repellents, wearing appropriate clothing, and avoiding vector-infested sites. Another option for prevention is changing habitats so that they are less attractive to host animals. Prompt removal of attached ticks also reduces disease transmission.

I. Rabies

Zoonoses are diseases that normally reside in the nonhuman world. In a sense, zoonoses are also vector-borne diseases, only that most of the vectors here are mammals. (Traditionally, however, only insects and ticks have been classified as "vectors.") Globally, the most important zoonosis is rabies, which causes a devastating viral infection of the central nervous system. Each year, rabies causes more than 50,000 deaths worldwide.[36] It affects people on every continent except Antarctica. It is mainly preventive medicine physicians who decide who should be immunized against rabies. Rabies reservoirs exist in two major forms:

- Urban rabies in domestic dogs
- Wildlife rabies in many mammals, including Canidae (foxes, coyotes), skunks, raccoons, and bats

Importantly, *any* mammal can develop rabies. The disease can take two forms:

- **Furious rabies.** Animals act unusually aggressive or affectionate. This form accounts for the majority of human bites.
- **Dumb rabies.** Animals act somnolent, paralyzed, and ataxic.

The rabies virus is highly neurotropic (targets nerve cells). In humans, rabies is almost always fatal once clinical signs develop. Suspicion of rabies is based on (1) a history of animal exposure, (2) suggestive clinical signs, and (3) a compatible disease course. Although a clinical diagnosis can be supportive, definitive diagnosis requires laboratory tests. Animal exposure does not require a bite mark. For example, bat bites can be small and difficult to detect, so the presence of a bat in a bedroom is enough to require postexposure prophylaxis. Wherever possible, the animal should be observed for 10 days, because clinical rabies will become apparent in animals in that period.[37]

PREEXPOSURE VACCINATION

Vaccination before exposure is only recommended for persons at risk of exposure to rabies, such as veterinarians, laboratory staff, and animal handlers. *Preexposure vaccination does not eliminate the need for postexposure prophylaxis,* but alters the schedule and obviates the need for immune globulin.

POSTEXPOSURE PROPHYLAXIS

The wound should be promptly cleaned. Postexposure prophylaxis (PEP) then requires that the patient receive both human rabies immune globulin (HRIG; if not previously vaccinated) and the rabies vaccine. Table 20-5 outlines the PEP schedule for rabies.[38]

To decide if PEP is warranted, the clinician must consider which animal is involved. If the bite is from a domestic

Table 20-5 **Rabies Postexposure Prophylaxis (PEP) Schedule—United States, 2010**

Intervention	Regimen*
Not Previously Vaccinated	
Wound cleansing	All PEP should begin with immediate thorough cleansing of all wounds with soap and water. If available, a virucidal agent (e.g., povidone-iodine solution) should be used to irrigate the wounds.
Human rabies immune globulin (HRIG)	Administer 20 IU/kg body weight. If anatomically feasible, the full dose should be infiltrated around and into the wound(s), and any remaining volume should be administered at an anatomic site intramuscularly (IM) distant from vaccine administration. Also, HRIG should not be administered in the same syringe as vaccine. Because HRIG might partially suppress active production of rabies virus antibody, no more than the recommended dose should be administered.
Vaccine	Human diploid cell vaccine (HDCV) or purified chick embryo cell vaccine (PCECV), 1.0 mL IM (deltoid area†); 1 each on days 0,‡ 3, 7, and 14.§
Previously Vaccinated‖	
Wound cleansing	All PEP should begin with immediate thorough cleansing of all wounds with soap and water. If available, a virucidal agent (e.g., povidone-iodine solution) should be used to irrigate the wounds.
HRIG	Should not be administered.
Vaccine	HDCV or PCECV, 1.0 mL IM (deltoid area†); 1 each on days 0‡ and 3.

From Advisory Committee on Immunization Practices (ACIP): Use of a reduced (4-dose) vaccine schedule for postexposure prophylaxis to prevent human rabies, *MMWR* 59(RR-2):1-10, 2010.
*These regimens are applicable for persons in all age groups, including children.
†The deltoid area is the only acceptable site of vaccination for adults and older children. For younger children, the outer aspect of the thigh may be used. Vaccine should never be administered in the gluteal area.
‡Day 0 is the day dose 1 of vaccine is administered.
§For immunosuppressed persons, rabies PEP should be administered using all 5 doses of vaccine on days 0, 3, 7, 14, and 28.
‖Any person with a history of preexposure vaccination with HDCV, PCECV, or rabies vaccine absorbed (RVA); prior PEP with HDCV, PCECV, or RVA; or previous vaccination with any other type of rabies vaccine and a documented history of antibody response to the prior vaccination.

animal that appears healthy and can be held for observation, the animal should be observed for 10 days. If it does not become sick in that time, no further action is necessary (for domestic animals, it has been established that rabies will become apparent in that timeframe). On the other hand, bats, raccoons, skunks, and foxes are considered rabid unless the animal is available for laboratory testing and proved negative. Observing these animals is not an option because it is unknown how long they would need to be observed to rule out rabies. Small mammals (squirrels, hamsters, guinea pigs, gerbils, chipmunks, rats, mice, rabbits, hares) are almost never rabid and rarely require rabies PEP.[38]

III. EMERGING THREATS

Microbes are continually evolving, so the threat of infectious disease is ever present. The situation is reminiscent of the Red Queen's race from *Alice in Wonderland*: "It takes all the running you can do to stay in the same place."

A. Antimicrobial Resistance and Health Care–Associated (Nosocomial) Infections

The term **health care–associated infection** (HAI) has replaced *nosocomial* (hospital-related) infections because it is now clear that any contact with the health care system (physician's office, dialysis center, or nursing home) can put patients at risk for infection. All antimicrobial-resistant organisms also cause problems in hospitals. However, in addition to microbial resistance, HAIs are also caused by infections from devices or replacement of the normal microbial flora with pathogenic organisms. Similarly, although antimicrobial resistance can result from antibiotic use in health care, the use of antibiotics in animal farming contributes significantly to resistance patterns.

Although causing significant morbidity and mortality, HAIs can be prevented in many patients. These infections occur because patients' normal defenses are weakened or breached by invasive procedures or devices; normal colonizing flora is altered by antibiotics or chemotherapy; and diseases spread from patient to patient through lack of barriers or insufficient handwashing. HAIs are estimated to occur in 4.5% of hospital patients. HAIs accounted for more than $30 billion in 2007 in direct costs and significantly affect length of stay, quality of life, and mortality after the event.[39] HAIs include the following:

Surgical site infections
Central line–associated infections
Ventilator-associated pneumonias
Catheter-associated urinary tract infections
Clostridium difficile–associated disease

Resistant organisms are increasingly found in the community, which complicates treatment of outpatients.

The ability of microbes to adapt and evolve leads to resistance. In any group of microbes, some will have mutated. Most mutations do not confer a survival advantage, but some allow a microbe to survive when all the other bacteria are wiped out by an antimicrobial drug. Bacteria can also share genes with other bacteria and acquire resistance this way (**horizontal evolution**). This can happen even between different species of bacteria. Through these mechanisms, strains of many bacteria have developed resistance to all or most classes of antibiotics. Such bacteria include the following[40]:

Vancomycin-intermittent *Staphylococcus aureus* (VISA)
Multidrug-resistant gonococci
Escherichia coli

Resistance increases if bacteria are exposed to drugs repeatedly, at suboptimal concentrations, or for inadequate time. Clinical examples include unnecessary use of antibiotics for viral colds or antimalarial agents for nonmalarial fever, patients stopping antibiotics before finishing an entire course, and the continuous low-level use of antibiotics in farm animals.

PREVENTION

Prevention of HAI begins with selective and judicious use of antimicrobials, both inside and outside the health care system. The Union of Concerned Scientists estimated that 70% of all antibiotics go toward nontherapeutic uses in livestock.[41] All clinicians should use antibiotics only when there is a high chance of a bacterial infection. If prescribed, an antimicrobial should be the narrowest antibiotic possible and should be used for a full course. Furthermore, people who are sick should be properly isolated (Table 20-6).

Hospitals are also required to have an **infection control program,** which includes the following:

- Active infection surveillance system, with reporting of results to staff members
- Presence of vigorous control measures once hazards are recognized
- Sufficient staff (1 infection control staff per 250 patients)
- Knowledgeable physician who is an active program participant

Historically, public health agencies have tried to decrease HAI by benchmarking facilities and requiring public reporting. More recently, the trend has been toward the following:

- "Bundle approaches," using multiple interventions based on evidence provided by the infection control community and implemented by a multidisciplinary team
- A culture of "zero tolerance"[42]
- Environmental solutions

For example, a hospital reduced HAI significantly by decreasing the number of items taken from room to room. Each patient's room had a blood pressure cuff, thermometer, and dedicated stethoscope. All patients were isolated, tested, and treated with contact precautions until they had been confirmed *not* to carry any multidrug-resistant organisms.[43] Other measures include hand hygiene awareness. For example, some systems have an alarm sounding if staff do not wash their hands on entering the room. However, the investment to make these changes is prohibitive for most institutions.

B. Emerging Infectious Diseases and Bioweapons

New infectious diseases continue to emerge as microbes mutate and move from animals to humans or travel from one continent to another. Other diseases thought to be controlled or eradicated reemerge, such as TB in the wake of HIV/AIDS. Other examples for emerging infectious diseases include hantaviruses, SARS, and avian influenza. These can be understood in the setting of the convergence model, discussed earlier.

Prevention of emerging infectious diseases requires investment in the capacity of the poorest countries to detect and address diseases as they arise before they become global epidemics. Most emerging diseases are zoonoses with a wildlife origin. They erupt where human population density increases in areas of high wildlife biodiversity. They also tend to develop in emerging infectious disease (EID) hotspots in tropical Africa, Latin America, and Asia.[44]

One of the most concerning developments is the use of microbes with an intent to harm, such as in biologic warfare (bioweapons) or bioterrorism. Certain organisms are particularly suitable for such use because 1) they can be easily transmitted from person to person or easily disseminated; 2) they can cause significant mortality and morbidity; 3) they might cause particular panic; 4) because the health care system is poorly prepared to deal with these organisms. Such organisms are called **category A** organisms and include the following[45]:

Anthrax *(Bacillus anthracis)*
Botulism *(Clostridium botulinum* toxin)
Plague *(Yersinia pestis)*

Table 20-6 **Isolation Measures for Select Infected Patients**

Target Patients	Type of Precaution	Measures
All	Universal precautions	Handwashing before and after every patient contact
		Gloves, gowns, and eye protection as indicated before exposure to body fluids
		Safe disposal/cleaning of instruments and linen
Tuberculosis, varicella, measles*	Airborne	Private room with negative air pressure
		Wearing of mask with HEPA filter†
Meningococcus, pertussis, pharyngeal diphtheria, pneumonic influenza, rubella, mumps, adenovirus, parvovirus B19*	Droplets	Private room
		Hospital personnel wear mask within 1 meter of patient†
Colonization with multidrug-resistant bacteria; enteric infections, scabies, impetigo*	Contact	Private room or cohorting
		Nonsterile gloves for all patient contact
		Gowns for direct substantial patient contact†

Modified from Wallace RB, editor: Maxcy-Rosenau-Last: *Public health and preventive medicine,* ed 15. II. Communicable diseases, New York, 2008, McGraw-Hill Medical, and http://www.cdc.gov/hicpac/2007IP/2007ip_appendA.html
HEPA, High-efficiency particulate air; *Hib, Haemophilus influenzae* B.
*Known or suspected measles, varicella, and draining TB also require contact precautions.
†In addition to universal precautions.

Box 20-5	Barriers and Opportunities in the History of Medicine
2000 BCE	Here, eat this root.
1000 CE	That root is heathen. Here, say this prayer.
1850	That prayer is superstition. Here, drink this potion.
1920	That potion is snake oil. Here, swallow this pill.
1945	That pill is ineffective. Here, take this penicillin.
1955	Oops ... bugs mutated. Here, take this tetracycline.
1960–1999	39 more "oops." Here, take this more powerful antibiotic.
2000	The bugs have won! Here, eat this root.

Modified from World Health Organization: Anonymous, 2000. http://books.nap.edu/openbook.php?record_id=11669&page=1

Smallpox (variola major)
Tularemia *(Francisella tularensis)*
Viral hemorrhagic fevers (filoviruses such as Ebola and Marburg; arenaviruses such as Lassa and Machupo)

C. Barriers and Opportunities

In the long history of interactions between humans and microbes, the period in the 20th century where antibiotics easily cured many infectious diseases may have been a short interlude (Box 20-5). Poverty, inequality, and disenfranchisement continue to fuel the evolution of new infectious diseases and the reemergence of others. The public health community has had some victories over infectious disease, such as the eradication of smallpox. However, future gains may require more than only becoming better at fighting "the war" against microbes. Perhaps this war can never be won, but becoming better at coexisting peacefully with microbes might be possible, through the use of probiotics, immune stimulation, and support of the natural colonizing flora of the gut.[46]

IV. SUMMARY

Infectious diseases emerge in a complex interplay of human and microbes and are affected by physical environmental factors, genetic and biologic factors, ecological factors, and social, political, and economic factors (convergence model). Understanding and controlling infectious diseases requires integrating many different prevention and public health skills. Tasks that preventive medicine physicians are frequently asked to do include interpreting hepatitis serology patterns and making decisions about rabies vaccination. Infectious disease and poverty reinforce each other. Globally, the burden of infectious disease falls heavily on developing countries and children. In some developing countries, HIV/AIDS, tuberculosis, and malaria together account for more than 50% of deaths. Successful infectious disease prevention strategies include treatment, addressing motivations, social norms, and behavior clusters, and aiming to empower high-risk populations. Of particular public health concern are emerging infectious diseases, multidrug-resistant organisms such as extensively resistant TB, and biowarfare agents. The war against microbes ultimately may be futile, but better coexistence with microbes may be possible.

References

1. Institute of Medicine, Board on Global Health: The causes and impacts of neglected tropical and zoonotic diseases: opportunities for integrated intervention strategies—workshop summary, 2011. http://www.iom.edu/reports/2011/causes-and-impacts-of-neglected-tropical-and-zoonotic-diseases-opportunities-for-integrated-intervention-strategies.aspx
2. Institute of Medicine, Board on Global Health: Microbial threats to health: emergence, detection, and response, 2003. http://www.nap.edu/openbook.php?record_id=10636&page=5
3. Wallace RB, editor: Maxcy-Rosenau-Last: *Public health and preventive medicine*, ed 15. II. Communicable diseases, New York, 2008, McGraw-Hill Medical.
4. Armstrong GL: Trends in infectious disease mortality in the United States during the 20th century. *JAMA* 281:61–66, 1999. doi:10.1001/jama.281.1.61
5. Lopez AD, Mathers CD, Ezzati M, et al: Global and regional burden of diseases and risk factors. *Lancet* 367:1747–1757, 2006.
6. Chomel BB, Sun B: Zoonoses in the bedroom. *Emerg Infect Dis* (Internet serial), 2011. http://dx.doi.org/10.3201/eid1702101070
7. US Centers for Disease Control and Prevention (CDC): Sexually transmitted diseases treatment guidelines, 2010. http://www.cdc.gov/std/treatment/2010/clinical.htm
8. California STD/HIV Prevention Training Center: A guide to sexual history taking. http://www.stdhivtraining.net/educ/training_module/docs/08v2-Guide-SexHist_Taking.pdf; National Network of STD/HIV Prevention Training Centers: The ask, screen, intervene curriculum. http://www.stdhivtraining.org/asi.html.
9. http://effectiveinterventions.org
10. http://www.niaid.nih.gov/about/whoWeAre/Documents/global.pdf
11. http://www.theglobalfund.org
12. UNAIDS: Report on the global AIDS epidemic, 2010. http://www.unaids.org/documents/20101123_globalreport_chap2_em.pdf
13. http://www.cdc.gov/hiv/resources/factsheets/PDF/HIV_at_a_glance.pdf.
14. http://www.cdc.gov/std/treatment/2010/clinical.htm
15. UNAIDS: 2010 Global Report on AIDS, Chapter 2, p 16.
16. CDC: Revised recommendations for HIV testing of adults, adolescents, and pregnant women in health care settings. *MMWR* 55(RR-14):1–17, 2006.
17. Screening for HIV in health care settings: a guidance statement from the American College of Physicians and HIV Medicine Association. http://www.acponline.org/mobile/clinicalguidelines/statements/hiv_screening_0109.html
18. Diagnosis of HIV infection. In Mandell GL, Bennett JE, Dolin R, editors: *Mandell, Douglas, and Bennett's principles and practice of infectious diseases*, ed 7, Philadelphia, 2010, Churchill Livingstone.
19. CDC: Reported tuberculosis, 2009. http://www.cdc.gov/tb/statistics/reports/2009/pdf/ExecutiveCommentary.pdf on 10/18/2011
20. World Health Organization (WHO): Global tuberculosis control, 2011. http://www.who.int/tb/publications/global_report/2011/gtbr11_main.pdf
21. Zager EM, McNerney R: Multi-drug resistant tuberculosis. *BMC Infect Dis* 2008. doi:10.1186/1471-2334-8-10

22. Pai M, Zwerling A, Menzies D: Systematic review: T-cell–based assays for the diagnosis of latent tuberculosis infection: an update. *Ann Intern Med* 149:177–184, 2008.

23. Clemens JD, Chuong JJ, Feinstein AR: The BCG controversy: a methodological and statistical reappraisal. *JAMA* 249:2362–2368, 1983.

24. Sterling TR: Three months of rifapentine and isoniazid for latent tuberculosis infection. *N Engl J Med* 365:2155–2166, 2011.

25. WHO: Pursue high-quality DOTS expansion and enhancement. http://www.who.int/tb/dots/en/

26. Bellin EY, Fletcher DD, Safyer SM: Association of tuberculosis infection with increased time in or admission to the New York City Jail System. *JAMA* 269:2228–2231, 1993.

27. WHO: World malaria report, 2010. http://www.who.int/malaria/publications/atoz/9789241564106/en/

28. WHO: Malaria fact sheets. http://www.who.int/mediacentre/factsheets/fs094/en/index.html

29. Distinguishing malaria from other illnesses with similar clinical presentations. In Mandell GL, Bennett JE, Dolin R, editors: *Mandell, Douglas, and Bennett's principles and practice of infectious diseases*, ed 7, Philadelphia, 2010, Churchill Livingstone.

30. Freedman DO, Weld LH, Kozarsky PE, et al: Spectrum of disease and relation to place of exposure among ill returned travelers. *N Engl J Med* 354:119–130, 2006.

31. Heffernan JM, Smith RJ, Wahl LM: Perspectives on the basic reproductive ratio. *J R Soc Interface* 2:281–293, 2005. doi:10.1098/rsif.2005.004

32. Bloomfield SF, Exner M, Fara GM, et al: The global burden of hygiene-related disease in the home and community: report for the International Forum of Home Hygiene, 2009. http://www.ifh-homehygiene.org/IntegratedCRD.nsf/f5236e2da2822fef8025750b000dc985/29858aa006faaa22802572970064b6e8?OpenDocument

33. CDC: A comprehensive immunization strategy to eliminate transmission of hepatitis B virus infection in the United States: recommendations of the Advisory Committee on Immunization Practices. Part I. Immunization of infants, children, and adolescents. *MMWR* 54(RR-16), 2005. http://www.cdc.gov/hepatitis/hbv/PDFs/SerologicChartv8.pdf

34. Scavia G, Morabito S, Tozzoli R, et al: Similarity of Shiga toxin–producing *Escherichia coli* O104:H4 strains from Italy and Germany (letter). *Emerg Infect Dis* 17:1957–1958, 2011.

35. http://www.cdc.gov/outbreaknet/outbreaks.html

36. http://www.cdc.gov/rabies/location/usa/index.html

37. http://www.cdc.gov/rabies/exposure/animals/domestic.html

38. Vaccine schedule for post-exposure prophylaxis to prevent human rabies. *MMWR* 59(RR-2):1–10, 2010.

39. Scott DR, II: The direct medical costs of healthcare-associated infections in U.S. hospitals and the benefits of prevention. Report to the CDC, 2009. http://www.cdc.gov/HAI/pdfs/hai/Scott_CostPaper.pdf

40. Tenover FC: Mechanisms of antimicrobial resistance in bacteria. *Am J Med* 119:S3–S10, 2006.

41. http://www.ucsusa.org/food_and_agriculture/science_and_impacts/impacts_industrial_agriculture/hogging-it-estimates-of.html

42. Jarvis WR: The United States approach to strategies in the battle against healthcare-associated infections, 2006: transitioning from benchmarking to zero tolerance and clinician accountability. *J Hosp Infect* 65(suppl 2):3–9, 2007.

43. Muder RR, Cunningham C, McCray E, et al: Implementation of an industrial systems–engineering approach to reduce the incidence of methicillin-resistant *Staphylococcus aureus* infection. *Infect Control Hosp Epidemiol* 29:702–708, 2008.

44. Janes KE, Patel NG, Levy MA, et al: Global trends in emerging infectious diseases. *Nature*, Feb 21, 2008. doi: 10/1038/nature06536

45. CDC: Bioterrorism agents. http://www.bt.cdc.gov/agent/agentlist-category.asp

46. Institute of Medicine: "Ending the war" metaphor: the changing agenda for unraveling the host-microbe relationship. Executive summary, 2006. http://books.nap.edu/openbook.php?record_id=11669&page=1

Select Readings

Institute of Medicine, Board on Global Health: The causes and impacts of neglected tropical and zoonotic diseases: opportunities for integrated intervention strategies—workshop summary, 2011. http://www.iom.edu/reports/2011/causes-and-impacts-of-neglected-tropical-and-zoonotic-diseases-opportunities-for-integrated-intervention-strategies.aspx

Institute of Medicine, Board on Global Health: Microbial threats to health: emergence, detection, and response, 2003. http://www.nap.edu/openbook.php?record_id=10636&page=5

Mandell GL, Bennett JE, Dolin R, editors: *Mandell, Douglas, and Bennett's principles and practice of infectious diseases*, ed 7, Philadelphia, 2010, Churchill Livingstone.

Wallace RB, editor: Maxcy-Rosenau-Last: *Public health and preventive medicine*, ed 15. II. Communicable diseases, New York, 2008, McGraw-Hill Medical.

Websites

www.cdc.gov [US Centers for Disease Control and Prevention]
www.istm.org/geosentinel/main.html [GeoSentinel network]
www.IDSA.org [Infectious Disease Society of America]
http://www.unaids.org/en/ [Joint United Nations Program on HIV/AIDS]
http://www.theglobalfund.org/en/ [Global Fund to Fight AIDS, TB, and Malaria]
www.who.int [World Health Organization]

Mental and Behavioral Health

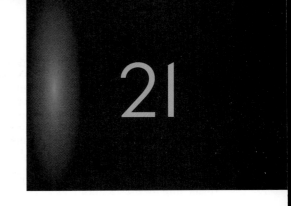

ELIZABETH C. KATZ, EUGENE M. DUNNE, SAMANTHA LOOKATCH, AND JOSHUA S. CAMINS

Depression, anxiety, schizophrenia, and substance abuse are prominent among the mental health and behavioral disorders. Affecting more than 450 million people worldwide and associated with substantial morbidity and mortality,[1] these disorders are critical targets for prevention efforts because of their toll on individuals and society.

I. MENTAL HEALTH/BEHAVIORAL DISORDERS AND SUICIDE

A. Definitions

MENTAL HEALTH DISORDER

Mental health disorder is a broad term that refers to a set of emotions, cognitions, and behaviors that cause distress to individuals or others, are abnormal from the perspective of the society or culture, and result in harm to self or others or in functional impairment in one or more domains (i.e.,

work, school, home).[2] Within the broader category of mental health disorder are *emotional disorders* that cross *Diagnostic and Statistical Manual for Mental Disorders* (DSM-IV-TR) diagnostic categories.[2] The most prevalent of the emotional disorders, and therefore the most costly to individuals and society, are depression and anxiety.[1] Table 21-1 outlines mood (depressive), anxiety, and trauma disorders, the mental health disorders that are the focus of this chapter.

BEHAVIORAL DISORDERS

Behavioral disorders involve substance use or participation in non-drug-related risky behaviors (e.g., gambling, overeating), also known as **behavioral addictions,** to such an extent that they appear *compulsive* ("out of control" of the individual) and pose serious threats to the participant's health and well-being. Behavioral disorders represent extreme cases of typical behaviors (e.g., alcohol dependence; overeating to point of obesity).

Substance use, both licit (e.g., alcohol, tobacco) and illicit (e.g., cocaine, heroin), varies along a continuum[3] (Fig. 21-1). *Misuse* of a substance is often indicative of a risk for more pathological use. *Pathological use* may be characterized by continued substance use despite serious consequences (e.g., HIV infection, incarceration), *tolerance* (need to take more of a substance to experience its customary effects), and withdrawal.[2]

Recent discussion has centered on whether other behaviors, such as overeating, excessive video game or Internet use, and sexual behavior, may be considered behavioral addictions. The following arguments favor the behavioral addiction concept:

- Such behaviors often appear compulsive (outside the individual's control).
- Participation is continued despite experiencing serious negative consequences.
- The same neural circuitry responsible for substance addiction is also involved in excessive pursuit of these behaviors.[4]

Research also suggests that substance and behavioral addictions are highly comorbid.[5] Although strong evidence supports the inclusion of pathological gambling and excessive Internet use within the broader category of addictive disorders, evidence supporting other behavioral addictions (e.g., kleptomania, sexual addiction) is less compelling.[5] However, others consider the evidence in support of the *food addiction* concept, specifically as it relates to compulsive overeating and bulimia,[4] to be compelling.[6] Obesity is discussed in Chapter 19.

Table 21-1 **Mood, Anxiety, and Trauma Disorders: Key Conditions and Description***

Category	Defining Conditions	Category Description
Mood (depressive) disorders	Major depressive disorder Dysthymic disorder	Pervasive and persistent feelings of sadness or loss of enjoyment or pleasure Weight loss/gain; decreased energy or agitation; poor self-concept; decreased attention/concentration
Anxiety disorders	Panic disorder with or without agoraphobia Specific phobia Social phobia Obsessive-compulsive disorder Generalized anxiety disorder	Adaptive emotional responses (e.g., fear, anxiety) triggered persistently and inappropriately Characterized by physical symptoms (e.g., heart palpitations; sweating); cognitive avoidance (e.g., distraction techniques or dissociation) and distortions; behavioral avoidance
Trauma disorders	Posttraumatic stress disorder Acute stress disorder	Anxiety disorder resulting from exposure to traumatic event (e.g., rape, war/combat, natural disaster, terrorism) Individual perceives self or other person to be at risk of incurring serious injury or dying. Individual reexperiences event through vivid dreams or memories, with dissociation and emotional numbing.

Modified from American Psychiatric Association: *Diagnostic and statistical manual of mental disorders,* ed 4 text revision), Washington, DC, 2000, APA.
*Descriptions refer to the general category rather than the specific disorders. Each disorder has an associated set of shared and unique criteria. The mood disorders category also includes *bipolar disorder,* which is not addressed in this chapter. The trauma disorders are included in the anxiety disorders category in DSM-IV-TR; however, because their prevention and treatment are often different from other anxiety disorders, they are treated as a separate category in this chapter.

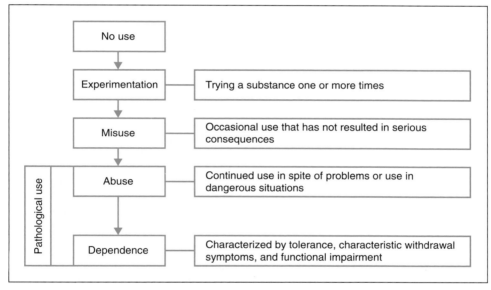

Figure 21-1 **Continuum of substance use.**

SUICIDE

Suicide is a purposeful act directed toward ending one's life. Whereas *suicide* is intended to refer to successful completion of the act, the term *suicide attempt* is intended to refer to any act of self-harm, including **parasuicidal behavior** such as cutting, regardless of the intent of the behavior or the outcome. **Suicidal ideation** refers to thoughts about killing or harming oneself.[7]

B. Epidemiology

MENTAL HEALTH DISORDERS

Mental health disorders affect a large segment of the U.S. population. Research suggests that about one in five adults

(age 18 or older) met criteria for a mental health disorder in the past year.[8] Table 21-2 outlines prevalence estimates for mood (depressive), anxiety, and trauma disorders.

BEHAVIORAL DISORDERS

Figure 21-2 presents rates of licit and illicit substance use. Among licit substances, alcohol is most often used, with 52% of individuals age 12 or older reporting tobacco use in the past year, followed closely by tobacco products, used by 28% of individuals age 12 years and older.[9] While not as prevalent as alcohol and tobacco, illicit substances are used at alarming rates and include marijuana, cocaine, heroin, and amphetamines. Evidence indicates abuse of prescription medications (i.e., use for nonprescribed purposes such as "getting high" or to help study) has been increasing in recent years.[10,11]

Table 21-2 **Prevalence Estimates for Depressive, Anxiety, and Trauma Disorders***

Disorders†	Prevalence
Mood (depressive)	11% for any mood disorder, all ages
	2.7%-10% for major depressive disorder, all ages
	6%-8% for any mood disorder, children and adolescents
	As many as 30% experience subclinical depressed mood lasting 2 or more weeks
Anxiety	17% for any anxiety disorder, all ages
	10% for any anxiety disorder, children and adolescents
	27%-70% of children experience anxiety that does not meet DSM-IV criteria for disorder
Trauma	3.6% for posttraumatic stress disorder (PTSD), all ages†
	5%-51% meet criteria for PTSD (lifetime) after exposure to trauma; variations in rates depend on severity of trauma and methodologic issues‡

*Rates reflect past year prevalence unless noted otherwise.
†Modified from Dozois DJA, Westra HA: In Dozois DJA, Dobson KS, editors: *The prevention of anxiety and depression: theory, research, and practice,* Washington, DC, 2004, American Psychological Association.
‡From Story TJ, Zucker BG, Craske MG: In Dozois DJA, Dobson KS, editors: *The prevention of anxiety and depression: theory, research, and practice,* Washington, DC, 2004, American Psychological Association.

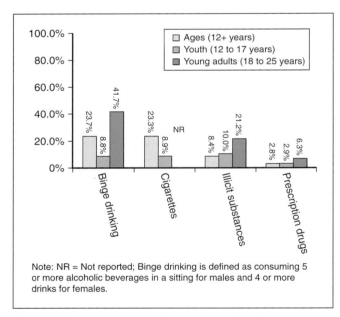

Note: NR = Not reported; Binge drinking is defined as consuming 5 or more alcoholic beverages in a sitting for males and 4 or more drinks for females.

Figure 21-2 **Past-month prevalence estimates for substance use, 2009.** Binge drinking, cigarette smoking, illicit substances, and prescription drug use in persons age 12 and older, adolescents age 12-17, and young adults 18-25. (Modified from Substance Abuse and Mental Health Services Administration: Results from the 2009 National Survey on Drug Use and Health, Rockville, Md, 2010, Office of Applied Studies; and National Institute of Alcohol Abuse and Alcoholism: NIAAA council approves definition of binge drinking.)

Among behavioral addictions, pathological gambling is estimated to affect 1% to 2% of the U.S. population. Sexual behavior considered pathological is estimated to affect 5%. In regard to problematic Internet use, whereas 6% of users can be considered addicted, this represents less than 1% of

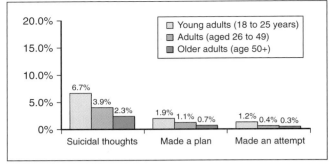

Figure 21-3 **Past-year prevalence estimates for suicidal ideation, 2008.** Serious suicidal thoughts, making plans for suicide, and suicide attempts in young adults age 18-24, adults age 26-49, and older adults 50 and older. (From Substance Abuse and Mental Health Services Administration: Suicidal thoughts and behaviors among adults: the NSDUH report, Rockville, Md, 2009, Office of Applied Studies. http://www.samhsa.gov/data/2k9/165/Suicide.htm)

the U.S. population. Eating or food addictions are believed to affect 3%, with women affected more often than men.[11]

CONCURRENT MENTAL HEALTH AND BEHAVIORAL DISORDERS

There is a high degree of comorbidity among mental health disorders and between mental health and behavioral disorders. Specifically, anxiety and depression are present concurrently in about 50% of patients.[12] Among substance-dependent individuals, 60% to 80% of adults and 60% of youth have a comorbid mental health disorder. Moreover, approximately 25% to 30% of depressed and anxious adults meet criteria for a substance use disorder.[13] Behavioral addictions (e.g., gambling, overeating, Internet overuse) are often associated with other behavioral and drug addictions, as well as psychiatric disorders.[11]

SUICIDE

Suicide accounted for more than 32,000 adult deaths in the United States in 2006. Many more adults have serious thoughts about killing themselves than make a suicide plan or attempt suicide. Research also suggests that for every one successful suicide, there are as many as 20 attempts.[1] Among youth, estimates suggest that between 9.4% (ages 12 to 13) and 12.7% (ages 14 to 17) were at serious risk for suicide by virtue of having had serious suicidal ideation or having made a previous attempt. Among those at *high risk,* 37% made a suicide attempt in the past year[14] (Fig. 21-3).

C. Costs

Mental health and behavioral disorders are extremely costly to society (Fig. 21-4). Whereas anxiety and depression costs primarily result from mental health care utilization, the costs associated with substance use disorders include both health care utilization (outpatient treatment; hospitalization) as well as incarceration and interdiction efforts.

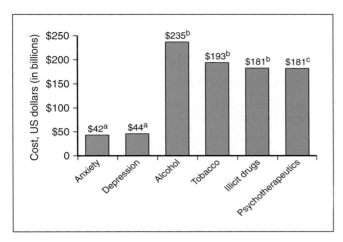

Figure 21-4 Overall economic impact of mental health and behavioral disorders. [a]Annual estimate; [b]year of estimate: 1998 (alcohol), 2007 (tobacco), 2002 (illicit drugs); [c]year of estimate: 2002. (*a* from Dozois D|A, Westra HA: In Dozois D|A, Dobson KS, editors: *The prevention of anxiety and depression: theory, research, and practice,* Washington, DC, 2004, American Psychological Association; *b* from Substance Abuse and Mental Health Services Administration: State estimates of substance use and mental health disorders from the 2008-2009 National Surveys on Drug Use and Health, NSDUH Series H-40, HHS Pub No SMA 11-4641, Rockville, Md, 2011, Office of Applied Studies; *c* from Manchikanti L: *Pain Physician* 9:289–321, 2006.)

MENTAL HEALTH DISORDERS

In addition to economic impacts, mental health disorders are associated with the following[1,12]:

- Educational and occupational impairment
- Difficult social relationships
- Stress and mental health problems in family members caring for an affected person
- Poor quality of life
- Development of, and impaired recovery from, medical conditions
- Substance abuse/dependence
- Death by suicide or other causes

BEHAVIORAL DISORDERS

Substance use disorders cause significant morbidity and mortality both in the United States and worldwide. Alcohol, tobacco, illicit substances, and prescription medications are all responsible for a substantial number of avoidable deaths because of their deleterious health effects. Specifically, excessive use of both licit and illicit substances is associated with cardiovascular disease and many different types of cancer.[1]

By impairing attention, concentration, and judgment, alcohol consumption is believed to be a causal factor in risky sexual practices,[15] increasing the risk of unwanted pregnancies and sexually transmitted infections (STIs), aggressive behavior, and fatal motor vehicle crashes.[1] Smoking during pregnancy is associated with premature birth as well as low birth weight, which increase the risk for attention-deficit hyperactivity disorder (ADHD), conduct problems, and poor school achievement.[9]

Nonprescription use of medications accounts for a substantial number of emergency department admissions and overdoses.[10] Illicit substance use significantly increases the risk of contracting infectious diseases (e.g., HIV, hepatitis B)

through injection/intravenous drug use (IDU)[16] or risky sexual practices with infected partners. Drug use during pregnancy is associated with withdrawal symptoms among infants after birth and an increased risk of offspring developing substance use disorders.[1]

SUICIDE

Following a successful suicide, bereavement of family and friends can be lengthy and complicated.[17] In addition to grief, surviving family members and friends feel guilty, confused, depressed, and anxious and may even experience suicidal thoughts or make suicide attempts themselves.[18]

II. RISK AND PROTECTIVE FACTORS

Factors that affect the development of mental and behavioral health disorders fall within several broad categories: biologic, psychological, social, environmental, and cultural.

Whereas some may be directly modifiable through education or treatment (e.g., negative thinking), other risk factors (e.g., temperament) may not. However, some suggest that a *diathesis-stress model* may serve as the most useful framework for understanding the development of mental health disorders[19] and behavioral problems. This model suggests that preexisting biologic and psychological vulnerabilities predispose a vulnerable individual to problematic emotions and behaviors when facing stress that exceeds one's ability to cope. Thus, it is important to be able to recognize these nonmodifiable factors because they may help identify those most in need of prevention and intervention efforts.

A. Biologic Risk Factors

Genetics have been found to account for 30% to 40% of an individual's risk for anxiety and depression[20,21] and 50% to 60% of risk for substance dependence (although heritability estimates for drug dependence are more variable than for alcohol dependence). Research on genetics of addiction suggests that although environmental factors play a more prominent role in the early stages of use (initiation and misuse), genetics is more influential in the progression to pathological use.[22]

Endophenotypes represent inherited traits that are risk factors for disorder and are both present and detectable before the disorder is expressed. Table 21-3 lists traits that represent possible endophenotypes for mental health and behavioral disorders. Other biologic factors associated with dysphoric mood (either anxiety or depression) include the following:

- Hormonal changes (e.g., mood disorder with postpartum onset)[2]
- Pediatric autoimmune neuropsychiatric disorders associated with streptococcal infections (PANDAS), associated with a rapid onset of tics, Tourette's syndrome, and obsessive-compulsive disorder in children[23]
- Amount of daylight (e.g., mood disorder with seasonal pattern)[2]
- Disturbances of the circadian rhythm[24]

The pharmacologic properties of drugs explain why they are used. In particular, users often report that they use substances "to feel good, to feel better, to alter consciousness,"[3]

Table 21-3   Inherited Temperaments or Traits Indicative of Risk for Anxiety, Mood (Depressive), and Substance Use Disorders

Disorder	Traits	Impact
Anxiety and depression*	Behavioral inhibition (tendency toward introversion, shyness, and caution in novel situations)	Increase risk
	Difficult temperament (tendency to be fussy, agitated, and irritable)	Increase risk
	Negative affect (tendency toward negative, depressed, irritable, or angry mood)	Increase risk
Alcohol dependence†	Facial flushing	Decrease risk†
	Decreased sensitivity to effects of alcohol	Increase risk
Alcohol and drug dependence†	Behavioral disinhibition, sensation seeking, impulsivity, impaired executive functioning (complex cognitive processes such as planning and judgment)	Increase risk
	Psychiatric disorders	Increase risk
Suicide‡	Impulsivity	Increase risk

*Modified from Dozois DJA, Dobson KS, editors: *The prevention of anxiety and depression: theory, research, and practice,* Washington, DC, 2004, American Psychological Association.

†Modified from Miller WR, Carroll KM, editors: *Rethinking substance abuse: what the science shows, and what we should do about it,* New York, 2006, Guilford.

‡Modified from Giegling I, Olgiati P, Hartmann AM, et al: Personality and attempted suicide. Analysis of anger, aggression and impulsivity, *J Psychiatr Res* 43:1262-1271, 2009.

and to do better (e.g., steroids to enhance physical performance; prescription stimulants to enhance academic performance).

The presence of one disorder may be a risk factor for another. Specifically, anxiety often precedes, and thus may be a causal factor in, the development of depression.[25,26] Externalizing disorders during childhood (e.g., conduct disorder, ADHD) are associated with an increased risk of substance use problems that persist into adulthood.[27] Other potential associations between psychiatric and substance use disorders include the following:

- Pathological substance use causes anxiety, depression, and other mental health disorders by increasing stress or impacting sensitive neural systems.
- Anxiety, depression, and other mental health disorders cause pathological substance use because substances help to regulate negative moods.
- Psychiatric and substance use disorders share genetic risk factors (e.g., difficult temperament, negative affectivity) and other risks (e.g., maladaptive responses to stress, lack of adequate coping mechanisms).
- Psychiatric and substance use disorders reciprocally influence one another.[13]

B. Psychological Risk Factors

Individuals' thoughts, beliefs, expectancies, and self-perceptions are shaped through an interaction of inherited temperaments, sensitive neural systems, hormones, and early learning experiences and thereby influence the development of mental health and behavioral disorders. Thus, both depression and anxiety are associated with maladaptive thought patterns, although the content of the maladaptive thoughts associated with anxiety and depression differs.[25,26] Similarly, beliefs about the effects of a substance, known as *outcome expectancies,* influence the age of onset and level of substance use. Positive expectancies (beliefs that drinking will produce positive outcomes) are associated with increased use, but negative expectancies do not appear to deter use.[27] Moreover, one explanation for the increase in nonmedical use of prescribed medications includes the perception that

such drugs are safer than illicit substances and pose no serious health risks.[10]

The extent to which an individual believes that others would benefit from the person's death ("perceived burdensomeness") and that the individual's basic needs for affiliation are not being met ("thwarted belongingness") are risk factors for suicidal ideation.[28] Suicide risk increases when suicidal thoughts are combined with an increased acceptance of suicide as a viable option and feelings of hopelessness. One of the best predictors of future suicide attempts is past suicidal behavior.[29]

C. Social Risk Factors

Among vulnerable individuals, exposure to anxious parents[30] or to substance-using peers[27] increases the risk of developing an anxiety or substance use disorder, respectively. Parental depression significantly increases the risk of depression among offspring, perhaps from poor communication, lack of emotional availability and bonding, or family disruption.[31] Direct exposure to a threatening stimulus (e.g., trauma, social evaluation) will also lead to the development of specific phobias and traumatic stress disorders.[30] Direct-to-consumer advertising of psychotherapeutics may play a role in perceptions of these drugs and nonmedical use.[10] Excessive attention and glorification of suicides in the media are believed to increase the risk for "copycat" behavior.[32]

D. Environmental Risk Factors

Stress and adverse early environments, such as those characterized by child abuse and neglect, domestic violence, discrimination, and poverty, are among the most significant risk factors for anxiety and depression,[12] behavioral problems,[1,27] and suicide.[29] Beyond stress, other environmental risk factors for mental and behavioral health disorders are as follows:

- Social isolation
- Inadequate transportation, housing, education, employment, and nutrition[1]
- Poor parenting practices

- Easy access to drugs and alcohol and exposure to drug-using peers[27]
- Increases in the number of prescriptions written for opioid and stimulant medications, as well as availability for purchase online[10]
- Poverty[1]

The following environmental risk factors are specific to suicide:

- Suicide among family or friends
- Inaccessibility of mental health services[1]
- Serious physical illness
- Communities where highly lethal means for committing suicide are readily available[32]

E. Culture/Diversity

Diversity, in terms of gender, race, age, socioeconomic status, and religious affiliation, is a critical factor in determining both risk and resilience for mental health and behavioral disorders. For example, research suggests that anxiety and mood disorders are more prevalent among women,[26] whereas substance use[22] and suicide[32] are more frequent among men. However, although men have an earlier onset of substance use and use more heavily than women, research suggests that rates of cigarette smoking are gender comparable. Moreover, women who do use substances may progress to pathological use more rapidly and have greater difficulty in quitting than men.[33]

Social injustice and *discrimination* are significant risk factors for mental health and behavioral disorders.[1] *Stigma* and discrimination may explain why mental and behavioral disorders are more prevalent among sexual minorities (lesbian, gay, transgendered).[34] *Age* is also a risk factor for the development of these disorders. Some argue that individuals over age 50 are at higher risk than their younger counterparts,[1] but others find that young adults are at greater risk for suicidal ideation and attempts.[35]

Minority status has also been implicated as a risk factor for experiencing traumatic events as well as for developing all mental health and behavioral disorders.[36] Onset of substance use is later among African Americans and Hispanics than among Caucasians.[27] Moreover, racial and ethnic groups experience different levels of substance use disorders, possibly because of genetic and social factors. For example, the increased risk of alcoholism among Native Americans may be caused by an inherited low-level response to alcohol, whereas the relatively low rates of alcoholism among Asians may result from an inherited flushing response.[22] Jewish people may experience lower rates of alcoholism because drinking occurs in the context of family and religious rituals.[27] Ethnic minorities are also at higher risk for committing suicide.[32] However, the relationship between ethnic/racial minority status and mental health/behavioral problems may largely be caused by the effects of poverty and lack of access to adequate mental health care[37] and behavioral health care.[36]

F. Protective Factors

Even among individuals predisposed to develop a mental health or behavioral disorder by virtue of one or more risk factors, the availability of protective factors can help mitigate that risk. Achieving developmental milestones at appropriate times, being physically healthy, and being physically active are associated with good mental health.[1] Possessing at least average cognitive ability is also associated with lower rates of anxiety and depression.[12,21]

Cognitive, social, environmental, and cultural factors that contribute to good mental and behavioral health outcomes include the following:

- Secure attachment during infancy, which contributes to the development of a positive self-image and adequate social skills[20,31]
- Strong attachments to family, school, and community among adolescents
- Social support and positive parenting practices[1,27]
- Adequate coping skills for managing stress
- High self-esteem[1]
- Strong religious beliefs[38]

III. PREVENTION AND HEALTH PROMOTION STRATEGIES

The Institute of Medicine (IOM) proposed a typology for prevention of mental health and behavioral problems based on that used for physical health problems. This typology comprises three categories: universal, selective, and indicated. Similar to primary prevention, **universal prevention** efforts are targeted toward an entire population, regardless of risk level. The other two IOM categories involve secondary prevention, because they are directed toward those at greater risk for mental health and behavioral disorders. These individuals possess risk factors such as anxious temperament or early childhood adversity (i.e., **selective prevention**), or they are experiencing subclinical symptoms that do not meet the criteria for disorder, such as anxious mood without functional impairment (i.e., **indicated prevention**). Selective prevention and indicated prevention are collectively referred to as **targeted prevention**.

Because the IOM classification does not address prevention of relapse or reduction of harm among individuals who are experiencing or have experienced a first episode of disorder, a fourth category, *treatment*, which is most similar to tertiary prevention, is also needed.[25]

A. Theoretical Framework

The **health belief model** provides a framework for understanding how people perceive themselves to be at risk for developing problems and factors associated with decisions to enact disorder prevention and health-promotion behaviors (see Chapter 15). The health belief model was created in the late 1950s in response to the lack of utilization of public health efforts to vaccinate people for tuberculosis. The model includes the following four cognitive dimensions that impact an individual's willingness to modify risky health behaviors.

1. *Perceived susceptibility* is the extent to which individuals recognize that they are at risk for developing an undesirable health outcome.
2. *Perceived severity* involves the extent to which associated consequences are perceived to be grave.

3. *Perceived benefits* of change
4. *Perceived barriers* to change

More recently, the health belief model was modified to include the concept of *perceived self-efficacy* in recognition of its importance in predicting the likelihood of behavior change. Self-efficacy refers to confidence or a belief in one's competence to do what is needed to enact health-enhancing behaviors.[39]

B. Public Policy

Universal prevention efforts include policy changes that are targeted toward an entire population and serve to reduce the incidence of mental health or behavioral disorders. Strategies shown to improve mental health outcomes include the following:

- Improving nutrition and housing
- Improving access to education and health care
- Improving access to work and reducing poverty[1]

Although legal approaches to substance use (e.g., incarceration of drug users; interdiction efforts) may prevent experimentation or initial use of substances, these efforts have been largely ineffective for stopping established use.[3] The following policies have led to decreases in rates of substance use and related problems:

- "Sin taxes" (increasing the cost of alcohol and cigarettes)
- Raising the legal age to purchase and drink alcohol
- Reducing the availability of alcohol by regulating number and open hours of places selling alcohol[1,27]
- Advertising bans
- Banning smoking in public places[1]

In addition to the efforts noted thus far, which would reduce suicide rates by reducing anxiety, depression, and substance use, other suicide prevention efforts might include:

- Reducing the toxicity of gasoline and car exhausts
- Minimizing access to high places such as rooftops and bridges
- Enforcing gun control policies
- Controlling the availability of pesticides and prescription medications[1,32]

Selective or indicated prevention efforts might include improving accessibility, affordability, and perceived helpfulness of mental health or substance abuse treatment, especially for groups with limited access.[3,36,37]

C. Media Campaigns

Universal prevention efforts may include media campaigns that highlight the consequences of substance use. The Legacy Foundation's "Truth" campaign links smoking with serious health consequences and death (http://www.thetruth.com/). Television advertisements are effective for reducing drunk-driving crashes and related trauma.[40] Similarly, countermarketing, or antitobacco advertisements, have been found to increase knowledge and negative beliefs about the use of tobacco.[41] Media campaigns can be similarly effective for reducing illicit substance use.[42]

D. Screening

Screening programs may be used as universal prevention efforts to identify individuals who would benefit from more targeted prevention efforts. Brief screening tools can be used in a variety of settings (e.g., primary care physician offices, schools, emergency rooms) to determine level of risk and type of intervention required. For example, the **psychosocial assessment tool** (PAT) is a 20-item self-administered questionnaire for families of chronically ill children that assesses 10 domains of risk factors. The PAT was found to be a valid tool, with most families requiring universal prevention (consisting of screening and support), many fewer requiring selective prevention (services targeted toward specific risk factor identified), and the fewest requiring indicated prevention (involving referral to behavioral health specialist).[43]

A list of measures is useful for identifying risk of developing *anxiety and depression* (e.g., cognitive biases; anxiety sensitivity), diagnosing anxiety or mood disorders, and assessing general mental health, functional impairment, and quality of life.[44] Among the most widely used risk factors measures are the 21-item Beck depression and Beck anxiety inventories, which provide criteria for determining the severity of symptoms (i.e., mild to profound); individuals scoring in the mild to moderate range could be candidates for selective or indicated prevention efforts whereas those scoring higher would likely need treatment. The *brief psychiatric rating scale* (BPRS) is a validated 24-item diagnostic screening tool assessing five domains of mental health problems: thought disorder, withdrawal, anxiety–depression, hostility-suspicion, and activity. Although its psychometric properties are good, diagnoses must be confirmed with a more thorough assessment.[44]

A number of brief screening tools have also been developed for assessing the presence and extent of substance use problems as well as motivation to quit. The four-item CAGE (cut down, annoyed, guilty, eye-opener) and 24-item Michigan Alcoholism Screening Test (MAST) are effective for identifying problematic levels of alcohol use.[45,46] The Rutgers Alcohol Problem Index (RAPI)[47] is an 18-item measure that assesses drinking-related consequences. A revision of the MAST, the drug abuse screening test (DAST), is a 20-item measure that can be used to identify individuals who are using or at risk for using illicit substances.[48]

Also, the **addiction severity index** (ASI, 5th edition) is a structured interview widely used in both substance abuse treatment clinics and treatment research.[49] The ASI assesses severity of problems in seven domains related to drug and alcohol use: medical, employment, alcohol, drug, legal, family/social, and psychiatric. Advantages include good psychometric properties and guiding treatment planning. Disadvantages of the ASI are that it takes 45 minutes to administer and interviewers must be trained to ensure it is administered properly.

A comprehensive assessment of *smoking* should include measures of motivation, nicotine dependence, past quit attempts, smoking history, other substance use, presence of psychiatric conditions, and treatment preferences.[50] All these factors will affect whether a quit attempt is made and whether that attempt is successful. Nicotine dependence can be assessed with the six-item Fagerstrom Test of Nicotine Dependence and two-item *heaviness of smoking* index. Both measures include a question regarding the amount of time

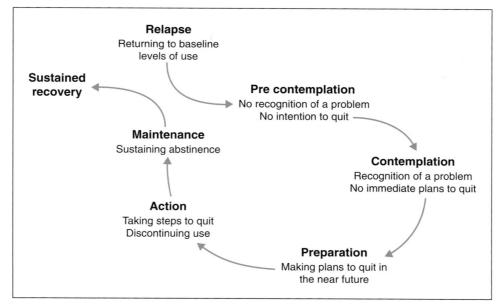

Figure 21-5 **Stages of change model.** (Modified from Prochaska JO, DiClemente CC: *Psychotherapy* 19:276-288, 1982.)

between waking and smoking the first cigarette, which is strongly associated with level of dependence. Motivation can be assessed using the *contemplation ladder,* which has smokers indicate their readiness to stop smoking on a scale of 0 to 10.[50] The contemplation ladder has its theoretical foundation in the **stages of change model,**[33] which is comprised of five stages and is reinitiated by a relapse (Fig. 21-5).[51] The contemplation ladder may also be useful for assessing motivation to quit among users of alcohol and other drugs.[52] These measures could be used in combination with a brief physician intervention (e.g., five "A" model described later) to enhance motivation to quit as well as to guide decisions about the most appropriate approach to encourage cessation.

While simply asking about thoughts of suicide and the presence of a plan is considered a reasonable strategy for identifying individuals at risk of killing themselves, using the **depressive symptom index** (DSI) **suicidality** subscale is recommended.[53] This four-item measure, with scores from 0 to 12 (higher scores indicate greater risk), assesses presence and frequency of suicidal ideation, presence of a plan, and pervasiveness of the desire to kill oneself. A cutoff score of 3 is recommended to ensure that all high-risk persons are identified while minimizing false positives.

E. Psychosocial Interventions

1. Brief Interventions

Few prevention programs specifically target *anxiety.* However, given the significant number of shared risk factors between anxiety and other mental health and behavioral problems, prevention programs aimed at other disorders will likely have a broad beneficial impact for preventing anxiety.[20] School-based programs are effective for improving coping and social skills and thereby reducing the risk of depression and anxiety.[1] One of the most well-known and widely used

universal school-based drug prevention programs delivered by police officers is Project DARE (Drug Abuse Resistance Education). Despite its popularity, meta-analyses show that DARE produces either no effect or possibly harmful effects in terms of youth drug use.[54] Conversely, school-based interventions that teach drug refusal skills and address outcome expectancies for drugs, delivered as either universal or selected prevention programs, can be effective for decreasing substance use.[55]

Universal efforts to prevent *suicide* involve psychoeducational programs targeted to increasing awareness of the symptoms of mental health disorders, their role in suicide, and available resources. In **gatekeeper training,** for example, selected individuals are trained to recognize warning signs of depression and suicide and to intervene with distressed persons. A systematic review found that gatekeeper training improved trainee's knowledge, skills, and attitudes toward intervening and, in specific populations, produced reductions in suicidal ideation and attempts.[56] Research on the efficacy of crisis centers and hotlines, both targeted prevention programs, is inconclusive.[1]

Targeted brief interventions and brief treatments for substance use and mental health disorders include **motivational interviewing** (MI), a brief intervention (1-4 sessions) developed to encourage internal motivation for change. MI has been effective for enhancing treatment retention and reducing substance use and related negative consequences.[57] Recently, MI has been effectively applied to the treatment of mental health disorders, either to increase motivation to engage in treatment or to encourage patients in treatment to take the steps necessary to achieve therapeutic change (e.g., exposure exercises)[58] (see Chapter 15).

In addition to MI, research suggests that advice by a physician may be sufficient to enhance motivation to change behavior and to enter treatment.[59] The U.S. Public Health Service and National Cancer Institute developed the five "A" program, a brief intervention designed to assist physicians in assessing patient smoking status and encouraging them to quit.[60] The **five "A" model**, based on research on persuasion and the health belief model, involves these five steps:

1. *Ask* all patients about their current smoking status.
2. *Advise* smoking patients to quit. Provide feedback about the role of smoking in causing or exacerbating their current health concerns, as well as personalized information about the benefits of quitting.
3. *Assess* their smoking and related health status.
4. *Assist* patients in their quit attempts. Refer them for psychosocial treatment, or discuss pharmacologic treatment options.
5. *Arrange* a follow-up appointment in the next 3 months.

The five "A'" program has been shown to be effective for motivating patients to quit smoking[61] (see Box 15-2).

2. Longer-Term Interventions

Consistent with the finding that insecure attachment is associated with poor psychosocial outcomes, early home-based interventions that help to facilitate maternal responsiveness and expression of positive affect, as well as teach effective parenting skills to reduce child abuse and neglect, are likely to enhance resilience of at-risk children (e.g., impoverished parents, teenage mother).[1] School-based and community-based programs that encourage prosocial behavior, foster expression of positive affect, and teach empathy and cognitive skills for effectively regulating negative emotions as well as problem-solving skills have been useful for improving general mental health and substance use. Programs that address substance use and other risky behaviors teach skills that are also effective for increasing resilience and preventing mental health disorders.[20]

Cognitive-behavioral therapy (CBT) is extensively used for the treatment of anxiety, depression, and substance use disorders. CBT focuses on restructuring maladaptive cognition and teaching effective strategies for coping with stress. In addition, it also identifies thoughts, feelings, and behaviors *(triggers)* that maintain substance use and teaches strategies for coping with triggers (people, places, things, thoughts, feelings). Exposure may be used as part of CBT to foster extinction of the learned association between environmental cues and fear as well as between triggers and drug craving. Research suggests that cognitive and behavioral approaches are effective for preventing a first depressive episode,[1,20] for encouraging drug abstinence during treatment, and for promoting sustained abstinence. Also, patients show continued reductions in substance use for as long as 1 year after CBT ends.[57] For anxiety, CBT is more effective than pharmacotherapy for producing symptom reduction and preventing relapse.[62] Research on the relative effectiveness of psychosocial treatment, pharmacotherapy, and their combination for substance use shows that both are equally effective when used as monotherapy and that their combination offers no advantage.[63]

After exposure to trauma, intervening with individuals exhibiting symptoms of acute stress disorder (ASD) might help to forestall the development of posttraumatic stress disorder (PTSD). However, research on **critical incidents stress debriefing** (CISD), a popular brief intervention for individuals exposed to trauma, has been mixed; some studies find it helpful, and others find it is iatrogenic (i.e., increasing

the risk of traumatic stress disorder symptoms). Conversely, cognitive restructuring and exposure therapies effectively reduce symptoms of PTSD and prevent relapse.[30]

Postsuicide intervention programs are based on the same principles as CISD and involve providing survivors with information about resources and with opportunities to share their thoughts and feelings about the suicide. As with CISD, however, such approaches either have no beneficial effects or may be harmful because the suicidal act is glorified, inspiring suicidal thoughts in participants and copycat behavior.[64]

Effective treatments for substance dependence include contingency management and social network and family models. **Contingency management** (CM) models operate on the premise that drug use is highly reinforcing and that motivation for abstinence can be increased when abstinence and participation in non-drug-related activities are reinforced. CM interventions use a variety of reinforcements, including vouchers with monetary value that can be exchanged for goods and services, retail items/gift certificates, and for heroin users, take-home methadone doses. Although CM is most effective for promoting drug abstinence when reinforcement is present (with high rates of relapse once the reinforcement is removed), it does seem to be an effective approach for improving compliance (counseling session attendance; taking medication as prescribed) during treatment, which may translate into longer-term posttreatment benefits.

Social network and family models are rooted in research showing that social support is critical for increasing the likelihood of treatment entry and engagement, abstinence, and sustained recovery. In addition to interventions that focus on involving drug-free family members and significant others in treatment, self-help groups (e.g., Alcoholics Anonymous, Narcotics Anonymous, Rational Recovery) are also effective for improving substance use outcomes.[57]

F. Medical/Pharmacologic Interventions

Pharmacotherapies, particularly selective serotonin reuptake inhibitors (SSRIs) and serotonin-norepinephrine reuptake inhibitors (SNRIs), are often used for the treatment of anxiety and depression with the goal of reducing symptoms and improving overall quality of life. However, research suggests that the effectiveness of SSRIs and benzodiazepines for treating anxiety are limited to the period of medication administration, with patients experiencing a relapse of symptoms on cessation.[26] Similarly, pharmacotherapy is less effective than cognitive therapy for preventing relapse after medication discontinuation, although relapse appears to be reduced if (1) the patient experiences full remission of symptoms (partial remission of symptoms increases the risk of relapse after discontinuing medication) and (2) medication is continued for at least 4 to 6 months after remission of symptoms.[65]

However, research does suggest that the increased risk of suicide associated with pharmacologic treatment can be mitigated by the addition of CBT.[66]

Pharmacologic interventions for substance use (Table 21-4) either encourage abstinence initiation or prevent relapse through the following:

■ Blocking the effects of drugs and thereby reducing their euphoric effects; such drugs will also instigate the onset of withdrawal symptoms (i.e., antagonists).

Table 21-4 Pharmacotherapies for Substance Use Disorders

Medication	Mechanism of Action	Use
Alcohol		
Benzodiazepines	GABA agonist	Effective for safely detoxifying alcohol-dependent patients
Disulfiram (Antabuse)	Inhibits breakdown of acetylaldehyde; produces headache, facial flushing, and nausea/vomiting	Discourages drinking; only effective if administration is supervised, otherwise patients are noncompliant
Naltrexone	Opiate antagonist	Discourages drinking; more effective than placebo
Acamprosate	Modulates glutamate receptor activity; reduces distress associated with withdrawal	Promotes maintenance of abstinence; more effective than placebo
Ondansetron	Reduces serotonin receptor activity	Discourages drinking; particularly effective for alcoholism with onset before age 25
Nicotine		
Nicotine replacement	Replaces nicotine obtained through smoking; prevents withdrawal	Effective for encouraging smoking abstinence initiation; recommended for short-term use only
Bupropion	Uncertain; presumably blocks the reinforcing effects of nicotine	Effective for promoting smoking abstinence initiation
Nicotine vaccine	Blocks nicotine from entering brain, reducing its euphoric effects	Currently under investigation
Opioids		
Methadone	Full opioid agonist	Effective as a maintenance medication if patients are compliant; patients must attend specialty clinics to obtain medication
Buprenorphine	Partial opioid agonist	Effective as a maintenance medication; more expensive than methadone, but lower risk of overdose death; available by prescription
Naltrexone	Opioid antagonist	Effective for reversing overdose Patient must be fully detoxified to begin medication; poor compliance Under investigation for use in rapid opioid detoxification

Modified from Miller WR, Carroll KM, editors: *Rethinking substance abuse: what the science shows, and what we should do about it,* New York, 2006, Guilford.
GABA, γ-Aminobutyric acid.

- Mimicking the effects of drugs and therefore preventing withdrawal as well as blocking their euphoric effects (agonists).
- Preventing drugs from entering the brain and thereby reducing their euphoric effects (vaccines).[63]

Although considerable research has been done to identify effective pharmacotherapies for stimulants, such as cocaine, none has received U.S. Food and Drug Administration (FDA) approval at present. However, ongoing research is testing the efficacy of a cocaine vaccine. Moreover, there are no FDA-approved pharmacotherapies for marijuana,[63] which is itself now a legal medical therapy in many states.

In addition to interventions that increase abstinence rates and prevent relapse, other medical interventions are designed to reduce harm and prevent overdose or death. For example, programs in which opioid-addicted individuals are prescribed and trained to use naloxone (opioid antagonist) are effective for reversing the effects of opiate overdose in as many as 96% of cases.[67] Needle exchange programs, in which injection drug users can safely exchange used for unused hypodermic needles, are designed to prevent transmission of infectious diseases as well as facilitate entry into treatment.[68] Prevention education and HIV testing, providing condoms, and drug substitution therapy may help reduce the spread of HIV and other transmissible infections.

IV. SUMMARY

Mental health/behavioral disorders and suicide are prevalent and exact significant tolls on individuals, families, and society. Research has begun to identify the shared and unique risk factors as well as protective factors associated with these disorders. Shared risk factors include poor parent-child bonding and inadequate parenting skills, parental mental health problems, poverty, and stress. Unique risk factors are behavioral inhibition for anxiety and depression versus disinhibition for behavioral disorders; anxious role models for anxiety disorders; and substance-using role models for substance use disorders. Shared protective factors include social support and social and emotional competence. Despite advances in the development of effective prevention and intervention approaches, further research is needed to ensure that prevention policies and interventions are grounded in theory, are culturally-informed and relevant, and reflect state-of-the-art (evidence-based) knowledge, to reduce the burden of these disorders while improving quality of life.

References

1. Hosman C, Jane-Llopis E, Saxena S: *Prevention of mental disorders: effective interventions and policy options—summary report,* Oxford, 2005, Oxford University Press.
2. American Psychiatric Association: *Diagnostic and statistical manual of mental disorders,* ed 4, text revision, Washington, DC, 2000, APA.
3. Miller WR, Carroll KM, editors: *Rethinking substance abuse: what the science shows, and what we should do about it,* New York, 2006, Guilford.
4. Holden C: "Behavioral" addictions: do they exist? *Science* 294:980–982, 2001.
5. Grant JE, Potenza MN, Weinstein A, et al: Introduction to behavioral addictions. *Am J Drug Alcohol Abuse* 36:233–241, 2010.

6. Katz DL: Unfattening our children: forks over feet. *Int J Obesity* 35:33–37, 2011.

7. US Centers for Disease Control and Prevention: Definitions: self-directed violence, 2011. http://www.cdc.gov/Violence Prevention/suicide/definitions.html

8. Substance Abuse and Mental Health Services Administration: *State estimates of substance use and mental health disorders from the 2008-2009 National Surveys on Drug Use and Health, NSDUH Series H-40, HHS Pub No SMA 11-4641*, Rockville, Md, 2011, Office of Applied Studies.

9. Substance Abuse and Mental Health Services Administration: *Results from the 2009 National Survey on Drug Use and Health. Vol I. Summary of national findings, NSDUH Series H-38A, HHS Pub No SMA 10-4856*, Rockville, Md, 2010, Office of Applied Studies.

10. Manchikanti L: Prescription drug abuse: what is being done to address this new drug epidemic? Testimony before the Subcommittee on Criminal Justice, Drug Policy, and Human Resources. *Pain Physician* 9:1533–3159, 2006.

11. Freimuth M, Waddell M, Stannard J, et al: Expanding the scope of dual diagnosis and co-addictions: behavioral addictions. *J Groups Addict Recov* 3:137–160, 2008.

12. Dozois DJA, Dobson KS, Westra HA: The comorbidity of anxiety and depression, and the implications of comorbidity for prevention. In Dozois DJA, Dobson KS, editors: *The prevention of anxiety and depression: theory, research, and practice*, Washington DC, 2004, American Psychological Association.

13. Mueser KT, Drake RE, Turner W, et al: Cormorbid substance use disorders and psychiatric disorders. In Miller WR, Carroll KM, editors: *Rethinking substance abuse: what the science shows, and what we should do about it*, New York, 2006, Guilford.

14. Substance Abuse and Mental Health Services Administration: *Substance use and the risk of suicide among youths: the NHSDA report*, Rockville, Md, 2002, Office of Applied Studies.

15. Corbin WR, Fromme K: Alcohol use and serial monogamy as risk for sexually transmitted diseases in young adults. *Health Psychol* 21:229–236, 2002.

16. Grigoryan A, Hall HI, Durant T, et al: Late HIV diagnosis and determinants of progression to AIDS or death after HIV diagnosis among injection drug users, 33 U.S. States, 1996–2004. *PLoS One* 4:e4445, 2009.

17. Mitchell AM, Kim Y, Prigerson HG, et al: Complicated grief in survivors of suicide. *Crisis* 25:12–18, 2004.

18. Runeson B, Åsberg M: Family history of suicide among suicide victims. *Am J Psychiatry* 160:1525–1526, 2003.

19. Clark DA: Design considerations in prevention research. In Dozois DJA, Dobson KS, editors: *The prevention of anxiety and depression: theory, research, and practice*, Washington, DC, 2004, American Psychological Association.

20. Hudson JL, Flannery-Schroeder E, Kendall PC: Primary prevention of anxiety disorders. In Dozois DJA, Dobson KS, editors: *The prevention of anxiety and depression: theory, research, and practice*, Washington, DC, 2004, American Psychological Association.

21. Sullivan P, Neale M, Kendler K: Genetic epidemiology of major depression: review and meta-analysis. *Am J Psychiatry* 157:1552–1562, 2000.

22. Hasin D, Hatzenbuehler M, Waxman R: Genetics of substance use disorders. In Miller WR, Carroll KM, editors: *Rethinking substance abuse: what the science shows, and what we should do about it*, New York, 2006, Guilford.

23. Coffey BJ, Rapoport J: Obsessive-compulsive disorder and Tourette's disorder: where are we now? *J Child Adolesc Psychopharmacol* 20:235–236, 2010.

24. Harvey AG: Sleep and circadian functioning: critical mechanisms in the mood disorders? *Annu Rev Clin Psychol* 7:297–319, 2011.

25. Dozois DJA, Dobson KS, editors: *The prevention of anxiety and depression: theory, research, and practice*, Washington, DC, 2004, American Psychological Association.

26. Dozois DJA, Westra HA: The nature of anxiety and depression: implications for prevention. In Dozois DJA, Dobson KS, editors: *The prevention of anxiety and depression: theory, research, and practice*, Washington, DC, 2004, American Psychological Association.

27. Hesselbrock VM, Hesselbrock MN: Developmental perspectives on the risk for substance abuse problems. In Miller WR, Carroll KM, editors: *Rethinking substance abuse: what the science shows, and what we should do about it*, New York, 2006, Guilford.

28. Joiner T: *Why people die by suicide*, Cambridge, Mass, 2005, Harvard University Press.

29. Joiner TE, Walker RL, Rudd EM, et al: Scientizing and routinizing the assessment of suicidality in outpatient practice. *Profession Psychol Res Pract* 30:447–453, 1999.

30. Story TJ, Zucker BG, Craske MG: Secondary prevention of anxiety disorders. In Dozois DJA, Dobson KS, editors: *The prevention of anxiety and depression: theory, research, and practice*, Washington, DC, 2004, American Psychological Association.

31. Essau CA: Primary prevention of depression. In Dozois DJA, Dobson KS, editors: *The prevention of anxiety and depression: theory, research, and practice*, Washington, DC, 2004, American Psychological Association.

32. Krug EG, Mercy JA, Dahlberg LL, et al: The world report on violence and health. *Lancet* 360:1083–1088, 2002.

33. DiClemente CC: Natural change and the troublesome use of substances: a life-course perspective. In Miller WR, Carroll KM, editors: *Rethinking substance abuse: what the science shows, and what we should do about it*, New York, 2006, Guilford.

34. Meyer I: Prejudice, social stress, and mental health in lesbian, gay, and bisexual populations: conceptual issues and research evidence. *Psychol Bull* 129:674–697, 2003.

35. Substance Abuse and Mental Health Services Administration: *Suicidal thoughts and behaviors among adults: the NSDUH report*, Rockville, Md, 2009, Office of Applied Studies.

36. Satcher D: Embracing culture, enhancing diversity, and strengthening research. *Am J Public Health* 99:S4, 2009.

37. Samaan RA: The influences of race, ethnicity, and poverty on the mental health of children. *J Health Care Poor Underserved* 11:100–110, 2000.

38. Wink P, Dillon M, Larsen B: Religion as moderator of the depression-health connection: Findings from a longitudinal study. *Res Aging* 27:197–220, 2005.

39. Rosenstock IM, Strecher VJ, Becker MH: Social learning theory and the health belief model. *Health Educ Q* 15:175–183, 1988.

40. Elder RW, Shults RA, Sleet DA, et al: Effectiveness of mass media campaigns for reducing drinking and driving and alcohol-involved crashes: a systematic review. *Am J Prev Med* 27:57–65, 2004.

41. Murphy-Hoefer R, Hyland A, Rivard C: The influence of tobacco countermarketing ads on college students. *J Am Coll Health* 58:373–381, 2010.

42. Carpenter CS, Pechmann C: Exposure to the Above the Influence antidrug advertisements and adolescent marijuana use in the United States, 2006–2008. *Am J Public Health* 101:948–954, 2011.

43. Kazak AE: Pediatric psychosocial preventive health model (PPPHM): research, practice, and collaboration in pediatric family systems medicine. *Fam Systems Health* 24:381–395, 2006.

44. Bieling PJ, McCabe RE, Antony MM: Measurement issues in preventing anxiety and depression: concepts and instruments. In Dozois DJA, Dobson KS, editors: *The prevention of anxiety and depression: theory, research, and practice*, Washington, DC, 2004, American Psychological Association.

45. Ewing JA: Detecting alcoholism: the CAGE questionnaire. *JAMA* 252:1905–1907, 1984.

46. Ross HE, Gavin DR, Skinner HA: Diagnostic validity of the MAST and the alcohol dependence scale in the assessment of DSM-III alcohol disorders. *J Stud Alcohol* 51:506–513, 1990.

47. White HR, Labouvie EW: Towards the assessment of adolescent problem drinking. *J Stud Alcohol* 50:30–37, 1989.

48. Cocco K, Carey K: Psychometric properties of the drug abuse screening test in psychiatric outpatients. *Psychol Assess* 10:408–414, 1998.

49. McLellan AT, Kushner H, Metzger D, et al: The fifth edition of the addiction severity index: historical critique and normative data. *J Subst Abuse Treat* 9:199–213, 1992.

50. Niaura R, Shadel WG: Assessment to inform smoking cessation treatment. In Abrams DB, Niaura R, Brown RA, et al, editors: *The tobacco dependence treatment handbook*, New York, 2003, Guilford.

51. Prochaska JO, DiClemente CC: Transtheoretical therapy: toward a more integrative model of change. *Psychotherapy* 19:276–288, 1982.

52. Hogue A, Dauber A, Morgenstern J: Validation of a contemplation ladder in an adult substance use disorder sample. *Psychol Addict Behav* 24:137–144, 2010.

53. Wingate LR, Joiner TE, Walker RL, et al: Empirically informed approaches to topics in suicide risk assessment. *Behav Sci Law* 22:651–665, 2004.

54. Ennett ST, Tobler NS, Ringwalt CL, et al: How effective is drug abuse resistance education? A meta-analysis of Project DARE outcome evaluations. *Am J Public Health* 84:1394–1401, 1994.

55. Griffin KW, Botvin GJ, Nichols TR, et al: Effectiveness of a universal drug abuse prevention approach for youth at high risk for substance use initiation. *Prev Med* 36:1–7, 2003.

56. Isaac M, Elias B, Katz LY, et al: Gatekeeper training as a preventative intervention for suicide: a systematic review. *Can J Psychiatry* 54:260–268, 2009.

57. Carroll KM, Rounsaville BJ: Behavioral therapies: the glass would be half full if only we had a glass. In Miller WR, Carroll KM, editors: *Rethinking substance abuse: what the science shows, and what we should do about it*, New York, 2006, Guilford.

58. Arkowitz H, Miller WR, Westra HA, et al: Motivational interviewing in the treatment of psychological problems: conclusions and future directions. In Arkowitz H, Westra HA, Miller WR, et al, editors: *Motivational interviewing in the treatment of psychological problems*, New York, 2008, Guilford.

59. Fiore MC, Keller PA, Baker TB, et al: Preventing 3 million premature deaths and helping 5 million smokers quit: a national action plan for tobacco cessation. *Am J Public Health* 94:205–210, 2004.

60. Fiore MC, Jaen CR, Baker TB, et al: Treating tobacco use and dependence: 2008 update. US Public Health Service clinical practice guideline: executive summary. *Respir Care* 53:1217–1222, 2008.

61. Stead LF, Bergson G, Lancaster T: Physician advice for smoking cessation. *Cochrane Database Syst Rev* 2:CD000165, 2008.

62. Dugas MJ, Radomsky AS, Brillon P: Tertiary intervention for anxiety and the prevention of relapse. In Dozois DJA, Dobson KS, editors: *The prevention of anxiety and depression: theory, research, and practice*, Washington, DC, 2004, American Psychological Association.

63. O'Malley SS, Kosten TR: Pharmacotherapy of addictive disorders. In Miller WR, Carroll KM, editors: *Rethinking substance abuse: what the science shows, and what we should do about it*, New York, 2006, Guilford.

64. Szumillas M, Kutcher S: Post-suicide intervention programs: a systematic review. *Can J Public Health* 102:18–29, 2011.

65. Dobson KS, Ottenbreit ND: Tertiary intervention for depression and prevention of relapse. In Dozois DJA, Dobson KS, editors: *The prevention of anxiety and depression: theory, research, and practice*, Washington, DC, 2004, American Psychological Association.

66. Treatment for Adolescents with Depression Study (TADS) Team: Fluoxetine, cognitive-behavioral therapy, and their combination for adolescents with depression. Treatment for Adolescents with Depression Study (TADS) randomized controlled trial. *JAMA* 292:807–820, 2004.

67. Bennett A, Bell A, Tomedi L, et al: Characteristics of an overdose prevention, response, and naloxone distribution program in Pittsburgh and Allegheny County, Pennsylvania. *J Urban Health* 88:1020–1030, 2011.

68. Kidorf M, King VL: Expanding the public health benefits of syringe exchange programs. *Can J Psychiatry* 53:487–495, 2008.

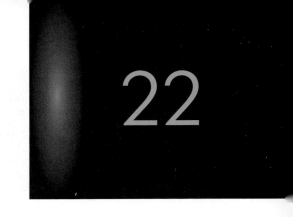

Occupational Medicine

Mark Russi

Occupational injuries and illnesses impact substantially the health of working adults. In 2010 the U.S. Bureau of Labor Statistics (BLS) reported almost 3.1 million workplace injuries and illnesses among those employed in the U.S. private sector, an incidence rate of 3.5 cases per 100 full-time workers.[1] More than half of these were serious enough to require days away from work, job transfer, or restriction of work activities. The majority of reported cases were injuries; illnesses accounted for a smaller proportion and included respiratory and skin conditions, poisonings, hearing loss, and a broad range of other conditions. Because years of exposure are required for many diseases to develop, and because many illnesses caused by work exposures may not be recognized initially as such, annual BLS statistics probably underestimate incidence.

Estimating the frequency of work-related medical conditions is further complicated by the fact that common illnesses such as asthma, bronchitis, hypersensitivity dermatitis, cancers, and musculoskeletal disorders may be caused by workplace exposures, lifestyle factors, or a combination of both. Because clinical manifestations of such diseases are rarely specific to the exposure that caused them, recognizing occupational illness requires a detailed occupational history from the patient, often enumerating decades of workplace exposure. Such detailed occupational history is not consistently incorporated into general medical practice. Other factors that predispose to underreporting include fears among workers of job loss or reprisal, hesitation among medical practitioners to engage with the complexities of workers' compensation insurance, and the lack of a requirement in many states for physicians to report occupational illnesses.

This chapter discusses the hazards of workplaces, the resulting injuries and illnesses, and the role of occupational medicine in assessing and preventing work-related medical conditions. A limited number of environmental exposures are described as well. Hazards can be broadly divided into those resulting from physical, chemical, biologic, and psychosocial factors. **Physical hazards** include direct trauma, repetitive strain, radiation, noise, and thermal stresses. **Chemical hazards** include organic solvents and related compounds; metals; mineral dusts such as coal, asbestos, silica and synthetic vitreous fibers; toxic gases; and a vast array of organic compounds, including pesticides and chemical-manufacturing intermediates. **Biologic hazards** include the blood-borne pathogens (e.g. HIV, hepatitis B and C); pathogens spread by the airborne, droplet, or contact route; pathogens spread by animal contact or arthropod vectors; and allergens. **Psychosocial stressors** include long hours and fatigue, limited social support, and jobs over which workers have little control.

I. PHYSICAL HAZARDS

One need only consider the range of human activity to imagine ways in which working people may sustain acute traumatic injuries. Industrial accidents, motor vehicle crashes, falls, and trauma involving farming or mining equipment (Fig. 22-1). In general, such events are addressed immediately and directly, and the link between workplace trigger and health outcome is minimally prone to dispute. When traumas occur more gradually, as from the repetitive strain of lifting, twisting, or manipulating loads in the workplace, establishing a causal link between exposure and health condition may be more challenging. Examples include *lumbar disc disease* in nurses and nurses' aides from decades of patient lifting, *carpal tunnel syndrome* among clerical workers, *Raynaud's disease* (vasospasm resulting in reduced blood flow to fingers) in workers who use vibratory tools, and *degenerative joint disease* in materials handlers. Such health conditions also occur in individuals without

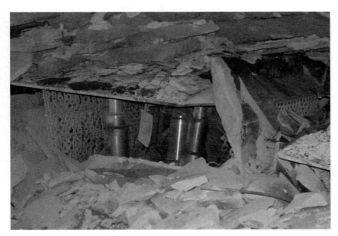

Figure 22-1 Mining tunnel cave-in. Underground mining has one of the highest fatal injury rates of any U.S. industry—more than five times the national average compared with other industries. Between 1999 and 2008, almost 40% of all underground fatalities were attributed to mine roof, rib, and face falls. (From http://www.cdc.gov/niosh/mining/topics/images/rockfall.jpg.)

workplace stressors, and a health care practitioner's decision regarding work-relatedness must incorporate a thoughtful approach to the relative importance of various stressors. Generally, the receipt of workers' compensation benefits requires that a physician state the condition "more probably than not" (>50%) is related to the workplace.

A. Radiation

As a physical hazard, radiation exposure is widespread, and occupations account for only a small portion of overall population exposures, most of which emanate from radon gas in homes, cosmic rays from the sun, and radioactive elements in the earth's crust. The largest occupational group monitored for radiation is health care workers, although for most, exposures do not exceed typical background levels. Other exposed groups include aircraft pilots and crews, nuclear industry workers, and miners.

Individuals exposed to extremely high levels of radiation, such as in a nuclear accident, may suffer acute radiation sickness with sloughing of the skin, damage and depression of bone marrow, ulceration and bleeding in the gastrointestinal tract, inflammation and scarring of the lungs, and a range of other effects. Survivors of very high acute radiation doses also have elevated risk of blood and solid-organ malignancies. More common radiation exposures may also result in elevated cancer risk; radon exposure in miners is strongly associated with increased risk of lung cancer, and nuclear workers have shown increased rates of leukemia and lung cancer.

B. Noise

Noise is one of the most prevalent physical hazards in workplaces. More than 10 million U.S. workers may be exposed to greater than 80 decibels (dB), and more than 1 million have occupational hearing loss. By age 50, an estimated half of heavily exposed construction workers and 90% of heavily exposed miners will have hearing impairment. Substantial

noise exposure occurs in almost every variety of manufacturing; exposures in mining, construction, and transportation may be equally hazardous. The U.S. Occupational Safety and Health Administration (OSHA) requires periodic monitoring of noise levels and periodic audiometry of workers with exposure of 85 dB or higher.[2] Control of noise in the workplace often involves a combination of engineering solutions to reduce noise sources, limiting exposure time in noise environments, and wearing hearing protection.

C. Heat and Cold

Thermal stress constitutes another physical stressor in workplaces. Excessive levels of heat are encountered in foundries, smelting operations, firefighting, and in many outdoor settings. Heavy work demands, heavy clothing, lack of air circulation, and high humidity may contribute to heat stress. Health effects may include lightheadedness, swelling of the extremities, muscle cramping, and in more severe cases, agitation and delirium, lysing of muscle cells, circulatory collapse, and kidney failure. Workers not accustomed to high-heat environments and those with other medical conditions are at particular risk.

Excessive **cold exposure** occurs among workers in cold-climate outdoor activities, divers and others in the maritime industry, military personnel, and workers in refrigerated environments. Although the potential for *hypothermia*, defined as a fall in body temperature to below 35° C (95° F), exists in such settings, localized cold effects are more common, such as frostbite, Raynaud's phenomenon, and cold-induced hives.

Cold exposure may also occur in high-altitude environments, although the principal hazard of such settings is *reduced oxygen content*. High altitude–associated conditions range from acute mountain sickness (AMS) to potentially life-threatening pulmonary and cerebral edema. AMS is characterized by fatigue, malaise, shortness of breath, disturbances of memory, concentration and sleep, and generally occurs within 24 hours of arrival at altitude. Pulmonary edema may be triggered by changes in the pulmonary blood vessels from decreased oxygen, rapid breathing, and the resulting alkalosis and pulmonary hypertension. Edema of the brain may result from hypoxia and may be both insidious and life threatening. Gradual ascent may prevent or moderate altitude-associated illnesses.

II. CHEMICAL HAZARDS

More than 80,000 chemicals are in common use. Although discussion of acute and chronic toxicities is beyond the scope of this chapter, categories of particular interest, due to high frequency of use or significant health impact, are solvents, metals, mineral dusts, polycyclic aromatic hydrocarbons, pesticides, and inorganic gases. Dedicated OSHA standards exist for only a few chemical exposures. For many others, guidance is in place from the National Institute for Occupational Safety and Health (NIOSH), American Conference of Governmental Industrial Hygienists (ACGIH), and other advisory groups. In the absence of a specific standard, OSHA may cite workplaces under the General Duty Clause, which requires employers to provide a workplace free of recognized hazards.

A. Solvents

Solvents are widely used in industrial processes. Major classes include aliphatic, aromatic, and halogenated compounds, all of which can cause acute encephalopathic effects, generally manifested by a sense of lightheadedness, disorientation, and irritability. Exposure occurs primarily by inhalation and skin absorption. Although symptoms generally resolve within hours following cessation of exposure, chronic encephalopathic changes, potentially with progression to dementia, may occur after years of heavy exposure. Most solvents may also irritate the skin, cause defatting of dermal tissue, and serve as carriers through the skin of other chemical substances. The following solvents have uniquely toxic properties:

- Both n-hexane and methyl-n-butyl ketone may cause a mixed motor and sensory neuropathy.
- Benzene is well established as a cause of aplastic anemia and acute myelogenous leukemia.
- Carbon tetrachloride is a potent toxin of the liver.
- Methylene chloride causes carboxyhemoglobinemia
- Carbon disulfide may cause acute psychosis, optic neuritis, peripheral neuropathy, and over time, atherosclerosis.
- Extremely heavy exposure to halogenated solvents has been associated with cardiac arrhythmias and sudden death.

Acute encephalopathic effects may result from exposure to a single solvent or a combination of solvents. Assessment of workplace exposure must consider the possibility of combined toxicity, and that measured air levels may not adequately account for dermal exposures. Biologic monitoring, generally the measurement of urinary solvent metabolites, has been used to account for body burden from different exposure pathways.

B. Metals and Mineral Dusts

Metal exposures occur in a variety of industrial settings and may trigger a broad range of health effects. Although **lead** exposure to the general population has been greatly reduced by the removal of lead as a gasoline additive in the 1970s, many occupational groups remain at high exposure risk, including construction workers, welders, solderers, pipe cutters, foundry workers, demolition workers, home renovators, and battery makers. Toxicities associated with lead exposure range from subtle behavioral and cognitive effects to hemolytic anemia, peripheral neuropathy, chronic encephalopathy, hypertension, and impotence (Fig. 22-2). The following metals also may cause a variety of acute and chronic effects:

- **Arsenic** exposure causes hyperpigmented skin lesions, peripheral neuropathy, and peripheral vascular disease and is a well-established risk factor for skin and lung cancer.
- Chronic exposure to **mercury** is linked to tremor, psychological disturbances, and neuropathy, whereas acute exposure may trigger a severe chemical pneumonitis.
- **Beryllium** may also cause acute pneumonitis and in certain individuals leads to chronic berylliosis, a syndrome similar to sarcoidosis, a systemic disorder often resulting in chronic lung disease.

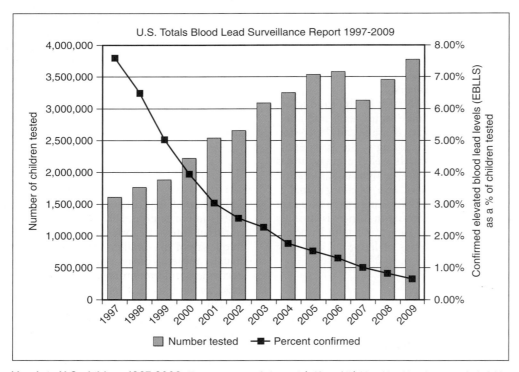

Figure 22-2 **Lead levels in U.S. children, 1997-2009.** The proportion of elevated (>10 μg/dL) blood lead levels in sampled children decreased from approximately 7.5% to less than 1%. (From http://www.cdc.gov/nceh/lead/data/StateConfirmedByYear_1997_2009.pdf.)

- **Cobalt** and **cadmium** may also affect the lungs. Cobalt causes asthma, giant cell pneumonitis, and scarring of the lungs of certain individuals; acute cadmium exposure is associated with pneumonitis. Cadmium may also severely damage the kidneys.
- **Chromium** and **nickel** have a number of skin effects and are risk factors for lung cancer.

Exposures to metal dusts and fumes in the workplace are better controlled now than in past decades, partly because of the establishment of applicable OSHA standards. For example, the OSHA standard for lead requires both air monitoring in lead-contaminated workplaces and biologic monitoring through blood testing of exposed workers. Workers are required to be removed from exposure without loss of pay if their blood level exceeds the threshold value of 50 μg/dL.[3]

Several widely recognized occupational diseases result from chronic exposures to mineral dusts. Long-term **asbestos** exposure may cause pleural plaques (areas of scarring along lung lining), as well as asbestosis, a diffuse scarring process in the lungs themselves that may lead to compromise of oxygenation (Fig. 22-3). Chronic **silica** exposure may also cause diffuse lung scarring (silicosis), which differs pathologically from asbestosis and tends to predominate in the upper lobes. Very heavy exposures to freshly fractured silica have been linked to severe and progressive lung disease (acute silicosis), which may cause death within 1 year of exposure. Coal worker's pneumoconiosis leads to scarring and weakening of the lung's connective tissue and formation of carbon-filled nodules, predominantly in the upper lung fields.

Several tumors have been linked with mineral dust exposure. Asbestos is a well-established cause of lung cancer and malignant mesothelioma, a rare tumor of high mortality affecting the pleural lining of the lung. Asbestos is also associated with other malignancies, particularly laryngeal cancer.[4] Silica appears to be a risk factor for lung cancer, whereas coal exposure does not.[5,6]

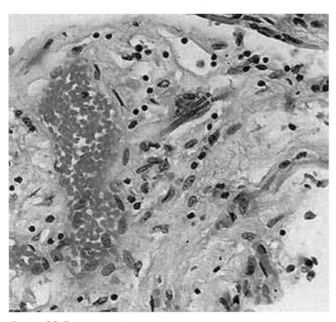

Figure 22-3 Asbestos fibers in lung tissue. (From http://www.atsdr. cdc.gov/asbestos/asbestos/health_effects/.)

C. Hydrocarbons and Pesticides

Another established risk factor for lung cancer is exposure to **polycyclic aromatic hydrocarbons** (PAH), a diverse group of substances formed from incomplete combustion of coal or oil. Occupational exposures in gas and coke works, iron and steel foundries, aluminum reduction plants, tar distillation facilities, chimney cleaning, and roofing and transportation industries have been linked to increased lung cancer risk. Risk of skin and bladder cancers has also been seen. PAH exposure is widespread in the general environment as well, deriving from tobacco smoke, fire fumes, ambient air pollution, and cooked food. Some studies show an association between lung cancer and urban air pollution, although it is not known whether risk is caused by PAH exposure. Studies in China of cooking and heating fumes have implicated PAH as a lung carcinogen.[7]

Pesticides comprise a broad category of chemicals used to control insect, plant, and fungal species. Exposures occur among farm and orchard workers, greenhouse and nursery workers, landscapers, chemical manufacturers, forestry workers, wood treaters, hazardous waste workers, and a range of others. Exposures to the general public are associated with household and lawn residues, termite control, food and water residues, accidental or intentional ingestions, and spills. Major classes of pesticides include organophosphates and carbamates, pyrethroids, organochlorines, and chlorophenoxy and nitroaromatic compounds.

Organophosphates and **carbamates,** which are linked with the largest proportion of acute systemic poisonings, act by inhibiting the enzyme acetylcholinesterase, which catalyzes breakdown of the neural transmitter acetylcholine. Depending on dose, the resulting clinical presentation may include nausea and vomiting, diarrhea and cramping, chest tightness, increased tearing and salivation, blurred vision, and profuse sweating. Muscle twitching and weakness, as well as anxiety, tremor, and impaired cognition, may also occur. Long-term effects are controversial; some studies suggest an increased risk of adverse reproductive outcomes. Specific pesticides have also been linked to chronic central and peripheral nervous system effects following heavy exposure. Several studies of farm workers show elevated cancer risk, particularly for leukemia and lymphoma, but it is not known whether this risk is caused by pesticide exposure (Fig. 22-4).

D. Inorganic Gases

Inorganic gases are encountered in a wide range of industrial settings and are a concern because of their acute toxicity in enclosed environments and long-term sequelae. Simple *asphyxiants,* such as **methane** and **nitrogen**, may dilute oxygen in an enclosed space but do not act as direct toxins. In contrast, **cyanide** and **carbon monoxide** interfere with cellular respiration and oxygen transport, respectively, and may be rapidly fatal at sufficient dose. The effects of irritant gases depend on water solubility and the chemical properties of the gas. **Ammonia** and **sulfur dioxide** are rapidly absorbed because of high water solubility and exert an irritant effect in the upper respiratory tract. In contrast, low-solubility gases, such as **phosgene** and **nitrogen oxide**, may cause profound and delayed effects in the lower respiratory tract, including bronchospasm, pneumonitis, and pulmonary

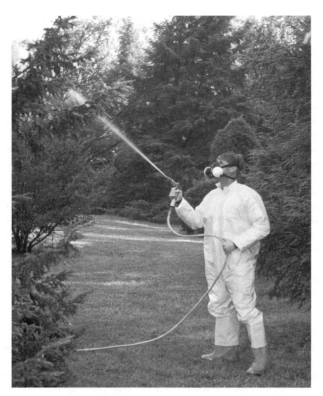

Figure 22-4 **Pesticide spraying.** This worker is using a cartridge respirator and skin protection while spraying. (From http://www.ars.usda. gov/is/graphics/photos/jan96/K7049-4.htm.)

edema. Long-term lung damage may occur in survivors of the acute toxicities of nitrogen oxide, phosgene, or *chlorine* gas exposures.

III. BIOLOGIC HAZARDS

Occupational biologic hazards are encountered in health care workplaces, areas of contact with animals or arthropod vectors, and locations in the general environment with exposure to an altered range of diseases. In health care facilities the blood-borne pathogens human immunodeficiency virus (HIV) and hepatitis B (HBV) and hepatitis C (HCV) viruses are of greatest concern; other infectious hazards include airborne or droplet-spread organisms (e.g., tuberculosis, varicella, measles, pertussis, parvovirus, influenza) and organisms spread by fecal-oral contact (e.g., enteroviruses, *Salmonella, Shigella,* hepatitis A virus). Outside the health care setting, animal breeders and handlers, farmers, and veterinarians are at risk for a range of illnesses that spread from animal to human (zoonoses). Workers in outdoor environments, such as groundskeepers, park rangers, and construction workers, may be at increased risk for diseases spread by arthropod vectors. Workers in the developing world may be at risk for tropical diseases.

A. Bloodborne Pathogens

Blood-borne pathogens are spread in health care settings by needlesticks or by splashes of blood or other infectious body fluids onto mucous membranes or abraded skin. Unfortunately, despite use of safety-engineered sharps, about half a million needlestick injuries still occur each year in the United States. Hollow-bore needles impart higher transmission risk, but exposures with suture needles are much more common. One study suggested that needlesticks may occur in up to 15% of surgical procedures.[8] An often-quoted risk for seroconversion after exposure to HIV is 0.3%, although this risk is clearly influenced by the quantity of blood delivered and the viral load in the source patient. Seroconversion risk after HCV exposure varies from study to study but is likely less than 2%, whereas risk of HBV seroconversion in an unvaccinated individual may be 1% to 6% if the source is e-antigen negative and as high as 22% to 31% from an e-antigen-positive source.[9] The U.S. Centers for Disease Control and Prevention (CDC) is aware of 57 individuals who have become HIV positive after workplace exposure. In the years before broad provision of HBV vaccination, thousands of health care workers, principally surgeons, contracted hepatitis B occupationally.

The OSHA Bloodborne Pathogen Standard requires annual training, engineering controls, personal protective equipment (PPE), and an exposure control plan in work settings with potential blood-borne exposure. Safety-engineered sharps have been shown to reduce needlesticks and must be used where feasible. Also, workers at risk for exposure must be provided hepatitis B vaccine, as well as appropriate medical follow-up after an exposure incident.[10] Such follow-up includes antiretroviral prophylaxis for those with HIV exposure. For those who contract hepatitis C, some support early institution of therapy with interferon alpha-2b.

B. Aerosol/Droplet-spread Infections

Infections spread by aerosols or droplets constitute another risk for health care workers. After years of declining tuberculosis (TB) incidence in the United States, a rise in case numbers during the mid-1990s prompted the CDC to issue new guidance for health care settings and the community. Enhanced systems for recognition of potentially infectious patients, construction of negative-pressure isolation rooms, use of fit-tested respirators, and yearly and postexposure monitoring of employees for TB have resulted in minimal rates of new TB infection among U.S. health care workers. Before such measures, several outbreaks were documented, and there continues to be significant risk to health care workers in areas of the world where TB prevalence is high. The presence in many such settings of multidrug-resistant or extensively drug-resistant strains augments the occupational hazard. As with measles and varicella, TB may spread on suspended aerosol particles over longer distances and does not appear to require face-to-face contact for transmission.

In contrast, other infections (e.g., influenza, pertussis, adenovirus, *Neisseria meningitidis,* hemorrhagic fever viruses, severe acute respiratory syndrome [SARS]) generally require closer contact for transmission and may be spread principally by droplets, which fall to the ground more quickly than aerosols. For several apparently droplet-spread infections, however, the rare outbreaks suggest transmission over greater distances. Such **opportunistic** airborne spread may be enhanced by low humidity levels and favorable patterns of air movement. Research is underway to better understand the role of disease spread through suspended aerosol particles. With influenza in particular, polymerase chain reaction (PCR) testing shows virus suspended on small aerosols, and animal studies suggest longer-range transmission. Such issues take on greater importance with the emergence of influenza strains with higher mortality, particularly among young persons (e.g., H1N1, highly pathogenic H5N1 avian).

Policies enacted during the 2009 novel H1N1 influenza pandemic, specifically those addressing protection of health care workers, illustrate well an important occupational health principle. As the pandemic began, neither the virulence of the virus nor its transmission characteristics had been fully characterized, and neither the general population nor hospital workers had been vaccinated against it. In the setting of a rapidly spreading virus with particular hazard to younger people, the CDC recommended use of fit-tested N95 respirators for health care workers caring for affected patients. (Such respirators generally are recommended only when caring for patients with diseases spread via the airborne route and are not used by health care workers caring for patients with seasonal influenza.) Although considerable controversy surrounded the policy, and many hospitals did not fully adhere to it, the recommendation was fundamentally grounded in the **precautionary principle:** if the level of harm may be high, action should be undertaken to prevent or minimize that harm even when the absence of scientific certainty makes it difficult to predict the likelihood of harm occurring, or the level of harm should it occur. Under this principle the need for control measures increases with both the level of possible harm and the degree of uncertainty. The precautionary principle relates to a broad range of decisions necessary to protect working populations whenever new and inadequately characterized hazards are introduced. Recommendations for use of airborne precautions when caring for patients with SARS or smallpox are consistent with it, as are recommendations for PPE use by health care workers caring for victims of biologic weapons when the infectious agent is unknown.

C. Animal Contact and Arthropod Vector

Outside of hospital settings, major groups at increased risk of occupational infectious diseases include those with frequent animal contact, those likely to have contact with arthropod vectors, and those working in other than their native microbiologic milieu, usually at sites in the developing world. Zoonotic diseases include brucellosis, cat-scratch disease, leptospirosis, plague, psittacosis, tularemia, cryptococcosis, histoplasmosis, ringworm, giardiasis, cryptosporidiosis, hantavirus, monkeypox, and rabies (see Chapter 20). Outside the usual occupational groups at risk for such diseases (farmers, veterinarians, animal handlers, cullers), anyone with regular animal contact, such as pet owners and those who keep livestock species near their home, may be at risk.

Diseases requiring an arthropod vector are a particular risk for those who work in outdoor settings and include West Nile virus, Rocky Mountain spotted fever, Lyme disease, babesiosis, ehrlichiosis, and several viral encephalitides. Malaria, typhoid, dengue, yellow fever, and a broad range of parasitic diseases constitute risks among those who work in the developing world. Important preventive medicine services for those who travel to tropical and subtropical destinations include the provision of vaccines, prophylactic medications, and advice on how to avoid insect vectors and hazardous food or water.

IV. PSYCHOSOCIAL STRESS

Long hours, rotating work shifts, demanding jobs, limited decision latitude, competing time demands, repetitive tasks, threat of violence, job insecurity, and poor management contribute to stress in the workplace. Importantly, chronic exposure to such work circumstances may have adverse physiologic effects. Jobs with excessive work hours have been associated with perception of poor health, with increased injury risk, and with increased cardiovascular disease: Cardiovascular risk is also associated with high-demand jobs in which the worker has limited control.[11]

The physiologic connection between stress and adverse health outcomes has not been completely elucidated. Possible etiologic links include elevated catecholamine levels and abnormalities of the pituitary-adrenocortical axis, both components of the body's response to acute and chronic stress. The resulting state may lead over time to increases in blood pressure and heart rate, constriction of blood vessels, increases in circulating lipid levels, and an increased tendency toward blood clotting. Effects on the immune system may occur as well. Animal studies show increased infections under stressful conditions; human studies suggest that circadian rhythm disturbance may elevate cancer risk.

V. ENVIRONMENTAL HAZARDS

The key distinguishing characteristic of environmental hazards versus workplace hazards is that although exposure levels are usually lower, environmental hazards may impact all age groups at all times. Environmental exposures result from the following:

- Water contamination from industrial effluents or toxic waste disposal
- Soil contamination from fallout of fumes or particulates released into the air
- Food contamination from compromised soils, water, or processing methods
- Air pollution from industrial or natural sources

Two important examples of environmental hazard with pervasive and significant health impact are domestic radon exposure and ambient air pollution (Fig. 22-5).

A. Radon Exposure

Radon (Rn) is a product of the radioactive breakdown of uranium. ^{222}Rn has a half-life of approximately $3\frac{1}{2}$ days and decays by release of an alpha particle to short-lived daughters, which themselves release alpha radiation. Radon is detectable in most environments because of the presence of uranium in rocks and soil and may become concentrated in indoor spaces, particularly in the lower levels of dwellings.

After epidemiologic studies of miners working underground showed elevated lung cancer risk, many studies examined whether exposures to radon in the home may also elevate cancer risk. Most were case-control studies

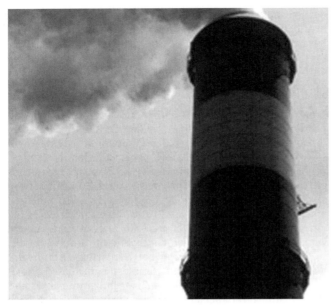

Figure 22-5 Pollution-emitting smokestack. Air pollution from multiple sources contributes to pulmonary and cardiovascular mortality in the general population. (From http://www.nrel.gov/data/pix/|pegs/00560.jpg.)

comparing measured radon levels in homes occupied over several decades by residents with and without lung cancer. The studies have been challenging because buildings inhabited by subjects may have been torn down or altered over the years in ways that could alter the radon measurement. In addition, because most residents have lived in many places throughout life, cumulative radon exposure tends to become similar from person to person, decreasing the number of study participants who have experienced cumulative exposures in excess of mean population levels. Because of this, and because the relative risk of exposure is small, large numbers of participants have been required to evaluate the impact of domestic radon exposure, necessitating meta-analytic techniques. These meta-analyses demonstrated statistically significant (10%-25%) elevations of lung cancer risk for those exposed to radon levels greater than 4 picocuries per liter (pCi/L), consistent with the risk estimates extrapolated from the studies of radon-exposed underground miners.[12-14]

The U.S. Environmental Protection Agency (EPA) has estimated that more than 20,000 lung cancer deaths per year in the United States may be caused by domestic radon exposure.[15] The EPA recommends retesting and mitigation of homes where basement radon levels exceed 4 pCi/L. From a public health perspective, radon mitigation of such homes is an important intervention; and because of population mobility, much of the mitigation benefit will pass to future residents. Systems to reduce indoor radon levels usually function by establishing a pressure gradient to reduce travel of radon into basements from surrounding soil and rock.

B. Ambient Air Pollution

Unlike radon, ambient air pollution is derived largely from human activity, principally industrial and vehicular combustion. Pollutants of major concern include **sulfur dioxide, nitrogen oxides, acid aerosols, particulates, volatile organic compounds, lead,** and **ozone.** In general, air pollution levels in developed countries have become better controlled in recent decades, while in the developing world, increased vehicular traffic, industrialization, and in some cases lack of regulation have resulted in less well-controlled levels. The U.S. Clean Air Act of 1970 requires the EPA to set standards to protect the general public, including those predisposed to harm from air pollution, such as asthmatics, the very young, and the very old.[16] National Ambient Air Quality Standards are in place in the United States for carbon monoxide, particulate matter, sulfur dioxide, nitrogen dioxide, lead, and ozone. The World Health Organization has set guidance for certain air pollutants as well and challenged governments worldwide to reduce exposures to below recommended levels.[17]

Health outcomes linked to air pollution include increased cardiopulmonary mortality; increased numbers of visits to emergency departments and physician offices; increased rates of hospitalization; exacerbations of asthma; and higher frequency of respiratory infection. Laboratory studies have revealed in response to specific air pollutants increases in airway inflammation, decreases in lung function, and increased upper respiratory irritation. A study of 100 U.S. counties showed an increase in cardiovascular mortality of 0.24% per 10-µg/m^3 increase in inhalable (PM10) particulate matter.[18] Effects may be enhanced in elderly persons and those exposed to fine particulate matter (i.e., particles small enough to be inhaled deeply into lungs).[19] The mechanisms by which air pollution may cause increased cardiopulmonary and other mortality remain incompletely understood. Beyond the capacity of respiratory irritants to exacerbate underlying chronic respiratory illness, studies have focused on the role of air pollution in inducing systemic inflammatory mediators, which over time may predispose to cardiovascular disease.[20]

VI. QUANTIFYING EXPOSURE

The distinguishing challenge of occupational epidemiology is exposure assessment. Modern workplaces are characterized by rapid turnover of personnel, changes over time in production methods and hygiene, and frequent job switching. Measurement of contaminant levels may be done for nonrandom reasons (e.g., workplace inspection, process change follow-up) and may not adequately represent exposures over time. Such measurements are also carried out relatively infrequently, and given the multitude of processes in many industrial facilities, may not reflect exposures of all workers. With the exception of settings in which significant radiation exposure requires daily use of personal dosimeters, there are few workplaces in which widespread and frequent personal exposure monitoring takes place. Such issues become more important when studying diseases of long latency and the possible causative exposures.

Assessing the impact of exposure on a working population also requires a suitable nonexposed group for comparison. The characteristic that working populations are generally healthier than the general population, known as the **healthy worker effect,** may result from less healthy individuals not entering the workforce, as well as attrition. A demographically similar working population without exposure to the contaminant under study may serve as a better basis for comparison than the general population.

Many smaller epidemiologic studies, such as community-, registry-, or hospital-based **case-control comparisons,** have relied on "job title" as a surrogate for exposure. Such an approach offers the advantage of simplicity and low cost. Work records are more often organized by job roles than by the exposures that accompany them, so personnel records or death certificates can be used to ascertain usual or most recent job title. Although occasionally revealing occupations at increased risk, serving as a basis both to target public health interventions and to explore the exposures likely associated with a job title, such studies have several weaknesses. Most reveal large numbers of job titles for comparison, increasing the likelihood of random associations. Jobs may also entail both variety and inconsistency of exposures, making it difficult to identify the specific hazard that may underlie an apparent job-based risk. For studies of cancer, in which decades of workplace exposure must be considered, studies must also tally decades of employment records. Although limited in scope, such investigations have served to develop and refine hypotheses, particularly when several studies have pinpointed the same job title in association with a disease outcome.

Cohort studies, in which hazards of concern are measured over time, can provide a greater detail of information than case-control studies. Because complete databases of personal exposure levels rarely exist, investigators employ a **job-exposure matrix,** which relies on measurement of the exposures most likely associated with a job title in order to assign exposure levels. Although the construction of a job-exposure matrix is a complex task requiring both professional judgment and measurement of contaminants, the exposure information it yields may be quite approximate. Hazards associated with a specific job may be classified merely as present or absent or at low, medium, or high level. Considerable heterogeneity may also exist within a job title, so that two workers assigned the same job in different parts of a factory may have different exposures. Splitting job titles into descriptions of greater specificity may mitigate that problem, but this often leads to more comparisons and fewer individuals in each comparison group, increasing the likelihood of a study to document spurious associations.

As investigators undertake study of lower-risk exposures, greater precision of both measurement and estimation may necessitate personal dosimeter measurements of larger samples of a workforce, carried out at greater frequency, and at times that best reflect typical hazard levels. Because many studies, particularly those examining long-latency diseases such as cancer, are of retrospective cohort design, reconstructions of past workplace conditions may be undertaken to estimate past exposures more accurately. Many studies have also moved beyond the relatively simple job-exposure matrix to more complex modeling in which exposure levels are tied to specific tasks, production levels, ventilation levels, and other potential predictors.

VII. SUMMARY

The practice of occupational and environmental medicine (OEM) exists at an interface of clinical medicine and public health. OEM physicians are required to have knowledge of the broad range of exposures associated with human disease, to understand the toxicologic principles that underlie disease risk for many exposures, to interpret and apply findings of epidemiologic studies to decisions about causality and prevention, and to possess the clinical skills to recognize signs of symptoms of occupational illness. They must engage with public health officials when inspecting workplace hazards, making decisions about removal of a patient or group of workers from exposure, instituting medical screening or surveillance programs, or formulating policies to ensure the safety of a workplace or other environment. Although the OEM field impacts the health of large numbers of workers, it remains grounded in the clinical skills required to care properly for the individual patient: taking a thorough history, performing an appropriate diagnostic workup, and intervening to reduce or eliminate hazardous exposure.

This chapter has outlined physical, chemical, biologic and psychosocial hazards encountered in workplaces, and described a range of clinical conditions associated with them. Prevention principles have been discussed for some exposures, as have specific mechanisms of prevention, such as OSHA Standards. Radon and air pollution were cited as examples of environmental hazards, which are generally characterized by lower level, but more widespread exposures than those encountered in workplaces. The challenge of studying links between occupational or environmental exposures and human health is substantial, particularly with respect to quantification of exposures over long latency periods. However, increasingly sophisticated job- or task-exposure matrices, more frequent and regular hygienic measurements, and complex exposure modeling have enhanced our capacity to perceive effects which may not have been evident in the past, particularly those which may persist despite the workplace hygienic improvements of recent decades.

References

1. http://www.bls.gov/news.release/osh.nr0.htm
2. http://www.osha.gov/pls/oshaweb/owadisp.show_document? p_table=STANDARDS&p_id=9735
3. http://www.osha.gov/pls/oshaweb/owadisp.show_document? p_table=STANDARDS&p_id=10030
4. http://monographs.iarc.fr/ENG/Monographs/vol14/volume 14.pdf
5. http://monographs.iarc.fr/ENG/Monographs/vol68/volume 68.pdf
6. http://monographs.iarc.fr/ENG/Monographs/vol68/mono68-12.pdf
7. http://www.ncbi.nlm.nih.gov/pubmed/16406110
8. http://www.ncbi.nlm.nih.gov/pubmed/1953115
9. http://www.ncbi.nlm.nih.gov/pubmed/11442229
10. http://www.osha.gov/pls/oshaweb/owadisp.show_document? p_table=STANDARDS&p_id=10051
11. http://www.ncbi.nlm.nih.gov/pubmed/15127782
12. http://www.ncbi.nlm.nih.gov/pubmed/16538937
13. http://www.ncbi.nlm.nih.gov/pubmed/8978406
14. http://www.ncbi.nlm.nih.gov/pubmed/9008203
15. http://www.epa.gov/radon/pubs/citguide.html
16. http://www.epa.gov/air/caa/
17. http://www.who.int/mediacentre/news/releases/2006/pr52/en/
18. http://aje.oxfordjournals.org/content/166/8/880.long
19. http://www.ncbi.nlm.nih.gov/pubmed/12762571
20. http://www.ncbi.nlm.nih.gov/pubmed/20056584

Birth Outcomes: A Global Perspective

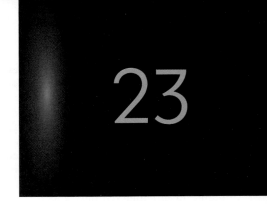

23

Joy E. Lawn, Elizabeth M. McClure, and Hannah Blencowe

I. BIRTH COUNTS

The estimated 135 million babies born worldwide[1] enter very different worlds in terms of the care that they and their mothers receive. Also, very different databases are associated with their birth and, if they die, their mortality.

Although celebrated in rich countries, childbirth in many poorer countries is accompanied by apprehension for the mother and newborn, who may remain hidden at home with limited access to care. More than 98% of neonatal mortality (death in first 28 days after birth)[2] and third-trimester stillbirths (death of fetus in utero at ≥1000 g birth weight or ≥28 completed weeks' gestation)[3] occur in low-income and middle-income countries, and approximately half occur at home. In poor communities, many babies die unnamed and unrecorded, the majority of these without record of birth or death.[4,5] Often the live-born baby is unnamed until several weeks have passed, reflecting a sense of fatalism and perceived inevitability of high mortality.[4,6]

For the 60 million women giving birth outside a health facility each year, physical distance is often a barrier to care

seeking.[6] In many cases, cultural norms also keep pregnancy hidden and preclude care seeking outside the home at birth or in the postnatal period, generally considered up to 6 weeks after birth.[7] Should complications occur, which may be understood as having a nonbiomedical cause, traditional remedies are often used.[8] Although many gaps exist in delivery of services, understanding and addressing the sociocultural context are also critical to accelerating demand and improving coverage of effective care.

In contrast, the 1% of neonatal deaths that occur in rich countries are the subject of confidential inquiries and public outcry if services are considered substandard.[9] The majority of published trials of neonatal interventions focus on these relatively few deaths in high-income countries.[10,11] The "inverse care law," first described in Britain in the 1960s, still holds true: the availability of good medical care tends to vary inversely with the need for it in the population served.[12] This law could appropriately be extended to the "inverse information and inverse care law": those communities with the most deaths have the least information on them and the least access to cost-effective interventions to prevent them.[4]

Birth is the time in the human life span with the greatest risk of death. Each year an estimated 720,000 babies die soon after birth from intrapartum-related injury, particularly childbirth complications, primarily in low- and middle-income countries.[13] These deaths are closely linked to at least 1.2 million stillbirths occurring during labor.[14] In addition, an unknown number of babies survive preterm birth and intrapartum or other insults, only to have long-term impairment and thus are not able to reach their full potential.[15] During this same period, the majority of the world's approximately 300,000 maternal deaths occur, as well as many more "near-miss" maternal deaths and significant maternal morbidity.[16-18] Therefore, a total of about 2 million deaths occur at birth, making this a critical time for programmatic focus and emphasizing the need for effective epidemiologic data[14,19] (Fig. 23-1).

II. DEFINING BIRTH OUTCOMES

A. Epidemiologic Definitions and Time Periods

Birth outcomes considered in this chapter include stillbirth, preterm birth, and neonatal mortality. Other important outcomes around the time of birth are those related to the mother, notably maternal mortality, near-miss maternal events, and maternal morbidity. Other important outcomes for the baby include low birth weight and small for gestational age, acute morbidities that may lead to subsequent

Figure 23-1 Deaths at the time of birth. (Modified from Lawn JE, et al: *Int J Gynaecol Obstet* 107:S5–S18, S9, 2009.)

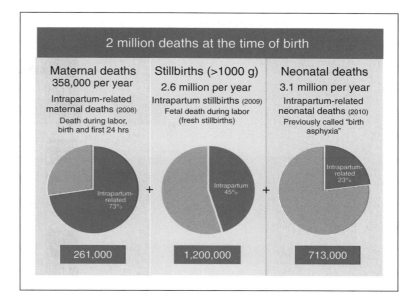

long-term impairment, and congenital abnormalities (not reviewed in detail here).

The term **perinatal mortality** refers to deaths occurring before or soon after birth, including stillbirths and neonatal deaths.[20] Historically, there was an advantage in combining these two mortality outcomes, because even in settings with skilled personnel present at birth, significant misclassification occurs between stillbirths and early neonatal deaths.[21] However, epidemiologists now prefer that the two specific outcomes of **stillbirth** and **neonatal death** are defined and reported as distinct outcomes for a number of reasons.[22] First, the combination hides the data issues associated with underreporting between the two outcomes.[23] Second, there is inconsistency in the use of the term "perinatal," which may refer to eight or more different time periods, depending on the definitions used. For example, stillbirths may be defined as fetal deaths occurring at 18, 20, 22, 23, 24, or 28 weeks' gestation, depending on the definitions used.[24,25] The neonatal component may include only "early" neonatal deaths (1-7 days) or "all" neonatal deaths (1-28 days).

The World Health Organization (WHO) *International Classification of Diseases* (ICD) is widely used as a standard to define conditions and causes of death.[26] Figure 23-2 shows the main definitions related to neonatal deaths and stillbirths.

I. Preterm Birth and Stillbirth

Preterm birth is defined by WHO as all births before 37 completed weeks of gestation, or fewer than 259 days since the first day of a woman's last menstrual period.[27] Preterm birth can be further subdivided based on gestational age: *extremely preterm* (<28 weeks' gestation), *very preterm* (28 to <32 weeks), and *moderate preterm* (32 to <37 completed weeks) (Figure 23-2).[25] Moderate preterm birth may be further split to focus on *late preterm* birth (34 to <37 completed weeks). Recent thinking has questioned this definition, noting that even babies born at 37 or 38 weeks have higher risks than those born at 39 to 41 weeks.[28,29]

Stillbirth is generally defined as a birth without signs of life (i.e., no breathing, movement, or heart rate after birth).[14] The international definition for stillbirth uses stillbirths greater than 1000 g or 28 weeks' gestation to differentiate stillbirth from **miscarriage**.[3,14] For the stillbirth rate, the denominator includes all births (live births plus stillbirths) using these standard cutoff points, improving the ability to compare rates across countries and over times.[3,14] In contrast, for preterm birth, the ICD encourages the inclusion of all live births.[26,30] This definition for preterm birth has no lower gestational age or birth weight boundary which complicates the comparison of reported preterm birth rates both between countries and within countries over time, since perceptions of viability of extremely preterm babies change with increasingly sophisticated neonatal intensive care.[31] In addition, some reports use nonstandard cutoffs for upper gestational age (e.g., including babies born at up to 38 completed weeks of gestation).[30]

About 80% of all stillbirths in high-income countries are born preterm, potentially accounting for 5% of all preterm births.[9] However, these are excluded from the international preterm birth rates. Thus, counting only live births underestimates the true burden of preterm birth in terms of effect on the health system and on families.

B. Real World Definitions

Although it is recommended that all newborns with any signs of life at birth count as live births, for extremely preterm babies, medical practice is variable and associated with *perceptions of viability* for extremely preterm babies and stillbirth registration thresholds.[32,33] In some high-income and middle-income countries, the official definitions of live birth or stillbirth have changed over time. Even without an explicit lower gestational age cutoff in national definitions, the medical care given and whether or not birth and death registration occurs may depend on these perceptions of viability. Therefore, even if no official lower gestational age cutoff is specified for recording a live birth, misclassification of a live birth to "stillbirth" is more common if the medical team perceives the baby to be extremely preterm and thus less likely to survive.[31,32]

Data quality is particularly affected by underregistration of extremely preterm births or their misclassification to

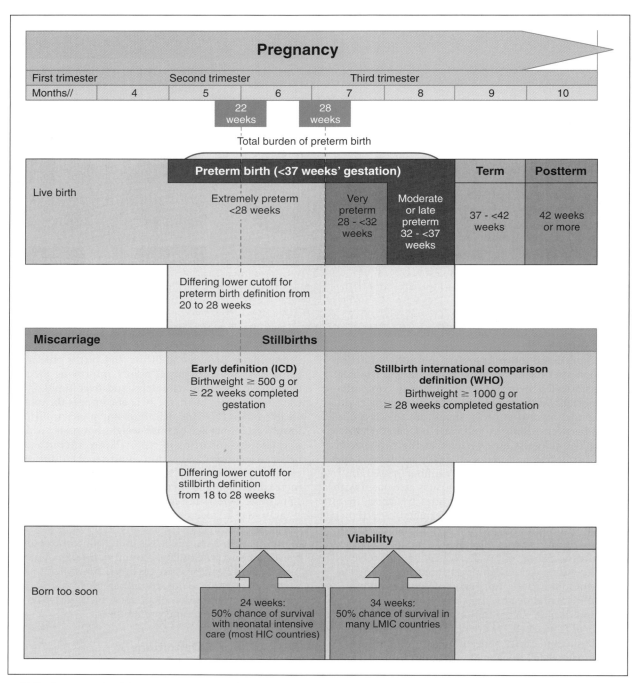

Figure 23-2 Overview of definitions for pregnancy outcomes related to preterm birth and stillbirths. *WHO*, World Health Organization; World Bank income groupings: *HIC*, high-income countries; *LMIC*, low- and middle-income countries. (From Blencowe H, Cousens S, Chou D, et al: 15 million preterm births: priorities for action based on national, regional and global estimates. In Howson C, Kinney M, Lawn JE, et al, editors: *Born too soon: the global action report on preterm birth.* March of Dimes, Partnership for Maternal, Newborn and Child Health, Save the Children, Geneva, 2012 World Health Organization; and www.data.worldbank.org/about/country-classifications/country-and-lending-groups.)

"stillbirths" near the thresholds of perceived viability and variable standards for stillbirth registration.[30] Countries using preterm birth definitions that include all births (both stillborn and live-born) from 20 weeks on report a higher proportion of preterm births under 28 weeks (~9%); other countries including live births only consistently report proportions of preterm less than 28 weeks of about 5% (Fig. 23-3).[34]

When thresholds are changed, it may take some time before recording of cases near the new threshold improves. For example, Denmark changed the lower threshold for registering preterm births from 28 to 22 weeks in 1997, but it was 5 years later when the proportion of all preterm births under 28 weeks increased (Fig. 23-4).[34]

In addition, some reports for birth outcomes exclude babies with congenital abnormalities, and others include

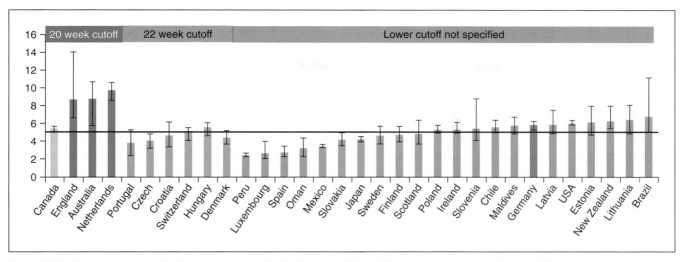

Figure 23-3 Mean percentage of all reported preterm births less than 28 weeks' gestation by country. Data from 32 countries with at least one reported data point providing information on the proportion of preterm births that are less than 28 weeks of gestation. Error bars show range of reported proportions. All these countries report using live births as numerator/denominator except for England, Australia, Netherlands, and Germany, who report using total births. (From Blencowe H, Cousens S, Oestergaard M, et al: National, regional and worldwide estimates of preterm birth rates in the year 2010 with time trends for selected countries since 1990: a systematic analysis and implications. *Lancet* 379:2162–2172, 2012.)

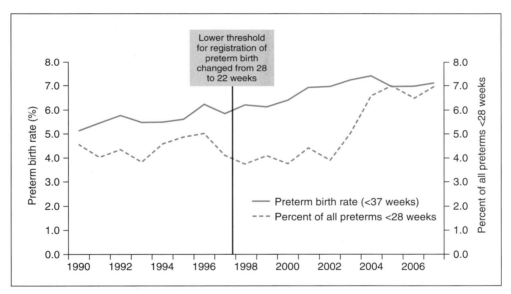

Figure 23-4 Variation in preterm birth rate and proportion of preterm births <28 weeks. With a reduction in the lower threshold for registration of preterm births from 28 to 22 weeks of gestation in Denmark. (From Blencowe H, Cousens S, Oestergaard M, et al: National, regional and worldwide estimates of preterm birth rates in the year 2010 with time trends for selected countries since 1990: a systematic analysis and implications. *Lancet* 379:2162–2172, 2012.)

only singleton births. These practices and perceptions vary between countries and over time, complicating the comparison of reported rates and interpretation of trends.[24] Furthermore, methods for assessing gestational age vary between high-income and low-income countries and at least in high-income countries, have improved over time. *Obstetric ultrasound* is generally considered the standard of care in high-income countries,[35] and although standardization remains a challenge, accuracy of gestational age assessment is better than in low-income countries.[36,37] These variations in gestational age measurement methods further complicate the interpretation of preterm birth rates both within and between countries.

III. DATA SOURCES

A. Vital Registration and Birth or Death Certificates

High coverage of vital registration through civil registration or certificates provides countries with data on numbers of births, deaths, and causes of death reasonably quickly. The time lag is usually 1 or 2 years.[38] About 60% of the world's births have a birth certificate, and while registration coverage has increased over the last decade, the countries with the most births and most deaths are least likely to have a high coverage of vital registration. However, vital registration coverage and quality have recently increased in some middle-income countries. About 81 countries now have vital registration systems with high coverage, accounting for only about 30% of the world's births and about 26% of all deaths, and lower for neonatal mortality.[39] Currently, birth certificates do not include "gestational age" and therefore cannot inform estimates of preterm birth rates.[34]

Death certificates are less often filled than birth certificates and less likely to be completed for stillbirths and early neonatal deaths compared to older children or adults. Until recently, many countries did not require stillbirth registration at all, and even in areas with high coverage, stillbirths are underreported.[14,40-42] Furthermore, the quality of death certificate data varies significantly. Despite efforts to standardize death certificates both within countries and internationally, studies consistently demonstrate significant variability in reporting.

Clearly, the long-term solution is to improve registration systems to achieve high coverage of births and deaths. In the interim, **demographic surveillance sites** are another valuable source of data on trends, especially if selected to be nationally representative. Such sample registration systems are now used in China and India.[43,44] In other countries, demographic surveillance sites that are not nationally representative may nevertheless provide useful data on mortality trends (http://www.indepth-network.org/). In the short-term, there is also a move to increase the frequency of UNICEF's Multiple Indicator Cluster Surveys, using fewer questions and focusing on coverage of selected interventions, to provide more responsive data on program if not on mortality outcomes.[45]

Who Counts? "Most people in Africa and Asia are born and die without leaving a trace in any legal record or official statistic. Absence of reliable data for births, deaths, and causes of death are at the root of this scandal of invisibility, which renders most of the world's poor as unseen, uncountable, and hence uncounted."

From Setel PW, Macfarlane SB, Szreter S, et al: A scandal of invisibility: making everyone count by counting everyone. *Lancet* 370:1569–1577, 2007.

B. National Household Surveys and Censuses

Thus, to account for three quarters of the world's births, we are dependent on other methods. The most important of these is the **household survey,** using a questionnaire to ask women about previous births and child deaths. This method has two major providers: DHS and MICS. **Demographic and health surveys** (DHS) are funded largely by U.S. government aid, but usually in partnership with national statistics offices,[46] with data and results open access (www.measure.dhs.com). DHS report "under-five" mortality (children <5 years of age) and neonatal mortality rates for more than 80 countries, which account for two thirds of the world's births.[47] Some surveys also report data on stillbirth rates, but the quality of this reporting is variable. For the most recent Child Health Epidemiology Reference Group (CHERG/WHO) stillbirth rate, only about 50 countries had

usable survey data, and 22 of 99 surveys were excluded based on quality criteria with implausible stillbirth rate/neonatal mortality rate (SBR/NMR) ratios. The United Nations International Children's Emergency Fund (UNICEF) **Multiple Indicator Cluster Surveys** (MICS) address under-five mortality and coverage of interventions in many of the same countries, but these do not routinely analyze or report on stillbirths or neonatal deaths. Summary results are available (www.childinfo.org), but not the data sets.

Without household surveys, epidemiologists would have little idea of global child mortality or coverage of priority interventions, and their importance makes recognition of survey limitations essential. One important limitation is frequency. The expense and challenge of data collection and analysis in low-resource settings, using a survey tool with over 700 questions in the case of DHS, means that in most countries, surveys are only conducted every 5 years.[48] Their ability to detect rapid changes in mortality or to disentangle contributory factors is therefore limited. This is important, especially in the context of the United Nations (UN) **Millennium Development Goals** (MDGs), which represent the widest commitment in history to addressing global poverty and ill (poor) health (http://www.un.org/millenniumgoals/).[38,49] With increasing investment in maternal, newborn, and child health, governments and donors seek data capable of detecting short-term trends, particularly in the years up to 2015, the target for the MDGs.[50] This would require huge increases in sample size. In Nigeria, for example, it would mean a fivefold expansion from the sample of 7225 households that already constitutes a major feat of organization.

Surveys, which depend on *recall,* also have particular limitations with respect to neonatal deaths and stillbirths, of which the most important is the potential for underascertainment of deaths compared with prospective surveillance. Systematic analyses of the extent of this problem are limited, but one study from rural India suggests that underreporting, especially in traditional societies, may halve the numbers of deaths reported.[51] Even in transitional societies, early neonatal deaths are often unregistered, and stillbirths rarely so.[52] Other issues of data quality include "age heaping" on certain days, notably days 7, 14, and 30, and miscoding between day 0 and day 1. Misclassification between stillbirths and early neonatal deaths, another important issue, was one of the arguments in favor of the combined measure of perinatal mortality, although expert opinion now favors separate reporting of stillbirths and neonatal deaths.[4] More systematic analytic work is required to develop objective scores of data quality and transparent methods to correct for underreporting.

The usefulness of household surveys to inform estimates of preterm birth rates has been limited, and data on gestational age have not routinely been included in most surveys.

C. Modeled Estimates

For most countries, the available data are not nationally representative or recent, so some modeling is used to adjust national data. For neonatal mortality, most countries do have national data as an input for modeling. A small group of countries accounting for about 5% of births have no nationally representative input data. These are either conflict or postconflict settings, or small nations such as Pacific islands. For these countries, under-five mortality and neonatal mortality are estimated annually by the UN and academic partners or by other groups.[2,47,49] Data gaps are even more marked for stillbirths and preterm birth, with no regular collation of rates by the UN, and no data available for 64 and 84 countries respectively in the most recent WHO estimates. Thus the uncertainty may be considerable, and one cannot merely use statistical confidence estimation methods, or the countries with no input data may appear to have less uncertainty. Detailed descriptions of inputs, methods, and uncertainty estimates are becoming the norm to which global health estimates aspire.[38]

IV. OVERVIEW OF BIRTH OUTCOMES

A. Stillbirths

The first systematic national, regional, and global estimates for stillbirth causes of death were published in 2011 in the *Lancet* Stillbirth Series.[3] Based on this analysis, in 2009 the total predicted number of stillbirths was 2.6 million (uncertainty range, 2.1-3.8 million), corresponding to a worldwide average stillbirth rate of 18.9 per 1000 births. In comparison, in 1995 the estimated rate was 22.1 per 1000 births (worldwide total, 3.0 million; uncertainty range, 2.4-4.2 million stillbirths), suggesting a 14.5% decline in the worldwide stillbirth rate between 1995 and 2009. The estimated declines varied significantly by region. For example, East Asia had a 47.5% decline in the stillbirth rate between 1995 and 2009, while the smallest percentage declines (<10%) were reported in Oceania and sub-Saharan Africa. In 2009 the regions with

the highest stillbirth rates were southern Asia and sub-Saharan Africa (Table 23-1). At a national level, the lowest stillbirth rates were in Finland and Singapore (2.0 per 1000 births), while Pakistan, Nigeria, and Bangladesh had estimated rates of over 35 per 1000 births (Fig. 23-5). In 2009 the 10 countries with the most stillbirths accounted for two thirds of all stillbirths (1.76 million, 67%) (Table 23-2).

Although both cause and timing of stillbirth are important, the data regarding the *timing* of stillbirths relative to birth are more widely available. **Intrapartum stillbirths** are generally defined as stillbirths occurring after the onset of labor, or as "fresh stillbirths" (with skin still intact, implying death occurred less than 12 hours before birth) weighing more than 1000 grams (g) and of 28 weeks or more of gestation, but exclude severe lethal congenital abnormalities.

Based on these estimates, 1.2 million intrapartum stillbirths occur annually (uncertainty bounds: 0.8-2.0), representing one third of stillbirths globally.[14] Despite the caveats inherent in the interpretation of the intrapartum stillbirth estimates, these estimates clearly highlight the magnitude of loss of life just minutes and hours before birth. Hospital-based studies suggest that 25% to 62% of intrapartum stillbirths are avoidable with improved obstetric care and more rapid responses to intrapartum complications, including reducing delays in seeking care from home.

Where data do exist, the lack of comparability across studies greatly inhibits interpretation. More than 30 different stillbirth classification systems have been identified in the literature,[53] with some encompassing up to 37 causes. Most of the international focus on stillbirths has been for those occurring in high-income countries, where determination of

Table 23-1 Stillbirth and Neonatal Mortality Rates by Region

Millennium Development Goal Region		Neonatal Mortality* (2009)	Stillbirth† (2009)	Preterm Birth‡ (2010)
Global	Rate	23.9	18.9	11.1
	Number in 1000s (% of global)	3,265 (100)	2,642 (100)	14,900 (100)
Developed	Rate	3.5	4.6	8.6
	Number in 1000s (% of global)	33 (1.0)	44 (1.7)	1,233 (8.3)
Southern Asia	Rate	34.0	26.5	13.3
	Number in 1000s (% of global)	1,349 (41.0)	1,080 (40.9)	5,159 (34.6)
Sub-Saharan Africa	Rate	36.6	28.4	12.3
	Number in 1000s (% of global)	1,172 (35.9)	935 (35.4)	3,937 (26.4)
Eastern Asia	Rate	11.5	9.9	7.2
	Number in 1000s (% of global)	216 (6.6)	188 (7.1)	1,262 (8.5)
Latin America	Rate	8.9	7.0	8.4
	Number in 1000s (% of global)	127 (3.4)	101 (3.8)	853 (5.7)
Southeastern Asia	Rate	17.3	13.9	13.6
	Number in 1000s (% of global)	191 (5.9)	156 (5.9)	1,497 (10.0)
Western Asia	Rate	16.4	12.5	10.1
	Number in 1000s (% of global)	78 (2.4)	60 (2.3)	488 (3.3)
Northern Africa	Rate	14.0	13.7	7.3
	Number in 1000s (% of global)	51 (1.6)	51 (1.9)	259 (1.7)
Caucasus and Central Asia	Rate	17.7	8.8	9.2
	Number in 1000s (% of global)	28 (0.8)	14 (0.5)	151 (1.0)
Caribbean	Rate	18.3	12.5	11.2
	Number in 1000s (% of global)	13 (0.4)	9 (0.3)	76 (0.5)
Oceania	Rate	22.8	14.5	7.4
	Number in 1000s (% of global)	6 (0.2)	4 (0.1)	19 (0.1)

*Neonatal mortality rates given per 1000 live births; from Oestergaard MZ, et al: *PLoS Med* 8:e1001080, 2011.[2]
†Stillbirth rates given per 1000 total births. From Cousens S, et al: *Lancet* 377:1319–1330, 2011.[3]
‡Preterm birth rates given per 100 live births. From Blencowe H, et al: *Lancet* 379:2162–2172, 2012.[34]

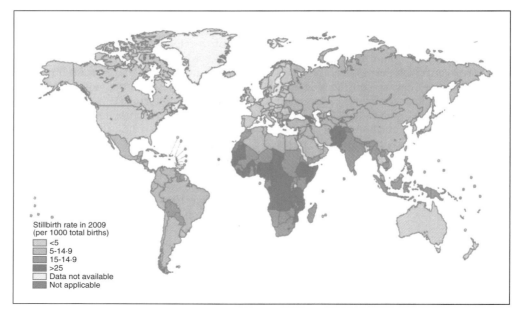

Figure 23-5 Global map showing stillbirth rates by country, 2009. (From Cousens S, Blencowe H, Stanton C, et al: National, regional, and worldwide estimates of stillbirth rates in 2009 with trends since 1995: a systematic analysis. *Lancet* 377:1319–1330, 2011.)

Table 23-2 Top 10 Countries for Absolute Numbers of Stillbirths, Preterm Births, and Neonatal Deaths

	Stillbirths* (2009)			Preterm Births† (2010)			Neonatal Deaths‡ (2009)	
1	India	605,230	1	India	3,519,100	1	India	907,824
2	Pakistan	264,550	2	China	1,172,300	2	Nigeria	236,546
3	Nigeria	264,390	3	Nigeria	773,600	3	Pakistan	225,447
4	China	182,150	4	Pakistan	748,100	4	China	208,415
5	Bangladesh	128,550	5	Indonesia	675,700	5	DR Congo	149,968
6	DR Congo	86,130	6	USA	517,400	6	Ethiopia	110,583
7	Ethiopia	82,370	7	Bangladesh	424,100	7	Bangladesh	100,422
8	Indonesia	62,290	8	Philippines	348,900	8	Indonesia	80,163
9	Tanzania	47,550	9	DR Congo	341,400	9	Afghanistan	69,560
10	Afghanistan	39,310	10	Brazil	279,300	10	Tanzania	60,878

*Data from Cousens S, et al: *Lancet* 377:1319–1330, 2011.[3]
†From Blencowe H, et al: *Lancet* 379:2162–2172, 2012.[34]
‡From Oestergaard MZ, et al: *PLoS Med* 8:e1001080, 2011.[2]

the most prevalent causes requires fetal surveillance and sophisticated diagnostics.[54] In contrast, the majority of stillbirths occurring in low-income countries may be prevented with known interventions that are not readily available to many women in these settings.

B. Preterm Births

The first set of national, regional, and global estimates of preterm births was published in 2012.[34] The worldwide total estimated in 2010 was 14.9 million (uncertainty range: 12.3-18.1 million), a global average preterm birth rate of 11.1% (9.1%-13.4%). More than 1 in 10 babies worldwide is born preterm.

The rate of preterm birth rates varies widely between countries and regions. The regions with the highest preterm birth rates in 2010 were southeastern Asia, south Asia, and sub-Saharan Africa (Fig. 23-6). At a national level, the estimated preterm birth rate was less than 10% in 88 countries

and less than 6% in 11 countries. Of the 11 countries with estimated rates of 15% or more in 2010, all except two were in sub-Saharan Africa. Rates are highest for low-income countries (11.8%), followed by lower middle–income countries (11.3%), and lowest for upper-middle and high-income countries (9.4% and 9.3%, respectively). However, in contrast to other perinatal outcomes, relatively high preterm birth rates are seen in many high-income countries, including the United States (12%) and Austria (10.9%). The United States accounts for 30% of live births in the developed region but more than 42% (0.5 million) of the 1.2 million preterm births.

In almost all high- and middle-income countries, preterm birth is the leading cause of neonatal and child deaths.[55] Very preterm birth in particular makes a large contribution to neonatal mortality rates in these countries, which can be greatly affected by differences in case ascertainment.[56]

More than 60% of all preterm births are estimated to have occurred in sub-Saharan Africa and south Asia, where 9.1

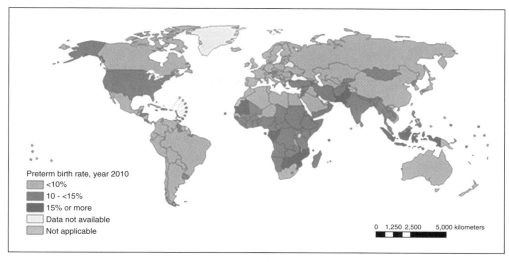

Figure 23-6 Global map showing preterm birth rate by country, 2010. (From Blencowe H, Cousens S, Oestergaard M, et al: National, regional and worldwide estimates of preterm birth rates in the year 2010 with time trends for selected countries since 1990: a systematic analysis and implications. *Lancet* 379:2162–2172, 2012.)

million births (12.8%) were estimated to be preterm in 2010 (see Table 23-1). These two regions account for 52% of live births worldwide. In 2010 the 10 countries with the most preterm births accounted for over half of all preterm (8.8 million, 59%) (see Table 23-2).

C. Neonatal Deaths

Global demand for information on neonatal deaths is growing with the recent recognition that an increasing proportion of global mortality for children under age 5 years occurs in the first 28 days of life. The Millennium Development Goals to address global poverty and "ill health" include **MDG 4,** for child survival, which aims for a two-thirds reduction in "under-five" mortality by the year 2015 compared to the baseline of 1990 (Fig. 23-7). This results in a target under-five mortality rate of 29 per 1000. The second half of the 20th century witnessed a remarkable reduction in child mortality, with a halving of the risk of death before age 5 years.[2]

The majority of this reduction, however, has been in lives saved after the first 4 weeks of life, with relatively little reduction in the risk of death in the neonatal period. Neonatal deaths now account for 41% of under-five deaths globally.[2] However, the global neonatal mortality rate is estimated to be 23.9 per 1000 live births; thus more than three quarters of the target for under-five mortality is currently taken up by neonatal deaths. If MDG 4 is to be achieved, reducing neonatal deaths must become a major public health priority, and the slower progress for reducing neonatal deaths needs to be addressed.[57]

Neonatal mortality rates also vary significantly by region with a pattern similar to stillbirths (see Table 23-1). Of the 40 countries with the highest neonatal mortality rate (NMR) in 2009, only six are from outside the African continent: Afghanistan, Pakistan, India, Bhutan, Myanmar, and Cambodia (Fig. 23-8). Among the 15 countries with the highest NMR (>39), 13 were from sub-Saharan Africa and two from southern Asia. Throughout the period 1990-2009, India has been the country with the largest number of neonatal deaths.

In 2009 the 10 countries with the most deaths accounted for two thirds of all neonatal deaths (2.15 million, 66%) (see Table 23-2).

Globally in 2010, the major causes of neonatal deaths were complications from preterm birth (35%), asphyxia (23%), and infections with sepsis and pneumonia (27%)[55] (Fig. 23-9). In countries with high NMR, about half of neonatal deaths result from infections, which are generally considered preventable or treatable. In countries with lower NMR, however, higher proportions of neonatal deaths are caused by preterm birth complications and congenital anomalies.[4]

V. ADVERSE BIRTH OUTCOMES

Major causes of maternal death also contribute to stillbirth and early neonatal morbidity or mortality, including hypertensive disease of pregnancy and obstetric complications (e.g., hemorrhage, obstructed labor)[58,59] (Table 23-3). Most of these conditions are preventable or can be treated with effective antenatal and obstetric care, so deaths related to these conditions have largely been eliminated in high-income countries.[60] In low-income countries, however, these maternal complications have a significant impact on women and babies.[58-63]

A. Importance of Maternal Health and Care

In addition, maternal health has an important effect on birth outcomes, notably existing chronic conditions such as hypertension and diabetes.[14] Infections during pregnancy, especially sexually transmitted infections (STIs) such as syphilis,[64] remain an important and treatable cause of stillbirths, as well as preterm birth and growth restriction.[63,65] Maternal human immunodeficiency virus (HIV) infection is a critical factor, especially in high-prevalence countries. Malaria in pregnancy is a risk factor for preterm birth, especially in areas of unstable transmission.[63,65]

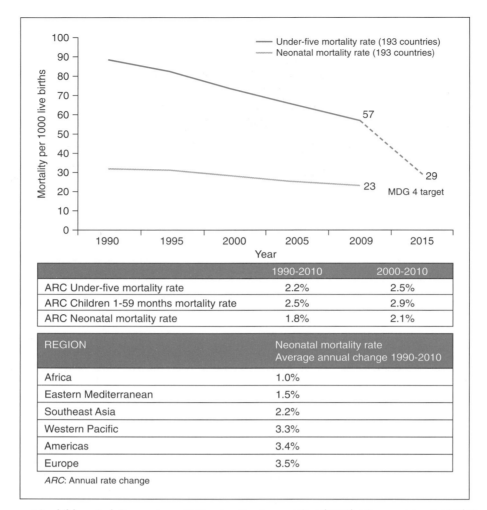

	1990-2010	2000-2010
ARC Under-five mortality rate	2.2%	2.5%
ARC Children 1-59 months mortality rate	2.5%	2.9%
ARC Neonatal mortality rate	1.8%	2.1%

REGION	Neonatal mortality rate Average annual change 1990-2010
Africa	1.0%
Eastern Mediterranean	1.5%
Southeast Asia	2.2%
Western Pacific	3.3%
Americas	3.4%
Europe	3.5%

ARC: Annual rate change

Figure 23-7 Improvement in child survival. Progress toward Millennium Development Goal (MDG) 4 for neonatal and child (<5 years) survival showing progress globally (193 countries). (Modified from Lawn | et al: *Health Policy Plan* 2012. Data from Oestergaard M, et al: *PLoS Med*, UNICEF, 2011. www.childinfo.org.)

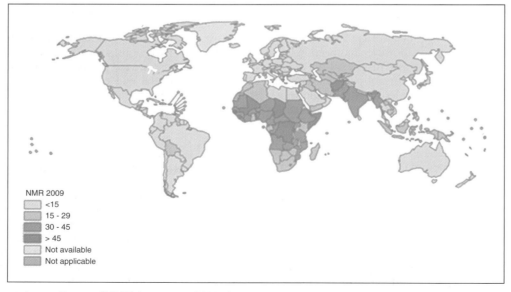

Figure 23-8 Neonatal mortality rate (NMR) by country, 2009. (From Oestergaard MZ, Inoue M, Yoshida S, et al: Neonatal mortality levels for 193 countries in 2009 with trends since 1990: a systematic analysis of progress, projections, and priorities. *PLoS Med* 8:e1001080, 2011.)

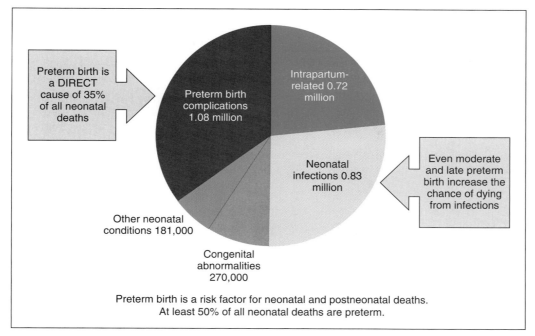

Figure 23-9 **Estimated distribution of causes of 3.1 million neonatal deaths in 193 countries, 2010.** (From Blencowe H, Cousens S, Chou D, et al: 15 million preterm births: priorities for action based on national, regional and global estimates. In Howson C, Kinney M, Lawn JE, et al, editors: *Born too soon: the global action report on preterm birth.* March of Dimes, Partnership for Maternal, Newborn and Child Health, Save the Children, Geneva, 2012 World Health Organization.)

Table 23-3 **Conditions that Affect Maternal Pregnancy Outcomes and Stillbirths/Neonatal Outcomes**

	Mother	Stillbirth	Neonate
Childbirth Complications			
Hemorrhage	X	X	X
Obstructed labor	X	X	X
Preterm labor or birth	—	X	X
Infection			
Intrauterine infection	X	X	X
Syphilis	—	X	X
Malaria	X	X	—
Maternal Disorders			
Preeclampsia or eclampsia	X	X	X
Diabetes	X	X	—
Fetal growth restriction	—	X	X
Congenital abnormalities	—	X	X

From Goldenberg RL, et al: *Lancet* 377:1798–1805, 2011[58]; Stillbirth Series Steering Committee.

One of the most cost-effective ways to improve maternal and birth outcomes is through **family planning,** addressing the unmet need for modern contraceptives.[66] Other maternal conditions, although more distal and lower risk, may be very prevalent and can play an important role in fetal growth and newborn outcomes.[67,68] *Undernutrition* is common among women in low-income countries, and the resulting deficiencies are exacerbated in pregnancy, leading to potentially adverse effects on the mother and fetal and neonatal outcomes.[67] Maternal conditions related to *obesity* such as diabetes also clearly have a role for perinatal mortality, especially in high-income countries and are increasingly common in middle-income countries[69] (Table 23-4).

VI. USING THE DATA FOR ACTION

The potential impact of evidence-based interventions to reduce neonatal mortality, stillbirths, and preterm birth have been found to be cost-effective.[62,70-73] Especially in low-resource settings, effective interventions often overlap with those to reduce maternal death.[69,74] Thus, although interventions are assessed individually, strategies are usually considered together as service delivery packages in the continuum of maternal newborn and child care.[75]

A. Preventive Medicine

As part of an assessment for Global Alliance to Prevent Preterm Birth and Stillbirths (GAPPS), a systematic assessment was performed of approximately 2000 potential interventions for preterm birth (or low birth weight), stillbirth, or perinatal mortality.[71] Each was classified and assessed by the quality of available evidence and its potential to treat or prevent preterm birth and stillbirth. Of the 82 interventions, 49 were relevant to low- and middle-income countries and had sufficient evidence for inclusion. Most interventions identified require additional research to improve the quality of evidence while others had little evidence of benefit.

Two interventions to reduce preterm birth rates in low-income countries, *smoking cessation* and *progesterone,* were

Table 23-4 Summary of Maternal Risk Factors for Adverse Birth Outcomes*

Risk Factors	Adjusted OR*
Life Cycle Factors	
Maternal Age	
<18 years	1.1-2.3
>35 years	1.3-2.0
Maternal Size	
Height <150 cm	1.3-4.8
Prepregnancy weight <47 kg	1.1-2.4
Parity	
Primigravida	1.3-2.2
Parity >6	1.4-1.5
Poor obstetric history (previous perinatal death or instrumental delivery)	1.6-3.5
Antenatal Factors	
Multiple pregnancy	2.0-6.8
Hypertensive disorders	
Preeclampsia	1.7-3.7
Eclampsia	2.9-13.7
Bleeding per vagina after 8th month	3.4-5.7
Maternal jaundice	2.0-7.9
Maternal anemia (PCV <0.21)	1.9-4.2
Maternal anemia (PCV <33%)	NS in 4 studies
Maternal malaria (blood test positive)	2.2-3.5†
Syphilis (perinatal death)	1.7-5.8
HIV (infant death)	7.2
Intrapartum Factors	
Malpresentation	
Breech	6.4-14.7
Other	8.3-33.5
Obstructed labor/dystocia	6.7-84.9
Prolonged second stage	2.6-4.8
Maternal fever during labor (>38° C)	9.7-10.2
Rupture of membranes >24 hours	1.8-6.7
Meconium staining of liquid	11.5

From Lawn JE, et al: *Lancet* 365:891–900, 2005.
HIV, Human immunodeficiency virus; *NS,* not significant; *PCV,* packed cell volume.
*From more distal life cycle factors to proximal, showing range of adjusted odds ratios (ORs) from population-based studies.
†Risk for low birth weight, not mortality.

supported by data. Interventions identified with evidence to prevent stillbirths included the following:

- Screening and treatment of syphilis
- Intermittent presumptive treatment for malaria during pregnancy
- Insecticide-treated mosquito nets
- Birth preparedness
- Emergency obstetric care
- Cesarean section for breech presentation
- Elective induction for postterm birth

Eleven interventions were highlighted to improve survival of preterm newborns in low-income countries, including the following:

- Antenatal steroids for women in preterm labor
- Antibiotics for premature rupture of membranes
- Vitamin K supplementation at birth
- Delayed cord clamping
- Neonatal resuscitation
- Hospital-based "kangaroo" mother care
- Early breastfeeding
- Thermal care
- Case management of neonatal sepsis and pneumonia

Surfactant therapy and application of continued distending pressure to the lungs for respiratory distress syndrome are other evidence-based strategies but require greater health system capacity.[76]

For the *Lancet* Stillbirth Series, evidence-based interventions to prevent stillbirth were evaluated, observing that the majority of these also reduced neonatal mortality and a number also improved maternal survival.[69,70] Interventions provided in basic antenatal care, advanced antenatal care, and childbirth care were evaluated for the number of lives saved at full (99%) coverage (Fig. 23-10). The greatest reduction was associated with deaths during the time of birth, particularly emergency obstetric care, antenatal corticosteroids for preterm labor, and neonatal resuscitation.[69]

B. Continuum of Care

Although individual preventive interventions may have important effects, ultimately a continuum of care from household to hospital is essential, especially for care around the time of birth.[77] For low-income settings especially, outreach can provide care close to home. Such services can encourage care seeking for danger signs during pregnancy and are associated with substantially increased use of skilled care during childbirth.[71] Protocol-based referral systems allow consultation or transfer of cases for appropriate clinical care, to the level of comprehensive emergency obstetric and advanced neonatal care. **Community care** comprises promotion and implementation of healthy practices—appropriate diet, avoidance of tobacco and indoor air pollution, family involvement, birth preparedness, and increasing demand for safe childbirth attended by properly trained health workers in an appropriately equipped facility—and neonatal care following birth.[78]

VII. IMPROVING THE DATA

Despite the huge burden of deaths around the time of birth, the associated loss to families and countries is rarely highlighted in global health policy and research agendas. In addition, the morbidity and long-term disability associated with perinatal insults are considerable.[15] Epidemiologists and researchers face formidable barriers in collecting and analyzing data about prevalence and interventions, particularly in south Asia and sub-Saharan Africa, where two thirds of this burden occurs.[79-81] The places with the highest risk currently have the least information available.

The quantity and quality of information could be improved, even in the short-term, by the following actions[79,82] (Table 23-5):

1. Use consistent definitions and classification systems across current data collection mechanisms, especially in vital registration, facility-based data, and research. Current ICD-10 codes for both stillbirth and preterm birth need to be updated to reflect definitions currently

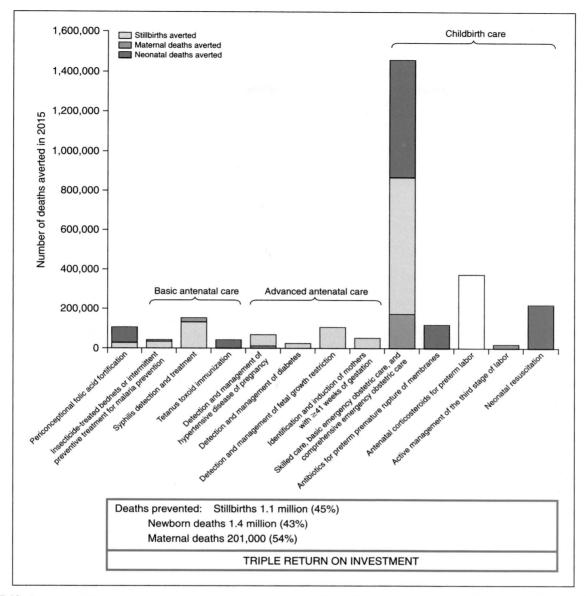

Figure 23-10 **Estimated stillbirths, newborn, and maternal deaths prevented by evidence-based strategies.** (From Pattinson R, Kerber K, Buchmann E, et al: Stillbirths: how can health systems deliver for mothers and babies? *Lancet* 377:1610–1623, 2011; Stillbirth Series Steering Committee.)

in use and advances made in the last decade. Research into etiologic mechanisms responsible for stillbirth and preterm birth has been hampered by the lack of standardized definitions and measurement protocols for assessing these outcomes.

2. Seize opportunities to add or test the measurement for birth outcomes linked to ongoing data collection mechanisms (e.g., household surveys, the main data source for the countries with 75% of global burden), and undertake validation studies. The expanded number of demographic surveillance sites currently functioning in various low- and middle-income countries (LMICs) offer excellent opportunities to compare prospective versus retrospective reporting on pregnancy outcomes.

3. Validate a simple, standardized classification system for stillbirth cause of death that is feasible through verbal autopsy but maps onto more complex causal classifications.

4. Improve systems and tools to capture gestational age, acute neonatal morbidity, and long-term impairment and chronic disease outcomes after preterm birth, small for gestational age, and other adverse pregnancy or neonatal events.

VIII. SUMMARY

The large numbers—more than 3 million neonatal deaths, 2.6 million third-trimester stillbirths, and 14.9 million preterm births—are similar to the issues considered the greatest priorities in global health today, and indeed, larger

Table 23-5 Improving Country-level Data for Neonatal Deaths: Recommendations and Research Questions

Category	Action to Improve Data		Research Questions*
	High-income Countries	Low-income Countries	
1. Counting pregnancy outcomes, including all births, maternal deaths, neonatal deaths, and stillbirths	Vital registration (VR) and use of specific death certificates for stillbirth and neonatal deaths Cross-link civil registration system and health system databases.	Household surveys (retrospective): use of pregnancy history, not birth history, in DHS to better capture early neonatal deaths and stillbirths; promote inclusion of key modules in UNICEF's MICS. Demographic surveillance sites (prospective): consider sentinel surveillance sites, especially in large countries (e.g., India, China), or network or study sites (e.g., INDEPTH). Improve VR: increase coverage and quality of births and deaths registration; cross-link civil registration system and health system databases.	Improving measurement of pregnancy outcomes in surveys (e.g., comparing pregnancy history and birth history for validity and additional time taken during survey) Developing a "quality score" to assess neonatal mortality data for representativeness, age heaping, etc. Novel use of facility data: can recognized biases in facility data be adjusted for using modeling?
2. Case definitions and hierarchical cause-of-death attribution	Consensus on consistent list of programmatically relevant, comparable categories, case definitions, and explicit hierarchy Data collected through: VR Confidential enquiry systems Special studies	Consensus on consistent list of programmatically relevant, comparable categories, case definitions, and explicit hierarchy Verbal autopsy studies with standard data collection tool and hierarchical attribution Data collected through: Follow up study after household surveys (e.g., DHS) Demographic surveillance sites (e.g., sentinel sites) Improved VR Special studies	Evaluation of standard verbal autopsy tool, case definitions, and hierarchy, mapping more complex subcategories from ICD onto basic list of programmatically relevant causes Effect of varying hierarchies on proportionate mortality Comparison of cause-of-death allocation by experts or by computer algorithm Inclusion of a standard social autopsy module
3. Neonatal morbidity and risk factors	Standardize case definitions for tracking morbidity (e.g., neonatal encephalopathy). Cross-link existing databases (e.g., perinatal follow-up and cerebral palsy registries).	Standardize case definitions for tracking morbidity (e.g., neonatal encephalopathy). Data collected through: Demographic surveillance sites (e.g., sentinel sites) Special studies	Improving gestational age data (e.g., weight as surrogate, simplified clinical assessment) Developing disability assessment standards and simpler tools across cultures (e.g., motor, IQ) and setting protocol for what to measure at what age
4. Counting avoidable factors and suboptimal care	National audit systems with regular reports on data and trends, as well as specific themes (e.g., intrapartum stillbirths) Consider confidential inquiry for maternal, infant deaths, and stillbirths.	Audit system for maternal, neonatal deaths, and stillbirths. Collate data nationally, and promote sentinel sites in varying regions and health systems so that information can be useful for policy prioritization while not representative. Consider focus on few indicators initially (e.g., intrapartum stillbirths, predischarge neonatal deaths in babies >2000 g).	Evaluation of simplified audit tools and mechanism to maximize resultant change in policy and programs

Modified from Lawn JE, et al: *BMC Pregnancy Childbirth* 10:S1, 2010.
DHS, Demographic and health surveys; *ICD*, *International Classification of Diseases* (WHO); *MICS*, Multiple Indicator Cluster Surveys.
*With focus on low-income countries.

than some that receive major attention, such as 2 million annual HIV/AIDS deaths or the 800,000 annual malaria deaths.[83] However, neonatal deaths, and particularly stillbirths, are not among global priorities. This invisibility is partly an issue of data, despite increasing quality and progress for global estimates. Another critical issue is the value put on a baby's life; a newborn remains the most vulnerable human, and a preterm newborn is even more vulnerable.

Yet each loss is bereavement for families and may leave a deeper scar than a death that is openly acknowledged and mourned. Long-term follow-up studies show that 20 years after a stillbirth, a woman may remain in a delayed grief response.[84] The societies where stillbirth and preterm birth have become priorities are those where such babies are expected to live, and women and families can express their loss. Indeed, the power of these families to use data for change may be likened to the power of individuals who lost loved ones from HIV/AIDS and advocated successfully for change. As Figure 23-11 depicts, data alone will not result in change until society and leaders recognize that these deaths are a loss that can and must count and be prevented.

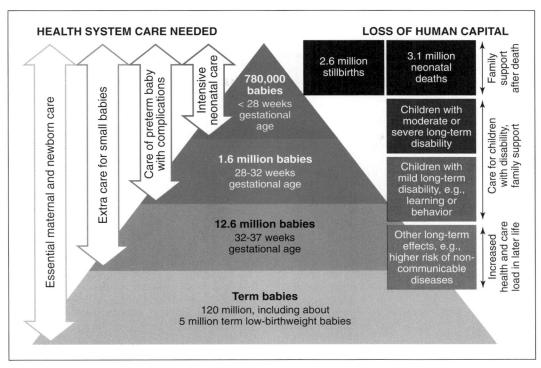

Figure 23-11 Pyramid of 135 million births showing health system care needed and loss of human capital. (From Lawn |E, Davidge R, Vinod P, et al: Care for the preterm baby. In Howson C, Kinney M, Lawn |E, et al, editors: *Born too soon: the global action report on preterm birth.* March of Dimes, Partnership for Maternal, Newborn and Child Health, Save the Children, Geneva, 2012 World Health Organization.)

References

1. UNICEF: State of the world's children. 2012. http://www.unicef.org/sowc/.

2. Oestergaard MZ, Inoue M, Yoshida S, et al: Neonatal mortality levels for 193 countries in 2009 with trends since 1990: a systematic analysis of progress, projections, and priorities. *PLoS Med* 8:e1001080, 2011.

3. Cousens S, Blencowe H, Stanton C, et al: National, regional, and worldwide estimates of stillbirth rates in 2009 with trends since 1995: a systematic analysis. *Lancet* 377:1319–1330, 2011.

4. Lawn JE, Cousens S, Zupan J: 4 million neonatal deaths: when? where? why? Neonatal Survival Steering Team. *Lancet* 365:891–900, 2005.

5. Bhutta ZA, Chopra M, Axelson H, et al: Countdown to 2015 decade report (2000-10): taking stock of maternal, newborn, and child survival. *Lancet* 375:2032–2044, 2010.

6. Darmstadt GL, Lee AC, Cousens S, et al: 60 million non-facility births: who can deliver in community settings to reduce intrapartum-related deaths? *Int J Gynaecol Obstet* 107:S89–S112, 2009.

7. Haws RA, Mashasi I, Mrisho M, et al: "These are not good things for other people to know": How rural Tanzanian women's experiences of pregnancy loss and early neonatal death may impact survey data quality. *Soc Sci Med* 71:1764–1772, 2010.

8. Kumar V, Mohanty S, Kumar A, et al: Effect of community-based behaviour change management on neonatal mortality in Shivgarh, Uttar Pradesh, India: a cluster-randomised controlled trial. *Lancet* 372:1151–1162, 2008.

9. Flenady V, Middleton P, Smith GC, et al: Stillbirths: the way forward in high-income countries. *Lancet* 377:1703–1717, 2011.

10. Simmons LE, Rubens CE, Darmstadt GL, et al: Preventing preterm birth and neonatal mortality: exploring the epidemiology, causes, and interventions. *Semin Perinatol* 34:408–415, 2010.

11. Ramsay S: No closure in sight for the 10/90 health-research gap. *Lancet* 358:1348, 2001.

12. Hart JT: The inverse care law. *Lancet* 1(7696):405–412, 1971.

13. Lawn J, Shibuya K, Stein C: No cry at birth: global estimates of intrapartum stillbirths and intrapartum-related neonatal deaths. *Bull WHO* 83:409–417, 2005.

14. Lawn JE, Blencowe H, Pattinson R, et al: Stillbirths: where? when? why? How to make the data count. *Lancet* 377:1448–1463, 2011.

15. Mwaniki MK, Atieno M, Lawn JE, et al: Long-term neurodevelopmental outcomes after intrauterine and neonatal insults: a systematic review. *Lancet* 379:445–452, 2012.

16. Hogan MC, Foreman KJ, Naghavi M, et al: Maternal mortality for 181 countries, 1980-2008: a systematic analysis of progress towards Millennium Development Goal 5. *Lancet* 375:1609–1623, 2010.

17. Tuncalp O, Hindin M, Souza J, et al: The prevalence of maternal near miss: a systematic review. *BJOG* 119:653–661, 2012.

18. Trends in maternal mortality: *1990 to 2008, WHO, UNICEF.* UNFPA, World Bank, 2010. http://whqlibdoc.who.int/publications/2010/9789241500265_eng.pdf.

19. Lawn JE, Lee AC, Kinney M, et al: Two million intrapartum-related stillbirths and neonatal deaths: where, why, and what can be done? *Int J Gynaecol Obstet* 107:S5–S18, S9, 2009.

20. World Health Organization (WHO): 2011. http://www.who.int/healthinfo/statistics/indneonatalmortality/en/.

21. Edmond KM, Quigley MA, Zandoh C, et al: Diagnostic accuracy of verbal autopsies in ascertaining the causes of stillbirths and neonatal deaths in rural Ghana. *Paediatr Perinat Epidemiol* 22:417–429, 2008.

22. Kramer MS: The epidemiology of adverse pregnancy outcomes: an overview. *J Nutr* 133(suppl 2):1592–1596, 2003.

23. Cartlidge PH, Stewart JH: Effect of changing the stillbirth definition on evaluation of perinatal mortality rates. *Lancet* 346:486–488, 1995.

24. Joseph KS, Liu S, Rouleau J, et al: Influence of definition based versus pragmatic birth registration on international comparisons of perinatal and infant mortality: population-based retrospective study. *BMJ* 344:e746, 2012.

25. Facchinetti F, Reddy U, Stray-Pedersen B, et al: International issues in stillbirth. *J Matern Fetal Neonatal Med* 21:425–428, 2008.

26. WHO: *International statistical classification of diseases and related health problems,* 10th revision, ed 2 (ICD-10). 2004. http://www.who.int/classifications/icd/ICD-10_2nd_ed_volume2.pdf.

27. WHO: Recommended definitions, terminology and format for statistical tables related to the perinatal period and use of a new certificate for cause of perinatal deaths: modifications recommended by FIGO as amended October 14, 1976. *Acta Obstet Gynecol Scand* 56:247–253, 1977.

28. Fleischman AR, Oinuma M, Clark SL: Rethinking the definition of "term pregnancy". *Obstet Gynecol* 116:136–139, 2010.

29. Marlow N: Full term: an artificial concept. *Arch Dis Child Fetal Neonatal Ed* 97:F158, 2012.

30. Kramer MS, Papageorghiou A, Culhane J, et al: Challenges in defining and classifying the preterm birth syndrome. *Am J Obstet Gynecol* 206:108–112, 2012.

31. Sanders MR, Donohue PK, Oberdorf MA, et al: Perceptions of the limit of viability: neonatologists' attitudes toward extremely preterm infants. *J Perinatol* 15:494–502, 1995.

32. Goldenberg RL, Nelson KG, Dyer RL, et al: The variability of viability: the effect of physicians' perceptions of viability on the survival of very low–birth weight infants. *Am J Obstet Gynecol* 143:678–684, 1982.

33. Morgan MA, Goldenberg RL, Schulkin J: Obstetrician-gynecologists' practices regarding preterm birth at the limit of viability. *J Matern Fetal Neonatal Med* 21:115–121, 2008.

34. Blencowe H, Cousens S, Oestergaard M, et al: National, regional and worldwide estimates of preterm birth rates in the year 2010 with time trends for selected countries since 1990: a systematic analysis and implications. *Lancet* 379:2162–2172, 2012.

35. Hadlock FP: Sonographic estimation of fetal age and weight. *Radiol Clin North Am* 28:39–50, 1990.

36. Landis SH, Ananth CV, Lokomba V, et al: Ultrasound-derived fetal size nomogram for a sub-Saharan African population: a longitudinal study. *Ultrasound Obstet Gynecol* 34:379–386, 2009.

37. Mikolajczyk RT, Zhang J, Betran AP, et al: A global reference for fetal-weight and birthweight percentiles. *Lancet* 377:1855–1861, 2011.

38. Boerma JT, Mathers C, Abou-Zahr C: WHO and global health monitoring: the way forward. *PLoS Med* 7:e1000373, 2010.

39. Mahapatra P, Shibuya K, Lopez AD, et al: Civil registration systems and vital statistics: successes and missed opportunities. *Lancet* 370:1653–1663, 2007.

40. Heuser CC, Hunn J, Varner M, et al: Correlation between stillbirth vital statistics and medical records. *Obstet Gynecol* 116:1296–1301, 2010.

41. Makelarski JA, Romitti PA, Caspers KM, et al: Use of active surveillance methodologies to examine over-reporting of stillbirths on fetal death certificates. *Birth Defects Res Clin Mol Teratol* 91:1004–1010, 2011.

42. Barfield WD: Standard terminology for fetal, infant, and perinatal deaths. *Pediatrics* 128:177–181, 2011.

43. Mari Bhat PN: Completeness of India's sample registration system: an assessment using the general growth balance method. *Popul Stud (Camb)* 56:119–134, 2002.

44. Yang G, Hu J, Rao KQ, et al: Mortality registration and surveillance in China: history, current situation and challenges. *Popul Health Metr* 3:3, 2005.

45. UNICEF: Multiple Indicator Cluster Surveys (MICS). http://www.unicef.org/statistics/index_24302.html.

46. ICF MACRO: Demographic health survey. http://www.measuredhs.com/.

47. UNICEF: Childinfo: monitoring the situation of children and women. www.childinfo.org.

48. Boerma JT, Sommerfelt AE: Demographic and health surveys (DHS): contributions and limitations. *World Health Stat Q* 46:222–226, 1993.

49. Lozano R, Wang H, Foreman KJ, et al: Progress towards Millennium Development Goals 4 and 5 on maternal and child mortality: an updated systematic analysis. *Lancet* 378:1139–1165, 2011.

50. Boerma JT, Bryce J, Kinfu Y, et al: Mind the gap: equity and trends in coverage of maternal, newborn, and child health services in 54 Countdown countries. *Lancet* 371:1259–1267, 2008.

51. Bang AT, Reddy HM: Child mortality in Maharashtra. *Econ Polit Wkly* 37:4947–4965, 2002.

52. Lumbiganon P, Panamonta M, Laopaiboon M, et al: Why are Thai official perinatal and infant mortality rates so low? *Int J Epidemiol* 19:997–1000, 1990.

53. Flenady V, Froen JF, Pinar H, et al: An evaluation of classification systems for stillbirth. *BMC Pregnancy Childbirth* 9:24, 2009.

54. Reddy UM, Goldenberg R, Silver R, et al: Stillbirth classification: developing an international consensus for research. Executive summary of a National Institute of Child Health and Human Development workshop. *Obstet Gynecol* 114:901–914, 2009.

55. Liu L, Johnson H, Cousens S, et al: Global, regional and national causes of child mortality: an updated systematic analysis. *Lancet* 379:2151–2161, 2012.

56. Field D, Draper ES, Fenton A, et al: Rates of very preterm birth in Europe and neonatal mortality rates. *Arch Dis Child Fetal Neonatal Ed* 94:F253–F256, 2009.

57. Lawn J, Kinney M, Oestergaard MZ: Newborn survival: a multi-country analysis of a decade of change. *Health Policy Plan* 27(Suppl 3):iii6–iii28, 2012.

58. Bhutta ZA, Lassi ZS, Blanc A, et al: Linkages among reproductive health, maternal health, and perinatal outcomes. *Semin Perinatol* 34:434–445, 2010.

59. Boama V, Arulkumaran S: Safer childbirth: a rights-based approach. *Int J Gynaecol Obstet* 106:125–127, 2009.

60. Goldenberg RL, McClure EM, Bhutta ZA, et al: Stillbirths: the vision for 2020. *Lancet* 377:1798–1805, 2011.

61. Khan KS, Wojdyla D, Say L, et al: WHO analysis of causes of maternal death: a systematic review. *Lancet* 367:1066–1074, 2006.

62. Goldenberg RL, McClure EM, Macguire ER, et al: Lessons for low-income regions following the reduction in hypertension-related maternal mortality in high-income countries. *Int J Gynaecol Obstet* 113:91–95, 2011.

63. Goldenberg RL, McClure EM, Saleem S, et al: Infection-related stillbirths. *Lancet* 375:1482–1490, 2010.

64. Blencowe H, Cousens S, Kamb M, et al: Lives Saved Tool supplement: detection and treatment of syphilis in pregnancy to reduce syphilis related stillbirths and neonatal mortality. *BMC Public Health* 11(suppl 3):9, 2011.

65. Goldenberg RL, Culhane JF, Iams JD, et al: Epidemiology and causes of preterm birth. *Lancet* 371:75–84, 2008.

66. Carvalho N, Salehi AS, Goldie SJ: National and sub-national analysis of the health benefits and cost-effectiveness of strategies to reduce maternal mortality in Afghanistan. *Health Policy Plan* 2012. [Epub ahead of print.].

67. Imdad A, Yakoob MY, Bhutta ZA: The effect of folic acid, protein energy and multiple micronutrient supplements in pregnancy on stillbirths. *BMC Public Health* 11(suppl 3):4, 2011.

68. Haider BA, Yakoob MY, Bhutta ZA: Effect of multiple micronutrient supplementation during pregnancy on maternal and birth outcomes. *BMC Public Health* 11 (suppl 3):19, 2011.

69. Pattinson R, Kerber K, Buchmann E, et al: Stillbirths: how can health systems deliver for mothers and babies? *Lancet* 377:1610–1623, 2011.

70. Bhutta ZA, Yakoob MY, Lawn JE, et al: Stillbirths: what difference can we make and at what cost? *Lancet* 377:1523–1538, 2011.

71. Barros FC, Bhutta ZA, Batra M, et al: Global report on preterm birth and stillbirth (3 of 7): evidence for effectiveness of interventions. *BMC Pregnancy Childbirth* 10:S3, 2010.

72. Darmstadt GL, Bhutta ZA, Cousens S, et al: Evidence-based, cost-effective interventions: how many newborn babies can we save? *Lancet* 365:977–988, 2005.

73. Lee AC, Cousens S, Darmstadt GL, et al: Care during labor and birth for the prevention of intrapartum-related neonatal deaths: a systematic review and Delphi estimation of mortality effect. *BMC Public Health* 11(suppl 3):10, 2011.

74. McClure EM, Goldenberg RL, Bann CM: Maternal mortality, stillbirth and measures of obstetric care in developing and developed countries. *Int J Gynaecol Obstet* 96:139–146, 2007.

75. Kerber KJ, de Graft-Johnson JE, Bhutta ZA, et al: Continuum of care for maternal, newborn, and child health: from slogan to service delivery. *Lancet* 370:1358–1369, 2007.

76. Howson CP, Kinney MV, Lawn JE, editors: *Born too soon: The Global Action Report on Preterm Birth. Eds. March of Dimes, PMNCH, Save the Children*, New York, World Health Organization, 2012 http://www.who.int/pmnch/media/news/2012/preterm_birth_report/en/index1.html.

77. Lawn JE, Kinney M, Lee AC, et al: Reducing intrapartum-related deaths and disability: can the health system deliver? *Int J Gynaecol Obstet* 107:S123–S140, 2009.

78. Lassi ZS, Haider BA, Bhutta ZA: Community-based intervention packages for reducing maternal and neonatal morbidity and mortality and improving neonatal outcomes. *Cochrane Database Syst Rev* 11:CD007754, 2010.

79. AbouZahr C, Cleland J, Coullare F, et al: The way forward. *Lancet* 370:1791–1799, 2007.

80. Hill K, Lopez AD, Shibuya K, et al: Interim measures for meeting needs for health sector data: births, deaths, and causes of death. *Lancet* 370:1726–1735, 2007.

81. Setel PW, Macfarlane SB, Szreter S, et al: A scandal of invisibility: making everyone count by counting everyone. *Lancet* 370:1569–1577, 2007 (Who counts? series).

82. Lawn JE, Gravett MG, Nunes TM, et al: Global report on preterm birth and stillbirth (1 of 7): definitions, description of the burden and opportunities to improve data. *BMC Pregnancy Childbirth* 10:S1, 2010.

83. Roll Back Malaria Partnership: The global malaria action plan for a malaria-free world, Geneva. 2008, RBM. http://www.rollbackmalaria.org/gmap/gmap.pdf.

84. Froen JF, Cacciatore J, McClure EM, et al: Stillbirths: why they matter. *Lancet* 377:1353–1366, 2011.

Select Readings/Organizations with Websites

Born Too Soon: *Global Action Report on Preterm Births* summarizes the first national estimates of preterm birth for 184 countries, time trends for 65 countries, and program solutions and research needs around the world. http://www.who.int/pmnch/media/news/2012/preterm_birth_report/en/index1.html.

Countdown to 2015 Initiative tracks country-level progress in achieving high, sustained and equitable coverage of effective interventions aimed at reducing maternal, newborn, and child mortality. http://www.countdown2015mnch.org/.

Healthy Newborn Network provides the latest information on newborn health statistics and care around the world. http://www.healthynewbornnetwork.org/.

Lancet Neonatal Survival Series in 2005 provided the first estimates on numbers and causes for 4 million neonatal deaths and analyzed cost and effect of solutions possible at the community level in low-income countries. http://www.thelancet.com/series/neonatal-survival.

Lancet Stillbirth Series in 2011 provided estimates of rates and of stillbirth and summarized analyses of effect and cost of varying health system approaches to prevent stillbirths (as well as maternal and neonatal deaths) and actions to halve stillbirth rates by 2020. http://www.lancet.com/series/stillbirth.

Lancet Who Counts? Series highlights the disparity in health outcome data around the world. http://www.who.int/healthinfo/statistics/LancetWhoCounts/.

United Nations Children's Fund (UNICEF) provides information on statistics about neonatal and child survival and coverage of interventions at its Childinfo, including a description of UN Interagency Group for Child Mortality Estimation and a link to its database, with information on newborn care (some information in several languages). http://www.childinfo.org.

World Health Organization also has information about the Millennium Development Goal 4, provides information on newborn mortality, with the latest estimates, and on demographic and health surveys.

Other Websites

http://www.indepth-network.org/.
http://www.measuredhs.com.
http://www.un.org/millenniumgoals/ [Millennium Development Goals].

Public Health

4

24 Introduction to Public Health

Thus far in this book, the discussion has focused mostly on what individuals and their clinicians can do to promote health and prevent disease and injury. Section 4 of this book focuses on public health. As the Institute of Medicine (IOM) indicated in its 1988 report *The Future of Public Health,*

"Public health is what we, as a society, do collectively to assure the conditions in which people can be healthy."[1]

To ensure better health, the responsibilities in public health are threefold: assessment, policy development, and assurance[1] (i.e., ensuring that appropriate services are available and accessible to meet the needs of the population). Chapter 2 provides tools for estimating the health of a population, and Chapter 14 discusses several definitions of health and their limitations. This chapter summarizes the current health of the U.S. population in the second decade of the 21st century and discusses data sources that public health practitioners can use to better understand the health issues in their communities. Injuries are also discussed in this chapter, both as a significant source of premature mortality, and as an example of how to think systematically about public health prevention efforts. Chapters 25 and 26 outline the U.S. public health system and how communities can improve their health. Chapters 27 and 28 address the specific public health topics of preparing for emergencies and ensuring the best quality of health care. Chapter 29 considers the complex and sometimes contradictory efforts of the medical care system to provide medical care, some of which can be considered preventive. Lastly, Chapter 30 outlines the important connections among environmental/ecological health, the health of other species, and human health and highlights new, integrative approaches for enhancing the "one health" we all share.

I. DEFINITIONS OF PUBLIC HEALTH

The term *public health* has the following two meanings:
- Health status of the public (i.e., a defined population)
- Organized social efforts to preserve and improve the health of a defined population

The best-known definition of public health in terms of this second meaning was written in 1920 by C.-E. A. Winslow[2] and is still remarkably current:

> Public health is the science and art of preventing disease, prolonging life, and promoting physical health and efficiency through organized community efforts for the sanitation of the environment, the control of community infections, the education of the individual in principles of personal hygiene, the organization of medical and nursing service for the early diagnosis and preventive treatment of disease, and the development of the social machinery which will ensure to every individual in the community a standard of living adequate for the maintenance of health.

This definition is especially significant in the following three ways:

1. It states the central emphasis of all public health work—promoting health and preventing disease.

2. It emphasizes the diverse strategies required to promote health and prevent disease, including environmental sanitation, specific disease control efforts, health education, medical care, and an adequate standard of living.

3. It clarifies that for these goals to be achieved, organized social action is required. This action is largely expressed in the policies of the federal, state, and local governments and in the activities of the agencies designed to promote and protect the health of the public.

II. HEALTH IN THE UNITED STATES

A. Major Sources of Mortality and Morbidity

All efforts to improve public health start with an assessment. Table 24-1 shows major *metrics* of public health in the United States. Overall metrics of mortality have been steadily improving since 1950. Life expectancy at birth has improved to 78.2 years, and overall infant mortality has declined to less than 7 per 1000 newborns.[3]

The three leading causes of death have changed recently. Historically, heart disease has been the number-one killer (which it remains), followed by cancer and stroke (cerebrovascular accident). As the mortality of all these diseases has decreased, mortality from chronic lower respiratory diseases has increased and is now third on the list. Mortality from Alzheimer's dementia has also increased, surpassing that from diabetes in 2009. The three leading cancers have long been lung, breast/prostate, and colorectal cancer. The trends over time have shown a large increase in lung cancer after the widespread use of tobacco. This peak has leveled off for men (Fig. 24-1). For women, the trend came later and has yet to level off (Fig. 24-2).

Globally, developing countries are undergoing a **demographic and epidemiologic transition.** Demographically, the population in these countries ages; epidemiologically, infectious diseases become less important as causes of death and chronic disease and cancers more important. In keeping with this trend, the global cancer burden is rising. Cancer trends in many developed countries are similar to U.S. trends. Developing countries have a larger burden of cancers from preventable infectious causes, such as cervical cancer.[4] Further data on global cancer statistics can be found online.[5]

Society should have an interest in reducing *all* mortality, but many public health officials have an appropriate and particular interest in reducing premature deaths. One way to account for the impact of mortality causes on premature death is to calculate **years of potential life lost** (YPLL). Figure 24-3 shows the 10 leading causes of YPLL before age 75 between 2000 and 2009. Analyzing the data in this way reverses first and second places on the mortality list; cancer is now the number-one cause of premature death because it affects more young people. Calculating the data this way also shows that chronic diseases such as chronic lower respiratory diseases and diabetes are less important in causing premature mortality. Intentional and unintentional injuries play a major role in premature death because they disproportionately affect younger people.

B. Actual Causes of Death

The previous death statistics are based on death certificates filled out by clinicians and do not account for the full causal pathway leading to death. One metric that attempts to account for this fact is **actual causes of death.** This metric was outlined for the first time in a landmark paper by McGinnis and Foege and last updated in 2004.[6] This analysis showed that *smoking, poor diet,* and *lack of physical activity* were the main drivers of mortality. However, analyzing actual causes of death should not be interpreted as a reduction of all mortality on individual behavior and an exoneration of structural determinants of health. As discussed in Chapters 14, 20, and 26, poverty, food environments, and safe environments all play an important role in shaping or enabling behavior.

C. Disability-adjusted Life Years

With death rates falling, many persons live with serious illness and disability for many years. To assess this burden of disease,

---

Table 24-1 Major Metrics and Sources of Mortality and Morbidity, United States

	1950	1980	2000	2006	2007	2009
Life Expectancy in Years						
At birth	68.1	73.9	76.8	77.7	77.9	78.2
At age 65	13.8	16.4	17.6	18.5	18.6	18.8
Infant Deaths per 1000 Live Births						
All infants	29.2	12.6	6.91	6.69	6.75	6.42
Deaths per 100,000 Population, Age-Adjusted						
All causes	1446.0	1039.1	869.0	776.5	760.2	741.0
Heart disease	586.8	412.1	257.6	200.2	190.9	179.8
Cancer	193.9	207.9	199.6	180.7	178.4	173.6
Stroke	180.7	96.2	60.9	43.6	42.2	38.9
Chronic lower respiratory diseases	—	28.3	44.2	40.5	40.8	42.2
Unintentional injuries	78.0	46.4	34.9	39.8	40.0	37.0
Motor vehicle	24.6	22.3	15.4	15.0	14.4	11.7
Diabetes	23.1	18.1	25.0	23.3	22.5	20.9

Data from Health, United States, 2005: chartbook on trends in the health of Americans (www.cdc.gov/nchs/data/hus/hus05.pdf); At a glance table, Health, United States, 2010 (http://www.ncbi.nlm.nih.gov/books/NBK54373/#ataglance.s1); and Deaths: preliminary data for 2009, *Natl Vital Stat Rep* 59:4, 2011 (http://www.cdc.gov/nchs/data/nvsr/nvsr59/nvsr59_04.pdf).

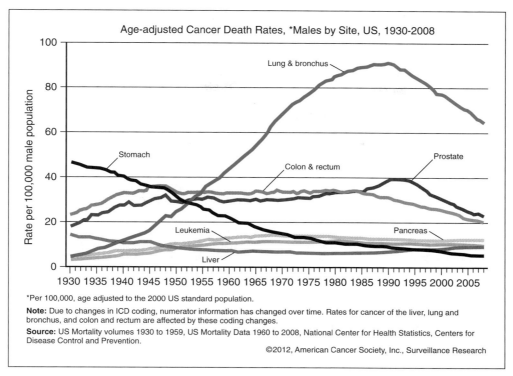

Figure 24-1 **Age-adjusted cancer death rates for males by cancer site, United States, 1930–2008.** (From American Cancer Society: *Cancer facts and figures: 2012*, Atlanta, 2012, ACS. http://www.cancer.org/acs/groups/content/@epidemiologysurveillance/documents/document/acspc-031941.pdf)

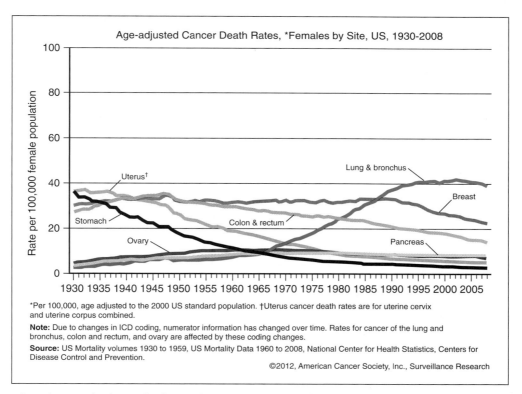

Figure 24-2 **Age-adjusted cancer death rates for females by cancer site, United States, 1930–2008.** (From American Cancer Society: *Cancer facts and figures: 2012*, Atlanta, 2012, ACS.)

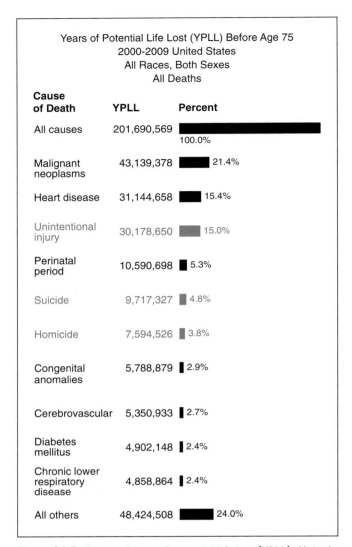

Figure 24-3 **Causes of years of potential life lost (YPLL), United States, 2000–2009.** (From National Center for Injury Prevention and Control, Atlanta, 2010, Centers for Disease Control and Prevention. http://webappa.cdc.gov/sasweb/ncipc/ypll10.html)

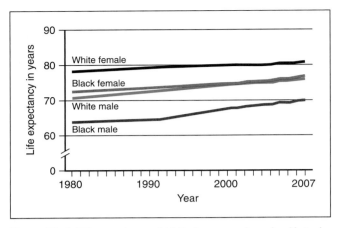

Figure 24-4 **Life expectancy at birth, by race and gender, United States, 1980–2007.** (From *Health of the United States 2010*, Washington, DC, 2010, US Department of Health and Human Services. http://www.cdc.gov/nchs/data/hus/hus10.pdf)

a metric called **disability-adjusted life years** (DALY) has been developed. This metric captures both the length of life lost from premature death and the time spent in poor health.[7] By this metric, the leading sources of premature death and disability were cardiovascular disease, cancer (especially breast and lung), depression, osteoarthritis, diabetes, and alcohol use. There were significant differences between genders and among ethnic groups. For example, for women, depression was the second leading cause of DALY (10 for males), whereas motor vehicle injuries and HIV-related deaths accounted for more DALY among ethnic minorities.

D. Health Care Disparities

The goal of public health is not just to decrease mortality and morbidity overall but also to decrease disparities. Historically, there has long been a gap between male and female life expectancy, as well as between whites and blacks. This gap has decreased somewhat but still exists; overall, white women live the longest, and black men are most likely to die

early (Fig. 24-4). In this analysis, race is likely not the causative agent but may be a correlate of proximate causes of decreased life expectancy, such as socioeconomic status and empowerment. Effective strategies to address health care disparities have been identified at the state and local level (see Chapter 26).

Health care disparities occur in all age groups but are exacerbated in particular groups. Although mortality rates and infant and child mortality all have improved significantly in the past five decades, this is not the case for young persons age 15 to 24.[8] The three leading causes of death in this age group include unintentional injuries (mainly motor vehicle crashes), homicide, and suicide (Fig. 24-5).

Even among young people, injury rates vary by region and ethnicity. Non-Hispanic black and American Indians/Alaska Natives have much higher mortality rates than the other races, largely because of higher rates of unintentional injuries (American Indian), homicides (non-Hispanic black), and suicide (American Indian).

See Figure 24-6 on studentconsult.com for youth mortality by causes of death and ethnicity.

Disparities in access to care, outcomes, and mortality persist, especially among poor and minority populations. The elimination of such disparities remains a public health priority and is the subject of dedicated institutes.

III. DATA SOURCES IN PUBLIC HEALTH

Public health data are used in research and in community assessment to evaluate, to plan, to foster accountability, and to spur change. To obtain and analyze **health indicator data,** epidemiologists rely on a variety of sources. Data for the rates used in epidemiologic studies can be discussed in terms of **numerator data,** which define the population experiencing events or conditions of concern, and **denominator data,** which define the population at risk. Statistics gathered from health, disease, birth, and death registries, as well as from other surveys, are used in the numerator. Census statistics are used in the denominator.

In clinical epidemiology, health-related data usually derive from patient examinations, clinical records, and

Figure 24-5 Mortality rates among youth ages 15 to 24 by race, 1935–2007. (From Singh GK: Youth mortality in the United States, 1935–2007, Rockville, Md, 2010, DHHS.)

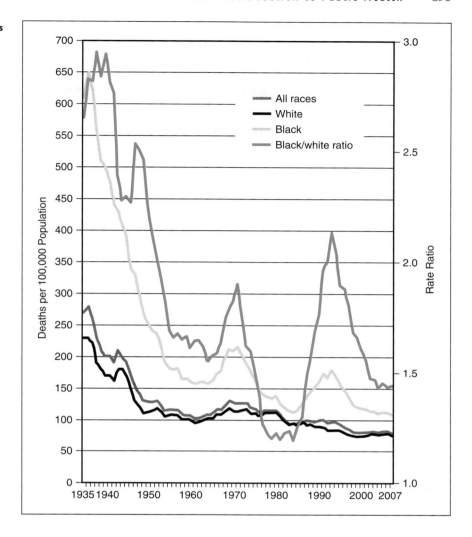

studies of specific clinical populations. When monitoring the health of large populations, epidemiologists use existing databases as much as possible to reduce costs and accelerate results.

The increasing availability of **electronic medical records** and other digitized repositories constitutes an explosion of public health data. The main challenge is no longer to find data, but to find *useful* data in a sea of sources. Box 24-1 illustrates an example of pulling information together for assessing the burden of disease from asthma in a community.

Public health planning in the United States benefits from many high-quality health-related surveys that are done regularly. With the growth of the Internet, social media, and applications that pinpoint the location of multiple people, new sources for surveillance have become available.

The most important uses of the data remain to foster *accountability* and to spur *change*. In an ideal world, everyone would use a coherent set of population health metrics to drive such change. To date, however, no coherent and consistent set is available.[9] Health knowledge should not devolve into its converse, morbidity and mortality (Fig. 24-7).[10] In keeping with theories of health and its determinants, such a consistent set of health indicators should measure not only disease burden but also health equity,

social determinants of health, environmental monitoring, quality of life, and aspects of health system performance.

A. Surveillance and Databases

Public health surveillance is defined as the ongoing systematic collection, analysis, and dissemination of data regarding a health-related event for use in public health action to reduce morbidity and mortality and to improve health.[11] Many entities on the local, state, and federal level are engaged in collecting such data. The data are usually used descriptively to do the following[12]:

- Measure the burden of disease or trends in the burden of disease.
- Educate the public.
- Guide action and develop priorities for public health action.
- Acquire resources (e.g., state grants).
- Develop policies.
- Guide the planning, implementation, and evaluation of programs.
- Provide a basis for research.

Public health databases usually track health-related events that affect large segments of the population. Some events

Box 24-1   **Using Data from Multiple Sources to Assess Level of Asthma Morbidity in a New York County**

In assessing the burden of disease in their community, public health planners need to access data from many sources. This involves an iterative process in which planners move between primary data collection in their community to publicly available data and back to more primary data collection. The following is a description of the steps a hypothetical public health planner might take to assess the disease burden from asthma in a county in New York State. Readers should note that New York has additional state-level resources. For states with a less active (or well-funded) state health department, planners may need to do more primary data collection. Because hospitalizations for asthma are considered preventable with optimal primary care, benchmark data are available from the Agency for Healthcare Research and Quality (AHRQ). This may not be true for other community health problems.

A. Describe the asthma prevalence and mortality among adults and children in the state, and describe trend.
  1. Assess the prevalence rate of adult asthma in certain subgroups (age, gender, race/ethnicity). (BRFSS)
  2. Compare the county adult asthma prevalence rate with the state. (BRFSS/EBRFSS)
  3. Assess the county adult asthma prevalence in population subgroups (age, gender, race/ethnicity). (BRFSS/EBRFSS)
  4. Compare the county population subgroup patterns to the state subgroups for adult asthma prevalence. (BRFSS/EBRFSS)
  5. Assess current asthma prevalence among children in the state. (National Asthma Surveillance—NY)
  6. Compare the state childhood asthma prevalence among population subgroups. (National Asthma Surveillance—NY)
  7. Perform primary data collection for county childhood asthma prevalence.
  8. Compare the county childhood asthma prevalence with the state prevalence.

9. Compare the asthma mortality rate for the state and county. (Vital Records—3 years)
B. Assess health care utilization resulting from asthma.
  1. Assess current rate of hospital discharge from asthma, and describe trends in different age groups (total, 0-17, 18-64, 65+; likely need to obtain from hospitals directly or from state hospital association).
  2. Compare the 3-year rates for state versus county by age.
  3. Compare hospitalization rate by zip code for 3 years; where are the high risk areas?
  4. Assess emergency room data—1-year cross-sectional; what percentage is asthma-related? Look at age, gender, race/ethnicity, and payment source distributions.
  5. Calculate the risk ratio for someone who lives in the _____ zip code being hospitalized/seen in the emergency room for asthma: ___; compared to other zip codes in the county.
  6. Compare county asthma hospitalization rate to benchmark. (AHRQ)
C. Describe overall health of the county.
  1. Assess median family income/per-capita income by zip code (from census).
  2. Assess county health ranking. (countyhealthranking or American Community Survey).
  3. Assess air quality (EPA).
  4. Could also assess adult and adolescent smoking rates (BRFSS and YBRFSS).
D. Perform primary data collection.
  1. Estimate sample size for sampling school asthma survey.
  2. Compare prevalence rates from school asthma data of four schools (two high-risk areas, one moderate-risk area, and one low-risk area).
E. Review primary data and determine if other data sources need to be accessed.

Modified from Epi Info Community Health Assessment Tutorial 2.0, 2005, Department of Health and Human Services, CDC, National Center for Public Health Informatics. ftp://ftp.cdc.gov/pub/Software/epi_info/EIHAT_WEB/EIHAT2.0.pdf
Note: The primary data collection will likely bring up more issues that require comparison to state and county averages.
BRFSS, Behavioral Risk Factor Survey System (*E*, Expanded; *Y*, Youth); *EPA*, Environmental Protection Agency.

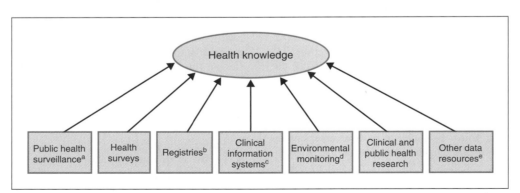

Figure 24-7 Knowing about health. [a]The ongoing, systematic collection, analysis, and interpretation of health-related data with the a priori purpose of identifying unusual events of public health importance, or preventing or controlling disease or injury, followed by their dissemination for public health action. For example:
[b]Vital registration, cancer registries, exposure registries.
[c]Medical and laboratory records, pharmacy records.
[d]Weather, climate change, pollution.
[e]Criminal Justice information, Lexis-Nexis, census. (From Lee LM, Thacker SB: Public health surveillance and knowing about health in the context of growing sources of health data, *Am J Prev Med* 41:636–640, 2011.)

may be important, however, even if they affect a small number of people, such as an outbreak of a severe or highly infectious disease (e.g., active tuberculosis).

Data from public health databases differ from research data in a variety of ways. The data are usually reported based on regulatory requirements or by law. Public health data come from a patchwork of local and state sources. Data may be incomplete or of low quality, and changes in data definition or wording of questions make it difficult to compare data over time. When reviewing any metric, it is important to ask the following questions to understand data attributes[13]:

- Is the survey based on a sample, or is it population-based?
- Are the data based on individual patients (e.g., mortality), events (e.g., hospitalizations), or local conditions (e.g., level of pollutants)?
- Do data points represent individual records or the aggregate?
- What are the criteria for reporting the location of the event?

For some events, such as motor vehicle deaths or hospitalization records, the database might report the location where an event was discovered (e.g., hospital where a food-borne illness was diagnosed). That county might be different from the county where the patient lives or where the exposure occurred.

B. Summary Measures of Health

Summary measures of health are usually mortality data for the general population (e.g., measures of neonatal health) and data on morbidity and mortality. As people live longer and more often develop chronic diseases, the focus has moved from mortality to more useful metrics of **health-adjusted life expectancy,** such as quality-adjusted life years and DALY (see earlier).

C. Census Data

Most countries conduct censuses periodically (e.g., every 10 years) to obtain data on the number and character-istics of their populations. They also use **continuous registration** (reporting) **systems** to collect data on the number and characteristics of births and deaths. Census data are the most fundamental data for a population. **Vital statistics registration systems** use recent census data for the denominators of birth and death rates. Access to recent statistics of various countries provides data for international comparisons of such data as infant mortality rates (see Chapter 23).

Not all countries have effective disease-reporting systems, however, and the accuracy of census and vital statistics data varies from country to country. The collection of these data is a national responsibility, but most countries also report their data to the United Nations (population, social, and economic data) and the World Health Organization (vital statistics and disease data). The best place to find census data on a specific country is the website of the country of interest. In addition, several websites are dedicated to collecting addresses of epidemiologic websites of global interest.[14]

1. U.S. Census

In the United States, public data systems collect many types of health-related statistics, including birth and death data.

Collecting such data frequently involves local, state, and national agencies. Data on births, deaths, causes of death, fetal deaths, marriages, and divorces are initially collected locally by the registrar of vital statistics for the municipality or county involved. Birth certificates are completed by a physician or other birth attendant, and death certificates are completed by a physician, medical examiner, or coroner. The local jurisdiction sends the original birth and death certifi-cates to the state government, which is responsible for main-taining permanent records. The state governments (often state health departments) prepare summaries of these data. The states also send copies of the birth and death certificates to the **National Center for Health Statistics** (NCHS), a branch of the U.S. Centers for Disease Control and Preven-tion (CDC), which prepares national summaries.

The federal government conducts the census. A complete population census, effective April 1, is performed in every year ending in 0. Census surveys are first distributed by mail; data collection is then supplemented by door-to-door inter-views. Findings from the census taken in 2010 are available online. Because the data are based on self-reporting, it might underestimate certain population groups, such as undocu-mented immigrants. Because some data are suppressed to maintain confidentiality, data may also be less reliable for some population groups.[15] States use projections to estimate the size of the population between censuses.

D. Numerator Data

1. U.S. Vital Statistics System

The federal government collates data on births, deaths, causes of death, fetal deaths, marriages, and divorces in the United States and its territories, as obtained by local and state officials. Because analyses are only as good as the data on which they are based, great care is taken to make the vital statistics system as accurate as possible. Nevertheless, there are many potential sources of error in these data, including unreported births and deaths, inaccurate death certificate diagnoses, and erroneous demographic and clinical data on birth and death certificates.

When the numbers of deaths in the United States are categorized by cause of death and reported in government publications, the cause provided is the **underlying cause of death,** not the **immediate cause of death.** The attending physician is responsible for completing the information on the cause of death. If a person dies without medical atten-tion, or if foul play is suspected, a medical examiner or coroner must decide the cause of death for that individual, sometimes aided by an autopsy.

2. Death Certificates

Death certificates usually do not suggest risk factors. For example, obesity is seldom mentioned on death certificates, despite its impact on mortality. There are fields (spaces) to document tobacco use, but these may not be filled in con-sistently or correctly. Either way, death certificates are unlikely to represent the full causal pathways leading to the individual's death.

Figure 24-8 shows the **cause-of-death** section of a death certificate. If a person dies of pneumonia after a cerebral hemorrhage, the physician probably would write "pneumo-nia" on line (a) and "cerebral hemorrhage" on line (b). The

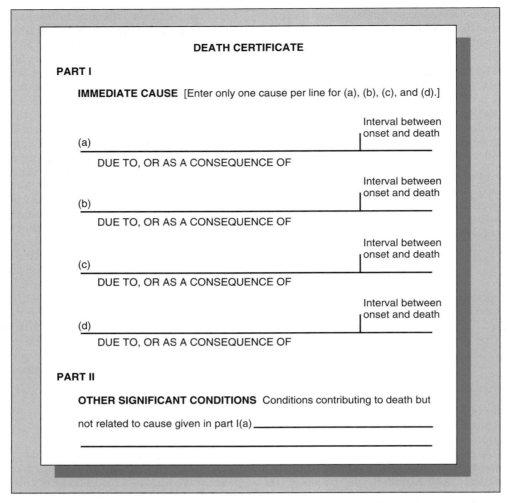

Figure 24-8 Facsimile of cause-of-death portion of death certificates. The form used in the United States also requests information regarding autopsy, referral to a medical examiner or coroner, and homicide investigation.

cerebral hemorrhage would be considered the underlying cause of death. If the physician decided that the person's coexistent hypertension caused the cerebral hemorrhage, however, "hypertension" would be recorded on line (c), and that would be considered the underlying cause of death. On the other hand, if the physician decided that the hypertension was too mild to cause the hemorrhage, he or she would enter "hypertension" under "Other significant conditions." In that case, "spontaneous cerebral hemorrhage" would be the underlying cause of death.

Crafting an accurate cause-of-death narrative may become more difficult when medical professionals other than the decedent's primary provider are called on to complete the death certificate, particularly when the death occurs in a hospital or other medical facility. Less accurate death certification may result when a provider unfamiliar with the patient's full medical history is asked to perform this function. Another source of inaccuracy is the translation of the narrative opinion on the death certificate to numerical codes using a set of complex rules. Vital statistics staff are trained to do this, but the added layer of interpretation remains another potential source of error. Once a death certificate is completed, errors, omissions, or inaccuracies can be corrected only through a formal process of amendment.

Although death certificate data on the underlying cause of death are sufficiently accurate for setting many national priorities in funding for research and health care, research suggests that the data are not accurate enough for robust epidemiologic research. One study focusing on test cases found only 56% agreement among physicians on diagnoses of underlying cause of death, with significant questions remaining among the rest.[16]

E. Leading Health Indicators

Important health indicators come from the *Healthy People 2020* process (see Chapter 26). These indicators are based on a multiyear process with input from many diverse groups and organizations. In *Healthy People 2020*, indicators focus on the following **foundational health measures:**

- General health status
- Health-related quality of life and well-being
- Determinants of health
- Disparities

Progress on these metrics can be accessed from an interactive website.[17]

Healthy People 2020 metrics are laudably extensive and very helpful to guide community health assessment efforts and program planning. They are also highly complex; it is difficult to synthesize overall progress. In 2009 the Institute of Medicine was directed to design a simpler and more comprehensive set of leading health indicators (Table 24-2).[18] Progress on these metrics is tracked on a dedicated website (www.stateoftheusa.org).

The United States is fortunate to have many large health surveys that regularly assess broad swaths of health and health behaviors. These surveys are large enough to have representative data on the state level. Researchers and public health activists can compare indicators over time. However, below the state level, these surveys usually only provide enough data for larger metropolitan areas.

I. National Notifiable Disease Surveillance System

Physicians, hospitals, clinics, and laboratories in the United States are required to report to local and state health departments all cases of many infectious diseases and certain noninfectious diseases, such as elevated lead levels in children. Local health departments in turn report this information to the CDC. Based on these reports, and as needed, local, state, or federal public health agencies perform epidemiologic investigations of possible disease outbreaks.

Although the states largely agree on which diseases must be reported, some variation persists. The list usually includes zoonoses (e.g., rabies), diseases that are highly infectious (e.g., measles), and those that might indicate an outbreak (e.g., salmonellosis) or bioterrorism (e.g., smallpox). Some states have added health care–associated infections to the list (see Chapter 20). Notifiable conditions are frequently updated if new diseases or disease entities (re-)appear (e.g., anthrax, dengue). Readers are encouraged to visit the CDC website and their state website for a current list.

Only a fraction of the actual disease cases are reported, largely depending on the seriousness of the disease. Most extremely serious diseases, such as paralytic poliomyelitis, tend to be reported if recognized, but even then, epidemiologists must be wary because numbers may be too low. In some cases the problem may be **underdiagnosis.** In others, clinicians may be hesitant to report a condition that could bring social isolation if discovered by others. Such illnesses include human immunodeficiency virus (HIV) infection, sexually transmitted diseases, and tuberculosis.

Underreporting is even more likely for common and less serious diseases. This does not mean that epidemiologic statistics have no value, particularly if the diseases are preventable by a vaccine. As long as the proportion of reported cases remains constant, the pattern revealed by reporting probably will reflect actual trends in disease occurrence and distribution.

Table 24-2 State of U.S. Health Indicators: Outcomes, Behaviors, Systems

Metric	Definition
Health Outcomes	
Life expectancy at birth	Number of years that a newborn is expected to live if current mortality rates apply
Infant mortality	Deaths of infants age under 1 year per 1000 live births
Life expectancy at age 65	Number of years of life remaining to a person at age 65 if current mortality rates continue to apply
Injury-related mortality	Age-adjusted mortality rates from intentional or unintentional injuries; includes deaths caused by motor vehicle crashes, poisoning, firearms, and falls
Self-reported health status	Percentage of adults reporting fair or poor health
Unhealthy days, physical and mental	Mean number of physically or mentally unhealthy days in the past 30 days
Chronic disease prevalence	Percentage of adults reporting one or more of six chronic diseases: diabetes, cardiovascular disease, chronic obstructive pulmonary disease, asthma, cancer, and arthritis
Serious psychological distress	Percentage of adults with serious psychological distress, as indicated by score of 13 or more on K6 scale
Health-Related Behaviors	
Smoking	Percentage of adults who have smoked more than 100 cigarettes in their lifetime and who currently smoke some days or every day
Physical activity	Percentage of adults meeting the recommendation for moderate physical activity: at least 5 days a week for 30 minutes a day of moderate activity, or at least 3 days a week for 20 minutes a day of vigorous activity
Excessive drinking	Percentage of adults consuming ≥4 drinks (women) or ≥5 drinks (men) on one occasion and/or consuming more than an average of one (women) or two (men) drinks per day during the past 30 days
Nutrition	Percentage of adults with a good diet, as indicated by score of ≥80 on the Healthy Eating Index
Obesity	Percentage of adults reporting a body mass index of ≥30
Condom use	Proportion of youth in grades 9-12 who are sexually active and who do not use condoms, placing them at risk for sexually transmitted infections
Health Systems	
Health care expenditures	Per-capita health care spending
Insurance coverage	Percentage of adults without health care coverage through insurance or entitlement
Unmet medical, dental, and prescription drug needs	Percentage of (noninstitutionalized) people who did not receive or who faced delays in receiving needed medical services, dental services, or prescription drugs during the previous year
Preventive services	Percentage of adults who are up-to-date with age-appropriate screening services and flu vaccination
Preventable hospitalizations	Hospitalization rate for ambulatory care-sensitive conditions
Childhood immunization	Percentage of children ages 19-35 months who are up-to-date with recommended immunizations

Modified from Institute of Medicine: *State of the USA health indicators,* Washington, DC, 2009, State of the USA.

2. National Center for Health Statistics

The NCHS performs many important studies on such topics as current levels of illness and disability, the practice of preventive health services, population use of preventive measures and medical care, and strategies to improve sampling methods and instrument design for health surveys. In addition, NCHS carries out its own surveys on a variety of topics. In the past, these have included hospital discharges, ambulatory medical care, and long-term care services. Other surveys include information about family growth and use of preventive health measures. Ongoing surveys include the following:

- National Health Interview Survey (NHIS), to determine yearly changes in acute and chronic illness and disability in the United States
- National Health and Nutrition Examination Surveys (NHANES), in which a large, random sample of the U.S. population participates in health interviews, physical examinations, and laboratory tests
- National Health Care Survey, which monitors the use of medical care in the United States

Data from most NCHS surveys can be found on the Internet, and detailed databases can be purchased from the NCHS. The NCHS also publishes a yearly chartbook of the nation's health.[19]

3. Behavioral Risk Factor Surveillance System

State health departments cooperate with the CDC on ongoing surveys of behavioral risk factors in the U.S. population. The largest example of this is the Behavioral Risk Factor Surveillance System (BRFSS). This is the world's largest telephone-based survey and is the primary source that most states use to assess health behaviors. In this survey, a random sample of the population is interviewed by telephone regarding a variety of behaviors that affect health, including exercise, smoking, obesity, alcohol consumption, drinking and driving, use of automobile seat belts and child restraints, and use of medical care.[7] The BRFSS is highly respected but often of limited use below state level. Also, its sampling depends on landlines. The Youth Risk Behavior Surveillance System is a special BRFSS effort that monitors high-priority health risk behaviors and the prevalence of obesity and asthma among youth and young adults.

4. National Health and Nutrition Examination Survey

The NHANES is a large survey by CDC that assesses the health and nutritional status of adults and children in the United States. The survey is the only large survey that combines interviews and physical examinations. NHANES includes interview questions about demographics, socioeconomic, dietary, and health-related topics. The examination component consists of medical, dental, and physiologic measurements as well as laboratory tests. NHANES therefore provides cross-sectional data on the relationships among activity, diet, and various laboratory markers.

F. Other Health-Related Registries

Many types of registries collect information about health and health care, including secondary data on patients who share a specific disease, symptom, medical regimen, or medical procedure. Depending on the registry, such reports can be used to assist individual patients, medical providers, insurance carriers, industry, and government. Many registries for chronic diseases (e.g., diabetes) allow public health managers to identify patients who need testing or who are not receiving a specified level of care. Measures tracked by these registries are often determined by panels of scientists and are defined by national organizations, such as the National Committee for Quality Assurance (see Chapter 28).

In some states and U.S. regions, government agencies or other authorities have established special registries to record information on specific conditions, such as cancer, tuberculosis, and birth defects. The oldest population-based cancer registry in the United States is the Connecticut Tumor Registry, which is maintained by the Connecticut State Department of Health. The name of every Connecticut resident in whom cancer has been diagnosed since 1935 has been reported to the registry, along with information from patient records, including extensive clinical, pathologic, and risk factor data. This registry and other cancer registries conduct extensive surveillance efforts to ensure complete reporting of cancers.

The National Cancer Institute sponsors the **Surveillance, Epidemiology, and End Results** (SEER) program and supports a network of U.S. cancer registries, including the Connecticut Tumor Registry and other regional, population-based registries. SEER currently collects and publishes data on cancer incidence and survival from registries covering approximately 28% of the U.S. population. Investigators involved in the SEER program study trends in the incidence and treatment of cancer and analyze treatment results over time.

Cancer registries are valuable aids for determining the effectiveness of cancer screening programs, allowing comparisons between death rates for patients who were and were not screened. The registries are also valuable for determining whether certain risk factors are linked with cancer. For example, the Connecticut Tumor Registry was used to study whether the introduction of alum-adsorbed allergenic extracts in "allergy shots" was associated with soft tissue sarcomas or other cancers at the injection sites. Study results showed that they were not related.[20]

Many states supplement national surveys with additional questions or state-level surveys (e.g., California Health Interview Survey). Private foundations (e.g., Kaiser Family) also allow state-by-state comparisons (see Websites at end of chapter). States that have active research organizations collaborating with statewide health foundations tend to have particularly rich databases. Because baseline data are needed to apply for grants and access other resources, disparities in available data will become exacerbated over time (data beget more data). Therefore, the best first step to address community health problems is often to collect data.

For public health professionals working at the *county* level, it can be difficult to obtain data with sufficient level of detail. Some health departments have taken the initiative to develop county-level surveys that focus on particular topics.[21]

The Georgia State Health Department focuses on health disparities, quality of and access to care, and health professional workforce. The New York City Health Department conducts surveys on health disparities based on social inequities. Seattle tracks living wage, affordable housing, homelessness, and other societal, environment, and art resources for health.

These surveys illustrate how collecting data is intertwined with community health action (see Chapter 26). These data were obtained because a community coalition identified these areas as a special interest. In turn, obtaining the data leads to action and more data. With help from private foundations, the Public Health Institute publishes a summary ranking of all U.S. counties by health factors and health outcomes.[22] For more help with county-level data, the Department of Health and Human Services (HHS) and CDC use the Community Health Data Initiative to pull data from various websites and provide a county's health status profile[23] (Table 24-3).

G. Other Data Sources

I. Third-party Payers and Insurance

Over the years, carriers of medical insurance and other third-party payers, such as Medicare, Medicaid, and the Veterans Administration, have collected increasing amounts of

Table 24-3 Selected National Data Sources of Health Indicators*

Survey	Examples of Measures	Geographic Availability			Approximate Sample Size	Administering Agency Source/link
		Nation	State	County		
Health Outcomes						
National Vital Statistics System—Birth File	Birth data (infant mortality, low birth weight, educational attainment of parents)	X	X	X	Data for most jurisdictions, but might be limited events for single years/subgroups	Local vital registration systems and NCHS http://www.cdc.gov/nchs/births.htm
National Vital Statistics System—Mortality	Cause-specific mortality, premature mortality (YPLL), life expectancy	X	X	X	Data for most jurisdictions; subgroup analysis and yearly data might be limited for some causes	Local vital registration systems and NCHS http://www.cdc.gov/nchs/deaths.htm
Behavioral Risk Factor Survey System (BRFSS)	Health-related quality of life, health conditions, use of recommended health care services, behaviors, access to care; **adults only**	X	X	Some	Annual sample size about 350,000; has some data for large metropolitan statistical areas	States with Division of Adult and Community Health; national (CDC) www.cdc.gov/brfss
Youth Risk Behavior Survey	Overweight, physical activity, diet, school foods	X	Some	Some large metro districts	>10,000 students	State, tribal, and local governments with CDC http://www.cdc.gov/HealthyYouth/yrbs/index.htm
Disease surveillance	Infectious diseases Cancer	X	X Some	X	Variable completeness of reporting	CDC http://www.cdc.gov/osels/ph_surveillance/nndss/phs.htm#data National Cancer Institute http://seer.cancer.gov/data/
Monitoring the Future	Risky behavior among youth (tobacco, drug, alcohol in grades 8, 10, 12)	X			About 48,000 students in 2006	Institute for Social Research, University of Michigan http://monitoringthefuture.org/
National Health Interview Survey (NHIS)	Illness, injuries, activity limitations, use of health services, vaccinations, screening	X			Adult and child data, about 35,000 households	CDC, U.S. Census Bureau http://www.cdc.gov/nchs/nhis.htm
National Health and Nutrition Examination Survey (NHANES)	Chronic diseases, mental health, oral health **combined with physiologic measurements** (BP, serum cholesterol)	X			Annual continuous sampling of about 10,000 participants	NCHS http://www.cdc.gov/nchs/nhanes.htm
National Immunization Survey	Childhood immunizations	X	X	Some	27,000 children age 19-35 months	NCHS http://www.cdc.gov/nchs/nis.htm

Continued

Table 24-3 Selected National Data Sources of Health Indicators—cont'd

Survey	Examples of Measures	Geographic Availability			Approximate Sample Size	Administering Agency Source/link
		Nation	State	County		
National Survey of Children's Health (NSCH)	Health and functional status; familial, social, and emotional environment; family function; neighborhood conditions	X	X		HRSA regions	NCHS http://www.cdc.gov/nchs/slaits/nsch.htm
National Survey on Drug Use and Health (NSDUH)	Use of illegal drugs, alcohol, and tobacco in people over age 12	X	X		Sample of about 70,000 non-institutionalized Americans over age 12	Substance Abuse and Mental Health Service Administration https://nsduhweb.rti.org/
Social and Environmental Health						
American Community Survey	Population and demographics (e.g., age, income, educational attainment)	X	X	X	65,000	U.S. Census Bureau http://www.census.gov/acs www.childstats.gov/americaschildren/survey.asp#acs
Current Population Survey	Children's health insurance coverage, income, etc.	X	X		State-based sample of >50,000 households	U.S. Census Bureau http://www.census.gov/acs
National Assessment of Educational Progress	Educational achievement	X	X		Large urban districts	National Center for Education Statistics http://nces.ed.gov/nationsreportcard/
American Housing Survey	Housing		X	X	Large metropolitan areas	U.S. Census Bureau http://www.census.gov/housing/ahs/
Physical Environment						
Air quality system	Outdoor air quality, suspended particulates	X	X	Some	Data from air quality–monitoring agencies	EPA http://www.epa.gov/ttn/airs/airsaqs/
NHANES	Indoor air quality	X			See above	See above
Toxic release inventory	Toxic chemical releases to the environment	X	X	Some	Reported by facilities	EPA http://www.epa.gov/tri/

Modified from Wold C: *Health indicators: a review of reports currently in use,* Washington, DC, 2008, State of the USA.
BP, Blood pressure; *CDC,* Centers for Disease Control and Prevention; *EPA,* Environmental Protection Agency; *HRSA,* Health Resources and Services Administration; *NCHS,* National Center for Health Statistics; *YPLL,* years of potential life lost.
*All the surveys are cross-sectional. It is therefore difficult to interpret causality and progress over time.

administrative and clinical data. These data often are used by clinical epidemiologists and health care researchers who are concerned with the patterns of health care utilization and the cost-effectiveness of medical care. Hospital discharge records are often aggregated and sold by state hospital associations.

2. Health of Special Populations

Population groups at both ends of life may experience health problems that are very different from the rest of the population. Because they can be underrepresented or not represented in national surveys, epidemiologists have designed dedicated data sets for children and elderly persons. For example, child health and development are highly dependent on safety, security, and social and emotional well-being, as well as developmental opportunities. Surveys dedicated to child health include the March of Dimes data on perinatal mortality and the America's Children and KIDS COUNT

surveys.[21] For the elderly population, who have problems with social support, ability to function independently, and availability of long-term care, the Older Americans Survey provides this specialized data.[24] Dedicated websites list resources for particular diseases or topics of interest, such as HIV or genomics.[25]

3. Environmental and Specialized Data

Environmental data are particularly challenging to interpret. Such data provide information on hazardous emissions into air, water, and soil and on the overall quality of the environment. Most environmental data are collected based on legislation (see Chapter 29). Not all regulations call for data on human health outcomes, or even data from human populations. Furthermore, data usually come from hourly or daily measurements at sampling stations, and results may not be reported unless they exceed a standard level. Levels are sometimes based on facility estimates rather than true samples.[26] Nevertheless, these sources provide rich data on the quality of the environment, emission of specific toxins (e.g., pesticides), weather data, and radiation levels. The information suggests areas of inquiry for the One Health approach (see Chapter 30), possible connections between hazard levels and poverty, and clustering of cancers. These databases are specialized and based on specific sampling methodologies, so readers should consult specialized literature.

In addition to data previously listed, and depending on area of interest, public health planners can access other databases. For example, the motor vehicle crash database from a state department of transportation shows crash frequencies by location; municipal data show clustering of emergency department (ED) visits or hospitalizations;[27] FBI crime databases assess an area's "walkable/bikable" status.[28] Other potential areas of interest may include legal databases listing international laws that protect vulnerable populations; animal health data for zoonotic diseases; U.S. Department of Agriculture data on access to healthy food; school-based data for measuring educational attainment and high-school completion rates in a community; and economic data on community infrastructure and economic opportunities.

IV. INJURIES

In the United States, injuries are the leading cause of YPLL before age 65. For people age 1 to 44, unintentional injuries are the leading cause of death. Intentional injuries also exert a major toll on the young. Homicide is the third and fourth leading cause of death for children age 1 to 4 years and 5 to 14, respectively, and becomes second for the age group 15-24. Suicide is also an important cause of death among young adults, especially age 25-34. Figure 24-9 outlines the 10 leading causes of death by age group.

Injuries can be categorized as follows: automobile (motor vehicle) crashes, home incidents (e.g., falls, burns, poisonings, electrocutions, drownings), occupational incidents, homicides, suicides, and miscellaneous injuries (e.g., plane/train crashes, building collapses).

This section discusses motor vehicle crashes and home incidents. Suicide and worksite incidents are discussed in Chapters 21 and 22. Specialists in the field of injury prevention do not refer to injuries sustained from automobile crashes or incidents in the home or worksite as "accidents," because the word carries the connotation that they are *not*

10 Leading Causes of Death by Age Group, United States – 2008

Rank	<1	1-4	5-9	10-14	15-24	25-34	35-44	45-54	55-64	65+	Total
1	Congenital Anomalies 5,638	Unintentional Injury 1,469	Unintentional Injury 835	Unintentional Injury 1,024	Unintentional Injury 14,089	Unintentional Injury 14,588	Unintentional Injury 16,065	Malignant Neoplasms 50,403	Malignant Neoplasms 104,091	Heart Disease 495,730	Heart Disease 616,828
2	Short Gestation 4,754	Congenital Anomalies 521	Malignant Neoplasms 457	Malignant Neoplasms 433	Homicide 5,275	Suicide 5,300	Malignant Neoplasms 12,699	Heart Disease 37,892	Heart Disease 66,711	Malignant Neoplasms 391,729	Malignant Neoplasms 565,469
3	SIDS 2,353	Homicide 421	Congenital Anomalies 170	Suicide 215	Suicide 4,298	Homicide 4,610	Heart Disease 11,336	Unintentional Injury 20,354	Chronic Low. Respiratory Disease 14,042	Chronic Low. Respiratory Disease 121,223	Chronic Low. Respiratory Disease 141,090
4	Maternal Pregnancy Comp. 1,765	Malignant Neoplasms 394	Homicide 113	Homicide 207	Malignant Neoplasms 1,663	Malignant Neoplasms 3,521	Suicide 6,703	Suicide 8,287	Unintentional Injury 12,782	Cerebro-vascular 114,508	Cerebro-vascular 134,148
5	Unintentional Injury 1,315	Heart Disease 186	Heart Disease 97	Congenital Anomalies 161	Heart Disease 1,065	Heart Disease 3,254	Homicide 2,906	Liver Disease 8,220	Diabetes Mellitus 11,370	Alzheimer's Disease 81,573	Unintentional Injury 121,902
6	Placenta Cord Membranes 1,080	Influenza & Pneumonia 142	Benign Neoplasms 59	Heart Disease 132	Congenital Anomalies 467	HIV 975	HIV 2,838	Cerebro-vascular 6,112	Cerebro-vascular 10,459	Diabetes Mellitus 50,883	Alzheimer's Disease 82,435
7	Bacterial Sepsis 700	Septicemia 93	Chronic Low. Respiratory Disease 55	Chronic Low. Respiratory Disease 64	Influenza & Pneumonia 206	Diabetes Mellitus 574	Liver Disease 2,562	Diabetes Mellitus 5,622	Liver Disease 8,526	Influenza & Pneumonia 48,382	Diabetes Mellitus 70,553
8	Respiratory Distress 630	Cerebro-vascular 63	Cerebro-vascular 41	Cerebro-vascular 56	Diabetes Mellitus 204	Cerebro-vascular 539	Cerebro-vascular 2,035	Chronic Low. Respiratory Disease 4,392	Suicide 5,465	Nephritis 39,921	Influenza & Pneumonia 56,284
9	Circulatory System Disease 594	Chronic Low. Respiratory Disease 54	Influenza & Pneumonia 40	Influenza & Pneumonia 49	Cerebro-vascular 189	Liver Disease 423	Diabetes Mellitus 1,854	HIV 3,730	Nephritis 4,803	Unintentional Injury 39,359	Nephritis 48,237
10	Neonatal Hemorrhage 556	Perinatal Period 51	Septicemia 25	Septicemia 36	Complicated Pregnancy 169	Congenital Anomalies 379	Septicemia 892	Viral Hepatitis 2,732	Septicemia 4,552	Septicemia 27,028	Suicide 36,035

Source: National Vital Statistics System, National Center for Health Statistics, CDC.
Produced by: Office of Statistics and Programming, National Center for Injury Prevention and Control, CDC.

CS227502

Centers for Disease Control and Prevention
National Center for Injury Prevention and Control

Figure 24-9 Leading causes of death by age group, 2008. (From Office of Statistics and Programming, National Center for Injury Prevention and Control, National Vital Statistics System, National Center for Health Statistics. Atlanta, 2008, Centers for Disease Control and Prevention. http://www.cdc.gov/Injury/wisqars/pdf/I0LCD-Age-Grp-US-2008-a.pdf.)

predictable. In fact, these injury-producing events are fairly predictable and partially preventable.

A. Motor Vehicle Crashes

Because prevention focuses on human factors and vehicle and environmental factors, it requires an understanding of human behavior and the types of behavioral interventions that do and do not work. Regulations regarding automobile construction have reduced injuries from crashes. Laws regarding human behavior (e.g., requiring drivers to use seat belts) have been less successful but still helped shift behavior to reduce injuries. It is not always clear when efforts to reduce injuries and their associated costs necessitate restrictions on behavioral freedoms. As medical care costs continue to rise, the balance may gradually shift in the direction of greater controls on behavior, especially on driving while intoxicated, as shown by efforts to reduce the allowable blood alcohol level to 0.08%.

Haddon, a founder of the field of automobile injury epidemiology, developed a detailed approach to injury prevention.[29] The **Haddon matrix** classifies the phases of injury and the factors involved (Table 24-4). This approach was originally developed for injury prevention but is also applicable to other fields of prevention[30] (see Chapter 26). The Haddon matrix is described here, with the *phases* classified as **preinjury** (preevent), **injury** (event), and **postinjury** (postevent) and the *risk factors* involved in motor vehicle injuries classified as **human, vehicle, physical environment,** and **social environment.**

I. Risk Factors in Preinjury Phase

HUMAN FACTORS

Drivers at increased risk for crashes include new drivers, young drivers, and drivers with alcohol intoxication, drug intoxication, fatigue, or a combination of these factors. In **new drivers** the excess risk of automobile crashes is related to the inability to anticipate and prevent developing hazards and the inability to recognize existing hazards and respond to them quickly and appropriately. New drivers often do not anticipate the dangers of taking curves at high speeds, particularly when roads are wet, and they often have difficulty coordinating manual actions, such as steering and braking, when it is necessary to respond to urgent driving demands. New drivers are at increased risk, regardless of the age at which they begin driving, but the excess risk decreases to zero over a few years of driving.

In the United States the high rates of serious injuries per mile of driving for **young drivers** are generally attributed to a combination of inexperience and immaturity factors. An emerging risk factor is the use of cell phones for talking or texting when driving. This practice tends to distract drivers, and it reduces the number of hands available to react quickly in an emergency. Different states have different rules forbidding some or all use of handheld phones while driving.[31]

Many proposals are in use to reduce the injury problems from teenage driving.[32] Many are now being used by numerous states, in different combinations. *Graduated licensing* requires new teenage drivers to graduate from a provisional or beginner's license to one or more intermediate licenses before receiving an unrestricted license. The major provisions of the restrictive licenses limit how late the driver can operate a vehicle (i.e., impose various curfews).

Driving while intoxicated with alcohol or drugs interacts with other factors to increase the risks late at night, such as fatigue, and reduce sensory input. This is one reason for considering a curfew of 11 PM or midnight for new teenage drivers, who are responsible for an excess number of fatal crashes in the United States, particularly single-vehicle crashes.[33] Although some groups advocated driver education programs in all U.S. high schools, a classic study showed that the rates of teenage crashes and injuries in counties providing in-school driver education were as high as or higher than the rates in counties without such education.[34] Apparently, the in-school driver education programs put significant numbers of young drivers on the road at an earlier age.

Laws concerning driving while intoxicated are already in place in the United States, as are regulations on the number of hours that professional drivers can operate trucks, buses, and other vehicles on the road per day and per week. Dozing and fatigue are responsible for numerous vehicle crashes, including those involving trucks. Many roads now have rumble strips in the breakdown lanes to awaken dozing drivers who veer off the primary lanes.

Table 24-4 Haddon Matrix of Injury Prevention Applied to Motor Vehicle Crash

Phases	Human Factors	Vehicle Factors	Environmental Factors Physical	Social
Preevent	Attitudes Knowledge Use of alcohol Driver experience	Vehicle condition Speed	Roadway design Traffic calming Pedestrian facilities	Traffic laws Cultural norms
Event	Use of seat belts Wearing fastened helmet	Seat belts Helmets	Shoulders, medians Guardrails	Helmet and seat belt laws
Postevent	First aid Medical treatment	Fire risk	Availability of trauma care equipment Traffic congestion	Standards of trauma care in hospitals

From Hazen A, Ehiri JE: Road traffic injuries: hidden epidemic in less developed countries. *J Natl Med Assoc* 98:73–82, 2006. http://www.ncbi.nlm.nih.gov/pmc/articles/PMC2594796/pdf/jnma00296-0083.pdf

VEHICLE FACTORS

The ability of vehicles to brake and other aspects of vehicle design, construction, and maintenance may influence the risk of injuries. Research has shown that a taillight pattern involving two lower red lights at the sides plus one higher red light in the middle of the rearview window catches the attention of drivers best and reduces rear-end collisions. All new passenger vehicles sold in the United States now have this taillight pattern.

ENVIRONMENTAL FACTORS

Rain, snow, and other bad weather can decrease visibility for drivers. Accordingly, drivers should slow down during periods of rain, snow, or poor visibility, but they do not always do so. Poor design and maintenance of roads and highways also increase the risk of vehicle crashes.

2. Risk Factors in Injury Phase

HUMAN FACTORS

The ability of humans to resist injury is influenced by the use of specific protection devices, such as seat belts and child seats in automobiles and helmets for motorcycle and bicycle riders. For children age 3 to 9 years, the risk of injury is decreased if booster seats are used and the chest strap of the seat belt is placed so it does not choke.

VEHICLE FACTORS

Vehicle design has been steadily improving because of federal regulations. Vehicle safety features include collapsible steering columns, energy-absorbing construction, in-door side protection, seat belts and air bags, and protected gasoline tanks. The need for further improvements in the design of vehicles and their accessories was nevertheless underscored in 2000 by reports about the tendency of sports utility vehicles to roll over because of their high center of gravity and, in some cases, the use of defective tires.

ENVIRONMENTAL FACTORS

The object into which a vehicle crashes affects the seriousness of the crash. Energy-absorbing barriers on the shoulder of the road reduce the risk that vehicles will go off the road, and median strip barriers reduce injuries from head-on collisions.

3. Risk Factors in Postinjury Phase

HUMAN FACTORS

The fate of crash victims may be influenced greatly by the ability of individuals at the crash scene to act quickly in summoning medical help and preventing other vehicles from becoming involved in the crash.

VEHICLE FACTORS

The construction of a vehicle, including the protection of the gas tank to prevent postcrash fire, may determine whether or not passengers survive a crash. A strong vehicle frame may reduce crushing and facilitate extraction of passengers by emergency response personnel.

ENVIRONMENTAL FACTORS

The extent of injury is influenced by the rapidity and quality of the emergency response. Advanced life support ambulance teams seek to stabilize the condition of injured persons at the crash scene before transport. Helicopter ambulance systems seem to improve outcomes, in part because they carry injured persons to trauma centers rather than to the nearest ED, which may not be adequately equipped for serious trauma.

4. Surveillance and Prevention of Injuries

An important factor in prevention is improved data on the nature of injuries, their rate of occurrence, and the circumstances. The Fatal Accident Reporting System was developed by the National Highway Traffic Safety Administration and provides valuable epidemiologic data.[35] Other injury surveillance systems depend on the use of the E-codes in the *International Classification of Diseases* (ICD) and the use of hospital ED and admission diagnoses.

B. Common Injuries in the Home

The many preventable injuries in the home include poisoning, fires, falls, and drowning. The victims of **poisoning** are usually toddlers and preschool children, who experiment with tasting or swallowing substances while exploring. Much has been accomplished in recent decades by developing childproof caps for containers of medicines and household products; by counseling parents to keep cleaning solutions, pesticides, medicines, and other hazardous substances out of the reach of their children; and by establishing poison control centers and hotlines.

The risk of **fires** has been reduced by tightening building codes, particularly the requirement for hard-wired smoke alarms in houses and sprinkler systems in public buildings. Nevertheless, many older buildings are not retrofitted with these devices. The reduction in the prevalence of cigarette smoking has reduced one source of fires, but arson is still common, either for insurance or revenge.

Although people of all ages can be the victims of **falls,** older people are at greater risk of serious injuries, such as hip fractures. A significant reduction in the incidence of hip fractures has been achieved in high-risk elderly persons by safety modification of their home environments, physical therapy, the use of devices such as walkers, and wearing padded hip protectors. In younger persons, falls are likely to be associated with activities such as climbing ladders, shoveling snow, or walking on an ice-covered surface. In older people, falls are frequently caused by environmental hazards combined with failing vision, loss of equilibrium or physical strength, and use of medications that decrease stability.[36] Multifactorial programs can reduce the incidence of falls in the elderly population if these address individual risk factors as well as environmental modifications, such as the provision of handrails in hallways and on stairs.[37]

Drowning occurs most often among school-age children, especially boys. Swimming lessons and water safety instruction at an early age may reduce the number of deaths and injuries associated with activities that occur in and near pools and other bodies of water.

C. Performance of Health Care Systems

Given rising health care costs, as well as more scrutiny on safety in health care, many researchers turn to databases identifying the performance variations in the health care system. For example, the Kaiser Family Foundation and *Dartmouth Atlas of Health Care* track unwarranted variations in spending to investigate opportunities to decrease health care spending (see below). Many organizations are involved in evaluating quality of health care (see Chapter 28). The following organizations are dedicated to tracking the progress on preventive health[21]:

- Trust for America's Health, a coalition of more than 130 organizations that publishes the 10 leading priorities for prevention
- Good Health Counts Report from the Prevention Institute
- Environmental Public Health Indicators project (CDC)
- National Center for Environmental Health
- Project Thrive (early childhood indicators)

D. Data for International Health

The World Health Organization (WHO) compares 193 countries in broad metrics of health and health care systems. The Commonwealth Fund publishes comparisons of health care systems across selected countries. In Europe the Organization for Economic Cooperation and Development (OECD) provides data for member countries on quality of life, life expectancy, infant mortality, and obesity. The European Union (EU) also conducts surveys on health care expenditures, and Self-Perceived Health in the EU[38] (see Websites).

V. FUTURE TRENDS

A. Self-reported Health and Well-being

Most surveys tend to underreport physical and social environments that optimize health[21] and instead focus on objective morbidity data. To counteract this trend, some surveys have sought to collect self-reported health and well-being data from a representative sample of the population. For example, the Gallup-Healthways Index measures life evaluation, emotional health, work environment, and basic access to safe living in addition to physical health.[39]

B. Informatics Concerns

In response to the Health Insurance Portability and Accountability Act (HIPAA; see Chapter 29), several public health agencies have worked together to make their systems more interchangeable. However, more data exchange increases the risk of accidental release of individually identifiable health data. In several cases, health care organizations have inadvertently released large amounts of patient data. For public health databases, confidentiality is at least as important.

C. Innovative Approaches

Data from different administrative or nontraditional data sources can also be combined to make connections. For example, **syndromic surveillance** in EDs measures the chief complaints of patients. A spike in patients with rashes or upper respiratory symptoms might signal the outbreak of smallpox or influenza, respectively. So far, however, the link of ED data with true outbreaks has not been validated. In one study, none of 40 signal investigations resulted in detection of an outbreak, and none of the localized outbreaks investigated by traditional methods revealed a syndromic signal.[40] Other useful data sources for the detection of an outbreak might be work or school absentee rates, pharmaceutical sales of over-the-counter cold medicines, or calls to emergency hotlines. In 2008, researchers investigated the link between Internet search data and influenza outbreaks.[41]

Other studies have connected data within or between different surveys. Examples include estimating deaths from health care–associated infections;[42] integrating data on nutrition and alcohol use with mortality statistics to delineate the mortality effects of various dietary or lifestyle risk factors;[43] and assessing the impact of different countries' policy on maternal leave on neonatal mortality.[44]

D. Genomics

Recent advances in the study of the genome (genomics) and pharmacogenomics are likely to affect public health databases. Already, genomic information has been integrated in NHANES.[45] One opportunity in the near-term is to explore the interaction of genetic and environmental factors influencing health in populations.

E. Maps

Visualization of data can provide insights that might otherwise be missed. Clusters of disease outbreaks, unintentional injuries, or health care utilization may not become apparent until these are mapped. Mapping of clusters dates back to the beginning of public health investigations with John Snow's maps of water sources and cholera cases (see Chapter 3, Fig. 3-15). Figure 24-10 shows a map of access to good nutrition in an Ohio neighborhood. More recently, however, the opportunities for such applications have increased exponentially. In an era of real-time data, when many citizens are equipped with mobile devices that can immediately upload pictures, it might become possible to shorten the time between surveillance and discovery and to *crowd-source* environmental monitoring.[46]

The evolving field of **geographic information systems** provides powerful tools to mine such data. Several data sources provide innovative use of maps. Most prominent is the Dartmouth Atlas, which shows potentially unwarranted variation in measures of health services and outcomes by geographic areas. One particularly famous map of health care spending by enrollee showed large variations that were not associated with underlying costs, comorbidities, or measurable difference in health outcomes (see the Websites list at the end of the chapter).

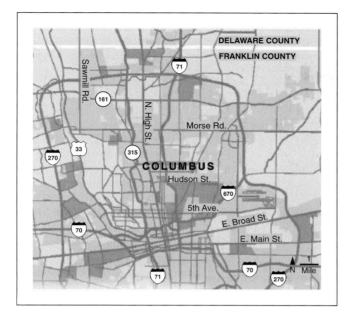

Figure 24-10 Closer to fast food. Columbus Public Health of Ohio has identified neighborhoods where the proximity to fast-food restaurants far outweighs the proximity to a large, full-service grocery. At least half the census blocks in these neighborhoods *(gray areas)* had worse access than average. (From Crane M: Lack of access to nutritious fare in poor areas contributes to obesity, other problems, Columbus Public Health, Ohio, 2010, *Columbus Dispatch.* http://www.dispatch.com/content/stories/local/2010/08/01/food-deserts.html.)

VI. SUMMARY

Important ways to view the health of a country come from census data, morbidity and mortality from major diseases, as well as years of potential life lost and disability-adjusted life years. Using measures of premature death and disability adjusting provides greater weight to the many lives lost to suicide and unintentional injuries and neuropsychiatric conditions, respectively. Significant disparities persist for all these metrics. Epidemiologists rely on a variety of sources for obtaining data to analyze health-related rates and risks. Data for the rates used in epidemiologic studies can be discussed in terms of denominator data, which define the population at risk, and numerator data, which define the population experiencing events or conditions of concern. Denominator metrics come from census data. Large, ongoing databases that provide numerator data include the BRFSS (telephone survey of behavioral risk factors), NHANES (survey of nutrition that includes biometric data), and SEER data (for cancer disease registries). A variety of other data sources inform health planning on state and county levels. In the future, mapping technology as well as connections between search data and real-time reporting might transform the field.

References

1. Institute of Medicine: The future of public health, Washington, DC, 1988, National Academy Press.
2. Winslow C-EA: The untilled fields of public health. *Science* 51:22–23, 1920.
3. At a glance table, Health, United States. 2010. http://www.ncbi.nlm.nih.gov/books/NBK54373/#ataglance.s1.
4. Jamal A: Global cancer statistics. *CA Cancer J Clin* 61(2), 2011. http://onlinelibrary.wiley.com/doi/10.3322/caac.20107/abstract.
5. http://www.who.int/topics/cancer/en; accessed 2/8/2012.
6. Mokdad AH, Marks JS, Stroup DF, et al: Actual causes of death. *JAMA* 291:1238–1245, 2004.
7. McKenna MT, Michaud CM, Murray CJ, et al: Assessing the burden of disease in the United States using disability-adjusted life years. *Am J Prev Med* 28:415–423, 2005.
8. Singh GK: Youth mortality in the United States, 1935–2007: large and persistent disparities in injury and violent death. A 75th Anniversary Publication, Health Resources and Services Administration, Maternal and Child Health Bureau. Rockville, Md, 2010, US Department of Health and Human Services. http://www.hrsa.gov/healthit/images/mchb_youthmortality_pub.pdf.
9. Institute of Medicine: For the public's health: the role of measurement in action and accountability, Washington, DC, 2011, National Academy Press.
10. Lee LM, Thacker SB: Public health surveillance and knowing about health in the context of growing sources of health data. *Am J Prev Med* 41:636–640, 2011.
11. Thacker SB, Berkelman RL: Public health surveillance in the United States. *Epidemiol Rev* 10:164–190, 1988.
12. CDC Guidelines Working Group: Updated guidelines for evaluating public health surveillance systems. *MMWR* 50(RR-13):1–35, 2001.
13. Ballard J: Concepts of data analysis for community health assessment. http://www.nwcphp.org/docs/bcda_series/data_analysis_mod1_transcript.pdf.
14. www Virtual Library: Medicine and health: epidemiology. www.epibiostat.ucsf.edu/epidem/epidem.html.
15. Alexander JT, Davern B, Stevenson B: Inaccurate age and sex data in the census PUMS files: evidence and implications. http://www.ifo.de/portal/pls/portal/docs/1/1185806.pdf.
16. Messite J, Stellman SD: Accuracy of death certificate completion. *JAMA* 275:794–796, 1996.
17. http://wonder.cdc.gov/data2010.
18. Institute of Medicine: State of the USA health indicators. 2009. www.stateoftheusa.org.
19. Health, United States. 2010. http://www.cdc.gov/nchs/data/hus/hus10.pdf.
20. Jekel JF, Freeman DH, Meigs JW, et al: A study of trends in upper arm soft tissue sarcomas in Connecticut following the introduction of alum-adsorbed allergenic extracts. *Ann Allergy* 40:28–31, 1978.
21. Wold C: Health indicators: a review of reports currently in use. Washington, DC, 2008, State of the USA. http://www.cherylwold.com/images/Wold_Indicators_July08.pdf.
22. Public Health Institute: Data sets, data platforms, data utility: resource compendium 2010. http://www.phi.org/pdf-library/PHI_Data_Resource_Compendium-Sept_2010.pdf.
23. http://www.cdc.gov/nchs/data_access/chdi.htm.
24. http://www.agingstats.gov/agingstatsdotnet/main_site/default.aspx.
25. http://phpartners.org/health_stats.html.
26. Act CA: White paper: overview of environmental data sources for environmental public health tracking. http://www.tulane.edu/publihealth/caeph/epht/upload/Environmental-Data-White-Paper.pdf.
27. Atul Gawande: The hot spotters, *New Yorker*, 2011.
28. http://www.fbi.gov/about-us/cjis/ucr/ucr.
29. Haddon W, Jr: A logical framework for categorizing highway safety phenomena and activity. *J Trauma* 12:197–207, 1972.
30. Runyan CW: Introduction: back to the future—revisiting Haddon's conceptualization of injury: epidemiology and prevention. *Epidemiol Rev* 25:60–64, 2003.

31. http://www.ghsa.org/html/stateinfo/laws/cellphone_laws.html.

32. Trempel RE: Graduated driver licensing laws and insurance collision claim frequencies of teenage drivers, Insurance Institute for Highway Safety Report. 2009. http://www.iihs.org/research/topics/pdf/h0101.pdf.

33. National Highway Traffic Safety Agency: Teen driver crashes: a report to Congress. 2009. http://www.nhtsa.gov/DOT/NHTSA/Traffic%20Injury%20Control/Articles/Associated%20Files/811005.pdf.

34. Robertson LS, Zador PL: Driver education and crash involvement of teenaged drivers. *Am J Public Health* 68:959–965, 1978.

35. http://www-fars.nhtsa.dot.gov/Main/index.aspx.

36. Rubenstein LZ: Falls in older people: epidemiology, risk factors and strategies for prevention. *Age Ageing* 35–S2, ii37–ii41, 2006. doi:10.1093/ageing/afl084.

37. Gillespie LD, Gillespie WJ, Robertson MC, et al: Interventions for preventing falls in elderly people. *Cochrane Database Syst Rev* 4:CD000340, 2003.

38. http://epp.eurostat.ec.europa.eu/portal/page/portal/health/public_health/data_public_health/database.

39. Gallup-Healthways: Well-being index. www.well-beingindex.com.

40. Steiner-Sichel L, Greenko J, Heffernan R, et al: Field investigations of emergency department syndromic surveillance signals. *MMWR* 53:184–189, 2004.

41. Polgreen PM, Chen Y, Pennock DM, et al: Using Internet searches for influenza surveillance. *Clin Infect* 47:1443–1448, 2008.

42. Klevens RM, Edwards JR, Richards CL, et al: Estimating health care–associated infections and deaths in U.S. hospitals, 2002. *Public Health Rep* 122:160–166, 2007.

43. Danaei G: The preventable causes of death in the United States: comparative risk assessment of dietary, lifestyle and metabolic risk factors. *PLoS Med* 6:e1000058, 2009.

44. Heymann J, Raub A, Earle A: Creating and using new data sources to analyze the relationship between social policy and global health: the case of maternal leave. *Public Health Rep* 126:127–134, 2011.

45. Chang M: Prevalence in the United States of selected candidate gene variants. Third National Health and Nutrition Examination Survey, 1991–1994. *J Epidemiol* 169:54–66, 2009.

46. Hesse BW: Public health surveillance in the context of growing sources of health data: a commentary. *Am J Prev Med* 41:648–649, 2011.

Select Readings

Act CA: Overview of environmental data sources for environmental public health tracking. http://tulane.edu/publichealth/caeph/epht/upload/Environmental-Data-White-Paper.pdf.

Boslaugh S: Secondary data sources for public health. St Louis, 2007, Washington University.

Friis RH, Sellers TA: Sources of data for use in epidemiology. In *Epidemiology for public health practice*, ed 4, Boston, 2009, Jones & Bartlett.

Indian Health Service, Portland Area: Injury prevention: the basics. http://www.ihs.gov/MedicalPrograms/PortlandInjury/about_ip.cfm.

Structure and function of the public health system in the United States: VII. Injury and violence. In Wallace RB, editor: Maxcy-Rosenau-Last: *Public health and preventive medicine*, ed 15. New York, 2008, McGraw-Hill Medical.

Websites

www.cdc.gov/brfss [Behavioral Risk Factor Surveillance System Survey Data].

http://www.cdc.gov/Injury/Publications/FactBook/ [Centers for Disease Control and Prevention Injury Factbook].

www.census.gov [U.S. Census Bureau].

www.countyhealthrankings.org.

http://www-fars.nhtsa.dot.gov/Main/index.aspx [Fatal Accident Reporting System].

www.fedstats.gov [Gateway for statistics from federal agencies].

http://www.healthyamericans.org [Information about state level: Trust for America].

www.statehealthfacts.kff.org [Kaiser Family Foundation].

www.marchofdimes.com/peristats.

www.nci.org [National Cancer Institute].

www.cdc.gov/nchs [National Center for Health Statistics].

www.nhtsa.gov [National Highway Traffic and Safety Administration].

http://www.cdc.gov/osels/ph_surveillance/nndss/phs/infdis2011.htm [Notifiable diseases].

http://phpartners.org/health_stats.html [Partners in Information Access for Public Health Workforce: health data tools and statistics].

www.phi.org [Public Health Institute].

www.stateoftheusa.org [State of the USA: leading health indicators].

http://www.dartmouthatlas.org/ [Dartmouth atlas of health care].

http://www.epibiostat.ucsf.edu/epidem/epidem.html [The www Virtual Library: Medicine and health: epidemiology].

http://www.americashealthrankings.org [United Health Foundation; America's Health Rankings].

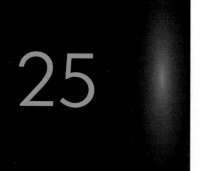

25 Public Health System: Structure and Function

The U.S. Institute of Medicine (IOM) describes the challenges inherent in organizing the public health system for the 21st century as follows[1]:

> The systems and entities that protect and promote the public's health, already challenged by problems like obesity, toxic environments, a large uninsured population, and health disparities, must also confront emerging threats, such as antimicrobial resistance and bioterrorism. The social, cultural, and global contexts of the nation's health are also undergoing rapid and dramatic change. Scientific and technological advances, such as genomics and informatics, extend the limits of knowledge and human potential more rapidly than their implications can be absorbed and acted upon. At the same time, people, products, and germs migrate and the nation's demographics are shifting in ways that challenge public and private resources.

The U.S. public health system was designed at a time when most threats to health were infectious, before computer information systems, and when local autonomy prevailed. This chapter describes the structure of the U.S. health system and discusses how it must respond to contemporary challenges. Public health systems in other countries are likely structured very differently but still need to adapt to the same challenges.

I. ADMINISTRATION OF U.S. PUBLIC HEALTH

A. Responsibilities of the Federal Government

The public health responsibility of the U.S. Federal Government is based on two clauses from Article 1, Section 8, of the U.S. Constitution. First, the Interstate Commerce Clause gives the federal government the right "to regulate Commerce with foreign Nations, and among the several States, and with the Indian Tribes." Second, the General Welfare Clause states that "the Congress shall have Power to lay and collect Taxes . . . for the common Defense and general Welfare of the United States." Federal responsibility also is inferred from statements that Congress has the authority to create and support a military and the authority to negotiate with Indian tribes and other special groups.

1. Regulation of Commerce

The regulation of commerce involves controlling the entry of people and products into the United States and regulating commercial relationships among the states. People may be excluded from entry to the United States if they have infectious health problems, such as active tuberculosis. Products may also be excluded from entry, such as fruits and vegetables if infested with certain organisms (e.g., Mediterranean fruit fly) or treated with prohibited insecticides or fungicides. In the past, similar prohibitions have been extended to the importation of animal products from cattle that might contain the prions of bovine spongiform encephalopathy and, as recently in 2011, produce that might be contaminated with *Escherichia coli*.

The regulation of commercial relationships between states has increased over time. Contaminated food products that cross state lines are considered to be "interstate commerce"; what crosses state lines are harmful microorganisms. The federal government takes the responsibility for inspecting all milk, meat, and other food products at their site of production and processing. (In contrast, the state or local government is responsible for inspecting restaurants and food stores.) Likewise, polluted air and water flowing from state to state are deemed to be "interstate commerce" in pollution and come under federal regulation.

2. Taxation for the General Welfare

The power to "tax for the general welfare" is the constitutional basis for the federal government's development of most of its public health programs and agencies, including the Centers for Disease Control and Prevention (part of the Department of Health and Human Services) and the Occupational Safety and Health Administration (OSHA, part of the Department of Labor); for research programs, such as those of the National Institutes of Health (NIH); and for the payment for medical care, such as Medicare and Medicaid (see Chapter 29).

3. Provision of Care for Special Groups

The federal government has taken special responsibility for providing health services to active military personnel, through military hospitals; families of military personnel, through military hospitals or the Civilian Health and Medical Program of the Uniformed Services; veterans, through the Veterans Administration hospital system; and Native Americans and Alaska Natives, through the Indian Health Service of the U.S. Public Health Service.

4. Funding Federal Legislation

Funding of federal legislation requires a two-step process. The initial bill provides an **authorization** of funds. An authorization bill only sets an *upper limit* to the amount of funds that can be spent. No monies can be spent, however, until they have been specifically **appropriated** for that bill's purposes in a subsequent appropriations bill. The authorization is a political fiction for which members of Congress can claim political gain. In practice, the amount *appropriated* tends to be about *half* the amounts *authorized* in the bills, and the amounts are usually appropriated for only one fiscal year at a time. It is in the funding bills that fiscal (and political) reality must be faced. Because a funding bill covers many items, the voters usually are unaware that the amount actually appropriated is much smaller than the amount promised in the authorization bill.

5. Coordination of Federal Agencies

In the United States the federal department most concerned with health is the Department of Health and Human Services (DHHS), which has four major operating units, described next[2] (Fig. 25-1).

ADMINISTRATION ON AGING

The Administration on Aging provides advice to the Secretary of the DHHS on issues and policies regarding elderly persons. It also administers certain grant programs for the benefit of the aging population.

ADMINISTRATION FOR CHILDREN AND FAMILIES

The Administration for Children and Families is responsible for administering child welfare programs through the states, Head Start programs, child abuse prevention and treatment programs, foster care, adoption assistance, developmental disabilities programs, and child support enforcement.

CENTERS FOR MEDICARE AND MEDICAID SERVICES

The Centers for Medicare and Medicaid Services (CMS) is responsible for administering two major programs of the

Social Security Act. **Medicare** is covered under **Title 18** of the Social Security Act and pays for medical care for the elderly population. **Medicaid** is covered under **Title 19** and pays for medical and nursing home care in cooperation with the states (see Chapter 29). CMS duties include setting standards for programs and institutions that provide medical care, developing payment policies, contracting for third-party payers to cover the bills, and monitoring the quality of care provided. CMS also supports graduate medical education, residency, and fellowship programs that provide care for individuals covered by Medicare or Medicaid.

PUBLIC HEALTH SERVICE

The U.S. Public Health Service (PHS) comprises the following eight constituent agencies:

1. The **Agency for Healthcare Research and Quality** (AHRQ) is the main federal agency for research and policy development in the areas of medical care organization, financing, and quality assessment. Since 2000, the agency has placed increasing emphasis on medical care quality.
2. The **Agency for Toxic Substances and Disease Registry** (ATSDR) provides leadership and direction to programs designed to protect workers and the public from exposure to and adverse health effects of hazardous substances that are kept in storage sites or are released by fire, explosion, or accident.
3. The **Centers for Disease Control and Prevention** (CDC) has the responsibility for "protecting the public health of the [United States] by providing leadership and direction in the prevention and control of diseases and other preventable conditions and responding to public health emergencies." The CDC directs and enforces federal quarantine activities; works with states on disease surveillance and control activities; develops programs for prevention and immunization; is involved in research and training; makes recommendations on how to promote occupational health and safety through the **National Institute on Occupational Safety and Health** (NIOSH); provides consultation to other nations in the control of preventable diseases; and participates with international agencies in the eradication and control of diseases around the world. The CDC has a complex organizational structure (Fig. 25-2).
4. The **Food and Drug Administration** (FDA) is the primary agency for regulating the safety and effectiveness of drugs for use in humans and animals; vaccines and other biologic products; diagnostic tests; and medical devices, including ionizing and nonionizing radiation–emitting electronic products. The FDA is also responsible for the safety, quality, and labeling of cosmetics, foods, and food additives and colorings.
5. The **Health Resources and Services Administration** (HRSA) is responsible for developing human resources and methods to improve health care access, equity, and quality, with an emphasis on promoting primary care. HRSA also supports training grants and training programs in preventive medicine and public health.
6. The **Indian Health Service** promotes the health of and provides medical care for Native Americans and Alaska Natives.

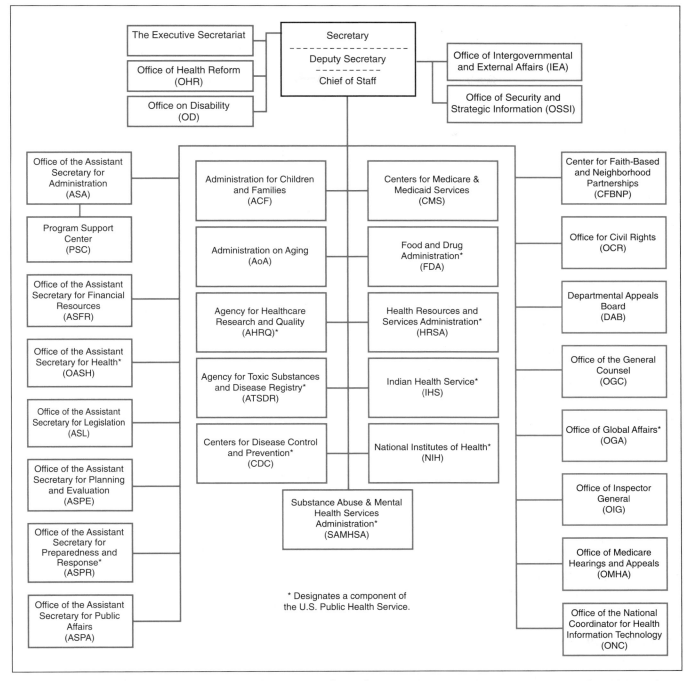

Figure 25-1 U.S. Department of Health and Human Services (DHHS) organizational chart. (From http://www.hhs.gov/about/orgchart.)

7. The **National Institutes of Health** (NIH) consists of 27 institutes, which perform *intramural* (in-house) research on their particular diseases, organ systems, or topics (e.g., National Cancer Institute; National Heart, Lung, and Blood Institute; National Human Genome Research Institute; National Center for Advancing Translational Science). The institutes also review and sponsor *extramural* research at universities and research organizations through competitive grant programs. Some of the institutes also undertake disease control programs and public and professional education in their area (e.g., National Library of Medicine, National Institute for Neurological Disorders and Stroke).

8. The **Substance Abuse and Mental Health Services Administration** (SAMHSA) provides national leadership in preventing and treating addiction and other mental disorders, based on up-to-date science and practices, and has four major operating divisions: Center for Mental Health Services, Center for Substance Abuse Prevention, Center for Substance Abuse Treatment, and Center for Behavioral Health Statistics and Quality.

The PHS is not the only important agency in public health. The other major federal organization is the **Office of Public Health and Science** (OPHS), which leads the *Healthy People* initiative through its Office of Disease Prevention and

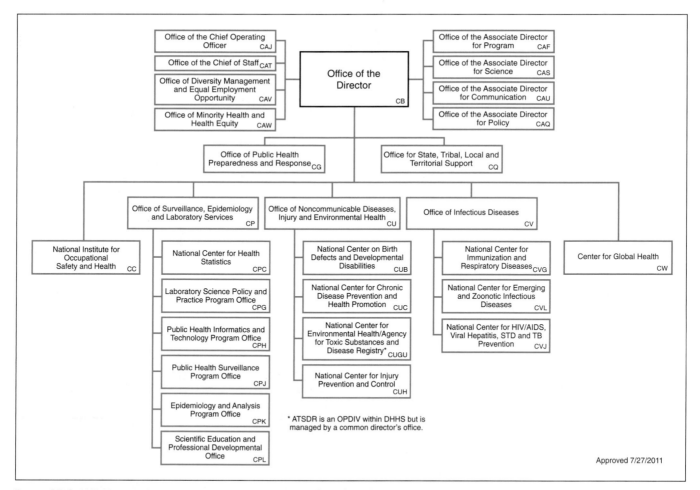

Figure 25-2 U.S. Centers for Disease Control and Prevention (CDC) organizational chart. *STD,* Sexually transmitted disease; *TB,* tuberculosis. (From http://www.cdc.gov/maso/pdf/CDC_Official.pdf.)

Promotion (see Chapter 26) and oversees the U.S. Surgeon General's office, President's Council on Bioethics, U.S. Public Health Service Commissioned Corps, and Office of Minority Health (Fig. 25-3).

B. Responsibilities of States

In the United States the fundamental responsibility for the health of the public lies with the states. This authority derives from the 10th Amendment to the Constitution: "The powers not delegated to the United States by the Constitution, nor prohibited by it to the States, are reserved to the States respectively, or to the people."

In 1988 the IOM stated that "the mission of public health is to ensure conditions in which people can be healthy", and that the three "core functions of public health agencies at all levels of government are assessment, policy development, and assurance."[3]

1. The **assessment** role requires that "every public health agency regularly and systematically collect, assemble, analyze, and make available information on the health of the community, including statistics on health status, community health needs, and epidemiologic and other studies of health problems."[3]

2. The **policy development** role requires that "every public health agency exercise its responsibility to serve the public interest in the development of comprehensive public health policies by promoting the use of the scientific knowledge base in decision-making about public health, . . . by leading in developing public health policy, and by taking a strategic approach, developed on the basis of a positive appreciation for the democratic political process."[3]

3. The **assurance** role requires that "public health agencies assure their constituents that services necessary to achieve agreed upon goals are provided, either by encouraging action by other entities (private or public sector), by requiring such action through regulation, or by providing services directly."[3]

Within these three core functions, 10 essential public health services have been defined (Box 25-1). Administrators and others involved in public health have been struggling to define how the mission and three core functions can best be fulfilled. As indicated by the assurance role, public health agencies enjoy considerable latitude. Although not required to provide all (or even most of) the services themselves, the agencies are expected to use all their authority and resources to ensure that needed policies, laws, regulations, and services exist.

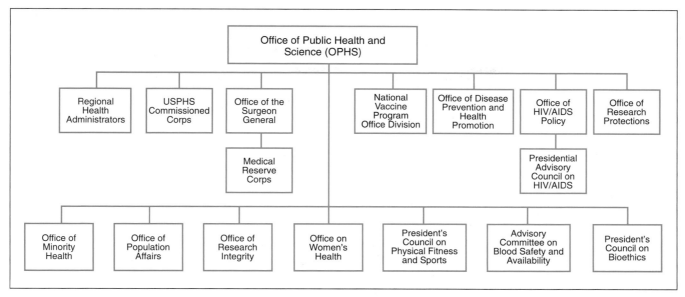

Figure 25-3 **U.S. Office of Public Health and Science (OPHS) organizational structure.** *HIV/AIDS,* Human immunodeficiency virus and acquired immunodeficiency syndrome. (From http://www.hhs.gov/about/orgchart/ophs.html.)

Each state has a health department to perform or oversee the performance of the 10 essential public health services. The state health department oversees the implementation of the **public health code,** a compilation of the state laws and regulations regarding public health and safety. (Laws are rules passed by a legislature. In contrast, **regulations** are technical rules added later by an empowered body with specific expertise, such as a state or local board of health.) In some states, responsibility for mental health services falls to the health department, whereas other states have separate departments of mental health services. Every state also licenses medical and other health-related practitioners and medical care institutions, such as hospitals, nursing homes, and home care programs.

C. Responsibilities of Municipalities and Counties

Although the states hold the fundamental police power to protect health, they delegate much of this authority to chartered **municipalities,** such as cities, or other incorporated areas. These municipalities accept public health responsibilities in return for a considerable degree of independence from the state in running their affairs, including property ownership and tax levies. In this respect, they differ from **counties** (called "parishes" in Louisiana). Counties are bureaucratic subdivisions of the state created to administer state responsibilities (with varying degrees of local control), such as health services, as well as courts of law, educational programs, highway construction and maintenance, and police and fire protection.

Local public health departments usually are administrative divisions of municipalities or counties, and their policies are established by a city or county **board of health.** These boards of health have the right to establish public health laws and regulations, provided that they are at least as strict as similar laws and regulations in the state public health code, and provided that they are *reasonable.* Anything that is too

---

Box 25-1   Governmental Public Health Infrastructure: The 10 Essential Public Health Services

Assessment

1. Monitor health status to identify community health problems.
2. Diagnose and investigate health problems and health hazards in the community.

Public Development

3. Inform, educate, and empower people about health issues.
4. Mobilize community partnerships to identify and solve health problems.
5. Develop policies and plans that support individual and community health efforts.

Assurance

6. Enforce laws and regulations that protect health and ensure safety.
7. Link people to needed personal health services, and assure the provision of health care when otherwise unavailable.
8. Ensure a competent public health and personal health care workforce.
9. Evaluate effectiveness, accessibility, and quality of personal and population-based health services.

Serving All Functions

10. Research for new insights, and innovate solutions to health problems.

Modified from Public Health Functions Steering Committee, 1994; American Public Health Association, Association of Schools of the Public Health Association of State and Territorial Health Officials, Environmental Council of the States, National Association of County and City Health Officials, National Association of State Alcohol and Drug Abuse Directors, National Association of State Mental Health Program Directors, Public Health Foundation, US Public Health Service.)

strict risks being overturned by the courts on the grounds that it is *unreasonable.*

The courts have generally upheld local and state health department laws and regulations when they pertain to the control of communicable diseases. The courts have also upheld laws relating to safe water and subsurface sewage disposal, immunization, regulation of restaurants and food stores, quarantine or treatment of persons with an infectious disease, investigation and control of acute disease outbreaks, and abatement of complaints relating to the spread of infectious disease (e.g., rabid animals).

Outside the area of communicable diseases, neither legislatures nor courts have been as supportive of laws and regulations. Laws requiring motorcyclists and bicyclists to wear helmets sometimes have not been enacted or have been repealed, despite abundant evidence of their benefits.[4] If an individual risk factor for disease can be shown to have a negative *public* impact, however, such as passive smoke inhalation, legislatures usually support controls, provided the direct fiscal impact is minimal (see Chapter 26).

D. Responsibilities of Local Public Health Departments

I. "Basic Six" to 10 Essential Services

The best-known description of the responsibilities of local health departments emerged in 1940, when six primary areas of responsibilities were defined as follows[5]:

1. Collecting vital statistics
2. Controlling communicable diseases
3. Protecting maternal and child health
4. Monitoring and protecting environmental health
5. Promoting health education
6. Maintaining public health laboratories

These functions of local health departments, later known as the "basic six," continue to influence the direction of local departments, despite the many changes in the nature of public health problems over time. However, these six functions are not fully adequate to deal with some more recent public health problems, such as environmental pollution crossing state lines and the increased incidence of chronic degenerative diseases. For a time, public health leaders debated the proper functions and responsibilities of health departments at the local and state level.[6,7] To help health departments in evaluating their work, the CDC has created a National Public Health Performance Standards Program.[8]

Public health departments cannot carry out their responsibilities without funding by legislative bodies. From the 1950s to the early 1970s, the danger of infectious diseases seemed to be waning. Consequently, and despite occasional warnings that communicable diseases were still major threats, legislatures saw infectious diseases as a diminishing threat, and funding for public health agencies decreased.[9] The emergence of legionnaires' disease and Lyme disease in the mid-1970s was soon followed by toxic shock syndrome, AIDS, multidrug-resistant tuberculosis, and the resurgence of other infectious diseases.[8,9] By the time society began to awaken to the problem of the emerging public health diseases, the IOM and others considered the public health

---

Box 25-2   Ten Greatest Public Health Achievements of 20th Century

1. Immunization
2. Motor vehicle safety
3. Improvements in workplace safety
4. Control of infectious diseases
5. Decline in deaths from coronary heart disease and stroke
6. Safer and healthier foods
7. Healthier mothers and infants
8. Family planning
9. Fluoridation of drinking water
10. Recognition of tobacco use as a health hazard

From US Centers for Disease Control and Prevention. http://www.cdc.gov/about/history/tengpha.htm

---

system to be in "disarray,"[3,10] and the "basic six" functions have reappeared as important functions of local health departments.

Public health agencies perennially struggle to garner enough popular and government support to promote health and prevent disease effectively. Nonetheless, Americans have benefited greatly from the many achievements of public health efforts, in conjunction with laboratory research, clinical medicine, and sanitary and safety engineering. Box 25-2 provides the CDC's list of the 10 leading public health achievements of the 20th century. For the 21st century, the following domains have been defined as "winnable battles," the public health priorities areas with proven effective interventions[11]:

- Food safety
- Global immunization against polio, measles, rubella, meningitis, pneumococci, and rotaviruses
- Health care–associated infections
- Human immunodeficiency virus (HIV) infection
- Lymphatic filariasis
- Mother-to-child transmission of HIV and congenital syphilis
- Motor vehicle injuries
- Nutrition, physical activity, and obesity
- Teen pregnancy
- Tobacco use (especially smoking)

2. Health Director's Duties

The programs run by a local health department vary by region or county and depend on available funding, state and local priorities, and availability of other providers and institutions. Some local health departments manage a complex set of services, including mental health and primary care for underserved populations, which involves managing teams and human resources, analyzing organizational performance, and overseeing budgeting analysis. Health directors must adhere to applicable federal and state rules when they hire, evaluate, and fire employees. Directors must also ensure that employees are supervised appropriately, including regular performance evaluation, pay equity to comparable jobs, and compliance with grievance process (see Chapter 28). Particular challenges arise if different staff members with similar responsibilities are paid from different payrolls (e.g., county, city, state, grant funders).

In addition to running these services, the health director serves as the *chief health policy advisor* to local elected officials for public health, community assessment, access to medical care, and financing of health and medical care.[12] The director also serves as the *chief public health educator* for politicians and the public, to ensure ongoing funding, grassroots support, and collaboration with community groups and health care institutions.

3. Environmental Protection

Among the functions of local health departments, protecting the public from food-borne illness and inspecting septic systems are among the most important.

RESTAURANT INSPECTION

Most contamination occurs through just a few breakdowns: unwashed hands, improper cooking, improper storage, unclean utensils, and contact between food and nonfood surfaces.[12] Local food regulations vary by county and district. However, most local health departments inspect restaurants episodically, assign points for violations of code depending on the gravity of violations, and provide grades to restaurants as a summary assessment (A-F or colors). Health inspectors particularly look at five critical items (sometimes called "red items") that pose an immediate health hazard, as follows[13]:

- Improper hand hygiene
- Food is not kept at temperatures high enough or low enough to inhibit bacterial growth
- Incorrect sanitizer concentrations of dishwasher or cleaning solutions
- Cross-contamination between raw and cooked products
- Plumbing hazards

If an establishment is found to pose an immediate hazard, or if it has a history of persistent failure to comply with recommendations, health inspectors can shut it down. In those cases, the establishment usually cannot reopen until the health inspector has returned to confirm that the violations have been corrected. Some departments also perform compliance inspections for restaurants with borderline scores to document improvement.[14]

WASTEWATER DISPOSAL

Many rural areas have no central sewage system. Every new building needs a septic tank and a "drain field," the size of which varies with the drainage pattern and depth of the topsoil. Otherwise, raw sewage may contaminate an aquifer and pollute everybody's drinking water. Given the amount of money involved in developing land and the potential for damage, the health director and environmental staff need to coordinate closely with local and county officials in planning and zoning and the granting of building permits.[12]

In an age of vanishing rain forests, receding polar ice caps, and progressive climate change, environmental protection has taken on new meaning. Such issues as conservation and biopreservation intersect meaningfully with public health, as addressed in Chapter 30.

II. BROADER DEFINITIONS OF PUBLIC HEALTH POLICY

The current view of public health policy in the United States is narrower than that in the world public health scene. According to the **Ottawa Charter for Health Promotion,** which guides much of the international work in this area, health promotion requires that *all* policies be reviewed for their health impact and adjusted to strengthen, rather than hinder, the effort to achieve good health, as follows[15]:

> Health promotion goes beyond health care. It puts health on the agenda of policy makers in all sectors and at all levels, directing them to be aware of the health consequences of their decisions and to accept their responsibilities for health.
>
> Health promotion policy combines diverse but complementary approaches including legislation, fiscal measures, taxation and organizational change. It is coordinated action that leads to health, income and social policies that foster greater equity. Joint action contributes to ensuring safer and healthier goods and services, healthier public services, and cleaner, more enjoyable environments.
>
> Health promotion policy requires identification of obstacles to the adoption of *healthy public policies* in non-health sectors, and ways of removing them. The aim must be to make the healthier choice the easier choice for policy makers as well.

The switch from *public health policy* to *healthy public policies* is subtle but important. The point of this approach was that *all* public policies must be evaluated and, if necessary, modified for their impact on public health.

III. INTERSECTORAL APPROACH TO PUBLIC HEALTH

So far, this chapter has emphasized the role of specific U.S. public health agencies at the federal, state, and local level. However, as the Ottawa Charter emphasizes, many duties with public health implications are carried out by government agencies that are not usually considered "health agencies." Departments of **agriculture** are responsible for monitoring the safety of milk, meat, and other agricultural products and controlling zoonoses (animal diseases that can be spread to humans). The U.S. Department of Agriculture (USDA) also administers the program for **Women, Infants, and Children** (WIC), which supports low-income women and children up to age 5 who are at nutritional risk by providing foods to supplement diets and financial support. This program has a substantial impact on food choices, childhood obesity, and oral health. Departments of **parks and recreation** must monitor the safety of water and sewage disposal in their facilities. **Highway** departments are responsible for the safe design and maintenance of roads and highways. **Education** departments are charged with overseeing health education and providing a safe and healthful environment in which to learn. Government departments that promote a **healthy economy** are crucial as well, because when an economy falters, the people's health suffers as well.

Because health is the result of the entire fabric of the environment and life of a population, a true public health approach must be **intersectoral;** that is, it must consider the health impact of policies in every sector of a society and government, not just in the health sector or medical care sector. Moreover, a true public health approach must also consider the health impact of policies on the planet more broadly, being mindful of the health of entire ecosystems (see Chapter 30). The perspectives of the Ottawa Charter and **intersectoral policy analysis** are foundations for the broader, more community action–oriented approach to public health currently emphasized in Europe and elsewhere. This approach is sometimes called "the new public health" or the "healthy communities" approach.[16] The healthy communities movement is also active in the United States[17] (see Chapter 26).

The United States is fortunate to be home to many voluntary health agencies and other nongovernmental organizations (NGOs) whose focus is to prevent or control diseases and promote health. Some focus on certain diseases (e.g., American Heart Association [AHA], American Lung Association [ALA]), and others confront a related group of diseases (e.g., American Cancer Society [ACS]). Sometimes groups join forces; cigarette smoking is a major risk factor for heart disease, lung disease, and cancer, so the AHA, ALA, and ACS have worked together to curtail smoking. These organizations raise money for research, public education, and preventive programs. Some NGOs even provide direct patient care, such as Planned Parenthood, which strives for a comprehensive approach to reproductive health. These agencies strive to fill the gaps left by the public health system. At the same time, these agencies form important stakeholders that can substantially influence the success or failure of public health initiatives.

IV. ORGANIZATIONS IN PREVENTIVE MEDICINE

Many organizations in the United States emphasize public health and preventive medicine; the largest is the **American Public Health Association** (APHA), with annual meetings typically bringing together 12,000 to 15,000 people. APHA has gradually changed from an organization focusing on science and the practice of public health to one emphasizing national public health and medical care **policy,** although some sections still emphasize science or practice. It publishes the *American Journal of Public Health* and welcomes as members anyone who is trained in, working in, or just interested in public health (www.apha.org).

Other organizations that promote the health of communities include **American College of Preventive Medicine** (ACPM) and **Association of Teachers of Preventive Medicine** (ATPM). With ATPM, ACPM copublishes the *American Journal of Preventive Medicine* and cosponsors a yearly conference on prevention science and policy. ATPM members include university faculty, preventive medicine residency program directors and faculty, and others interested in teaching health promotion and disease prevention in schools of medicine, public health, and other health professions. The goal of ATPM is to improve research, training, and practice in preventive medicine and to support the funding for

training programs. Chapter 15 provides more details on training for physicians.

V. ASSESSMENT AND FUTURE TRENDS

In its 2002 report the IOM assessed the state of the U.S. public health system as follows[1]:

> The governmental public health infrastructure has suffered from political neglect and from the pressure of political agendas and public opinion that frequently override empirical evidence. Under the glare of a national crisis [attacks of 9/11/2001], policy makers and the public became aware of vulnerable and outdated health information systems and technologies, an insufficient and inadequately trained public health workforce, antiquated laboratory capacity, a lack of real-time surveillance and epidemiological systems, ineffective and fragmented communications networks, incomplete domestic preparedness and emergency response capabilities, and communities without access to essential public health services. These problems leave the nation's health vulnerable—and not only to exotic germs and bioterrorism.

In response to this report and other voices, DHHS has disseminated sample policies, established grant programs to upgrade and integrate information systems, and developed an accreditation system for public health providers and local health departments. However, much remains to be done so that the public health system can maintain the gains made in the 20th century and prepare for the challenges of the 21st century.

VI. SUMMARY

Public health services in the United States are provided by the federal, state, and local levels of government, although the primary authority for health lies with the states. The federal government becomes involved in health mostly by regulating international and interstate commerce and by its power to tax for the general welfare. Local governments become involved in health as the states delegate authority for health to them. The fundamental health responsibilities have expanded greatly from the "basic six" minimum functions, when infectious diseases were the greatest concern, to a large and diverse set of functions that now include the control of chronic diseases, injuries, and environmental toxins (preventive medicine). In the intersectoral approach to public health, all public policies are scrutinized for their impact on health.

References

1. Institute of Medicine (IOM): *The future of the public's health in the 21st century*, Washington, DC, 2002, National Academies Press. http://books.nap.edu/catalog/10548.html on 1/25/.
2. US Department of Health and Human Services: 2012. http://www.hhs.gov.
3. IOM: *The future of public health*, Washington, DC, 1988, National Academy Press.
4. Centers for Disease Control and Prevention (CDC): Injury control recommendations: bicycle helmets. *MMWR* 44:1–17, 1995.

5. Jekel JF: Health departments in the U.S., 1920–1988: statements of mission with special reference to the role of C.-E. A. Winslow. *Yale J Biol Med* 64:467–479, 1991.

6. Hanlon JJ: Is there a future for local health departments? *Health Serv Rep* 88:898–901, 1973.

7. Terris M: The epidemiologic revolution, national health insurance, and the role of health departments. *Am J Public Health* 66:1155–1164, 1976.

8. National Public Health Standards. 2012. http://www.cdc.gov/nphpsp.

9. Jekel JF: Communicable disease control in the 1970s: hot war, cold war, or peaceful coexistence? *Am J Public Health* 62:1578–1585, 1972.

10. Garrett L: *Betrayal of trust: the collapse of global public health*, New York, 2000, Hyperion.

11. CDC: Winnable battles. http://www.cdc.gov/winnablebattles/FocusAreas.html.

12. Buttery CMG: *The local health department*. 2012. Chapter 1. Accessed at http://www.commed.vcu.edu/LOCAL/2012/Ch1_local_health_director_12.pdf.

13. What health inspectors look for. http://www.foodservicewarehouse.com/education/health-safety/what-inspectors-look-for.aspx.

14. New York City Department of Health and Mental Hygiene: Letter grading for sanitary inspections. http://www.nyc.gov/html/doh/downloads/pdf/rii/restaurant-grading-faq.pdf.

15. Ottawa Charter for Health Promotion: *Report of an International Conference on Health Promotion, sponsored by the World Health Organization, Health and Welfare Canada, and the Canadian Public Health Association, Ottawa*. 1986.

16. Ashton J: *The new public health*, Buckingham, UK, 1988, Open University Press.

17. Duhl LJ, Lee PR, editors: Focus on healthy communities, *Public Health Rep* 115:114–289, 2000.

Select Readings

Douglas FD, Keck CW: Structure and function of the public health system in the United States. In Wallace RB, editor: *Maxcy-Rosenau-Last: Public health and preventive medicine*, ed 15, New York, 2008, McGraw-Hill Medical.

Duhl LJ, Lee PR, editors: Focus on healthy communities, *Public Health Rep* 115(2 and 3):114–289, 2000 [special issues].

Fallon FL, Zgodinski EJ: *Essentials of public health management*, Boston, 2008, Jones & Bartlett.

Garrett L: *Betrayal of trust: the collapse of global public health*, New York, 2000, Hyperion.

Institute of Medicine: *For the public's health: revitalizing law and policy to meet new challenges*, Washington, DC, 2011, National Academies Press.

Novick LF, Mays GP: *Public Health Administration*, Gaithersburg, Md, 2001, Aspen.

Websites

www.apha.org [American Public Health Organization].
www.acpm.org [American College of Preventive Medicine].
www.atpm.org [Association of Teachers of Preventive Medicine].

Public Health Practice in Communities

With Thiruvengadam Muniraj

Chapters 24 and 25 discuss the organization and health of the public health system overall. This chapter discusses the theory and practice of improving community health. Theories are important because a theory-based program is more likely to be effective (see Chapter 15). The technical term for attempts to improve community health is *community/ program planning*.

Community planning is defined as an organized process to design, implement, and evaluate a clinic or community-based project to address the needs of a defined population.[1] Community planning is often the province of personnel in a public health agency, such as the commissioner of health or agency staff. However, the principles of community planning and evaluation pertain to any person who has a stake in improving the community (stakeholders, policy makers), including an employee of a foundation, school, mayor's office, or political party and any interested citizen. Although there are many ideas on how to improve the health of a community, many good ideas fail. Reasons include lack of community or organizational support, lack of coordination, "turf battles," inefficient and duplicative efforts, and failure to use evidence-based interventions. Careful planning before a project begins can make a significant impact on the success of the project.[2]

This chapter discusses the steps involved in planning and evaluating a program, highlighting two special applications of community planning: (1) tobacco prevention, as an example of multiple successful community interventions (Box 26-1), and (2) health disparities, one of the greatest public health problems. A community is only as strong as its weakest link. Therefore, public health practitioners should aim not just to raise health overall, but to raise most the health of the vulnerable populations. Box 26-2 lists some examples how health disparities have been successfully addressed.

Many models and acronyms describe the steps of community planning (Box 26-3). They all have their strengths and weaknesses. We follow mainly the steps outlined in the Centers for Disease Control and Prevention (CDC) model, Community Health Assessment and Group Evaluation (CHANGE).[3] Other models are described in the section that addresses their main emphasis. Any other model of community planning likely works equally well as long as planners follow the following basic principles:

- Assemble community stakeholders and, in collaboration with them, define the agenda, values, and priorities.
- Perform a needs assessment.
- Design measurable objectives and interventions.
- Choose multilevel approaches rather than single interventions.
- Build evaluation into the entire process.

Table 26-1 provides an overview of the process and possible resources for each step.

I. THEORIES OF COMMUNITY CHANGE

When behavioral factors are a threat to health, improving health requires behavior change. Unhealthy behaviors (e.g., sedentariness) need to be replaced by healthy ones (e.g.,

Box 26-1   Prevention Efforts: Tobacco Use (Cigarette Smoking)

The decrease in tobacco use has been called one of the 10 great public health achievements in the 20th century. This success illustrates what is required to change community health practices. Several historic factors came together to enable significant improvements in this important public health problem.

A. Credible evidence and effective interventions led to medical consensus:

1. Changes in understanding of the genesis of tobacco addiction reframed the problem as not one of individual control and choice, but of addiction. Evidence for harm to nonsmokers (secondary tobacco exposure) strengthened the case for regulation.
2. Behavioral and pharmacologic treatments became available, making it easier to support smokers desiring to quit.

B. Trusted experts and grassroots groups provided effective advocacy:

3. The American Cancer Society, American Lung Association, and American Heart Association were each advocating against tobacco independent from each other. In 1981 they formed a coalition on smoking, which was later joined by the American Medical Association. This broad coalition led legitimacy to the argument against smoking.
4. Grassroots efforts in many communities and from many sources changed cultural norms about smoking. Examples include flight attendants advocating for their right for a smoke-free workplace and the *Reader's Digest* series educating its readers. These grassroots groups framed their issues as part of the broader environmental protection movement and increased consumer health consciousness.

C. Political will on many levels and available funds led to effective tobacco control.

5. On a federal level, Congress passed several laws addressing tobacco labeling, advertising on TV and radio, smoking bans on airlines and buses, and changes to FDA rules for more oversight over tobacco production and marketing.
6. *States' action.* States used excise tax on tobacco to fund smoking control programs, which led to the development and evaluation of community-level approaches to tobacco control.
7. New litigation strategies opened up even more monies and created willingness in industry to agree to changes.

Because of this high level of attention at all levels and significant funding for community prevention programs, multiple effective interventions to reduce smoking were developed, evaluated, and disseminated. The U.S. Community Preventive Services recommends a three-pronged approach combining strategies to:

■ Reduce exposure to environmental tobacco smoke.
■ Reduce tobacco use initiation, especially among adolescents.
■ Increase tobacco use cessation.

Recommended interventions include:

■ Smoking bans and restrictions in public areas, workplaces, and areas where people congregate
■ Increasing the unit price for tobacco products
■ Mass media campaigns of extended duration using brief, recurring messages to motivate children and adolescents to remain tobacco free
■ Provider reminders to counsel patients about tobacco cessation
■ Provider education combined with such reminders
■ Reducing out-of-pocket expenses for effective cessation therapies
■ Multicomponent patient telephone support through a state quit line

Modified from Institute of Medicine: Ending the tobacco problem: a blueprint for the nation, 2007; Task Force on Community Preventive Services (TFCPS): Recommendations regarding interventions to reduce tobacco use and exposure to environmental tobacco smoke, *Am J Prev Med* 20(2 suppl):10–15, 2001; and Tobacco. In Zaza S, Briss PA, Harris KW, editors: *The guide to community preventive services: what works to promote health?* Atlanta, 2005, Oxford University Press, http://www.thecommunityguide.org/tobacco/Tobacco.pdf.

Box 26-2   Addressing Health Disparities

Health in the U.S. population is characterized by pervasive and persistent health care disparities, sometimes also called *health inequities.* Despite the deeply rooted and intractable nature of many health care disparities, many states and communities have successfully implemented intervention to reduce them. Characteristics of successful programs include:

■ Strong data skills with geographic mapping of premature death clusters and other determinants of health
■ Strong coalitions among agencies, community leaders, and other stakeholders
■ Assessment of the community environment as a whole and addressing the social determinants at the root of health inequities (e.g., poverty, low rates for high school graduation, violence)

■ Empowering communities to a sense of increased ownership and leadership
■ Emphasizing community participation
■ Addressing environmental factors such as safe walkability, bikeability of environment, and access to high-quality food
■ Making health equity a component of all policies, including housing, youth violence, transportation, and agriculture

Interventions against health inequities can be successful even on a very small scale. Examples for such successful interventions include librarians who visit schools to give each child a library card; public housing directors who address lead and mold; and safe route to school initiatives with "human school buses" (group of parents who take turns in walking children to school).

Modified from Centers for Disease Control and Prevention: Health disparities and inequalities report (CHDIR), 2011. http://www.cdc.gov/minorityhealth/CHDIReport.html#ExecSummary. IOM reports on unequal treatment and reducing healthcare disparities. http://www.iom.edu/Reports/2011/State-and-Local-Policy-Initiatives-To-Reduce-Health-Disparities-Workshop-Summary.aspx

Box 26-3	Frequently Used Acronyms in Program Planning
CBPR	Community-Based Participatory Research
CHANGE	Community Health Assessment and Group Evaluation
DEBI	Diffusion of Effective Behavioral Interventions
DOI	Diffusion of Innovations
HEDIS	Healthcare Effectiveness Data and Information Set
IOM	Institute of Medicine
MAP-IT	Mobilize, Assess, Plan, Implement, Track
MAPP	Mobilizing for Action through Planning and Partnerships
NACCHO	National Association of County and City Health Officials
NCQA	National Committee for Quality Assurance
NPHPSP	National Public Health Performance Standards Program
P.L.A.N.E.T.	Plan, Link, Act, Network with Evidence-based Tools
PAR	Participatory Action Research
PATCH	Planned Approach to Community Health
PRECEDE	Predisposing, Reinforcing, and Enabling Constructs in Educational Diagnosis and Evaluation
PROCEED	Policy, Regulatory, and Organizational Constructs in Educational and Environmental Development
RTIP	Research Tested Intervention Program
RE-AIM	Reach, Efficacy, Adoption, Implementation, Maintenance
SCT	Social Cognitive Theory
SMART	Specific, Measurable, Attainable, Relevant, and Timely
SPARC	Sickness Prevention Achieved through Regional Collaboration
VERB	Not an acronym, but a program emphasizing *verb* as a part of speech, meaning an *action* word

Table 26-1 Overview of Steps for Community Program Design, Implementation, and Evaluation

Step/Description	Suggested Resources*
1. Create strategy and elicit community input.	Community Health Assessment and Group Evaluation (CHANGE) http://www.cdc.gov/healthycommunitiesprogram/tools/change.htm
2. Identify primary health issues in your community.	Community Health Assessment and Group Evaluation County Health Rankings: http://www.countyhealthrankings.org/ National Public Health Performance Standards: http://www.cdc.gov/nphpsp/ Mobilizing for Action through Planning and Partnerships (MAPP): http://www.naccho.org/topics/infrastructure/MAPP/index.cfm
3. Develop measurable process and outcome objectives to assess progress in addressing these health issues.	*Healthy People 2020* leading health indicators http://www.healthypeople.gov/2020/default.aspx HEDIS (Healthcare Effectiveness Data and Information Set) performance measures http://www.ncqa.org/tabid/59/default.aspx
4. Select effective interventions to help achieve these objectives.	*Guide to Community Preventive Services* *Guide to Clinical Preventive Services* http://www.uspreventiveservicestaskforce.org National Guideline Clearinghouse: http://guidelines.gov/ Research-Tested Intervention Programs http://rtips.cancer.gov/rtips/index.do
5. Implement selected interventions.	Partnership for Prevention: http://preventioninfo.org/ CDCynergy http://www.cdc.gov/healthcommunication/CDCynergy/ http://rtips.cancer.gov/rtips/index.do
6. Evaluate selected interventions based on objectives; use this information to improve program.	Framework for program evaluation in public health http://www.cdc.gov/mmwr/preview/mmwrhtml/rr4811a1.htm CDCynergy www.re-aim.org

Modified from *The community guide,* Atlanta, 2011, Centers for Disease Control and Prevention. http://www.thecommunityguide.org/uses/program_planning.html.
*For all steps, 1 through 6: Community health promotion handbook: Action guides to improve community health: http://www.prevent.org/Action-Guides/The-Community-Health-Promotion-Handbook.aspx; Cancer Control P.L.A.N.E.T.: http://cancercontrolplanet.cancer.gov/; Community tool box: http://ctb.ku.edu/en/default.aspx; DEBI: http://www.effectiveinterventions.org/en/Home.aspx.

exercise). Individual behavior, however, does not occur in a vacuum; it is strongly influenced by group norms and environmental cues. Practitioners aiming to change group norms and environmental cues should be aware of theories of community changes. This is because, as with any behavior change, practitioners will have a higher chance of success if they intervene in accordance with a valid theory of

behavior change (see Chapter 15 for theories of individual behavior change.) A number of theories have been developed to describe how individual change is brought about through interpersonal interactions and community interventions. These theories can be broadly characterized as **cognitive-behavioral theories** and share the following key concepts:

- Knowledge is necessary, but is not in itself sufficient to produce behavior changes.
- Perceptions, motivations, skills, and social environment are key influences on behavior.

Some well-known theories governing social change are social cognitive theory, community organization and other participatory approaches, diffusion of innovations, and communication theory. Taken together, these theories can be used to influence factors within a social-ecological framework, as follows:

Interpersonal: Family, friends, and peers provide role models, social identity, and support.

Organizations: Organizations influence behavior through organizational change, diffusion of innovation, and social marketing strategies.

Community: Social marketing and community organizing can change community norms on behavior.

Public policy: Public opinion process and policy changes can change the incentives for certain behaviors and make them easier or more difficult (e.g., taxes on high-sugar beverages).

Although behavior can be changed directly through any of these levels, the physical, regulatory, and political environments also have a powerful impact on behavior.

A. Social Cognitive Theory

Social cognitive theory (SCT) is one of the most frequently used and robust health behavior theories.[4] It explores the reciprocal interactions of people and their environments and the psychosocial determinants of health behavior (see Chapter 15).

Environment, people, and their behavior constantly influence each other (**reciprocal determinism**). Behavior is not simply the result of the environment and the person, just as the environment is not simply the result of the person and behavior.[5] According to SCT, three main factors affect the likelihood that a person will change a health behavior: (1) self-efficacy (see Chapter 15), (2) goals, and (3) outcome expectancies, in which people form new norms or new expectations from observing others (**observational learning**).

B. Community Organization

A heterogeneous mix of various theories covers community organization. The **social action theory** describes how to

increase the *problem-solving ability* of entire communities through achieving concrete changes towards social cause. The theory includes several key concepts. **Empowerment** is a social action process that improves community's confidence and life skills beyond the topic addressed. Empowerment is any social process that allows people to gain mastery over their life and their community. For example, individuals in a community may feel more empowered as they work together to strengthen their cultural identity and their community assets. Empowerment builds community capacity.

Community capacity is the unique ability of a community to mobilize, identify, and solve social problems. It requires the presence of leadership, participation, skills, and sense of community. Community capacity can be enhanced in many ways, such as through skill-building workshops that allow members of the community to become more effective leaders.

Critical consciousness is a mental state by which members in a community recognize the need for social change and are ready to work to achieve those changes. Critical consciousness can be built by engaging individuals in dialogues, forums, and discussions that clearly relate how problems and their root causes can be solved through social action.

Social capital refers to social resources such as trust, reciprocity, and civic engagement that exist as a result of network between community members. Social capital can connect individuals in a fragmented community across social boundaries and power hierarchies and can facilitate community building and organization. Social networking techniques and increasing the social support are vital methods that build social capital.[6]

Media advocacy is an essential component of community organizing. It aims to change the way community members look at various problems and to motivate community members and policy makers to become involved. This occurs through a reliable, consistent stream of publicity about an organization's mission and activities, including articles and news items about public health issues. Media advocacy relies on mass media, which make it expensive. In the 21st century, *social media* and games can generate extensive publicity with minimal investment. Table 26-2 summarizes how social marketing, public relations, and media advocacy complement each other.

1. Participatory Research

Immigrants and racial or ethnic minorities often distrust the health care system, making it more difficult for researchers

---

Table 26-2 Relationship of Social Marketing, Public Relations, and Media Advocacy

	Social Marketing	Public Relations	Media Advocacy
Message focus	"Look at you." Know about risk. Change your behavior.	"Look at me." Enhance image and relationship with public.	"Look at us." Sets agenda. Shapes debate. Advances policy.
Target audience	Individuals at risk General public	Funders Clients	Stakeholders Policy makers
Effect	Individuals	Individuals	Social environment
Benefits	Motivates individual behavioral change.	Develops strategic relationships. Generates support for cause.	Community change through policy

Modified from Media Advocacy to Advance Public Health Policy, UCLA Center for Health Policy Research, 2002. http://www.healthpolicy.ucla.edu/healthdata/tw_media2.pdf

and health practitioners to identify and address the health needs of these communities. For these groups, as well as for building community capacity in general, various participatory research methods have been proposed. Participatory efforts combine community capacity–building strategies with research to bridge the gap between the knowledge produced and its translation into interventions and policies.[7]

Participatory action research (PAR) and **community-based participatory research** (CBPR) are two participatory research approaches that have gained increasing popularity since the late 1980s.[8] Both PAR and CBPR conceptualize community members and researchers working together to generate hypotheses, conduct research, take action, and learn together. PAR focuses on the researcher's direct actions within a participatory community and aims to improve the performance quality of the community or an area of concern.[9-12] In contrast, CBPR strives for an action-oriented approach to research as an equal partnership between traditionally trained experts and members of a community. The community members are partners in the research, not subjects.[13] Both approaches give voice to disadvantaged communities and increase their control and ownership of community improvement activities.[10,13,14]

The guidelines for participatory research in health promotion[15] describe seven stages in participation, from passive or no participation to **self-mobilization.** For both approaches, the process is more important than the output, goals and methods are determined collaboratively, and findings and knowledge are disseminated to all partners.[10,13] Participatory research is more difficult to execute because of greater time demands and challenges in complying with external funding requirements.[16-18] For example, if actions require a negotiated process with the community, they may divert from a project plan previously submitted to a funder.

Engaging the community in research efforts is essential in translating research into practice. However, there are still large gaps in translating conclusions from well-conducted randomized trials into community practice. The **Multisite Translational Community Trial** is a research tool designed to bridge the gap. This trial type explores what is needed to make results from trials workable and effective in real-world settings and is particularly suited to practice-based research networks such as the Prevention Research Centers.[19]

C. Diffusion of Innovations Theory

To be successful, a community strategy needs to be disseminated. Successful dissemination is called **diffusion.** Diffusion of innovations (DOI) theory is characterized by four elements: innovations, communication channels, social systems (the individuals who adopt the innovation), and diffusion time. The DOI literature is replete with examples of successful diffusion of health behaviors and programs, including condom use, smoking cessation, and use of new tests and technologies by health practitioners.[20] Although DOI theory can be applied to behaviors, it is most closely associated with devices or products.

Groups are segmented by the speed with which they will adopt innovations. *Innovators* are eager to embrace new concepts. Next, *early adopters* will try out innovations, followed by members of the *early majority* and *late majority.* *Laggards* are the last to accept an innovation. Consequently, innovations need to be marketed initially to innovators and early adopters, then need to address each segment in sequence. The relevant population segments are generally referred to as innovators 2.5% of the overall population), early adopters (13.5%), early majority (34%), late majority (34%), and laggards (16%).[20]

The speed of adoption by any group depends on *the perceived characteristics* of the innovations themselves. **Relative advantage,** the degree to which an innovation is perceived as being better than the idea it supersedes, is a consequence of the following:

- *Compatibility,* the degree to which an innovation is perceived to be consistent with the existing values, current processes, past experiences, and needs of potential adopters
- *Low complexity,* the degree to which an innovation is perceived as easy to use
- *Trialability,* the opportunity to experiment with the innovation on a limited basis
- *Observability,* the degree to which the results of an innovation are visible to others

I. Social Marketing in Public Health

Social marketing is typically defined as a program-planning process that applies commercial marketing concepts and techniques to promote behavior change in a **target audience.** Social marketing has also been used to analyze the social consequences of commercial marketing policies and activities, such as monitoring the effects of the tobacco and food industries' marketing practices.[21] As in commercial marketing, social marketing depends on the following:

Audience segmentation. Dividing markets into small segments based on sociodemographic, cultural, or behavioral characteristics.[22]

Tailoring messages to individuals. Tailored messages address specific cognitive and behavioral patterns as well as individual demographic characteristics. Therefore, tailored materials are more precise, but also more limited in population reach and more expensive. For example, the CDC's VERB campaign ("It's what you do") specially promoted the benefits of daily physical activity to children age 9 to 13 years.[23]

Branding. Public health branding is the application of commercial branding strategies to promote health behavior change.[24] For example, a study recruited highly regarded peers to make condom use "cool" among a group of men at risk for human immunodeficiency virus (HIV) infection.[25]

Marketing mix. Addressing the four Ps of marketing (product, price, place, promotion) and redefining them for social marketing (see next).

Product is the desired type of behavioral change and includes not only the behavior being promoted but also the benefits that go with it. **Price** is an exchange of benefits and costs and refers to barriers or costs involved in adopting the behavior (e.g., money, time, effort). **Place** (making new behaviors easy to do) is about making the "product" accessible and convenient, delivering benefits in the right place at the right time. **Promotion** (delivering the message to the audience) is how the practitioner informs the target market of the product, as well as its benefits, reasonable cost, and convenience. Social marketing techniques have been used successfully in many communities that seemed impervious to traditional health promotion messages.[26]

D. Communication Theory

Communication theory describes the use of communication to effect change at the community level and in society as well. Communication influences community and societal change in areas such as building a community agenda of important public health issues, changing public health policy, allocating resources to make behavior change easier, and legitimizing new norms of health behavior.

1. Delphi Technique

The Delphi technique is a method for structuring a group communication process so that it is effective in allowing a group of individuals, as a whole, to deal with a complex problem.[27] Furthermore, it is a method for the systematic solicitation and collation of judgments on a particular health topic through a set of carefully designed sequential questionnaires, interspersed with summarized information and feedback of opinions from earlier responses. The Delphi technique is used most frequently to integrate the judgments of a group of experts on guidelines if there is insufficient evidence. It can also be used to help decision making in a disparate group such as a community coalition.

2. Role of Media Communication

Media institutions play a crucial role in health behavior change because of their role in disseminating information. As agents of socialization, media also have a powerful impact in legitimizing behavioral norms. Popular and academic perspectives both hold that media communication plays a powerful role in promoting, discouraging, or inhibiting healthy behaviors. Public health managers need to be aware of how messages are produced and how they impact people. In particular, media can play a major role in how a problem is *framed*. This framing influences how the public understands it, how much attention people will pay, and which actions individuals or communities are likely to take. For example, the Harvard School of Public Health mounted a successful campaign to persuade television producers to include messages about designated drivers with their ads.[28]

Knowledge and behavior change can each precede the other. In **dissonance-attribution,** behavior change comes before attitude change and knowledge, whereas in the **low-involvement** hierarchy, increased knowledge leads to behavior change and finally attitude change. Early studies focused on opinion or attitude change based on the credibility of the information source, fear, organization of arguments, the role of group membership in resisting or accepting communication, and personality differences. Since the 1960s, however, research has emphasized cognitive processing of information leading to persuasion.

Table 26-3 summarizes key concepts and potential change strategies for communication. Table 26-4 outlines theories of behavior change at the community level.

E. Environmental Influences on Behavior

Many health promotion campaigns seek to reduce high-risk behaviors such as unhealthy eating, alcohol and drug abuse, and smoking. Such programs should not ignore the material, social, and psychological conditions in which the targeted behaviors occur. For example, a strong association exists among material hardship, low social status, stressful work or life events, and smoking prevalence.[29] Many strategies that include modifications of the regulatory environment (e.g., taxes on tobacco products) and "built" environment (e.g., impact of an environment that is conducive to exercise or obesity) seem to be at least as effective as those directly aimed at behaviors. The structural as well as the political and socioeconomic environment influences how people interact, behave, and recover from noxious stimuli. This interaction has been described extensively by D. William Haddon for the field of injury prevention (see Chapter 24). However, Haddon's concept of countermeasures to injury is equally

---

Table 26-3 Concepts in Communication: Agenda Setting

Concept	Definition	Potential Change Strategies
Media agenda setting	Institutional factors and processes influencing how the media define, select, and emphasize issues	Understand media professionals' needs and routines for gathering and reporting news.
Public agenda setting	The link between issues covered in the media and the public's priorities	Use media advocacy or partnerships to raise public awareness of key health issues.
Policy agenda setting	The link between issues covered in the media and the legislative priorities of policy makers	Advocate for media coverage to educate and pressure policy makers about changes to the physical and social environment needed to promote health.
Problem definition	Factors and process leading to identification of an issue as a "problem" by social institutions	Community leaders, advocacy groups, and organizations define an issue for the media and offer solutions.
Framing	Selecting and emphasizing certain aspects of a story and excluding others	Advocacy groups "package" an important health issue for the media and the public.

From Glanz K, Rimer BK, Viswanath K: *Health behavior and health education: theory, research, and practice,* Bethesda, Md, National Cancer Institute at National Institutes of Health, 2008. http://www.cancer.gov/cancertopics/cancerlibrary/theory.pdf

Table 26-4 Overview of Community-Level Theories of Behavior Change

Theory	Description	Key Factors
Community organization	Community-driven approaches to assessing and solving health and social problems	Empowerment Community capacity Participation Relevance Issue selection Critical consciousness
Diffusion of innovations	How new ideas, products, and practices spread within a society or from one society to another	Relative advantage Compatibility Complexity Trialability Observability
Communication theory	How different types of communication affect health behavior	Media agenda setting Public agenda setting Policy agenda setting Problem identification and definition Framing

From Glanz K, Rimer BK, Viswanath K: *Health behavior and health education: theory, research, and practice,* Bethesda, Md, National Cancer Institute at National Institutes of Health, 2008. http://www.cancer.gov/cancertopics/cancerlibrary/theory.pdf

Table 26-5 Application of Haddon Countermeasures to Gun Injury and Cancer Prevention

Countermeasure	Preventing Injury by Handguns	Preventing Cancer Associated with Smoking
1. Prevent the creation of the hazard.	Eliminate handguns.	Eliminate cigarettes.
2. Reduce the amount of hazard brought into being.	Limit the number of handguns allowed to be sold or purchased.	Reduce the volume of tobacco production by changing agricultural policy.
3. Prevent the release of the hazard.	Install locks on handguns.	Limit sales of tobacco to certain age groups.
4. Modify the rate of release of the hazard from its source.	Eliminate automatic handguns.	Develop cigarettes that burn more slowly.
5. Separate the hazard from that which is to be protected by time and space.	Store handguns only at gun clubs rather than at home.	Establish shutoff times for vending machines and earlier closings of convenience stores and groceries.
6. Separate the hazard from that which is to be protected by a physical barrier.	Keep guns in locked containers.	Install filters on cigarettes.
7. Modify relevant basic qualities of the hazard.	Personalize guns so they can be fired only by the owner.	Reduce the nicotine content of cigarettes.
8. Make what is to be protected more resistant to damage from the hazard.	Create and market bulletproof garments.	Limit exposure to other potential synergistic causes of cancer (e.g., environmental carcinogens) among smokers.
9. Begin to counter the damage done by the hazard.	Provide good access to emergency care in the prehospital period.	Set up screening to detect cancer in the early stages.
10. Stabilize, repair, and rehabilitate the object of damage.	Provide high-quality trauma care in hospitals.	Provide good-quality health care for cancer patients.

Modified from Runyan CW: *Epidemiol Rev* 25:60–64, 2003.

applicable to harmful behaviors such as smoking[30] (Table 26-5). Structural interventions for patients with HIV infection have been categorized into the following three dimensions:

1. **Social change.** These approaches focus on factors affecting multiple groups (e.g., a region or country as a whole), such as legal reform, stigma reduction, and efforts to cultivate strong leadership on acquired immunodeficiency syndrome (AIDS).
2. **Change within specific groups.** These approaches address social structures that create vulnerability among specific populations (e.g., men who have sex with men, mine workers, disadvantaged women). Examples include efforts to organize and mobilize sex workers, microfinance programs for poor women, and interventions to change harmful sexual norms.
3. **Harm reduction or health-seeking behavior change.** These approaches work to make harm reduction technologies available to those in need and to change rules, services, and attitudes about these technologies. Examples include efforts to provide safe housing for drug users and "100% condom use" campaigns.

Using a theoretical model of the interactions between behavior and environment (such as those just listed) allows planners to think through the interaction of people, harmful substances, and their environment. It opens up new ways of thinking about prevention in a more comprehensive way.

II. STEPS IN DEVELOPING A HEALTH PROMOTION PROGRAM

One model of program planning comes from the CDC's **Community Health Assessment and Group Evaluation.** CHANGE is a comprehensive data collection tool and resource for community program planning with the following steps (see Table 26-1):

1. Define a strategy and assemble a team.
2. Identify primary health issues.
3. Develop objectives to measure progress.
4. Select effective interventions.
5. Implement innovations.
6. Evaluate.

Some of the specific programs relevant to each of these steps are explained in detail next. Again, other planning resources/programs are described under those headings where they have a strong emphasis.

A. Define Strategy and Assemble Team

Broad-based participation in the planning process from the start is critical to the success of a project.[31] Possible coalition participants include physicians, nurses, social workers, teachers, emergency medical services (EMS) personnel, health educators, parents, and police. However, partners can also come from churches, businesses, dental clinics, and unions. It is important to stress that building a coalition should come *before* gathering any data. There is no reason to gather data on problems nobody is willing or able to change. *Sustainable coalitions* are those that utilize preexisting partnerships, have access to at least minimal levels of funding, are perceived as well functioning, and plan for sustainability.[32,33]

B. Identify Primary Health Issues

The second step in program planning is to identify the primary health issues concerning the community. This involves a **needs assessment** (areas for improvement) as well as **asset mapping** (identifying the people, institutions, available funds, and capacity to solve problems). Tools used in screening and identifying overall problems in the community include the following:

- PRECEDE-PROCEED model
- Planned Approach to Community Health (PATCH)
- Mobilizing for Action through Planning and Partnerships (MAPP)
- National Public Health Performance Standards Program (NPHPSP)
- Data sources (see Chapter 25)
- Tools within the CHANGE process

Examples for a needs assessment that emphasizes the environmental factors of diet, exercise, and smoking include the following questions[34]:

Do sidewalks make walking (walkability) and biking (bikeability) easy and safe? Are they connected, continuous, free from barriers, and safe from traffic and crime?

Are healthier food options in grocery stores available and affordable? Are they of good quality?

How many homes, parks, hospitals, and schools have easy access to tobacco and are exposed to tobacco advertising?

Are there tobacco-free campus policies in hospitals, on college campuses, and in multiunit housing?

I. PRECEDE/PROCEED Model

The PRECEDE-PROCEED tool, a planning model developed by Green and Kreuter, provides a comprehensive structure for (1) assessing health and quality-of-life needs and (2) for designing, implementing, and evaluating health promotion and other public health programs to meet those needs. The PRECEDE part—**Predisposing, Reinforcing, and Enabling Constructs in Educational Diagnosis and Evaluation**—outlines a diagnostic planning process to assist in the development of targeted and focused public health programs. The second part, PROCEED, provides an implementation and evaluation program—**Policy, Regulatory, and Organizational Constructs in Educational and Environmental Development**—for the program designed using PRECEDE. The process starts with desired outcomes and works backward to identify a mix of strategies for achieving objectives[35] (Fig. 26-1).

PRECEDE comprises the following five steps[36]:

Step I: **Social assessment.** Determining the quality of life or social problems and needs of a given population. To conduct a social assessment, the practitioner may use multiple data collection activities (e.g., key informant interviews, focus groups, participant observation, surveys) to understand the community's perceived needs.

Step II: **Epidemiologic assessment.** Identifying the health determinants of these problems and needs. The epidemiologic assessment may include secondary data analysis or original data collection to prioritize the community's health needs and establish program goals and objectives.

Step III: **Behavioral and environmental assessment.** Analyzing the behavioral and environmental determinants of the health problems. This step identifies factors, both internal and external to the individual, that affect the health problem. Reviewing the literature and applying theory are two ways to map out these factors.

Step IV: **Educational and ecological assessment.** Identifying the factors that predispose to, reinforce, and enable the behaviors and lifestyles. Practitioners can use individual, interpersonal, or community-level change theories to classify determinants of behavior into one of these three categories and rank their importance. Because each type of factor requires different intervention strategies, classification helps practitioners consider how to address community needs.

Step V: **Administrative and policy assessment.** Ascertaining which health promotion, health education, and policy-related interventions would best be suited to encourage the desired changes.

PROCEED comprises four additional phases, as follows[36]:

Step VI: **Implementation.** Carrying out the interventions from step V.

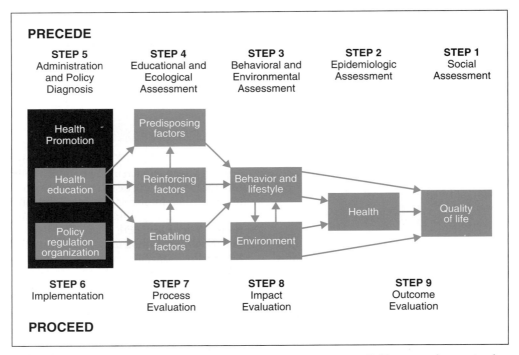

Figure 26-1 **The PRECEDE/PROCEED model.** (Redrawn and modified from Green L, Kreuter M: *Health program planning: An educational and ecological approach,* ed 4, New York, 2005, McGraw-Hill. Slide 8 from http://www.lgreen.net/hpp/chapters/Chapter01.htm.)

Step VII: **Process evaluation.** Evaluating the process for implementing the interventions.

Step VIII: **Impact evaluation.** Evaluating the impact of the interventions on the factors supporting behavior and on behavior itself.

Step IX: **Outcome evaluation.** Determining the ultimate effects of the interventions on the health and quality of life of the population.

In reality, when implemented in a program, PRECEDE and PROCEED interact as a continuous cycle, since feedback data from the PROCEED steps indicate how programs may be modified to more closely reach their goals and targets.[37]

2. Planned Approach to Community Health

The Planned Approach to Community Health (PATCH) was developed by the CDC in the mid-1980s. The primary goal of PATCH was to create a practical mechanism through which effective community health education action could be targeted to address local-level health priorities. A secondary goal was to offer a practical, skills-based program of technical assistance in which health education leaders in state health agencies could work with their local counterparts to establish effective community health education programs.[38] Those interventions included mobilizing the community, collecting and organizing data, choosing health priorities, developing a comprehensive intervention plan, and evaluation.

Historically, the most demanding and time-consuming step in PATCH has often been the gathering and analysis of local area data to facilitate program planning and evaluation. On average, communities spent about a year collecting and analyzing data. This energy appears to be well spent, however. With information to document the magnitude and extent of

their health problems and to set measurable health priorities for health promotion and disease prevention, communities have additional leverage to strengthen their requests for resources. With more data becoming available online (see Chapter 25), this step may become less demanding in the future.

3. Mobilizing for Action through Planning and Partnerships

Mobilizing for Action through Planning and Partnerships (MAPP) is a program sponsored by the National Association for County and City Health Officials (NACCHO) in cooperation with the Public Health Practice Program Office of the CDC. It is a community-driven strategic planning process for improving community health. The seven principles of MAPP are as follows:

1. **Systems thinking**—to promote an appreciation for the dynamic interrelationship of all components of the local public health system required to develop a vision of a healthy community.
2. **Dialogue**—to ensure respect for diverse voices and perspectives during the collaborative process.
3. **Shared vision**—to form the foundation for building a healthy future (visioning).
4. **Data**—to inform each step of the process.
5. **Partnerships and collaboration**—to optimize performance through shared resources and responsibility.
6. **Strategic thinking**—to foster a proactive response to the issues and opportunities facing the system.
7. **Celebration of successes**—to ensure that contributions are recognized and to sustain excitement for the process.

In addition to these seven principles, MAPP also emphasizes identifying community strengths and assessing current forces of change (Fig. 26-2).

C. Develop Objectives to Measure Progress

One of the most important parts in planning change is to define objectives. **Objectives** are defined as specific

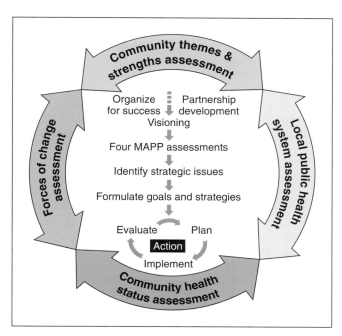

Figure 26-2 Mobilizing for Action through Planning and Partnerships (MAPP). (From National Association of County and City Health Officials, Washington, DC, with Centers for Disease Control and Prevention, Atlanta. http://www.naccho.org/topics/infrastructure/MAPP/index.cfm)

measurable parameters; each objective should be specific, relevant, measurable, and associated with a time frame. Objectives can cover structure, processes, or outcomes (see Chapter 28). When writing objectives, health planners should follow the acronym SMART: **specific, measurable, attainable, relevant, and timely.** One source of SMART objectives is the *Healthy People* database.[39]

I. Healthy People 2020

During the 1970s, representatives from many public health and scientific organizations began to develop national health promotion and disease prevention objectives. Their efforts resulted in the publication of objective, science-based, national 10-year objectives to improve the health of all Americans. The most recent version of these is *Healthy People 2020.* Although the federal government acted as coordinator and facilitator of these efforts and supported the goals and objectives outlined, the documents themselves were "not intended as a statement of federal standards or requirements."[40] They do represent, however, a national consensus strategy of the government, public health organizations, and public-spirited citizens. The reports have had a major impact on the way government and other institutions in the United States direct their resources in public health. For example, most federal grants require possible grantees to describe how proposals will advance *Healthy People 2020* goals.

Healthy People 2020 proposed the following four overarching goals (Table 26-6):

1. Attain high-quality, longer lives free of preventable disease, disability, injury, and premature death.
2. Achieve health equity, eliminate disparities, and improve the health of all groups.
3. Create social and physical environments that promote good health for all.

Table 26-6 *Healthy People 2020:* Goals, Foundational Health Measures, and Progress

Overarching Goals	Foundational Health Measures Category	Measures of Progress
Attain high-quality, longer lives free of preventable disease, disability, injury, and premature death.	General health status	Life expectancy Healthy life expectancy Physically, mentally unhealthy days Self-assessed health status Limitation of activity Chronic disease prevalence International comparisons (where available)
Achieve health equity, eliminate disparities, and improve the health of all groups.	Disparities and inequity	*Disparities/inequity to be assessed by:* Race/ethnicity Gender Socioeconomic status Disability status Lesbian, gay, bisexual, and transgender status Geography
Social and physical environments that promote good health for all.	Social determinants of health	*Determinants can include:* Social and economic factors Natural and built environments Policies and programs
Promote quality of life, healthy development, and healthy behaviors across all life stages.	Health-related quality of life and well-being	Well-being/satisfaction Physical, mental, and social health-related quality of life Participation in common activities

From *Healthy People 2020,* U.S. Department of Health and Human Services: http://healthypeople.gov/2020/TopicsObjectives2020/pdfs/HP2020_brochure_with_LHI_508.pdf

4. Promote quality of life, healthy development, and healthy behaviors across all life stages.

Four **foundational health measures** serve as an indicator of progress: (1) general health status, (2) health-related quality of life and well-being, (3) determinants of health, and (4) disparities (see Table 26-6). Each foundational health measure is further divided into submeasures. *Healthy People 2020* contains 42 topic areas with almost 600 objectives (with others still evolving), encompassing 1200 measures. A smaller set of objectives, called **leading health indicators,** has been selected to communicate high-priority health issues and actions that can be taken to address them (Table 26-7).

The document includes measurable indicators of progress, which are helpful in tracking progress or documenting the lack of progress. For each leading indicator, an objective is described and appropriate background information provided. Each focus area objective is broken into many subobjectives, each of which has baseline values and target values for subgroups of the population (age, gender, ethnic, and other subgroups).[40]

Mobilize, assess, plan, implement, track (MAP-IT) is a framework that can be used to plan and evaluate public health interventions in a community using the *Healthy People 2020* objectives (Fig. 26-3). Using MAP-IT, a step-by-step, structured plan can be developed by a coalition and tailored to a specific community's needs. The phases of mobilize-assess-plan-implement-track provide a logical structure for communities to address and resolve local health problems and to build healthy communities.

D. Select Effective Interventions

I. Community Preventive Services

The U.S. Preventive Services Task Force (USPSTF) *Guide to Clinical Preventive Services* championed a rigorous, evidence-based approach to **clinical** preventive services. Modeled on this process, the Department of Health and Human Services (DHHS) tasked the CDC to develop a parallel guide to **community preventive services** (CPS).[41] The *Guide to Community Preventive Services* is a free, online resource to help choose programs and policies to improve health and prevent disease in the community.[42]

METHODS

Systematic reviews are used to answer questions such as: Which program and policy interventions have proved

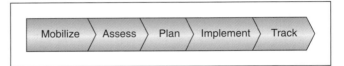

Figure 26-3 MAP-IT. This framework to help set objectives for the health of the U.S. population is from *Healthy People 2020*, a joint effort of the U.S. Department of Health and Human Services with representatives from the departments of Agriculture; Education, Housing and Urban Development; Justice; the Interior; and Veterans Affairs, as well as the Environmental Protection Agency.

Table 26-7 *Healthy People 2020:* **Leading Health Indicators**

12 Topic Areas	26 Leading Health Indicators
Access to health services	Persons with medical insurance
	Persons with a usual primary care provider
Clinical preventive services	Adults who receive colorectal cancer screening based on most recent guidelines
	Adults with hypertension whose blood pressure is under control
	Adult diabetic population with Hb A_{1c} value greater than 9%
	Children age 19-35 months who receive recommended doses of diphtheria, tetanus, and pertussis; polio; measles, mumps, and rubella; *Haemophilus influenzae* type b; hepatitis B; varicella; and pneumococcal conjugate vaccines
Environmental quality	Air Quality Index exceeding 100
	Children age 3-11 years exposed to secondhand smoke
Injury and violence	Fatal injuries
	Homicides
Maternal, infant, and child health	Infant deaths
	Preterm births
Mental health	Suicides
	Adolescents who experience major depressive episodes
Nutrition, physical activity, and obesity	Adults who meet current federal physical activity guidelines for aerobic physical activity and muscle-strengthening activity
	Adults who are obese
	Children and adolescents who are considered obese
	Total vegetable intake for persons age 2 years and older
Oral health	Persons age 2 years and older who used oral health care system in past 12 months
Reproductive and sexual health	Sexually active females age 15-44 who received reproductive health services in past 12 months
	Persons living with HIV infection who know their serologic status
Social determinants	Students who graduate with a regular diploma 4 years after starting ninth grade
Substance abuse	Adolescents using alcohol or any illicit drugs during past 30 days
	Adults engaging in binge drinking during past 30 days
Tobacco	Adults who are current cigarette smokers
	Adolescents who smoked cigarettes in past 30 days

Modified from *Healthy People 2020*, U.S. Department of Health and Human Services: http://healthypeople.gov/2020/TopicsObjectives2020/pdfs/HP2020_brochure_with_LHI_508.pdf effective? Are there effective interventions suited for that community? What might effective interventions cost? What is the likely return on investment?

Recommendations address a wide variety of topics, such as the following:

- Worksite health promotion (e.g., tobacco policy, physical inactivity, health risk appraisal)
- Supporting local community health (e.g., community water fluoridation, school vaccination program, school-based physical education)
- Addressing social determinants of health

After balancing the evidence and cost-effectiveness of recommendations, the guide provides the following ratings: recommended, recommended against, and insufficient evidence.

RECOMMENDATIONS

Changing Risk Behaviors Commensurate with policy successes, data is abundant to rate tobacco interventions (see Box 26-1), but much less for other less-funded topics, such as high-calorie foods and firearms. There are also sometimes heterogeneous results for identical interventions on various diseases, such as patient reminders for breast cancer screenings versus other cancers. Examples for community interventions aimed at changing risk behaviors[43] include community-wide campaigns to promote the intake of folic acid among women of childbearing age and restricted hours for teenage drivers (see Chapter 24).

Addressing the Environment Commensurate with the influence of environment on behavior, many community guide recommendations address the importance of the environment. Examples include laws mandating seat belt use, community-level urban redesign to make neighborhoods more walkable and bikeable, and community water fluoridation to decrease caries. Other agencies have also published numerous strategies to improve diet and exercise (e.g., improving school food policies to make healthy choices available for lunches and snacks), adopting worksite wellness policies that promote healthy lifestyle choices for staff and the community, establishing smoke-free environments in parks, and establishing farmers' markets and community gardens.

Reducing Disease, Injury, and Impairment Community guide recommendations addressing the reduction of disease, injury, and impairment include early-childhood home visitation programs for violence and injury prevention, influenza vaccination programs for health care workers, and partner notification for HIV-positive individuals.

2. Cultural Congruence of Interventions

It is important to balance evidence-based interventions with those that are culturally congruent with the community. Health program evaluators have long known that a particular program may be an outstanding success in one community, place, and time, yet fail miserably in another community or even in the same community at another time. Even strong evidence is not a substitute for common sense and sensitivity to local culture. Evidence supports that interventions with community support and perceived as culturally congruent are more effective.[44] Lastly, any intervention needs to be tailored to individual patients' needs for maximum engagement, especially for hard-to-reach populations.[45]

E. Implement Innovations

Implementation of interventions poses its own challenges, mainly managing people's reaction to change (see Chapter 28). The role of the environment and community capacity should not be underestimated. The *Guide to Community Preventive Services* evaluates the effectiveness of types of interventions (vs. individual programs) by conducting systematic reviews of all available research in collaboration with partners. One such innovation is the **Research Tested Intervention Program** (RTIP), a searchable database of cancer control interventions with detailed program materials. RTIP is designed to provide program planners and public health practitioners with easy and immediate access to research-tested materials.

F. Evaluate

Evaluation should be built into the entire process of any project. The evaluation must be planned at the start of the planning process. If left until the end of the project, important opportunities to understand what did and did not work may be lost. The overall structure of an evaluation program was outlined by the CDC in 1999 with 30 standards for effective program evaluation guided by the following overarching principles[46] (Fig. 26-4):

Utility. Evaluations should serve the practical information needs of a given audience. Questions for this domain include: Is the purpose of your evaluation clear? Who needs the information, and what information do they need? Will the evaluation provide relevant, useful information in a timely manner?

Feasibility. Evaluations take place in the field and should be realistic, prudent, diplomatic, and frugal. Questions for this domain include: How practical is your evaluation? How much money, time, and effort can you invest? Is the planned evaluation realistic, given the time, resources, and expertise available?

Propriety. The rights of individuals affected by evaluations should be protected. Questions for this area include: What steps need to be taken for your evaluation to be ethical and legal? Does it protect the rights and welfare of the individuals involved? Does it engage those affected by the program and the evaluation?

Accuracy. Evaluations should produce and convey accurate information about a program's merit and value. Questions for this area include: Have you documented your program clearly and accurately? What design will provide accurate, valid, and reliable information? Have you demonstrated that your measures are valid and reliable? Have you used appropriate analyses, and are your conclusions justified? Is your report impartial?

Other examples of domains to think through in evaluation include the RE-AIM model: **reach, efficacy, adoption, implementation, maintenance.**[47]

For evaluating, it can sometimes be helpful to structure evaluation of a project in the logic model. The **basic logic**

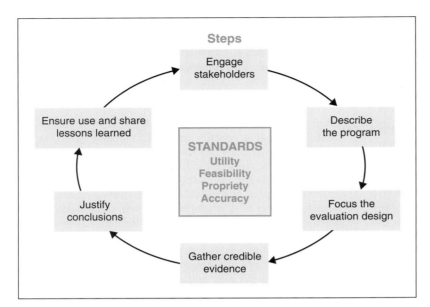

Figure 26-4 Program evaluation in public health.
(Modified from Baker QE, Davis DA, Gallerani R, et al: *An evaluation framework for community health programs,* Durham, NC, 2000, Center for the Advancement of Community Based Public Health. http://www.doh.state.fl.us/ COMPASS/documents/Community_Health_Programs_ Eval.pdf)

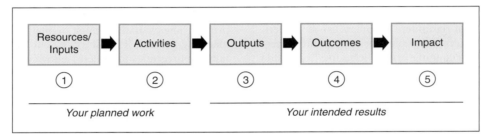

Figure 26-5 **Basic logic model.** (Modified from *The logic model development guide,* 1998, WK Kellogg Foundation. http://www.wkkf.org/knowledge-center/resources/2006/02/WK-Kellogg-Foundation-Logic-Model-Development-Guide.aspx)

model distinguishes resources, input, output, outcomes, and impact (Fig 26-5).

Evaluations can be done using qualitative or quantitative methods and can be formative or summative type. Questions for a **formative** evaluation include: Was the process implemented? Which activities, meetings, or training sessions were implemented, and when? A **summative** evaluation attempts to assess if the program had the expected impact/outcome. In practice, most evaluations are *quantitative* (e.g., surveys, screening, data collections, chart reviews, computer-generated reports). They use numerical data to evaluate objectives. However, quantitative evaluation will not provide information about why an intervention did or did not work, and whether participants were satisfied with the interventions. *Qualitative* methods can answer those questions; examples include direct observations, satisfaction surveys, focus groups, and interviews with providers or program participants (Fig. 26-6).

III. FUTURE CHALLENGES

Multiple challenges are inherent in the program planning process and are likely to become worse with decreasing resources and an environment less and less conducive to healthy lifestyles. A few of these challenges are outlined here.

A. Integrating Clinical Care and Prevention

Interventions that address multiple levels simultaneously are much more effective than interventions aimed at one group (e.g., tobacco quit rates among adolescents are higher if parents and adolescents are targeted at the same time).[48] Although some health problems might be best addressed by either a clinical prevention approach *or* a community approach, the theories listed at the beginning of this chapter teach us that an integrated and combined approach is usually most effective.[49] Interventions on both levels usually reinforce each other and also leverage existing resources for maximum impact.

B. Integrating Community-Based Prevention with Other Community Services

Another approach to prevention is to integrate it with other community services. This has been demonstrated successfully with the **Sickness Prevention Achieved through Regional Collaboration** (SPARC) model,[50] which integrates preventive services with voting booths and home-delivered meals. Other examples include school-based health clinics, and work-based incentives and competitions (see Chapter 22).

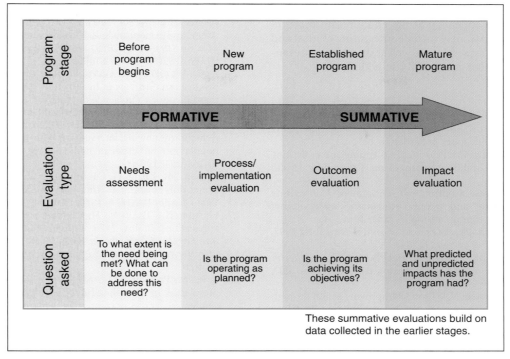

Figure 26-6 **Summary of evaluation procedures.** (Modifed from Norland E: From education theory ... to conservation practices. Annual Meeting of the International Association for Fish & Wildlife Agencies, Atlantic City, NJ, 2004; Pancer SM, Westhues A: A developmental stage approach to program planning and evaluation, *Eval Rev* 13:56–77, 1989; and Rossi PH, Lipsey MW, Freeman HE: *Evaluation: a systematic approach*, Thousand Oaks, Calif, 2004, Sage.)

C. E-Health

Electronic health information (e-health) includes the use of traditional media for new uses (e.g., TV series to promote healthy eating among Hispanic viewers),[51] as well as new media. Newer communication strategies include, but are not limited to, health information on the Internet, online support groups, online collaborative communities, information tailored by computer technologies, educational computer games, computer-controlled in-home telephone counseling, and patient-provider e-mail contact. Major benefits of e-health strategies follow:

- Increased reach (ability to communicate to broad, geographically dispersed audiences)
- Asynchronous communication (interaction not bounded by having to communicate at the same time)
- Ability to integrate multiple communication modes and formats (e.g., audio, video, text, graphics)
- Ability to track, preserve, and analyze communication (computer records of interaction, analysis of interaction trends)
- User control of the communication system (ability to customize programs to user specifications)
- Interactivity (e.g., increased capacity for feedback)

Examples for such successful use of new media include a video game series to improve children's and adolescents' self-care behaviors for asthma;[52] texting adolescents with sexual health test messages;[53] and the use of Internet tools to increase diagnosis of hepatitis C.[54]

Social media and emerging technologies will likely blur the line between expert and peer health information. Monitoring and assessing the impact of these new media (e.g.,

mobile health) on public health will be challenging. Further challenges arise with changes in health care quality and efficiency resulting from the creative use of health communication and information technology (IT). Capturing the scope and impact of these changes—and the role of health communication and health IT in facilitating them—will require multidisciplinary models and data systems. Such systems will be critical to expanding the collection of data to better understand the effects of health communication and health IT on population health outcomes, health care quality, and health disparities.[39]

IV. SUMMARY

Community program planning is defined as an organized process to design, implement, and evaluate a community-based project to address the needs of a defined population. Community planning should be guided by theories (social cognitive, diffusion, communication). Changing the structural, social, and political environment to be more conducive to healthy behavior is crucial. Multiple models to guide community planning are available, including PRECEDE/ PROCEED, PATCH, CHANGE, and MAPP. Community planning includes these steps: assemble a team, assess community health status, define objectives, select effective intervention, implement the intervention, and evaluate. The *Healthy People 2020* objectives provide science-based objectives for 26 leading health indicators. The *Guide to Community Preventive Services* evaluates community interventions in a rigorous, science-driven process, providing science-based recommendations on interventions proved effective. Evaluations can be formative or summative, and the evaluation process should be built into the entire program process rather than appended at the end. Future trends in community prevention may include integrating clinical and community preventive services as well as integrating preventive services with other community activities.

References

1. McKenzie J, Pinger R, Kotecki J: *An introduction to community health*, Boston, 2005, Jones & Bartlett, p 127.
2. Frazier PJ, Horowitz AM: Priorities in planning and evaluating community oral health programs. *Fam Community Health* 3:103–113, 1980.
3. Centers for Disease Control and Prevention: Community health assessment and group evaluation. www.cdc.gov/healthycommunitiesprogram/tools/change.htm
4. Bandura A: *Self-efficacy: the exercise of control*, New York, 1997, WH Freeman.
5. Glanz K, Rimer BK, Lewis FM: *Health behavior and health education: theory, research and practice*, San Francisco, 2002, Wiley & Sons.
6. Minkler M, Wallerstein N, Wilson N: Improving health through community organization and community building. In Glanz K, Rimer BK, Lewis FM, editors: *Health behavior and health education: theory, research, and practice*, San Francisco, 2008, Wiley & Sons.
7. Jacobs G: Conflicting demands and the power of defensive routines in participatory action research. *Action Res* 8:367, 2010.
8. Cornwall A, Jewkes J: What is participatory action research? *Soc Sci Med* 41:1667–1676, 1995.
9. Dick B: Action Research and Action Learning for community and organizational change, 2002. http://www.aral.com.au/resources/aandr.html
10. Reason P, Bradbury H, editors: *Handbook of action research: participative inquiry and practice*, Thousand Oaks, Calif, 2001, Sage.
11. Hult M, Lennung S: Towards a definition of action research: a note and bibliography. *J Manage Stud* 17:242–250, 1980.
12. McNiff J: Action research for professional development, ed 3. http://www.jeanmcniff.com/ar-booklet.asp
13. Minkler M, Wallerstein N, editors: *Community-based participatory research for health: from process to outcomes*, ed 2, San Francisco, 2008, Jossey-Bass.
14. Stoecker R: Making connections: community organizing, empowerment planning, and participatory research in participatory evaluation. *Sociol Pract* 1:209–232, 1999.
15. Green LW: Ethics and community-based participatory research: commentary on Minkler. *Health Educ Behav* 31:698–701, 2004.
16. Kur E, DePorres D, Westrup N: Teaching and learning action research: transforming students, faculty and university in Mexico. *Action Res* 6:327–349, 2008.
17. Sankaran S, Hase S, Dick B, et al: Singing different tunes from the same song sheet: four perspectives of teaching the doing of action research. *Action Res* 5:293–305, 2007.
18. Ospina S, Dodge J, Godsoe B, et al: From consent to mutual inquiry: balancing democracy and authority in action research. *J Action Res* 2:47–69, 2004.
19. Katz DL, Murimi M, Gonzalez A, et al: Controlled trial to community adoption: the Multisite Translational Community Trial. *Am J Public Health* 101:e17–e27, 2011.
20. Rogers EM: *Diffusion of innovations*, ed 5, New York, 2003, Free Press.
21. Hastings G, Saren M: The critical contribution of social marketing: theory and application. *Mark Theory* 3:305–322, 2003.
22. Forthofer MS, Bryant CA: Using audience-segmentation techniques to tailor health behavior change strategies. *Am J Health Behav* 24:36–43, 2000.
23. Huhman M, Berkowitz JM, Wong FL, et al: The VERB campaign's strategy for reaching African-American, Hispanic, Asian, and American Indian children and parents. *Am J Prev Med* 34:S194–S209, 2008. http://www.ajpmonline.org/article/S0749-3797(08)00261-4/fulltext
24. Evans WD, Hastings G: Public health branding: recognition, promise, and delivery of healthy lifestyles. In Evans WD, Hastings G, editors: *Public health branding: applying marketing for social change*, London, 2008, Oxford University Press.
25. Kelly JA, St Lawrence JS, Diaz YE, et al: HIV risk behavior reduction following intervention with key opinion leaders of population: an experimental analysis. *Am J Public Health* 81:168–171, 1991.
26. Gibson DR, Zhang G, Cassady D, et al: Effectiveness of HIV prevention social marketing with injecting drug users. *Am J Public Health* 100:1828–1830, 2010.
27. Linstone HA, Turoff M: The Delphic methods: techniques and applications. *Boston, 1975, Addison-Wesley. Available at http://is.njit.edu/pubs/delphibook*, 2002.
28. http://www.hsph.harvard.edu/research/chc/harvard-alcohol-project/
29. Osler M, Prescott E, Gottschau A, et al: Trends in smoking prevalence in Danish adults, 1964-1994: the influence of gender, age, and education. *Scand J Soc Med* 26:293–298, 1998.
30. Runyan CW: Introduction: back to the future—revisiting Haddon's conceptualization of injury. Epidemiology and prevention. *Epidemiol Rev* 25:60–64, 2003.
31. Hanlon JJ, Pickett GF: *Public health administration and practice*, St Louis, 1984, Mosby.
32. Feinberg ME, Bontempo DE, Greenberg MT: Predictors and level of sustainability of community prevention coalitions. *Am J Prev Med* 34:495–501, 2008.
33. Porterfield DS, Hinnant L, Stevens DM, et al: The diabetes primary prevention initiative interventions focus area: A case study and recommendations. *Am J Prev Med* 39:235–242, 2010.
34. Cowlitz County healthy communities assessment workbook, Pub No 345–296, Washington State Department of Health.
35. http://depts.washington.edu/waaction/action/n2/DOH-HC_Workbook_Cowlitz.pdf
36. Gold R, Green LW, Kreuter MW: *EMPOWER: enabling methods of planning and organizing within everyone's research*, Sudbury, Mass, 1997, Jones & Bartlett.
37. Green LW: Prevention and health education. In Last JM, Wallace RB, editors: *Maxcy-Rosnau-Last: Public health and preventive medicine*, ed 13, Norwalk, Conn, 1992, Appleton & Lange.
38. Nelson CF, Kreuter MW, Watkins NB, et al: A partnership between the community, state and federal government: rhetoric or reality? *Hygiene* 5:27–31, 1986.
39. http://healthypeople.gov/2020/topicsobjectives2020/overview.aspx?topicid=18
40. http://www.healthypeople.gov/2020/LHI/2020indicators.aspx.
41. Benedict I, et al: Developing the *Guide to community preventive services*: overview and rationale. *Am J Prev Med* 18(1 suppl):18–26, 2000.
42. www.thecommunityguide.org
43. http://www.nrpa.org
44. Plescia M, Herrick H, Chavis L: Improving health behaviors in an African American community: the Charlotte racial and ethnic approaches to community health project. *Am J Public Health* 98:1678–1684, 2008.
45. Lee E, Mitchell-Herzfeld SD, Lowenfels AA, et al: Reducing low birth weight through home visitation: a randomized controlled trial. *Am J Prev Med* 36:1554–1560, 2009.
46. http://www.cdc.gov/mmwr/pdf/rr/rr4811.pdf
47. http://cancercontrol.cancer.gov/is/reaim/
48. Guillamo-Ramos V, Jaccard J, Dittus P, et al: The Linking Lives health education program: a randomized clinical trial of a parent-based tobacco use prevention program for African American and Latino youths. *Am J Public Health* 100:1641–1647, 2010.

49. Ockene JK: Integrating evidence-based clinical and community strategies to improve health. *Am J Prev Med* 32:244–252, 2007.

50. http://www.cdc.gov/aging/states/sparc.htm

51. Hinojosa MS, Nelson D, Hinojosa R, et al: Using fotonovelas to promote healthy eating in a Latino community. *Am J Public Health* 101:258–259, 2011.

52. Lieberman DA: Management of chronic pediatric diseases with interactive health games: theory and research findings. *J Ambulatory Care Manage* 24:26–38, 2001.

53. Levine D, McCright J, Dobkin L, et al: Sexinfo: a sexual health text messaging service for San Francisco youth. *Am J Public Health* 98:393–395, 2008.

54. Zuure FR, Davidovich U, Coutinho RA, et al: Using mass media and the Internet as tools to diagnose hepatitis C infections in the general population. *Am J Prev Med* 40:345–352, 2011.

Select Readings

Public health management tools. In Wallace RB, editor: *Maxcy-Rosenau-Last: Public health and preventive medicine*, ed 15, New York, 2008, McGraw-Hill Medical.

Yarbrough DB, Shulha LM, Hopson RK: *The program evaluation standards: a guide for evaluators and evaluation users*, ed 3, Thousand Oaks, Calif, 2011, Sage. American Evaluation Association. http://www.eval.org/

Websites

http://www.ahrq.gov
http://www.thecommunityguide.org
http://www.countyhealthrankings.org/
http://www.effectiveinterventions.org
http://www.healthypeople.gov
http://www.naccho.org/
http://www.prevent.org
http://www.wkkf.org/knowledge-center

Disaster Epidemiology and Surveillance

LINDA DEGUTIS

I. OVERVIEW

Before discussing disaster epidemiology and surveillance, it is important to define what is meant by disaster. A **disaster** is generally considered to be an event that puts an overwhelming stress on a system such that the resources used on a daily basis are inadequate for dealing with the impact of the event. The resources may be inadequate because of the number of people affected by the event, or because the resources themselves have been damaged or limited as a result of the event. Disasters may be further categorized by *intent* or *cause*. Whereas **natural disasters** are events such as tsunamis, hurricanes, tornadoes, earthquakes, and floods, **man-made disasters** are related to human-developed technology and may be *unintentional*, such as a train crash, or *intentional*, such as a terrorist attack or the intentional distribution of a toxic agent (e.g., 1995 sarin gas release in Tokyo subway, 2011 anthrax letters sent in U.S.). In either case, the epidemiology and surveillance needs in a disaster may be impacted by the type of event that has occurred.

Disaster epidemiology and surveillance are rooted in epidemiologic principles that apply to other diseases, but unique challenges and concerns need to be considered in the context of disaster epidemiology. Investigators use disaster epidemiology to assess the short-term and long-term health effects

of disasters. In addition, disaster epidemiology is important in allowing epidemiologists to understand how to prevent deaths, injuries, and disease spread in disaster situations. Despite advances in disaster epidemiology, however, there is still a need to refine the approaches to surveillance and epidemiology in disaster situations, as Noji[1] stated in 1992.

Unlike in other types of events, when we perform epidemiologic studies and surveillance in disasters, we focus on not only the inhabitants of a community affected by the disaster, but also the workers and volunteers who respond to a disaster. These responders are often at risk for injury or disease because of their involvement in the response (e.g., an NYC Fire Department chaplain responding on 9/11 was killed by a falling object). In other situations, workers may be exposed to infectious diseases or injury risks.

A. Burden of Disaster

The World Health Organization (WHO) reports that 385 natural disasters killed more than 297,000 people in 2010. An additional 217 million people were affected by the disasters, at a cost equivalent to $123.9 billion in economic damages.[2] In the United States, there has been a steady increase in the number of official disaster "declarations" from 1990 to 2011, with 100 declarations in 2011 (Fig. 27-1).

II. DEFINITIONS AND OBJECTIVES

To have a basis for understanding the issues associated with disaster epidemiology and surveillance, it is important to understand the definitions commonly used in the study of disasters. First, a disaster could be considered to be an event that places a strain on the health or public health system such that additional resources are needed in order to respond. Disasters may occur within an institution, in a community, or on a broader scale. Disasters can be classified in a number of ways, but are usually described as natural or man-made, as previously noted. Natural disasters encompass a range of situations that put people at risk for significant health effects.

Disaster epidemiology is defined as the use of epidemiology to assess the short-term and long-term adverse health effects of disasters and to predict consequences of future disasters. It brings together various topic areas of epidemiology, including acute and communicable disease, environmental health, occupational health, chronic disease, injury, mental health, and behavioral health. Disaster epidemiology provides *situational awareness*; that is, it provides information that helps responders understand what the needs are, plan the response, and gather the appropriate resources.

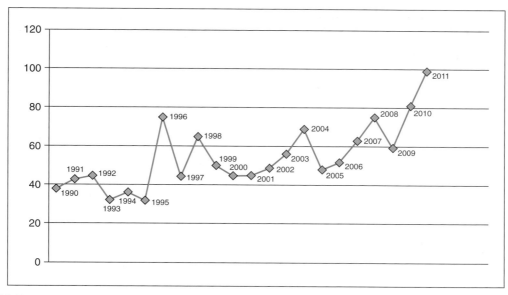

Figure 27-1 Disaster declarations by year, United States, 1990-2011. (From http://www.fema.gov/news/disaster_totals_annual.fema.)

The main objectives of disaster epidemiology are as follows:

- Prevent or reduce the number of deaths, illnesses, and injuries caused by disasters.
- Provide timely and accurate health information for decision makers.
- Improve prevention and mitigation strategies for future disasters by collecting information for future response preparation.

As with other types of epidemiology, disaster epidemiology focuses on identifying disease and injury patterns and risk factors to the population and community affected by the disaster. This information serves as the basis for developing prevention and mitigation strategies that are driven by three contexts of disasters: *time, place,* and *person.* For example, hurricane season on the U.S. East Coast, as well as in the Caribbean, is June 1 through November 30.[3] In addition, the geographic area generally at risk is defined. Although people who live on or near the coast are at increased risk of injury or death during a hurricane, evacuation from the hurricane zone minimizes or eliminates this risk. In contrast, the usual season for flu occurrence is over the winter months in the United States, and flu risk is related to exposure, immunization status, and other factors such as age; generally, elderly and very young populations, people with chronic illness or immunocompromise, and pregnant women are at increased risks for complications and mortality, depending on the flu strain that is active in a given year.[4] Prevention strategies would focus on immunization of highest-risk populations, and depending on the severity of an outbreak, isolation of people who have contracted flu or who have been exposed and are likely to expose others to risk.

In a disaster situation, three types of epidemiology generally are used: descriptive, analytic, and evaluative. Each contributes to the understanding of the disaster event, as well as the prevention and mitigation of harm from future events.

A. Descriptive Epidemiology

Epidemiologists use descriptive epidemiology to identify the distribution of disease or injury among the population groups affected by the disaster. This includes identifying the health-related issues that occur among people who are responding to the event.

After the World Trade Center disaster on 9/11, responders to the scene were exposed to various types of particulate matter, as well as larger pieces of debris, some of which fell from the collapsing towers. Other responders have complained of resulting respiratory problems. The epidemiology of the health aftermath of the disaster continues to emerge; longitudinal surveys are providing information on various health outcomes. A study of 2960 disaster workers found that 70% did not meet criteria for posttraumatic stress disorder (PTSD), but at 6 years after the event, 4.2% of nonrescue disaster workers still exhibited symptoms of PTSD or partial PTSD. Risk factors for ongoing PTSD included major depressive disorder 1 to 2 years after the event, history of trauma, and extent of occupational exposure.[5] Asthma rates are increased in the disaster responders as well, with a lifetime prevalence by 2007 that was almost twice (19% vs. 10%) that of the general population.[6] On a larger scale, the World Trade Center Health Registry at the New York City Department of Health and Mental Hygiene will provide a 20-year follow-up through periodic contact with the enrollees[7] (Box 27-1).

B. Analytic Epidemiology

Analytic epidemiology can provide information about differences between people who were injured or became ill during an event and those who did not. The benefit is that analytic epidemiology gives information about the **risk and protective factors** related to a disaster event. For example, an ongoing investigation of deaths and injuries after the 2011 tornado outbreak in Alabama can provide data about where people were when they were killed or injured, the types of

The current survey includes over 41,000 respondents as of February 28, 2012, and is split between survivors (>38,000) and responders (>31,000). Through the overall survey and special surveys, the Registry is being used to investigate the following:

- Cardiovascular disease
- Skin rash
- Alcohol use
- Posttraumatic stress disorder (PTSD) among police
- Unmet mental health care needs
- Cancer rates among enrollees
- Health of Staten Island landfill and barge recovery workers
- Respiratory and behavioral health of children
- Impact of 9/11 injuries on long-term enrollee health
- Coexistence, or comorbidity, of respiratory and mental health conditions experienced by many enrollees

Data from New York City Department of Health and Mental Hygiene, World Trade Center Registry, Survey response rate. http://www.nyc.gov/html/doh/wtc/downloads/pdf/registry/wave3-survey-response-rate.pdf. Accessed March 15, 2012.

injuries sustained, and whether protective factors had an impact on the occurrence of injuries. These may be environmental or behavioral factors. This type of study allows informed recommendations for interventions to help protect people from injury caused by tornadoes.

C. Evaluative Epidemiology

In using evaluative epidemiology, investigators can determine the effectiveness of specific interventions that have been implemented and identify factors that have resulted in their success or failure. It allows them to modify strategies and develop new interventions. This allows epidemiologists to determine, for example, if specific immunization strategies are effective in preventing spread of flu, or whether environmental changes (building standards) are effective in decreasing building collapses, and therefore deaths and injuries, in earthquakes.

III. PURPOSE OF DISASTER EPIDEMIOLOGY

Disaster epidemiology allows investigators to identify the priority health problems in the community affected by a disaster. Although the primary focus is on health problems related to the disaster itself, epidemiologists can also learn about preexisting health problems that impact a community's resilience and create needs for specific services during a disaster. In a disaster or public health emergency, it is also important to identify the causes of disease and injury and associated risk factors in the context of the event. This may include examining the results of laboratory testing of biologic and other specimens to identify specific disease agents or toxic substances involved in the event.

Various methods of classifying severity of injury or illness can aid in determining priorities for health interventions.

The epidemiologic assessment of health problems allows for a rapid needs assessment that leads to planning for interventions; identification of the need for additional help; and modifications as well as additional support for the infrastructure. As an event evolves, continued surveillance and epidemiology allow tracking of the course of diseases, as well as identification of emerging issues. For example, although many people were killed and injured in the 7.0 earthquake in Haiti on January 12, 2010, it took several days to identify the emergence of cholera, which presented a significant risk to the survivors. Epidemiology was used to identify cases and the spread of the disease. In January 2011 the Pan American Health Organization[8] released a report on the health impact of the earthquake, highlighting lessons that could be applied to the next major disaster event. In this way, the epidemiology and surveillance from one disaster can be used to inform planning and response for future events.

A. Forensic Epidemiology

Forensic epidemiology is not discussed as often as it might be with respect to disaster epidemiology. The field of forensic epidemiology brings together public health and a legal investigative approach to examining a disaster or emergency situation. This is especially important in cases of suspected bioterrorism and other intentionally created events. Forensic epidemiology explores the intent, persons involved, degree of harm, and risk factors, to form a complete picture of an intentional disaster. The 1985 investigation of intentional contamination of salad bars in Oregon led to the prosecution of the religious group responsible.[9]

IV. DISASTER SURVEILLANCE

As with other parts of epidemiologic practice, surveillance plays a critical role in epidemiologic investigations during and after a disaster. One of the major challenges of surveillance in disasters is that many routine surveillance systems may not provide the information necessary to assess needs or identify disease or injury patterns. This occurs in both natural and human-made disasters and creates difficulty for all types of disaster epidemiology. Disasters present special circumstances in which surveillance may be difficult, and during which routine surveillance systems may not be functional or accessible, because of the circumstances of the disaster.

A. Syndromic Surveillance

Syndromic surveillance uses indicators of population and individual health that may appear before widespread disease is confirmed through clinical or laboratory diagnosis. This type of surveillance is often set up as a routine surveillance mechanism that is in place to monitor for specific diseases. For example, a sharp increase in sales of over-the-counter cold remedies might indicate the emergence of a new respiratory virus. Across the United States, emergency departments participate in syndromic surveillance systems designed to detect clusters of events in the early phases of an outbreak, such as gastrointestinal illness caused by food poisoning or disaster. Syndromic surveillance systems may be based on existing data systems, particularly when electronic health records are available in real time. If the focus is looking for a specific disease, case criteria for surveillance are identified, whereas in a more general syndromic surveillance strategy, data may be monitored for unusual patterns that could indicate emerging disease. The Centers for Disease Control and Prevention (CDC) has developed definitions for diseases associated with critical bioterrorism agents.[10] In addition, syndromic surveillance may be implemented on a short-term basis during specific events when there is a possibility of either disease transmission or an intentional act that results in illness. For example, during the 2002 Kentucky Derby Festival, 12 hospitals successfully participated in the surveillance system that was set up.[11]

B. Challenges in Disaster Surveillance and Epidemiology

To perform disaster surveillance activities, it is important to predefine the variables and data points that would be of interest during a particular type of disaster. Although a core set of variables is important in any disaster event, each type of event has unique circumstances that need to be documented to understand fully the impact of the event. For example, the spread of a newly emerging strain of flu would necessitate identification of the strain causing infections in the population of interest, at least to the extent that one can assume the cases beyond a certain point in time could be attributable to the agent that has already been identified. In the case of a tornado or earthquake, the specific location of victims, with details about the type of building, the force of the tornado or earthquake, and the injuries sustained and their severity, and the outcome for each person injured are all important data to collect. In an infectious disease outbreak, the trajectory of the impact on the population is very different, and there may be more time to collect data in order to plan for the resources and interventions that will be needed. These are data points in addition to demographic data.

Surveillance is also important after the disaster, particularly if there are risks for the development and increased transmission of infectious diseases due to the nature of the event. Events that disrupt water supplies and sanitation place the communities affected at risk for the spread of infectious disease from contaminated water sources. Other postdisaster outcomes of interest include recovery status of injured disaster victims. An understanding of the severity of injuries sustained, as well as long-term rehabilitation and support needs, will aid in community planning.

C. Designing a Disaster Surveillance System

As much as possible, a disaster surveillance system should not require a large amount of additional resources during a disaster event. Because personnel will be consumed with responding to the disaster and implementing interventions, requirements for collecting large amounts of additional data are likely to create difficulties for the personnel involved. The number of skilled staff may be insufficient to collect the data needed, or the staff responding may not have a good understanding of basic epidemiologic principles and measurement. There may be limited access to the population of interest. If a sample of the population is surveyed, it may not be representative of the overall population affected by the

disaster. Cultural and language barriers pose additional problems, along with the difficulty in investigating the long-term needs of the affected population.

A core set of data points can be used in surveillance in most disaster events. Demographic data as well as simple outcome data for both victims and responders are useful in tracking the impact of the disaster as well as identifying the need for resources. A data system design that allows for a *modular* approach, depending on the type of event as well as the phase of the event, may be useful. System design requires consideration of the data collection methods that are routinely available and that may be available after the disaster. In addition, it is important to consider the burden that data collection will present to an already-stressed system. Whenever possible, it is important to use existing data systems rather than creating new systems that have not been tested or accepted by those involved in a disaster response; the simpler the data collection, the better. It is also possible to collect postdisaster data and interview people who were at the scene, but this is not always optimal because of the potential for *recall bias* and for data to be missing from patient records. Data collection during and after a disaster must take into account existing data sets and information; the size, demographics, and baseline health status of the population affected; and available resources. Geographic mapping can be useful in examining the impact of environmental factors in a disaster.

When there is an urgent need for information or acquisition of resources, a rapid survey may be done. In this scenario, only the minimum information necessary to meet the surveillance goals is collected. Only information that is not already available or cannot be collected in another way is obtained, and the goal becomes to collect as representative a sample as possible to ensure generalizability to the population affected. This type of survey is sometimes repeated and refined over the course of the event and postevent period.

In the postdisaster period, surveys of persons who were present during the event may be helpful, as may surveys of those who were injured or who became ill during the event. Key informant interviews can provide information about risks and mitigating factors experienced in the community and can help identify approaches to planning for future events. As previously described, longitudinal surveys of survivors and responders provide information about long-term health and social impacts.

V. ROLE OF GOVERNMENT AGENCIES AND NONGOVERNMENTAL ORGANIZATIONS

Preparedness for and response to disasters and pandemics require a coordinated effort from multiple agencies and organizations. Although an in-depth discussion is beyond the scope of this chapter, a brief summary of the role of federal agencies and nongovernmental organizations (NGOs) is helpful in understanding the multifaceted nature of preparedness and response.

Public health focuses on overall population health and ensuring that population-based measures are in place for disaster preparedness and response. Surveillance activities are in the realm of public health, as is disease reporting and investigation of disease and injury occurrence. **Emergency**

management agencies, which exist at various governmental levels, focus on the overall management of a disaster response and coordination of recovery services, and may be responsible for allocation of resources. The U.S. Federal Emergency Management Agency (FEMA), now in the Department of Homeland Security, works to plan for disasters and terrorism, makes recommendations to the public on how to prepare for events, provides education for responders, and reviews disaster declaration requests from governors to ensure that resources are appropriately allocated and distributed.[12]

Various other agencies are involved in preparing for and responding to disasters at the local, state, and federal levels. The private sector and NGOs, such as the American Red Cross,[13] have an important role as well, providing services such as shelter, food, and clothing. NGOs also respond to disasters that occur around the world, providing emergency and long-term shelter, health care, food, clothing, and other services.

VI. SUMMARY

Disaster epidemiology and surveillance are critical components of a disaster response and can contribute to understanding the nature of an event as well as the implications for planning for future events. There are unique challenges presented in performing surveillance during disasters, but the efforts made at surveillance and epidemiology provide valuable contributions to our understanding of disasters and planning for future events.

References

1. Noji EK: Disaster epidemiology: challenges for public health action. *J Public Health Policy* 13:332–340, 1992.

2. Guha-Sapir D, Vos F, Below R, et al: *Annual disaster statistical review 2010: the numbers and trends*, Brussels, 2011, Centre for Research on the Epidemiology of Disasters.

3. National Oceanic and Atmospheric Administration: National Weather Service. National Hurricane Center, 2012. http://www.nhc.noaa.gov/

4. Centers for Disease Control and Prevention: Key facts about flu vaccine. http://www.cdc.gov/flu/protect/keyfacts.htm

5. Cukor J, Wyka K, Mello B, et al: The longitudinal course of PTSD among disaster workers deployed to the World Trade Center following the attacks of September 11th. *J Trauma Stress* 24:506–514, 2011.

6. Kim H, Herbert R, Landrigan P, et al: Increased rates of asthma among World Trade Center disaster responders. *Am J Ind Med* 55:44–53, 2012.

7. New York City Department of Health and Mental Hygiene: 9/11 health, WTC Health Registry. http://www.nyc.gov/html/doh/wtc/html/registry/registry.shtml

8. Pan American Health Organization: *Health response to the earthquake in Haiti: January 2010*, Washington, DC, 2011, PAHO.

9. Török TJ, Tauxe RV, Wise PR, et al: A large community outbreak of salmonellosis caused by intentional contamination of restaurant salad bars. *JAMA* 278:389–395, 1997.

10. Syndrome definitions for diseases associated with critical bioterrorism-associated agents, Oct 23, 2003. http://www.bt.cdc.gov/surveillance/syndromedef/

11. Carrico R, Goss L: Syndromic surveillance: hospital emergency department participation during the Kentucky Derby Festival. *Disaster Manage Response* 3:73–79, 2005.

12. FEMA's role in winter weather. http://blog.fema.gov/2010/12/femas-role-in-winter-weather.html

13. American Red Cross. http://www.redcross.org/

28

Health Management, Health Administration, and Quality Improvement

Improving an organization first requires understanding it, and managerial skills are universally important. The requirements to run a project successfully are the same for managing a local health department, a clinic for underserved groups, leading a small quality improvement (QI) team, or running a large health care system. Health managers must understand the environment in which they operate; be able to assess organizational performance in regard to finance, clients or patients, and other stakeholders; know how to keep improving; and understand how to hire, promote, and fire the right people. This chapter explores these issues, as in other chapters, through a few of the important concepts. The goal is not to transform the reader into a human resource manager or an accountant. The goal is to familiarize readers with the basics so that they can have an educated conversation with such staff members and understand how each person's work influences the other. Readers who want to know more should consult the specialized literature (see Select Readings).

Health care delivery is ultimately a system involving multiple players: health care organizations, government agencies, for-profit companies, not-for-profits, and elements of various industries, from biotechnology and information technology, to medical devices and pharmaceuticals. The performance of the "health care system" and how it generates its principal outcome (health) relate in part to the structures, processes, and functioning of the system as a whole, along with its component parts. There is a growing awareness that the endeavor to improve the quality, efficiency, and equity of the health care system is a matter of great concern for public health practitioners. This effort is usually called quality improvement.

Long cultivated in other industries, methods of management and quality improvement have been applied more diligently and comprehensively to health care over recent decades. This chapter draws on a literature that is increasingly specific to health care, but originating with industrial applications, to examine the issue of health care delivery from the perspective of **systems management.** An understanding of how systems are structured, managed, monitored, and improved is important to all involved in such systems.

I. ORGANIZATIONAL STRUCTURE AND DECISION MAKING

The basic functions of management include planning, organizing, controlling, and leading. Often, the first three functions are called management or **operational skills,** summarized as "doing things right." In contrast, leadership or **strategic skills** are defined as "doing the right things." To thrive, an organization needs both.

What needs to be done depends on the organization. In the United States, there are for-profit corporations, public agencies, and not-for-profit organizations. Not-for-profits are also called "tax-exempt organizations," or sometimes **501(c)(3)s,** after the federal tax code provision that grants them their tax-exempt status. In any organization, it is vital to understand how revenues and expenses flow through the organization. Despite their name, even not-for-profit organizations need to make a profit to be financially viable. Not-for-profit organizations that do not generate sufficient financial resources will be unable to invest in infrastructure, new technology, or personnel development; consequently, they will eventually close or become obsolete.

To qualify as a **not-for-profit,** an organization's purpose must meet one of the *exempt purposes* in the federal tax code, which include charitable, religious, educational, and scientific endeavours. Many companies, including not-for-profits, also articulate that purpose in a *mission statement* that guides the overall strategy of the organization. Such a mission might be "to improve the health of the population of town X" or to "end cancer." Not-for-profits are governed by a **board of trustees;** in for-profits, such an oversight committee is called the **board of directors.** A board of trustees is the body ultimately responsible for setting the organization's policies and strategies. One of the board's most important jobs is to hire and fire the **chief executive officer** (CEO). The board also approves budgets and oversees the organizational performance. Underneath the CEO is a vice presidential suite, usually the **chief financial officer** (CFO), in charge of finances, and the **chief operational officer** (COO), who oversees day-to-day operations. Most organizations have additional chief officers, depending on their mission and size, such as **chief nursing officer** (CNO), **chief medical officer** (CMO), and **chief information officer** (CIO). In other organizations, such positions might be called **vice president** (VP, e.g., VP of Nursing, VP of Medical Affairs).

Organizations need to do more than just please their boards. They also have **stakeholders.** A stakeholder is anybody who is interested in or affected by the organization's operations. Stakeholders can include patients, community members, local employers, churches, and unions. Most organizations cannot reach major public health goals by themselves and need to build coalitions with other stakeholders to leverage resources and build political will. Organizations applying for grants must show they can build and work with coalitions and partnerships.

Managers and leaders seeking ways to build such coalitions must motivate their staff. For these tasks, it is important to understand how to motivate people. It is customary to distinguish between **extrinsic motivation** (money, status, job perks) and **intrinsic motivation** (desire to do good, sense of accomplishment, desire to be in control). Often, managers must rely mostly on their employees' intrinsic motivation. Fortunately, as long as people's basic safety needs are met, intrinsic motivation is usually enough "to keep people going."

Not everybody responds to the same motivations, however. Key motivators may be caring about doing a job well, job security, job title, the ability to mold things, the chance to learn new things, and the pleasure of working with likable people. These differences in motivators stem from personality types. There have been many ways of distinguishing different personality styles, such as the Myers-Briggs Personality Inventory that famously established *introverts* and *extroverts*. One popular rubric divides people into four types: the **architect** (interested in how things are put together), the **strategist** (interested in the "big picture"), the **diplomat** (interested in how things will be perceived and affect relationships), and the **fact finder** (interested in data, deadlines, and the bottom line).[1] Whatever system one prefers, what is most important is to recognize that such differences exist, and that effective managers address a performance challenge and its possible solutions in ways that meet as many of these dimensions as possible. In any case, when supervising employees, it is better to ask them what is important to them rather than to rely on a theoretical construct of what they ought to care about.

Public health is also a moral pursuit. This requires that the management of a public health agency should be *ethical,* and that the organization's mission should be reflected in its management methods.

II. ASSESSING ORGANIZATIONAL PERFORMANCE

If an organization is to survive, it must periodically assess various dimensions of its performance: finances, processes, people, and mission. Usually, assessment begins with the organization's mission as the basis for goals and measurable objectives. Performance measurement is a cyclical process with these four steps[2]:

1. **Setting performance standards.** The organization identifies relevant standards, selects indicators, sets goals and targets, and communicates expectations.
2. **Performance measurement.** The organization defines measures and valid indicators. It establishes systems for data collection.
3. **Performance reporting.** Data are analyzed and reported to managers, staff, policy makers, and constituents.
4. **Quality improvement.** Based on the analysis, the organization refines or reworks policies and programs and manages the human side of change.

A. Measurement Tools and Budgeting

An important way to assess operational organizational performance is **benchmarking.** To benchmark, an organization conducts a self-assessment and then compares itself to other, similar organizations to gauge its relative performance. For public health agencies, the National Public Health Performance Standards Program has developed such standards, for both state and local health agencies.[3] The Joint Commission provides similar guidance for health care providers (see later).

Instruments to report performance include dashboards and balanced scorecards. **Dashboards** are operational management tools that track many indicators together. For each indicator, there are benchmarks; indicators outside acceptable benchmarks may be shaded red or yellow, whereas acceptable ones may be green. This allows managers and personnel to see immediately which domains are working well and which are not. **Balanced scorecards** provide similar feedback but present a more holistic picture of an organization to link strategic and operational domains. In balanced scorecards an organization's vision, mission, and strategy are followed down into performance measures and initiatives, so that a mission goal can be followed all the way to a specific output and outcome metric[4] (Fig. 28-1).

In addition to providing a visual summary of certain benchmark indicators, balanced scorecards sometimes "weigh" dimensions by how much they contribute to the mission, providing a snapshot of the performance of the entire organization.

The main tool for assessing financial performance is a **budget,** because it can be used to plan, evaluate, and control expenditures. Most public health managers will encounter budgets, both in the planning process and when they are comparing actual performance to budgets. Budget planning is extremely important, since it is pointless to analyze variance from an unrealistic budget. However, all budgeting is based on *assumptions* and therefore represents a "best guess." Such planning can use **incremental budgeting.** For example, a department with five salaried employees the previous year would budget for the next year for the same five employees,

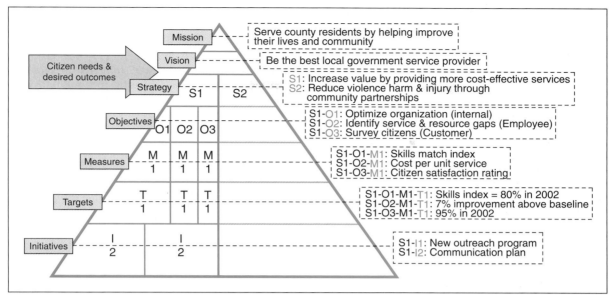

Figure 28-1 Example of balanced scorecard for a local government. (From Rohm H: *Perform* 2[2]. Available at www.balancedscorecard.org/LinkClick.aspx?fileticket=ph%2b8b3YMoBc%3d&tabid=56)

possibly with their salaries adjusted for any cost-of-living increases. The alternative to this is **zero-based budgeting**, in which an organization pretends it starts from zero. All expenditures must be justified not based on precedent, but rather by current need. Incremental budgets are easy to generate, but they may not serve an organization well if its conditions and environment have changed significantly. Zero-based budgeting allows optimal matching of recourses to current needs, although it can be disruptive to employees, stakeholders, and clients.

B. Variance Analysis

The act of comparing actual performance to budgets is called *variance analysis.* This is an extremely important step, because it allows managers to decide if they need to take action now to spend more or less in the future.[5] Budget variances are traditionally called *favorable* and *unfavorable*.

Table 28-1 provides a simple example of budget variance analysis. Budget variance can be caused by unexpected changes in clients, client mix, reimbursement, or expenses. Variance analysis needs to account for fixed and variable costs. As the name implies, *fixed costs* do not change with volume. For example, if one receptionist handles all the calls to an agency, that person's salary is a fixed cost; the pay will not change, whether the receptionist answers 1 or 100 calls per day. In contrast, *variable costs* change with volume (e.g., test strips needed for exam, mileage costs for car).

Other types of variance include the following:

- **Volume variance.** There were fewer or more people served (e.g., more homeowners requested water safety assessment).
- **Quantity** (use) **variance.** It took more of a certain resource to deliver a certain service (e.g., restaurant inspector needed double the number of test strips per restaurant inspection than anticipated).

Table 28-1 Variance Analysis, Unadjusted

	Budget	Actual
Sales volume	100	90
Sales value	1000	990
Variable costs	500	495
Fixed costs	200	210
Profit	300	285

From Palmer DA: Financial management development, No 213. © David A. Palmer 2012. http://www.financialmanagementdevelopment.com/Slides/handouts/213.pdf

Table 28-2 Variance Analysis, with Adjusted Variance

	Original Budget	Revised Budget	Actual	Variances
Sales volume	100	90	90	
Sales value	1000	900	990	90
Variable costs	500	450	495	[45]
Fixed costs	200	200	210	[10]
Profit	300	250	285	35

From Palmer DA: Financial management development, No 213. © David A. Palmer 2012. http://www.financialmanagementdevelopment.com/Slides/handouts/213.pdf

- **Price** (spending, or rate) **variance.** This variance occurs if the price of an input is different from the budgeted price. Price could be the price of a supply item such as radiology equipment.[6]

Table 28-2 provides another way to look at variances. Although the example shows a simple part of a budget from a company, the variance in a public health agency's budget could be analyzed similarly. When analyzing budget variances, it is important to identify *expected* fluctuations from *unexpected* fluctuations. Unexpected fluctuations can usually be found by comparing revenue or expense fluctuations to previous years. If the differences are real, a manager needs to look for reasons. However, it is important first to make sure that there are no faulty calculations in the original budget and no errors in the actual results. It is also important *not* to respond to budget variances that are caused by singular, unexpected events (e.g., natural or man-made disasters). The most common reason for budget variance is a difference between assumptions and reality. Since budgets are informed guesses, it is easy to guess wrong. However, such differences require managerial action *before* the organization is in trouble.[7]

For a public health agency, the budget in Table 28-2 might represent the fees brought in for new home inspections. By custom, favorable variances are shown as positive numbers; negative variances are shown in brackets. Since the revenue was below what was budgeted, one would expect a variance. However, since sales were below expected, the costs have to be adjusted for actual sales volume before further analysis.

Table 28-2 shows the budget revised for the actual volume. Now it is apparent that the sales value was actually higher (a good thing), but that both variable costs and fixed costs were also higher than expected (a bad thing). Armed with these numbers, the manager can investigate further and put fixes in place. For example, the manager might investigate why there is a different demand for the service, commend the salesperson for getting higher prices, and investigate why the fixed and variable costs were higher.

I. Break-even Calculation

Before buying new equipment or starting a new service line, it is important to model out how the new equipment or service would become profitable under various assumptions. Given that most people are too optimistic, it is important to have break-even calculations that recoup money under all or most realistic scenarios. The simplest way to view break-even calculations is to calculate the **break-even point.** For this calculation, one sums up the costs of the equipment and the fixed costs associated with it, then divides it by the expected volume times the profit margin of the procedure (i.e., the charge minus the costs):

$$\text{Break-even point} = \frac{\text{Costs of equipment} + \text{Other fixed costs (staff)}}{\text{Volume} \times \text{Profit margin}}$$

In reality, the calculation needs to take many other factors into consideration. The most important other economic consideration would be the **opportunity cost** of this investment. Opportunity cost describes the next best use of the money and energy. Any investment needs to be better than doing nothing, but also better than the next best use. Other considerations include if the procedure would replace others currently done, if it would require remodeling of space, and how it would change referral patterns.

Box 28-1 outlines the process for buying a new piece of equipment for a physician's office.

III. BASICS OF QUALITY IMPROVEMENT

The quality of medical practice has been a major concern since the early 20th century. In 1910 the historic Flexner Report advocated for higher standards in medical education.[8] After World War II, investigators began to define more clearly the dimensions of quality. In 1969, Donabedian[9] pioneered the study of health care quality by proposing that quality should be examined in terms of **structure** (the physical resources and human resources that a hospital or HMO possesses for providing care), **process** (the way in which the physical and human resources were joined in the activities of physicians and other health care providers), and **outcome** (the end results of care, such as whether the patients actually do as well as would be expected, given the severity of their problems). Another important pioneer of medical quality research was Wennberg, who developed a method of determining population-based rates for the utilization and distribution of health care services. This method, called **small-area analysis,** revealed large variations in health care usage among different areas and was important in determining which procedures or diagnoses most needed standardization or improvement.[10]

Several institutions and programs evaluate the quality of health institutions. State accreditation of facilities usually emphasizes structural and procedural issues. **The Joint Commission**[11] (TJC), formerly the Joint Commission on Accreditation of Healthcare Organizations (JCAHO), is an independent, not-for-profit organization that evaluates the quality and safety of most health care institutions in the United States. Quality review programs of the past, including the programs of **professional review organizations** (PROs), tended to focus on particular aspects of process called *procedural end points* and offered a detailed review of the methods of care provided and an analysis of how well certain disease-specific treatment criteria were met. In contrast, current quality improvement efforts emphasize *quality monitoring* and focus increasingly on outcomes.

One of the primary national data sets on quality of care focuses on the services provided by **managed care organizations** (MCOs), with particular attention to prevention and health maintenance aspects of their health plans. Called the **Healthcare Effectiveness Data and Information Set (HEDIS),**[12] this includes the following areas of prevention:

- Providing immunizations.
- Counseling patients to quit smoking.
- Screening for breast cancer, cervical cancer, hypercholesterolemia, and *Chlamydia* infections.
- Providing prenatal and postpartum care.
- Instituting measures to manage mental illness, menopause, and chronic conditions such as asthma, depression, diabetes, and hypertension.
- Counseling patients regarding the proper use of medications for several diseases.

Several federal agencies play an important role in defining and fostering high-quality health care. The **Health Resources and Services Administration** (HRSA)[13] is unique in that it finances not only quality work but also graduate medical education and direct patient care for underserved populations. The **Centers for Medicare and Medicaid Services** (CMS)[14] financed health care for 100 million people in 2012 through Medicare, Medicaid, and the Children's Health

| Box 28-1 | Break-even Calculations for Buying a Piece of Medical Equipment |

Estimate the number of procedures you will perform with the new medical equipment:

How many of your current patients go to another physician to have the procedure done?

How many of your current patients who otherwise would not have had the procedure done at all will now have you perform the procedure?

How many new patients will you attract by offering the procedure?

On average, how many procedures will each of these patients have per year?

What growth percentage do you expect each year in the number of procedures performed?

Estimated number of procedures for the first year:

Estimate the additional net revenue you expect to receive from the new procedure:

How much will you charge for the procedure?

What percentage of your practice is Medicare?

What is your discount rate for Medicare?

What percentage of your practice is Medicaid?

What is your discount rate for Medicaid?

What percentage of your practice is capitated managed care?

What is your discount rate for capitated managed care?

What percentage of your practice is discounted fee-for-service?

What is your discount rate for fee-for-service?

What percentage of your practice is self-pay?

What is your discount rate for self-pay?

What percentage of your practice is some other payer?

What is your discount rate for those payers on average?

Payer mix:

Estimated gross revenue:

Estimated adjustments to revenue:

Estimated total net revenue:

Estimated net revenue per procedure:

Estimate the lost revenue per year:

What is the amount of revenue you will lose by doing this procedure instead of what you normally do?

Estimated lost revenue per year:

Estimate the acquisition costs of the equipment:

What is the purchase price of the equipment (including any interest paid)?

What is the transportation cost of obtaining the equipment?

What are the remodeling costs associated with installation of the equipment?

Estimated acquisition costs:

Estimate the fixed costs of the equipment:

What is the cost of additional salaried personnel you will hire to use the equipment?

What is the cost of additional space you will acquire to use the equipment (including rent and property tax)?

What is the additional cost of insurance associated with the equipment (i.e., malpractice insurance, property insurance for the equipment, business hazard/loss of use insurance)?

Estimated fixed costs per year:

Estimate the variable costs of the equipment:

What is the additional wage and benefit cost for hourly personnel associated with each procedure?

What is the per-procedure cost of additional supplies you will use to perform this procedure?

Estimated variable costs per procedure:

Estimated total variable costs per year:

Estimate the rate of return on your alternative investments:

What percent return do you expect to make on your other investments during the duration of the analysis?

Modified from Willis DR: How to decide whether to buy new medical equipment. *Fam Pract Manage* 11:53–58, 2004. http://www.aafp.org/fpm/2004/0300/p53.html

Insurance program. As the largest payer in health care, CMS makes decisions on how to pay (DRGs; see Chapter 29), which preventive services to pay for (Chapter 18), and which quality initiatives to pursue, impacting the entire health care system. A good example is the CMS decision in 2011 to reimburse counseling for obesity.[15]

The **Agency for Healthcare Research and Quality** (AHRQ)[16] is the lead federal agency to improve the quality, efficiency, safety, and effectiveness of U.S. health care. The AHRQ website hosts the U.S. Preventive Services Task Force (USPSTF, see Chapter 18) recommendations and the National Guideline Clearinghouse (NGC), as well as survey data on the Medical Expenditure Panel Survey (MEPS) and the Healthcare Cost & Utilization Project (HCUP, see Chapter 25). AHRQ also finances projects to study the comparative effectiveness of various interventions and publishes technology reports that synthesize the status of the evidence on various health care topics. (Box 28-2 lists common health administration organizations and related terms by their acronym.)

In addition, the following **nongovernmental organizations** (NGOs) play an important role in defining and promoting high-quality health care:

The **National Quality Forum** (NQF)[17] convenes expert panels to study and endorse quality and performance metrics. In the prevention area, NQF collaborates with the Department of Health and Human Services (DHHS) to promote homogeneous reporting of adverse events and to align with other organizations in improving the care of people with chronic conditions.

The **Baldrige Program** educates organizations in performance excellence management and administers the Malcolm Baldrige National Quality Award. The organization is a public-private partnership dedicated to improving the performance of U.S. organizations by identifying and sharing best management practices, principles, and strategies.[18]

The **Institute for Healthcare Improvement** (IHI)[19] is an independent not-for-profit organization based in Cambridge, Massachusetts. It focuses on motivating and building the will for change by setting concrete goals and deadlines; identifying and testing new models of care in partnership with both patients and health care professionals; and ensuring the broadest possible adoption of best practices and effective innovations. IHI's highly

Box 28-2	Frequently Used Acronyms in Health Administration
AAFP	American Academy of Family Physicians
ACO	Accountable care organization
AHRQ	Agency for Healthcare Research and Quality
CEO	Chief executive officer
CFO	Chief financial officer
CIO	Chief information officer
CMO	Chief medical officer
CMS	Centers for Medicare and Medicaid Services
CNO	Chief nursing officer
COO	Chief operational officer
DRG	Diagnosis-related group
EEOC	Equal Employment Opportunity Commission
FMEA	Failure Mode and Effects Analysis
FMLA	Family and Medical Leave Act
HCAHPS	Hospital Consumer Assessment of Healthcare Providers and Systems
HCUP	Healthcare Cost & Utilization Project
HEDIS	Healthcare Effectiveness Data and Information Set
HMO	Health maintenance organization
HRSA	Health Resources and Services Administration
IHI	Institute for Healthcare Improvement
IOM	Institute of Medicine
MCO	Managed care organization
MEPS	Medical Expenditure Panel Survey
NCQA	National Committee for Quality Assurance
NGC	National Guideline Clearinghouse
NGO	Nongovernmental organization
NQF	National Quality Forum
PCMH	Patient-Centered Medical Home
PDSA	Plan-do-study-act
PRO	Professional review organization
QI	Quality improvement
RCA	Root cause analysis
SPC	Statistical process control
TJC	The Joint Commission*
USPSTF	U.S. Preventive Services Task Force
VP	Vice president

*Formerly Joint Commission on Accreditation of Healthcare Organizations (JCAHO).

publicized "5 Million Lives" campaign involved recruiting 4050 hospitals to implement bundles of proven improvement tools. A focus in 2012, its Triple Aim program involves improving health care quality with lower costs and increased patient satisfaction.

The **National Committee for Quality Assurance** (NCQA)[20] recognizes and accredits health care institutions and providers for implementing programs such as the Patient-Centered Medical Home (PCMH), accountable care organizations (ACOs; see Chapter 29), and various disease management programs.

Efforts to measure the quality of medical outcomes in a fair manner pose significant methodologic problems. Unless outcomes are adjusted for the severity of patients' illnesses, hospitals treating the sickest patients will be at an unfair disadvantage. The process of adjusting for the severity of illness usually is referred to as **case-mix adjustment.** The question arises as to whose judgment of outcome—the judgment of patients or that of professionals—should be used to evaluate outcomes, and how to account for patient compliance.

The federal government now rates hospitals by giving a **case mix–adjusted mortality** rate for each hospital. Although controversial, this process has generally provided reproducible results. Hospitals that have initiated measures to improve health care have been successful in lowering their case mix–adjusted mortality rates. In addition, the federal government has increased pressure on hospitals to improve the quality of their care by mandating that they report certain indicators about care of patients with pneumonia, heart failure, and acute myocardial infarction to the Centers for Medicare and Medicaid Services (**CMS quality indicators**)[21] and by tying part of reimbursement to good performance.

One major concern about current efforts to reduce costs is whether reducing cost would reduce quality of care as well. Clinicians and epidemiologists continue to address this question in ongoing studies. The Institute of Medicine (IOM) Reports on Safety and Quality of Care highlighted the pervasiveness of *medical errors* in the health care system and the need to redesign the whole system of care.[22] IOM proposed the following six aims for high-quality health care in the 21st century: **safe, effective, patient-centered, timely, efficient,** and **equitable**[23] (see later).

A similar process of systems thinking led the MacColl Institute for Healthcare Innovation to develop the **chronic care model,** which posits that the current health care system is designed to deal with acute episodes of infectious disease. Successfully treating chronic diseases requires that an *activated* patient be treated by an *activated* team who provides engagement, coaching, and links to community resources.[24] The chronic care model aims to empower, prepare, and train patients to manage their own health. This requires a collaborative approach between the care team and patient to define goals and establish treatment plans. The chronic care model stresses the importance of designing the delivery of care for a proactive, planned approach to keep patients healthy, as well as encouraging patients to participate in effective community programs.

All processes of quality improvement follow a few basic principles.[25] Each process has a certain amount of random fluctuation. It is important to distinguish *random fluctuation*, which likely cannot be changed, from other changes that can be managed. Also, most projects are best improved by *small increments* of change with **rapid cycle improvement,** which means that any possible interventions are tested and retested with repeated improvements within a small setting (e.g., with one nurse or on one floor). It is much better to test and tweak solutions to a problem than to roll out a grand strategy throughout the organization and then realize that it does not work optimally.

A. Model of Improvement

As developed by Deming,[26] the basic model of improvement has the structure shown in Figure 28-2. The first step is to describe the goal: "What are we trying to accomplish?" Examples include *reduce* patient complaints, *reduce* waiting time, and *decrease* expenses from overtime.

Second, and most importantly, managers must ask. "How will we know that a change is an improvement?" In simple systems, it is easy to see if a change is an improvement. For most systems, however, it is important to choose a metric that represents the interest of the "end consumer" (e.g., patient, client), and that is rapidly available and easy to measure. Simple histograms and scatter plots can provide much information about variation in the process and what drives the variation. If numbers change over time, they can be shown in a **run chart.**

A **statistical process control** (SPC) chart is a way to analyze data over time, taking into account random fluctuation. SPC charts have been successfully used to improve processes in public health settings[27] (Fig. 28-3). An SPC chart allows a manager to distinguish random fluctuation from that directly caused by interventions. For workflow issues (e.g., wait times in a clinic, delays in access to testing),

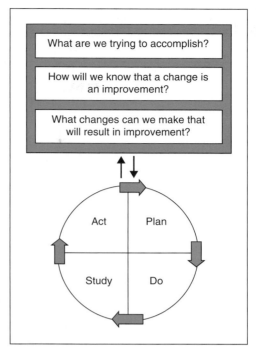

Figure 28-2 Basic principle of quality improvement. (From Ryvicker M, Schwartz T, Sobolewski S, et al: The Home Health Aide Partnering Collaborative: *Implementation manual*, Washington, DC, 2007, US Department of Health and Human Services. Diagram modified from Langley G| et al: *The improvement guide*, San Francisco, 1996, Jossey-Bass.)

workflow mapping often works well, too. In a graph, each step in the process is written down with measurements of the time spent on each step. Once the process is graphed in this way, it is often easy to pinpoint bottlenecks and repeat loops and to map out an alternative, easier process.

In the third step, the manager must ask, "What changes can we make that will result in improvement?" For most problem categories, certain changes have a good chance of succeeding. For example, for workflow issues with bottlenecks, the following changes can be helpful[25]:

- Eliminate multiple data entry.
- Remove intermediaries.
- Match staffing to demand spikes.
- Smooth workflow.
- Do tasks in parallel.

In the fourth step, each possible solution is then evaluated in a **plan-do-study-act** (PDSA) **cycle.** The "plan" part describes exactly who will do what, where, and when, and how data will be collected. In the plan part, it is also important to make predictions how any changes are expected to impact the problem. In the "do" part, the plan is carried out, problems and unexpected developments are documented, and data analysis is begun. In the "study" stage, data analysis is completed and compared to predictions, and learning points are summarized. These learning points lead to new changes to be made in the next cycle. This process is repeated until an intervention has been tried out in different environments and circumstances and the change seems robust enough to be broadly implemented.

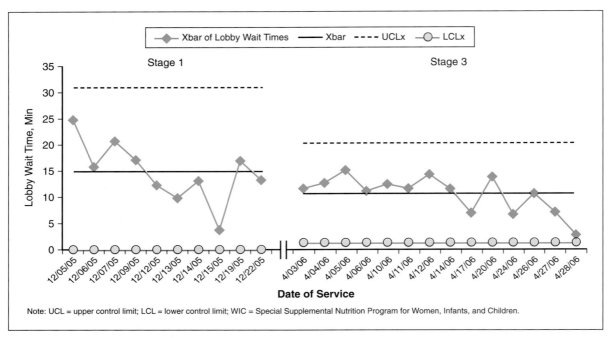

Figure 28-3 **Example of statistical process control (SPC) chart for wait times in WIC clinic.** *WIC*, Special Supplemental Nutrition Program for Women, Infants, and Children. (From Boe DT, Riley W, Parsons H: *Am J Public Health* 99(9), 2009. http://ajph.aphapublications.org/doi/pdf/10.2105/AJPH.2008.138289)

Some methodologies in quality improvement address individual dimensions of quality. These are discussed here especially in the context of the IOM's six aims for quality improvement.

Safe: Specific tools to increase safety include **failure mode and effects analysis (FMEA)** and **root cause analysis (RCA).** FMEA was originally developed by the U.S. military as a tool to predict the effect of system and equipment failures. It has since been successfully used in health care to identify vulnerabilities proactively and deal with them effectively.[28] In RCA, a safety team drills into the system issues behind mistakes by asking "what" and "why" multiple times until all aspects of the process are reviewed and the contributing factors considered.[29]

Timely/efficient: The **LEAN** approach was originated by the Japanese automobile manufacturer Toyota. Its central aims are to avoid waste and to concentrate on activities that bring value to the customer. Important concepts in LEAN include defining value from the consumer perspective, identifying value streams, smoothing out the flow of steps, and removing waste and activities that do not add value.[30] **Six Sigma** methodology concentrates on decreasing variation. The first steps are defining the project goals and requirements of internal and external customers, measuring and determining customers' needs and specifications, and then setting benchmarks to meet industry standards. The next steps include analyzing if the process meets the customer needs, then redesigning it if necessary. Lastly, the process is standardized until it shows only minimal variability.[31]

Patient-centered: The patient-centered dimension of care quality is built on patient feedback. Although patient information can come from informal surveys and focus groups, patient feedback usually is obtained through standardized surveys such as the Hospital **Consumers Assessment of Healthcare Providers and Systems** (HCAHPS).[32] It is important to pay attention to such standardized metrics because these will soon determine part of an institution's Medicare reimbursement. **Value-based purchasing** describes a Medicare initiative to be implemented in 2013, under which a hospital's reimbursement is decreased for failing to meet certain quality metrics.

Effective: This usually means **evidence-based.** Evidence-based treatment guidelines come from many sources. Good guidelines follow a format similar to the USPSTF (see Chapter 18), with clear questions, explicit guidelines for identifying and summarizing literature, and organized decision making. Sources of respected guidelines include the AHRQ, Cochrane database, and the National Guideline Clearinghouse (see Websites).

Equitable: This dimension is often the most difficult to operationalize. The main strategy here is to analyze outcomes for disparities among ethnic or socioeconomic minorities, then reduce or eliminate any disparities identified.

Managers also need to consider the **human side of improvement.** Machiavelli deftly described the difficulties this entails: "There is nothing more difficult to carry out, nor more doubtful of success, nor more dangerous to handle, than to initiate a new order of things. For the reformer has enemies in all those who profit by the old order, and only lukewarm defenders in all those who would profit by the new."[25] Most changes will not succeed without the support of people, and most improvement efforts require teamwork. People need to cooperate in new ways to effect change.

Change often results in some people losing control, power, or privileges. Concerns regarding such losses should be elicited and addressed. Managers must distinguish among subtly different reactions to change, as follows:

- Hostility ("I don't like it, and I will say so.")
- Apathy ("I don't care and will neither fight nor hinder.")
- Compliance ("I won't fight but will disagree privately.")
- Conformance ("It's a good idea, but not my fight.")
- Commitment (implementing and advocating a change)

People are not really allies until they reach the last stage, and they do this in the same way that patients change behavior. Changes always have a **physical aspect** (how a form or an office changes), a **logistical implication** (why this needs to happen), and **emotional impact** (how one feels about this change, and how it makes one appear).

Initial hesitation should not be viewed as resistance. However, ambivalence can easily become resistance. The main pitfall is to underestimate the resistance that does emerge, and to think of changes as only technical in nature. All changes have a human side, and that human side needs to be managed along with the other aspects of the change. The following strategies can help:

1. Communicating persistently why the change is needed and why the status quo is no longer an option. Such communication is most powerful if it relates back to the organization's mission and speaks with the voice of the patient, client, or consumer.
2. Gathering input about the ideas from those affected by the change. Those most affected often understand best what will or will not work. They should have significant say and their preferences taken into account when possible. This will help for them to buy into the end result.
3. Informing everyone about progress made during testing.
4. Sharing specific information as early as possible about how the change will affect people.
5. Designing the system so that making the correct choices is easy.

Most people can be brought around by following these strategies and by well-conducted improvement cycles. Ideally, a process should not be introduced without frontline staff having perfected the process under real-life conditions. Apart from making for a better intervention, this process also allows doubters to see that people like them have tried and adopted the intervention.

B. Implementation

It is important not to underestimate the work that still needs to be done after a workable solution has been identified. Implementation of a change requires a new set of strategies. Many successful solutions have been set aside because managers underestimate the energy and persistence necessary to hardwire a process broadly. Here are a few pointers:

- Implementation cycles take longer than testing cycles.
- During an implementation cycle, there is increased awareness of and resistance to a change.
- The implementation team needs increased managerial support to effect permanent change.
- Some form of staff training is usually required to implement a change.

- The implementation process needs to be monitored, adjusted, and sustained for a significant time before it can be trusted to be permanent.

Most resistance will come in the implementation phase. The same strategies for overcoming resistance as previously listed should be followed. If people continue to resist and oppose a change, this needs to be addressed as a performance issue (see later). Managers need to meet with employees, set behavioral expectations around changes, possibly offer incentives, and spell out consequences of continued noncompliance. Managers then must ensure those expectations are fulfilled. If not, a disciplinary process needs to be put into place.

C. Current State of Health Care Quality/Disparities

The current state of health care quality in the United States continues to show large variability, unequal improvement, and continued disparities. Particularly striking are the disparities in **social determinants of health,** such as high school noncompletion and poverty, which have not improved between 2005 and 2009. The Centers for Disease Control and Prevention (CDC) calls for communities to follow USPSTF recommendations on **community preventive services** to promote healthy social environments for low-income children and families and to reduce risk-taking behaviors among adolescents[33] (see Chapter 26).

Health care quality and access also continue to be suboptimal, especially for minorities.[33] This observation again illustrates the basic frustration of prevention in general and quality improvement in particular. Many established interventions would improve outcomes, but most of them are underused. Still, most research energy in the United States goes toward finding still more *new* solutions. If just a fraction of that energy were instead focused on implementing established effective care consistently, the gains in averted mortality and morbidity would be breathtaking.

D. State of Quality Improvement Research

There are important distinctions between quality improvement and research. Research involving human subjects is overseen by institutional review boards, whereas QI is usually exempt from such oversight. The state of QI and improvement research shows that the field is still disparate, with a need for more standardization and more attention to identifying which environmental factors contribute to effective and sustained improvement.[34]

However, some lessons from the literature seem to be emerging. Most initiatives leading to sustained and measurable improvement combine multiple interventions at multiple levels. Also, care provided in integrated models of care, such as the chronic care model described earlier or the patient-centered medical home (see Chapter 29), seem to provide the best chance of leading to meaningful patient behavioral changes.[35-37] Organizations that ensure open communication and constant learning will likely be able to survive in the new quality era with payment for outcomes.[38] Combining education with behavioral strategies such as feedback and increased self-monitoring is more effective than either alone.[39] Sustained QI requires leadership commitment, availability of infrastructure and staff support, and strategic partnerships.[40] Successful QI within practices and public health agencies is even more successful when combined with community initiatives.[41] Successful research, however, establishes more than only the effective interventions. Given the growing scarcity of resources in health care, some of the most helpful studies pinpoint which minimal interventions are needed for sustained change.[42]

V. MANAGING HUMAN RESOURCES

Employment Law is a patchwork of different federal, state, and local laws. Federal law mainly plays a role around antidiscrimination laws.[43] Employees enjoy many protections to be free from discrimination on various grounds (see also Chapter 29).

- The **Civil Rights Act** from 1981 forbids discrimination based on race and ethnicity. It was expanded in 1983 to include discrimination based on religion, sex, and national origin, and to forbid discharge due to exercising freedom of expression.
- **Title VII of the Civil Rights Act** prohibits all employers from discriminating against employees in hiring, promotion, and termination decisions based on race, color, religion, sex, or national origin. The Civil Rights Act is also interpreted to forbid **harassment** because of any of the protected categories, or the fostering of a hostile work environment.
- The **Age Discrimination in Employment Act** protects workers over age 40.
- The **Americans with Disabilities Act** requires employers to make reasonable accommodations to disabled workers.
- Federal employees can challenge employers directly over any discrimination, but private-sector employees must file complaints with states' **Equal Employment Opportunity Commission** (EEOC) or other state gatekeeping agency. Apart from being discriminated against in hiring decisions, employees have the right not to be subjected to adverse consequences for certain protected actions, such as speaking about matters of public interest, or alerting the public about a major problem (**whistleblower statute**).
- The **Occupational Safety and Health Act** requires employers to provide a workplace that is free from avoidable hazards.
- Under the **Family and Medical Leave Act** (FMLA), employers need to provide up to 16 weeks of unpaid leave to employees who leave because of medical needs or family emergencies. Small employers are exempt from this law, and it does not apply to executive-level employees.

Beyond such categories, employers have broad discretion. They can require workers to alter their dress, grooming habits, statements at work, or even affiliation with a political party, if party membership is necessary for a particular job. Public-sector employees also often have standards for "off-duty conduct" and can be disciplined for "behavior unbecoming a public employee" outside work hours. Unless covered by other contracts or union agreements, most employees are employed **at will.** This means they can be fired without cause, notice, or explanation, as long as the reason is not unlawful. However, many public employees are considered to have a **property interest** in continued employment (after completing a specified probationary period), thereby affording public employees due process rights before their jobs can be taken from them. This usually means they have the right to a hearing for an **adverse action,** meaning a suspension, demotion, salary decrease, or termination. Also, courts and states have created multiple exceptions to the "at will" doctrine, including requiring a certain amount of notice and due process for various-sized employers and for various reasons.

For optimal performance, it is necessary to generate task-based job descriptions. A job description should be sufficiently detailed so that employees are able to understand if they are meeting expectations. Once a job description is done and the job posted, managers need to recruit suitable candidates. The same antidiscrimination laws apply to recruiting as already outlined. Employers are not obligated to interview all candidates applying but cannot discriminate against applicants based on any of the protected categories. Most people recommend **behavior-based interviewing** as a best predictor of performance at the job; possible behavior-based interview questions include: "Tell me about a time where you felt you were treated unfairly," and "Tell me about a time where you had a conflict with a coworker."

Once employees have been hired, they need to be oriented, trained, and retained. Retaining includes periodic performance evaluation and appraisals. Powerful tools to motivate performance improvement include clear expectations, ideally based on written behavioral contracts[44] (Fig. 28-4), and rapid feedback. To be effective, managers should provide feedback in a safe setting and describe in specific terms the behavior that did not meet expectations, and which behaviors they want to see instead.[45] If such behavioral interventions do not lead to any improvement, supervisors should consult with the organization's human resource (HR) department to pursue discipline and possibly termination.

VI. SUMMARY

There is a growing awareness that the quality and efficiency of the U.S. health care system in general is a public health concern. Many higher-level public health jobs also require a degree of managerial skills and understanding of organizational decision making. Organizations are accountable to their boards, employees, clients, and community stakeholders. In a well-managed organization, the operational details (doing things right) flow from the overall strategic goals (doing the right things). Responsibility for not-for-profit organizations is vested in a board of trustees, which hires and fires the chief executives and oversees day-to-day operations.

Tools to measure organizational performance include identifying relevant standards, benchmarking, dashboards, and balanced scorecards. The main tools to assess financial performance are budget planning and variance analysis. Budgets can be planned in an incremental or zero-based manner. For budget variance analysis, actual revenue and expenses are compared to budget and favorable and

From: Director of Health

To: Health Department Administrator

Budget Management.

Review the total agency budget and that of your management area monthly. Whenever you are concerned about potential overspending, consult with me immediately. Where you see possible underspending, consult with the management team at its next meeting. I expect our data system and the city's to be able to provide similar status reports. Continue to oversee development of a system which ensures that deputies and office managers receive timely accurate data on the status of their budgets - at least monthly.

Take the lead in preparing the annual budget analysis and fiscal summary for the Board of Health, City Council, and appropriate committees. Consult with other managers; prepare data for director and present financial data as requested.

Figure 28-4 **Part of an employee performance contract.** (From Buttery CMG: http://www.commed.vcu.edu/LOCAL/2012/ch2_Admin_Org_I2.pdf)

unfavorable variances identified. Sources for variance include volume, sale, and price variances. Quality of care can be measured for structure, processes, and outcomes. The Institute of Medicine has defined the following aims for high-quality health care: safe, effective, patient-centered, timely, efficient, and equitable. The basis of a quality improvement process is the basic plan-do-study-act cycle. Changes should be tested in small increments with rapid improvement cycles before implementation. When planning an implementation process, managers should plan for and address staff resistance. Strategies to decrease resistance include constant communication of the need for change, involvement of frontline staff, and high-level support.

Many laws regulate the relationship between employer and employees. Employers are forbidden from discriminating against employees in hiring, disciplining, and firing in several protected categories. Most employees are employed at will, meaning they can be fired without cause, although in many cases an opportunity for a hearing and reasonable notice need to be provided.

References

1. The Advisory Board Company: Physician boot camp: leadership fundamentals for physicians. Board research and analysis, 2007.
2. Turning Point Performance Management National Excellence Collaborative 2004: Performance management-self assessment tool. http://www.turningpointprogram.org/toolkit/pdf/PM_Self_Assess_Tool.pdf
3. National Public Health Standards Program: http://www.cdc.gov/NPHPSP/theInstruments.html
4. Rohm H: Performance measurement in action: a balancing act. *Perform* 2(2). Available at www.balancedscorecard.org/LinkClick.aspx?fileticket=ph%2b8b3YMoBc%3d&tabid=56
5. Palmer DA: Financial management development. http://www.financialmanagementdevelopment.com/Slides/handouts/213.pdf
6. Variance analysis and sensitivity analysis. In *Tools to plan, monitor, and manage financial status*, Boston, Jones & Bartlett. Available at http://samples.jbpub.com/9780763778941/78941_18_CH17_189_204.pdf
7. Kavanagh SC, Swanson CJ: Tactical financial management: cash flow and budgetary variance analysis. From CBS Interactive Business Network Resource Library, 2009. http://findarticles.com/p/articles/mi_hb6642/is_5_25/ai_n45060500/
8. Flexner A: *Medical education in the United States and Canada.* A report to the Carnegie Foundation for the Advancement of Teaching, Buffalo, NY, 1910, Heritage Press.
9. Donabedian A: *A guide to medical care administration.* Vol 2. Medical care appraisal, New York, 1969, American Public Health Association.
10. *Dartmouth atlas of health care.* http://www.dartmouthatlas.org
11. http://www.jointcommission.org
12. http://www.ncqa.org/tabid/1415/Default.aspx
13. http://www.hrsa.gov
14. http://www.cms.gov
15. http://www.cms.gov/medicare-coverage-database/details/nca-decision-memo.aspx?&NcaName=Intensive%20Behavioral%20Therapy%20for%20Obesity&bc=ACAAAAAAIAAA&NCAId=253&
16. http://www.ahrq.gov
17. http://www.qualityforum.org
18. http://www.nist.gov/baldrige/about/what_we_do.cfm
19. www.ihi.org
20. http://www.ncqa.org
21. https://www.cms.gov/QualityInitiativesGenInfo
22. Institute of Medicine: *To err is human: building a safer health system*, Washington, DC, 2000, National Academies Press.
23. Institute of Medicine: *Crossing the quality chasm: a new health system for the 21st century*, Washington, DC, 2001, National Academies Press.
24. http://www.improvingchroniccare.org/index.php?p=Model_Elements&s=18
25. Langley GJ, Moen R, Nolan KM, et al: *The improvement guide*, ed 2, San Francisco, 2009, Jossey-Bass.
26. Deming WE: The new economics for industry, government, education, Cambridge, Mass, MIT, 1993.
27. Boe DT, Riley W, Parsons H: Improving service delivery in a county health department WIC clinic: an application of statistical process control techniques. *Am J Public Health* 99:1619–1625, 2009.
28. Veterans Administration handbook on safety topics. http://www.patientsafety.gov/SafetyTopics/HFMEA/PSQHarticle.pdf
29. http://www.index.va.gov/search/va/va_search.jsp?SQ=&TT=1&QT=NATIONAL+PATIENT+SAFETY+IMPROVEMENT+HANDBOOK+&searchbtn=Search
30. http://www.lean.org
31. http://www.sixsigmaonline.org
32. http://www.hcahpsonline.org

33. Agency for Healthcare Research and Quality: Highlights from the National Healthcare Quality and Disparities Reports. http://www.ahrq.gov/research/iomqrdrreport

34. Institute of Medicine: The state of quality improvement and implementation research, 2007. http://www.nap.edu/catalog/11986.html

35. Battersby M, von Korff M, Schaefer J, et al: Twelve evidence-based principles for implementing self-management support in primary care. *Joint Comm J Qual Safety* 36:561–570, 2010.

36. Parchman M, Kaissi AA: Are elements of the chronic care model associated with cardiovascular risk factor control in type 2 diabetes? *Joint Comm J Qual Safety* 35:133–138, 2009.

37. Hung DY, Glasgow RE, Dickinson LM, et al: The chronic care model and relationships to patient health status and health-related quality of life. *Am J Prev Med* 35:S398–S406, 2008.

38. Wynia MK, Johnson M, McCoy TP: Validation of an organizational communication climate assessment toolkit. *Am J Med Qual* 25:436–443, 2010.

39. Wing RR, Crane MM, Thomas JG, et al: Improving weight loss outcomes of community interventions by incorporating behavioral strategies. *Am J Public Health* 100:2513–2519, 2010.

40. Bray P, Cummings DM, Wolf M, et al: After the collaborative is over: what sustains quality improvement initiatives in primary care practices? *Joint Com J Qual Pt Safety* 35:502–508, 2009.

41. Etz RS, Cohen DJ, Woolf SH, et al: Bridging primary care practices and communities to promote healthy behaviors. *Am J Prev Med* 35:S390-S397, 2008.

42. Gierisch JM, DeFrank JT, Bowling JM, et al: Finding the minimal intervention needed for sustained mammography adherence. *Am J Prev Med* 39:334–344, 2010.

43. Gertz S: Legal rights and responsibilities: the law of the workplace. In Berman EM, Bowman JS, West JP, et al, editors: *Human resource management in public service: paradoxes, processes, and problems*, ed 4, Thousand Oaks, Calif, 2011, Sage.

44. Buttery CMG: The health director handbook. http://www.commed.vcu.edu/LOCAL/2012/ch2_Admin_Org_12.pdf

45. Patterson K, Grenny J, McMillan R, et al: *Crucial conversation tools for talking when stakes are high*, ed 2, New York, 2011, McGraw-Hill.

Select Readings

Adams K, Corrigan JM: *Priority areas for national action: transforming health care quality*, Washington, DC, 2003, National Academies Press.

Committee on Quality of Health Care in America and Institute of Medicine: *Crossing the quality chasm: a new health system for the 21st century*, Washington DC, 2001, National Academies Press.

Fallon LF, McDonnell CR: *Human resource management in health care: principles and practice*, Sudbury, Mass, 2007, Jones & Bartlett.

Fallon LF, Zgodzinksi EJ: *Essentials of public health management*, ed 2, Sudbury, Mass, 2008, Jones & Bartlett.

Institute of Medicine: *Priority areas for national action: transforming health care quality*, Washington, DC, 2003, National Academies Press.

Institute of Medicine: The state of quality improvement and implementation research, 2007. http://www.nap.edu/catalog/11986.html

Swartzmann RH, Sewell RH: *Principles of public health management*, New York, 2010, Wiley.

Websites

http://www.ahrq.gov [Agency for Healthcare Research and Quality]
http://www.nist.gov/baldrige/about/what_we_do.cfm [Baldrige program]
http://www.cms.gov [Centers for Medicare and Medicaid Services]
http://www.hrsa.gov [Health Resources and Services Administration]
www.ihi.org [Institute for Healthcare Improvement]
http://www.jointcommission.org [The Joint Commission]
http://www.ncqa.org [National Committee for Quality Assurance]
http://www.ncqa.org/tabid/1415/Default.aspx [National Guideline Clearinghouse]
http://www.qualityforum.org [National Quality Forum]
http://www.dartmouthatlas.org [Dartmouth Atlas of Health Care]
http://www.patientsafety.gov [Veterans Administration: Safety topics]

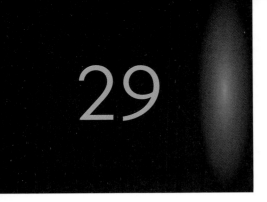

29

Health Care Organization, Policy, and Financing

I. OVERVIEW

All health care systems strive to reconcile seemingly unlimited health care needs with limited resources. In an ideal world, health care systems would achieve three goals: universal access, high quality, and limited costs. In the real world, there are tradeoffs; at best, health care systems can attain only two of these three goals at any one time[1] (Fig. 29-1).

This chapter examines the fundamental legal, social, and political framework underlying health care in the United States, how it is organized, and how it can provide the greatest value given limited resources. Although the legal and organizational framework of the health care delivery system is different in other countries, the challenges and need to distribute scarce resources are the same.

A. Terminology in Health Policy

Health care policy and financing require the use of economic terminology, including concepts such as needs and demand, utilization, and elasticity, often with an array of acronyms (Box 29-1). The **need for health care** usually is considered a professional judgment. Although the term "felt need" is sometimes used to describe a patient's judgment about the need for care, more frequently the **demand for health care** is actually studied. *Demand* has a medical and an economic definition. The medical definition of demand is the amount of care people would use if there were no barriers to care. The problem with this definition is that there almost always are barriers to care: cost, convenience, fear, or lack of real availability (see later). The economic definition of demand is the quantity of care that is purchased at a given price. For this economic definition to work, there must be an assumption of **price elasticity** (i.e., an assumption that as prices increase, the demand for a given service will decrease).

This assumption has been tested in one of the largest social science experiments, the **Health Insurance Experiment** conducted by the RAND Corporation in the 1970s. In this study, 5809 enrollees were randomly assigned to different insurance plans providing different levels of coverage, deductibles, and copayments. The study found that patients *did* change their utilization of health care somewhat in response to different insurance levels (i.e., there was some elasticity of health care to price). However, this elasticity was fairly small compared with that of demand for nonmedical goods and services. Furthermore, health care spending was reduced for *both* necessary care and unnecessary care, which led to worse blood pressure control, vision, and oral health.[2] These results call into question the suitability of market-based solutions for health care problems. It also demonstrates how almost any health policy solution usually has negative side effects, called **unintended consequences.**

Because of the difficulties of measuring demand, what is usually studied is the effective (realized) demand, called

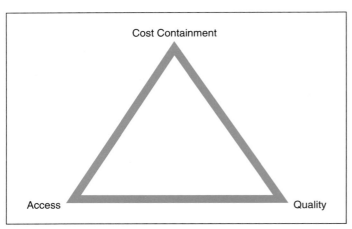

Figure 29-1 **The "iron triangle" of health care.** (From Kissick W: *Medicine's dilemmas: infinite need versus finite resources,* New Haven, Conn, 1994, Yale University Press.)

Box 29-1	Frequently Used Acronyms in Health Policy with Descriptions
ACO	**Accountable Care Organization** New care model that includes providers and hospitals cooperating together for better outcomes and taking financial risk for outcomes.
ADA	**Americans with Disabilities Act** Forbids discrimination based on disabilities and requires employers to make reasonable accommodations for disabled workers.
CAA	**Clean Air Act** Regulates emissions from area, stationary, and mobile sources.
CERCLA	**Comprehensive Environmental Response, Compensation, and Liability Act** Also called **Superfund Act,** established a trust fund for cleanup of abandoned and uncontrolled hazardous waste sites.
CMS	**Centers for Medicare and Medicaid Services** U.S. federal agency that administers Medicare, Medicaid, and the State Children's Health Insurance Program.
COBRA	**Consolidated Omnibus Budget Reconciliation Act of 1985** Allows employees to continue their insurance after job termination.
CWA	**Clean Water Act** Established pollution control for discharges into U.S. waterways; does not address drinking water (see SDWA).
EMR	**Electronic medical record**
EMTALA	**Emergency Medical Treatment and Active Labor Act** Law that requires emergency departments to provide initial evaluation and stabilization of all patients regardless of their ability to pay.
EPA	**Environmental Protection Agency**
ERISA	**Employee Retirement Income Security Act** Regulates the content of established employee health plans.
FIFRA	**Federal Insecticide, Fungicide, & Rodenticide Act** Enacted in 1996, controls the distribution, use, and sale of pesticides.
FQHC	**Federally qualified health centers** Community health centers that qualify for special federal grants to treat Medicare and Medicaid patients.
HIPAA	**Health Insurance Portability and Accountability Act** Calls for standards in implementing a national health information infrastructure and for regulation of the protection of individual health information in such a system.
HSA	**Health savings account** Individual tax-preferred savings account for health expenses, usually coupled with a high-deductible insurance plan.
MCO	**Managed care organization**
PCMH	**Patient-centered medical home** Care model in which patients are cared for by a physician-directed team that provides comprehensive care with enhanced access and responsibilities for patient engagement, coordination, and population management.
PPACA	**Patient Protection and Affordable Care Act** Health care reform bill passed in 2010 under President Obama in an effort to enact universal health care; Supreme Court ruled it constitutional in 2012.
PRO	**Peer review organization** Also formerly called *professional review organization;* group of medical professionals or a health care company that contracts with CMS to ensure that services covered by Medicare meet professional standards.
RCRA	**Resource Conservation and Recovery Act** Established that the Environmental Protection Agency should control hazardous waste "from cradle to grave."
SARA	**Superfund Amendments and Reauthorization Act** Expanded CERCLA and established a community's right to obtain information about hazards.
SDWA	**Safe Drinking Water Act** Protects surface water and groundwater designated as drinking-water sources.
TRI	**Toxic Release Inventory** Publicly available database on toxic chemical releases and other waste management activities.

utilization. Utilization is usually less than need, so the concept of unmet need was developed. **Unmet need** can be defined by the following equation:

$$\text{Unmet need} = \text{Need} - \text{Utilization}$$

B. Factors Influencing Need and Demand

Demographic factors are among the most important influences on the need and demand for medical care. Foremost is the age of the population, as well as mortality rates and fertility patterns. In the United States a rather sudden decline in birth rates occurred around 1970 with the wide availability of oral contraceptives, and when abortion was legalized (1973). This decline in birth rates accelerated the process of aging of the population due to longer life expectancy. Fertility levels have remained low. The long-term result of reduced fertility may be an extended period in which the proportion of workers in the U.S. population will be the smallest in history. This phenomenon is expected to peak around 2015, when large numbers of the "baby boom" children will reach retirement age. A major concern is whether the smaller number of workers will be able to support the large, older population with such benefits as Medicare and Social Security retirement payments. The expected shortage of workers will also put upward pressure on wages, making care more expensive.

Other factors that influence medical needs and demands include advances in medical technology, especially pharmaceutical and medical devices. As new methods of prevention, diagnosis, and treatment become available and prove to be useful, more providers and more patients will want to use them.

One might expect that the unmet need for medical care would be greatest among the poorest members of society, but that is not always true. People with income below some percentage of the poverty line are eligible for Medicaid (see later). People whose incomes are too high to be eligible for Medicaid are those who do not receive medical insurance in their jobs and are not able to pay for individual medical care insurance policies, and who are considered the **medically indigent.** They may be able to support themselves until a medical catastrophe strikes, but then they are unable to pay their bills. Many of the **medically uninsured** (those who have no health insurance) and **medically underinsured** (those whose health insurance is inadequate) are medically indigent. They are not on welfare, but they cannot financially tolerate major medical bills. In 2011 the medically uninsured population in the United States numbered about 49.9 million people, about 17% of the U.S. population.[3]

C. International Comparison

The United States has a higher growth of health care costs than other countries; it spends almost 50% more on health care than other industrialized countries, including Germany, Canada, and France, which provide health insurance to all citizens.[4] In 2008 the United States spent 16% of its gross domestic product (GDP) on health care, more than any other country. Sadly, these higher expenditures do not lead to uniformly superior outcomes[5] (Fig. 29-2). What is worse, the United States has made much less progress than other industrialized countries in improving overall life expectancy in the past 40 years.[6]

A study comparing the quality of health care across industrialized countries found that, as in past years, the United States ranks last or next to last on five dimensions of a high-performance health care system: quality, access, efficiency, equity, and healthy lives.[7] The mismatch between health expenditures and health and the inexorable rise of health cost are driving a push to control (i.e., reduce) health care spending.

To understand why we pay so much for so little health and how that could change, it is important to understand the underlying laws and functions of the health care system. Laws build the underpinnings of the health system and the complex environment that generates the conditions for health.[8]

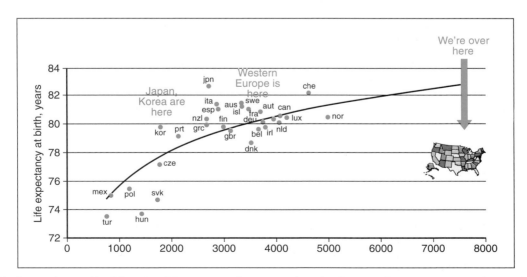

Figure 29-2 **Total expenditure of health against life expectancy by country.** (Modified from http://www.theatlantic.com/business/archive/2011/04/oecd-us-outspends-average-developed-country-141-in-health-care/237171.)

II. LEGAL FRAMEWORK OF HEALTH

A. U.S. Public Health System

Government's public health responsibilities exist at three levels: federal, state/tribe, and local/municipal.[8] Local public health agencies can report to a centralized state health department, to local governments, or to both.

The responsibility for public health below federal level is usually scattered through multiple agencies, and each state and locality has its own framework of laws and regulations. Most of the existing legislation was enacted at a time when infectious diseases were the main threat to public health. Frequently, these laws have not been meaningfully updated to account for new threats, such as chronic diseases, bioterrorism, or emerging epidemics, nor has the ability to share data kept pace with technologic innovations[8] (see Chapter 26).

For all states, surveillance and required reporting are exercises of state police powers.

B. Environmental Laws

The U.S. Congress passed most important environmental regulations in the 1970s. The **Clean Air Act** (CAA), passed in 1970 and amended in 1990, regulates emissions from area, stationary, and mobile sources, with recent discussions on whether its scope should include regulation of greenhouse gases. The CAA also established **National Ambient Air Quality Standards.**

The **Federal Water Pollution Control Act,** established in 1972 and amended in 1977 to become the **Clean Water Act** (CWA), established pollution control standards for discharges into U.S. waterways. The **Safe Drinking Water Act** (**SDWA**) was passed in 1974 to protect surface water and groundwater designated as a drinking water source. It regulates water and underground injection of waste, protecting groundwater.

The **Resource Conservation and Recovery Act** (RCRA) gave the **Environmental Protection Agency** (EPA) control over hazardous waste "from cradle to grave." It focused only on active and future facilities, not on defunct sites. These inactive sites are addressed through the **Comprehensive Environmental Response, Compensation, and Liability Act** (CERCLA), also called the **Superfund Act.** This law created a tax on industries and established a trust for cleanup of abandoned and uncontrolled hazardous waste sites. CERCLA was amended in 1986 through the **Superfund Amendments and Reauthorization Act** (SARA), which established the community's right to obtain information about hazards and the **Toxic Release Inventory** (TRI). The **Federal Insecticide, Fungicide, & Rodenticide Act** (FIFRA), enacted in 1996, controls the distribution, use, and sale of pesticides.[9]

C. Duties of Health Care Providers and Hospitals

Title VI of the Civil Rights Act of 1964 states, "No person in the United States shall, on the ground of race, color, or national origin, be excluded from participation in, be denied the benefits of, or be subjected to discrimination under any program or activity receiving Federal financial assistance." This act has been interpreted to mean that facilities have to provide qualified interpreter services. Similarly, the **Americans with Disabilities Act** (ADA) of 1990 forbids discrimination based on disabilities. The **Hill-Burton Act** financed construction of public and not-for-profit community hospitals. It established a "community services obligation" in exchange for receiving funds that requires hospitals to demonstrate how they serve their communities. The **Emergency Medical Treatment and Active Labor Act** (EMTALA) requires emergency departments to evaluate and treat patients regardless of their ability to pay.

The **Health Insurance Portability and Accountability Act** (HIPAA) was enacted in 1996. HIPAA required the Department of Health and Human Services (DHHS) to develop national standards for an information system and for the protection of health information in such a system. These standards were published as the Privacy Rule in 2000 and mandate that all entities that handle identifiable health information implement standards that protect against the misuse of such information.

D. Health Care Financing and Insurance

The **Employee Retirement Income Security Act** (ERISA) from 1974 regulates the content of established employee health plans. It was later amended by the **Consolidated Omnibus Budget Reconciliation Act** of 1985 (COBRA), which enables employees to purchase employer-sponsored health insurance for a limited time after termination.

1. Patient Protection and Affordable Care Act

The **Patient Protection and Affordable Care Act** (PPACA) became law in 2010 and may be the most comprehensive health care legislation since Medicare in 1965. The act offers a mix of regulations covering a wide swath of topics.[10] In broad strokes, PPACA does the following:

- Requires most U.S. citizens and legal residents to have health insurance *(individual mandate),* and provides tax penalties if they do not.
- Expands Medicaid, provider payments in Medicaid, and Children's Health Insurance Program coverage.
- Provides subsidies to individuals at certain income levels to obtain insurance.
- Establishes *state-based insurance exchanges* for employers and individuals to obtain coverage.
- Imposes rules on insurance plans, requiring them to provide basic preventive services at no cost and insurance coverage for dependent children up to age 26, and forbidding them to exclude patients because of preexisting conditions (see Chapter 28).
- Provides funds for various initiatives to explore innovative care approaches, such as accountable care organizations, comparative effectiveness research, and other attempts to reduce health care costs without jeopardizing quality.
- Establishes an **Independent Payment Advisory Board** to provide recommendations to reduce Medicare costs; these recommendations become binding unless Congress finds similar cost reductions elsewhere.
- Decreases expenses by penalizing readmissions, taxing high-end plans, cutting provider payments, and establishing a value-based purchasing program that penalizes hospitals for low rates on established quality metrics.

■ Increases funds for employer-based wellness programs and preventive services with an A or B rating from the U.S. Preventive Services Task Force (USPSTF).

The PPACA closely mirrors the health reform law passed in Massachusetts in the early 2000s. Not surprisingly, given the political stakes, opinions differ about what the Massachusetts experience has shown. Most analysts agree that the health care reform has expanded the insured pool and increased access to providers, perhaps more so for disadvantaged citizens.[11] Views on the impact on costs are more mixed. The reform has resulted in a net cost rather than net savings and has led to an influx of more newly insured patients without expanding the provider pool, which may have increased wait times. Also, the reform has not changed patient behavior or convincingly slowed the growth of health care costs in Massachusetts.[12] In June 2012 the U.S. Supreme Court ruled on the balance of federal and state powers in regards to health care, and the extent of federal powers under the commerce clause to enforce the individual mandate (see Chapter 25). The Court held that the individual mandate exceeded Congress' power to regulate commerce, but was constitutional under the power to levy taxes.[13]

III. THE MEDICAL CARE SYSTEM

A. Historical Overview

Until the late 1800s, most medical care was ambulatory. Patients paid local practitioners on a fee-for-service basis. The hospital tended to be viewed as a "death house" and a place for the sick poor, often supported by the church or other benevolent organizations. In the early 1900s, as medicine became more scientific and more surgical procedures available, the hospital came to be seen as the "doctors' workshop." The technology and ancillary personnel and services were usually provided at no charge to the physicians, which helped them practice their craft. In turn, physicians kept the hospitals in business by bringing in patients. With the founding of the National Institutes of Health (NIH) in 1948 came a push for improved biomedical technology. The research done since then has made the practice of medicine not only much more effective but also far more complex and costly. This increased complexity has resulted in increasing specialization of physicians and other health care workers and has required an increasing rationalization and control of the levels of care.

B. Levels of Medical Care

In an effort to maximize the effectiveness and efficiency of the process, health care professionals have proposed an integrated system of graded levels of care. The levels range from treatment in the patient's home, the least complex level, to treatment in a tertiary medical center, the most complex level of care (Box 29-2). A patient is initially assigned to an appropriate level of care and is reassigned to another level whenever there is an improvement or setback in the patient's condition. Although the movement from one level to another should be easy, rapid, and smooth, often this is not the case. Transitions in care are risky, and transfers require particular care to accurate communication of medication changes, treatment plans, and follow-up tests.

Box 29-2	Levels of the Medical Care System*

1. **Acute, general hospital facilities**
   Tertiary medical center (with all or most of the latest technology)
   Intermediate hospital (medium to large community hospital with considerable amount of the latest technology)
   Local community hospital
2. **Rehabilitation or convalescent care facilities**
   Special unit in a regular hospital
   Rehabilitation hospital
3. **Extended care facilities**
   Skilled nursing facility (nursing home)
   Intermediate care facility
   Hospice
4. **Organized home care**
   Public agencies (local health departments or visiting nurse associations)
   Private organizations
5. **Self-care in the home**

*1 = Most complex; 5 = Least complex.

At the top of the scale of complexity are three types of **acute, general hospital facilities.** The first type is the **tertiary medical center,** which has most or all of the latest technology and usually participates actively in medical education and clinical research. Within this facility, different units offer different levels of care, including intensive care units, special units for observation of patients, and standard units for the care of patients. The second type of hospital facility is the **intermediate hospital,** which is a medium to large community hospital that has a considerable amount of the latest technology but less research and investigational activity. The intermediate hospital may support cardiac bypass surgery, for example, but not necessarily organ transplantation. The third type is the **local community hospital,** which provides services such as routine diagnosis, treatment, and surgery but lacks the personnel and facilities for many complex procedures.

Moving down the scale of complexity, there are two types of *rehabilitation* or *convalescent* care facilities: a **special unit** in a regular hospital and a **rehabilitation hospital.** In particular, patients recovering from trauma or from neurologic diseases or surgery may benefit from physical therapy, occupational therapy, and other methods of tertiary prevention (see Chapter 17).

If patients are not discharged from the hospital directly to their homes, they are most likely discharged to one of three different types of **extended care facilities** (ECFs). The first type is the **skilled nursing facility** (SNF), often called a nursing home. It provides 24-hour nursing care and special forms of care, such as intravenous fluids, medicines, and rehabilitation. The second type is the **intermediate care facility** (ICF), which is suitable if the patient's primary need is for help with the activities of daily living (eating, bathing, grooming, transferring, toileting). Unlike an SNF, an ICF is not required to have a registered (skilled) nurse on duty at all times. Some nursing homes provide both skilled and intermediate levels of care. The third type is the **hospice,** a nursing home that specializes in providing *palliative* (comfort) *care* for terminally-ill patients, such as patients with cancer.

Organized home care may be necessary for patients who are discharged from the hospital to their homes, where they continue to receive treatment or follow-up procedures that require specialized skills. Examples of care include placing and monitoring intravenous lines for therapy and drawing blood for tests.

The least complex level of medical care is **self-care** in the home. In fact, the majority of medical care decisions are not made by professionals but instead by people for themselves, for friends, or for members of their families. Home diagnostic tools, such as blood pressure cuffs and blood glucose testing equipment, have given patients greater power to monitor their health. In keeping with other trends in U.S. society, patients increasingly are expected to take control over their own health care. With the Internet and direct-to-consumer marketing of drugs, patients have a wealth of information about (and therefore more control over) their own health and illnesses. The tremendous amount of health information now available has been a major force for empowering people regarding their own health. However, this information is usually not *peer-reviewed* and may contain incorrect or misleading statements. Also, to make informed decisions, patients need to be able to read and understand medical information, a capability called **health literacy** (see Chapter 15). Some patients may be overwhelmed by providers' expectations that they share or make important decisions about their health care.

IV. HEALTH CARE INSTITUTIONS

A. Hospitals

Although the term *hospital* is generally thought to refer to an institution providing acute, general care to persons with a wide range of health problems, there are various types of hospitals. Some focus on a special group of patients (e.g., children's hospital), whereas others focus on a special type of medical problem (e.g., psychiatric hospital) or a particular type of service (e.g., rehabilitation hospital).

Hospitals may be for-profit or not-for-profit. A for-profit hospital may be independent or part of a for-profit chain of hospitals. Not-for-profit hospitals may be sponsored by various institutions, such as the local community churches; the city, county, or state government; or a university (see Chapter 28).

B. Physician Practices

Historically, most U.S. physicians were in **solo medical practice,** although they might share night and weekend coverage with other solo practitioners. This type of practice could be emotionally rewarding but exhausting. Gradually, U.S. physicians began to develop **practice partnerships,** to solve the problem of sharing weekend and nighttime coverage and to achieve efficiencies and economies by sharing the cost of office space, equipment, and staff. In a partnership, each physician still works only for himself or herself.

A logical extension of the partnership was the formation of a **group practice** consisting of three or more (often many more) physicians. This increased the efficiencies of sharing office space and staff and increased the free time available to physicians. It also had the advantage of providing built-in

consultation with other physicians concerning complex cases. In a group practice, physicians are employees of the practice. Group practices could be of the single-specialty or the multispecialty type. Although most group practices initially operated on a fee-for-service basis, some began to develop the concept of **prepaid group practice,** in which the practice collects money from patients or employers and commits to providing all the care needed for these patients. On the West Coast the Kaiser Corporation set up its own multispecialty group practice before World War II to care for its workers. Membership has since been opened to the general public, and it is now known as Kaiser Permanente. This was the first example of a large, prepaid group practice in the United States.

C. Health Maintenance Organizations

During the Nixon administration, prepaid group practices that met certain standards and contractual arrangements were named **health maintenance organizations** (HMOs). The national HMO law passed in 1973 encouraged the large-scale development of HMOs. People who enrolled in an HMO were usually part of some economic group, such as workers in a company or industry, but their enrollment had to be voluntary. They paid a fixed monthly fee, which varied depending on the size of the group. In return, the HMO had the contractual obligation to *provide* the types of medical care specified in the contract (rather than to provide *financial reimbursement*, as in the case of an insurance company), or at least to ensure that the stipulated care was provided. The HMO assumed some of the risk when income was less than expenses and made a profit when income was greater than expenses.

Structurally, an HMO has three main components: (1) legal and fiscal entity that develops contracts and handles financial transactions, (2) physicians, and (3) hospitals and ancillary service providers. The HMO is defined as the organization that collects prepaid capitation premiums for medical services provided to its enrollees, monitors the service pattern, and approves and pays bills for services from physicians, hospitals, and others.

Health maintenance organizations can be organized in three different models: staff, group, and network. In the **staff model** HMO, most of the physicians are salaried, full-time employees who either work exclusively in the health plan or (as is typical in Kaiser Permanente) belong to a physician group that contracts to provide all the medical services in the health plan. A staff model HMO may own its hospitals; however, in most cases, the HMO contracts with one or more local hospitals for all hospital care. In the staff model the full-time physicians' time and effort are directed mainly or exclusively toward care of the HMO patients; these physicians serve as **gatekeepers**, coordinating care to patients and controlling referrals to specialists. A **group model HMO** provides the physician services through contracts with one or more organized groups of physicians. The HMO also contracts with one or more area hospitals for hospital services at predetermined rates. A **network model HMO** is similar to a group model HMO but is looser in structure. The network model HMO has contracts with many physician groups (single-specialty and multispecialty groups) and sometimes also with individual physicians. It may have a contract with one or more hospitals. The more providers an

HMO has in a geographic area, the more attractive it is to patients because they are usually able to choose their preferred physicians and hospitals.

An **independent practice association** (IPA) is a legal entity, usually an organization of physicians, that solicits enrollees and their premiums (from HMO payers or companies) and also contracts with office-based fee-for-service physicians in private practice to provide the required care, at a discounted rate. In addition, the IPA contracts with hospitals to provide inpatient care. (The **physician-hospital organization** [PHO] is a variant of IPA that is associated with a single hospital, which usually does the administrative work.) In IPAs the practitioners are supposed to perform the gatekeeper function (although they are usually less effective in controlling costs than are practitioners in other HMOs), and the IPA monitors utilization for appropriateness. Enrollees must receive their care from an IPA-affiliated hospital and from members of the IPA's **physician panel** (primary care physicians and specialists who have a contractual arrangement with the IPA). A physician may be a member of the panel of several IPAs, which makes the referral process quite confusing.

Currently, the most dominant model is the **preferred provider organization** (PPO). A PPO is a variation on the IPA theme; it is not usually approved as a federally qualified HMO because it lacks tight cost-control procedures. A PPO is formed when a third-party payer (e.g., insurance plan or company) establishes a network of contracts with independent practitioners. As with the standard IPA, the PPO has a panel of physicians who have contracted to provide services at agreed-on (reduced) rates. A major difference between the standard IPA and a PPO, however, is that the patients in a PPO can see physicians who are not on the PPO panel, although they will have to pay extra to do so (**point-of-service** [POS] **plan**).

In the past, many HMOs have used financial incentives for providers to shape provider behavior and avoid unnecessary costs. Important ethical problems can arise, however, if the compensation plan puts physicians' financial incentives in conflict with their patients' interests, such as when primary care physicians receive a bonus if they keep referral rates to specialists low. In response to these ethical dilemmas, the American College of Physicians has published an **Ethics in Practice Statement** advocating for transparency in managed care, open and participatory processes in resource allocation policy, and an obligation for individual providers to enter into agreement only if they can ensure that these agreements do not violate professionalism and ethical standards.[14]

D. Ambulatory Care

Outside of physicians' offices, ambulatory care can be through hospital outpatient clinics, surgicenters (freestanding surgical centers), walk-in clinics inside pharmacies, and urgent care clinics. Of particular importance for underserved patients are **community health centers.** Federal health programs in the 1960s and 1970s encouraged the development of community health centers. Many of these centers were supported partly through federal and state grants, and most were placed in underserved areas in big cities or rural locations. These **federally qualified health centers** (FQHCs) are eligible for federal grant support and enhanced reimbursement for Medicare and Medicaid patients and can provide free immunizations for uninsured children and reduced fees to other patients.

V. PAYMENT FOR HEALTH CARE

A century ago, physicians were paid directly by patients for their services. As medicine became more scientific, technical, and expensive, the out-of-pocket payment method became inadequate. One solution to the cost problem was to create a third-party payer, such as an insurance company. The third-party payer collected money regularly from a large population in the form of medical insurance premiums and paid the hospitals and physicians when care was required.

A. Physician Payments

Currently, physicians are usually paid in one of three ways: fee-for-service, capitation, or salary. Each of these payment systems provides incentives for providers to maximize or minimize certain types of care. None contains in itself incentives to maximize the quality of health care.

In the **fee-for-service** method, physicians are paid for each major item of service provided. Charges are established on the basis of the type and complexity of service (complete workup, follow-up visit, hospital visit, major surgical procedure). The amount charged by a physician may exceed the amount that a third-party payer is willing to reimburse, in which case the patient is expected to pay the difference. This payment system provides an incentive to provide more services than might be necessary, because each service brings in a fee.

Sometimes primary care physicians are paid on a **capitation** ("per head") basis. Regardless of the number of services needed by their patients, providers receive the same amount of money per month or per year. This method of payment has much lower administrative costs than the fee-for-service method and is thought to promote physicians' efforts in preventive care, although it provides an incentive to do as little as possible. It also may lead to poor gatekeeping, because clinicians may find it easier to refer a patient to a specialist than to provide a service themselves. The capitation method is sometimes used in the United States to pay practitioners working in HMOs; it is commonly used in Great Britain to pay general practitioners.

The third method of payment is a **salary.** Physicians who work full-time for HMOs, hospitals, universities, companies, or some group practices may be paid a *flat salary*. Although this method does not provide an incentive to provide either too little or too much care, it also does not provide incentives for productivity or high-quality care. Providers receive the same amount of money regardless of the amount or quality of care they provide. Recently, **pay-for-performance** methods and paying for outcomes have been explored. However, designing payment systems to reward quality also has drawbacks. It requires systems to measure quality of care and complex adjustments for comorbidities, which divert money and energy to measurement or documentation of care and away from the care itself (see Cost Containment).

B. Insurance and Third-Party Payers

Modern U.S. hospital insurance had its foundation in 1929 in Dallas, when a group of schoolteachers entered into a contract with Baylor University Hospital. Each teacher paid the hospital 50 cents per month. In turn, the hospital promised to cover the cost of any hospital stay. This scheme led to the development of **Blue Cross,** which is a form of insurance that covers only hospital care. Later, in response to recommendations from physicians and others, **Blue Shield** was developed as a parallel organization that allowed members to pay in advance for physician services.

To understand how insurance companies work, it is necessary to review a few concepts concerning benefits. If an insurance policy covers **indemnity benefits,** this means that the insurance company (carrier) will reimburse the insured patient a fixed number of dollars per service, regardless of the actual charges incurred; the patient must pay the difference. In contrast, if an insurance policy covers **service benefits,** the carrier must pay the full amount of the contracted payment for the needed services, regardless of their costs.

Actuaries, the statisticians who estimate risks and establish premiums for insurance companies, have a standard set of *actuarial principles* that guide the process of *underwriting* (insuring) medical risks and other risks such as fire and flood. Actuaries make sure that an insurance carrier does not collapse financially. Originally, insurance was designed to pool the risk from large groups to protect individuals from rare but devastating losses, such as fires in their homes or businesses. However, the actuarial principles developed to accomplish this objective do not adapt well to all medical care, for three reasons. First, medical care involves both frequent, and fairly predictable, costs and rare, catastrophic costs. Second, those at greatest risk of ill health and hospitalization can least afford the cost of insurance, although according to actuarial principles, they should be charged the most. Third, although homeowners may not be able to prevent fires and floods, many factors that affect health can be greatly influenced by personal behavior. Therefore, medical insurance requires adaptations to achieve a just and equitable system for financing medical care.

So far, one of the primary solutions for this dilemma in health care has been *pooling risk.* If all of the people in a large, natural community (i.e., a community consisting of people of various ages and degrees of health) were to be insured by the same carrier and were to pay the same monthly premium rate, the law of averages would work so as to protect the carrier from excessive loss. In effect, the low-risk people in the population would help pay the premiums for the high-risk people; the risk would be averaged according to the *community rating* or *experience rating* of the entire group. This is not a complete solution, because poor persons still might not be able to pay the established premium.

Initially, Blue Cross plans began to cover large segments of communities, and the community pooling of risk appeared to work. However, problems emerged as many insurance carriers sought to attract the business of low-risk individuals and companies by offering lower premiums. As the people with low risks were lured away from the community pool ("cream skimming" or "cherry picking"), those remaining in the pool were, on average, at higher risk. Consequently, they had to be charged a higher premium, making the community pool still less attractive. The phenomenon by which the people most attracted to purchasing health insurance are those who cost most to insure is called **adverse selection,** and occurs in any insurance system.

I. Benefit Design

All benefit plans offered by a third-party payer, including HMOs of various types, seek provisions to attract the patients they want to recruit to the plan, while at the same time limiting the financial exposure of the insurer. First, the plan may try to reduce premiums and costs by enlisting the patients themselves in reducing costs through such traditional methods as deductibles and copayments. Second, a common practice is to exclude or at least limit the amount of certain benefits. For instance, as previously mentioned, plans frequently limit or exclude benefits for mental health and dental health. A serious problem for many patients forced to change insurers is that the insurer may refuse to cover the cost of certain **preexisting conditions,** thus limiting the company's financial exposure for many chronic diseases and disorders. Legislation to control these loopholes is part of the Affordable Care Act (see earlier).

C. Social Insurance

Compulsory insurance for a population group is often called **social insurance** or **public insurance**. Most people employed in the United States must make payments into the Social Security Trust Fund for two national social insurance programs: Medicare and retirement benefits.

Medicare is authorized under Title 18 of the Social Security Act and is administered by the federal government (although it uses insurance carriers as fiscal intermediaries for managed Medicare plans, discussed later). The people eligible for Medicare include most individuals 65 years or older and most individuals who receive Social Security benefits because of disability. Part A and Part B of Medicare provide partial coverage for hospitalization and physician fees. Part A is paid by the Medicare Trust Fund, a separate government account funded by payroll taxes. Parts B and D (prescription drug coverage) are financed through premiums from enrollees and from general tax revenues. Part C of Medicare established managed care plans for Medicare enrollees (**Managed Medicare** or **Medicare Advantage**). In essence, Medicare pays an HMO to manage the Medicare recipient. Although Social Security beneficiaries do not pay premiums for Part A coverage after age 65, they do pay premiums if they elect to have Part B coverage. Medicare also will pay for a certain amount of home care or nursing home care for a medical problem that follows directly from a Medicare-covered hospitalization. However, Medicare does not pay for long-term nursing home care. Because Medicare does not cover all hospital expenses, patients are billed for the portion of charges not covered by Medicare.

More recently, insurance companies have started to offer **long-term care insurance** to cover nursing home costs. So far, these insurance plans are neither mandatory nor widely used.

D. Social Welfare

Medicaid is authorized under Title 19 of the Social Security Act. Unlike Medicare recipients, Medicaid recipients have not previously paid money into a trust fund. Medicaid is paid from general tax revenues of the federal and state governments. Therefore, the benefits of Medicaid are considered to be social welfare instead of social insurance.

The people covered by Medicaid are poor and usually receive additional assistance, such as **Aid to Families with Dependent Children** (AFDC). Unlike Medicare, which is entirely federally administered, Medicaid is administered by the states, which share the costs of the program with the federal government. Although the federal government usually reimburses a state for approximately half its Medicaid costs for a given year, poorer states receive slightly more. The federal government stipulates a minimum set of standards for Medicaid; beyond this, the eligibility criteria and covered services vary from state to state.

Medicaid basically covers two areas. First, it pays for medical care expenses, including both hospital and physician bills. The amount of reimbursement is often far below the customary charges of physicians, making the program unpopular with many providers and making it difficult for many patients to find physicians, especially specialists. Second, Medicaid pays for long-term nursing home care, but only after people have largely exhausted their personal resources, a process called "spend-down."

Under Title 21 of the Social Security Act, most states have established **Children's Health Insurance Programs** (CHIP) to provide health insurance to families whose income is too high to qualify for Medicaid. As with Medicaid, these programs are funded jointly by DHHS and the states and have various eligibility requirements and benefits.

VI. COST CONTAINMENT

The cost of medical care has long been a topic of concern in the United States. The first Committee on the Costs of Medical Care was established in 1929 and published its landmark report in 1932 that recommended the development of prepaid group practices (the forerunners of HMOs) as the most effective and efficient means to provide and finance medical care.[15] Until recent decades, the most common forms of cost containment were simple and straightforward. The pressure to control health care costs is driven by the rising national debt and the inability of employers to shoulder the burden of increasing health insurance premiums. Eventually, this pressure will require drastic action. Different policy makers will prefer different policy tools, but all will push to bring overall health care costs down and significantly decrease the growth in costs.

A. Reasons for Rapid Increase in Cost of Medical Care

Many of the controls over medical practice that were developed over the last half century were intended to limit the rapidly increasing costs of medical care. These costs were increasing much faster than the general inflation rate; in 2011, health care spending represented about 17% of GDP. Although managed care was able to reduce the rate of medical care inflation for a time in the 1980s, inflation rose to double digits again toward the end of the 20th century. Among the reasons for this rapid increase in costs were the following:

- Rapid innovations in costly new technologies, driven by a health care financing system that rewards expensive new technologies
- Increases in the wages for health care personnel
- Reliance on complex but only partially effective medical technology
- Increases in the demand for care because of population changes and changing expectations
- Inefficiencies in the delivery of care, stemming from such factors as underuse of facilities, fragmented care, inadequate insurance, and misuse of emergency rooms

The fee-for-service payment system, which was the norm in the United States through the 1970s, provided no incentive to providers to decrease costs. In fact, it rewarded *overuse* of services because revenues could be generated simply by performing more procedures. It also encouraged use of complex technologies and specialists and had no mechanism to ensure that new, more expensive technologies provided cost-effective care.[16] Medical costs have been and continue to be increased by the use of complex but only partially effective technology for the diagnosis and treatment of disease. Before polio vaccines were developed, for example, iron lungs were used to extend the lives of paralytic poliomyelitis victims. In contrast to the polio immunization program, which has proved to be highly cost-effective, the iron lung was an expensive and ineffective (only partially effective or *halfway*) technology. A more recent example of partially effective technology is surgery for cervical cancer compared with the human papillomavirus (HPV) vaccine, which prevents cervical cancer from developing.

I. Inefficiencies in Health Care Delivery

Not providing medical insurance for everyone is more costly than providing it. Lack of insurance leads to inappropriate use of emergency departments and to delayed care. This results in increased expenses because disease is found at a later, and less treatable, stage and in a more costly setting. The costs of this care eventually must be borne by society. Frequently, hospitals shift the costs of providing care for uninsured persons to society by charging insured persons more, often by shifting costs in some hidden fashion from those who cannot pay to those who can.

Planning failures have also contributed to increasing costs of medical care. Beginning in the mid-1960s and continuing for almost 20 years, the federal government supported official health planning strategies, largely in an effort to control costs. Among the primary strategies it supported were the appointment of rate-setting authorities within states and the issuance of a **certificate of need** (CON) for the construction of new hospitals or purchase of expensive equipment. Planning efforts were often ineffective in preventing the duplication of facilities and expensive equipment. In some areas, however, the regulatory efforts were reasonably effective. For example, the number of beds per 1000 population varies considerably in the United States, with no related changes in outcomes. If there is an empty hospital bed, somebody will try to fill it. Similar inefficiencies in care have been amply documented by the Dartmouth Atlas Project (see Websites and Chapter 24).

2. Decreasing Ability of Employers to Fund Health Care

Among the most important external forces that push costs to the consumers is the globalized operating environment for U.S. businesses. With global competition and the deregulation of many industries, fewer U.S. firms still have enough profits to subsidize health insurance for their workers.[17]

In the United States, most workers receive their health insurance through their employers. Employers essentially subsidize the cost of health insurance for their employees but have found doing so increasingly difficult. This has prompted employers to resort to shifting costs to employees, whether through high deductibles or in the so-called tax-preferred health savings accounts, which hand over almost all the responsibility for financing health care to individuals, as discussed next.

B. Strategies Targeted at Consumers or Services

The first and most basic method of discouraging the overuse of health care was to create **deductibles,** which are out-of-pocket payments made by the patient, often at the beginning of the care process. Medical deductibles work in much the same way as automobile or home insurance deductibles: they discourage the use of insurance for *unimportant* problems and reduce the amount of paperwork for the insurance companies. Deductibles are usually applied for an entire year (the patient might have to pay the first $5000 of yearly costs) or to each physician visit (the patient might have to pay $25 for each visit), with the insurance company paying the remainder of the eligible charges after the deductible is met. In general, physicians have worried that deductibles might discourage patients from coming in for early symptoms of serious disease, a concern substantiated by the findings of the RAND Health Insurance Experiment mentioned earlier. Recently, deductibles have started to range between $5000 and $10,000. At that rate, the deductible is so high that patients basically pay for their entire health care costs (**high-deductible plans**). Even though, in theory, the high-deductible plan covers expenses once the deductible is met, many patients may not exhaust their deductible unless they have a catastrophic illness.

The second basic cost-control method was **copayments**. In copayments, patients pay a given percentage of medical expenses. This provides an incentive for patients to contribute to keeping expenses low because copayments apply linearly to all costs. In contrast to deductibles, copayments were thought to *discourage* patients from staying in hospitals longer than necessary. Some health economists use the term **coinsurance** instead of copayments for payments that vary with the underlying cost of the service. As with deductibles, this cost-containment method discourages overutilization. In addition, and unlike deductibles, it also encourages patients to seek out low-cost settings because the patient is paying a fixed percentage of the entire cost of care.

The third common method was **exclusions** in the insurance. Some insurance policies totally excluded psychiatric care and dental care from coverage, whereas others severely restricted the reimbursement for these types of care. Psychiatric care, in particular, was perceived by third-party payers as a potentially bottomless pit that could consume large amounts of money in endless visits.

In the early 2000s, policy makers experimented with market-based health care policy solutions. Examples for such policy instruments are private long-term care insurance for nursing home care and **health savings accounts** (HSAs), also called "consumer-driven health care." HSAs were established in the **Medicare Modernization Act** of 2003. They consist of a high-deductible health plan (minimum of $1000 per person) and an individual, "tax-preferred" savings account from which individuals would directly finance their health care without a third-party payer. Monies not used in 1 year roll over to the next year. In effect, such an account delegates the responsibility of dealing with foreseeable health care expenses to the individual consumer and limits health insurance for catastrophic events. In order to work, such a model requires sophistication and much decision making by patients. Therefore, most proponents of market-based health policy solutions advocate for sponsors (employers or health care purchasing cooperatives) to act for a large group of subscribers to establish equity, manage risk selection, and create price-elastic demand.[18]

C. Strategies Targeted at Providers and Systems

If resources for medical care are inadequate to meet demand, there are three basic methods of responding: increase resources, decrease demand (or at least utilization), and increase efficiency. Given the many resources already devoted to financing health care, the recent emphasis is on *decreasing demand* and *increasing efficiency* through "bundling." One of the oldest bundling methods and the blueprint for newer versions is the **prospective payment system,** based on diagnosis-related groups, and the ambulatory payment classification system for the outpatient setting (see below). More recent efforts of bundling include episode-based payments, accountable care organizations, and the patient-centered medical home.

1. Prospective Payment System Based on Diagnosis-Related Groups

Developed in the 1970s, **diagnosis-related groups** (DRGs) have changed the way hospitals provide care. Each hospital admission is classified into major diagnostic categories based on organ systems, as outlined in the *International Classification of Diseases* (ICD), and then these diagnostic categories are further subdivided into DRGs. A DRG may consist of a single diagnosis or procedure, or it may consist of several diagnoses or procedures that, on average, have similar hospital costs per admission. An uncomplicated delivery of an infant, for example, is coded as DRG 775, and a percutaneous cardiovascular procedure with a non-drug-eluting stent without complications is coded as DRG 249.[19]

The federal government began to use DRGs in the treatment of Medicare patients in October 1983. Note that the hospital is actually reimbursed *after* a specific type of care is given; however, the amount of payment for the specific care is decided in advance. If a hospital can find a way to reduce the costs and provide the care for less than the amount reimbursed, it can retain the excess amount. If a hospital is inefficient and has higher-than-average costs, it loses money on that admission. The average cost for each of the more than 700 DRGs is set prospectively for each region of the country and adjusted for region; comorbidities, severity of illness, and risk of mortality.[19] Although extra amounts are added for tertiary hospitals and for hospitals engaged in medical education, these adjustments do not always fully cover the costs of providing care to indigent persons and paying for hospital-based medical education. Because hospitals with the strongest administrative teams and data systems are best able to keep costs below reimbursements, the strong hospitals tend to become stronger and the weak hospitals weaker.

The **prospective payment system** (PPS) added urgency to an already-growing trend to move as much medical care as possible out of acute, expensive, and poorly reimbursed general hospitals and into ambulatory surgery and diagnostic centers. Because it does not apply to ambulatory procedures, providers in ambulatory settings could set their own rates. In addition, many hospitals and staff model HMOs began to develop infirmaries, where patients who did not need acute, intensive care could be given moderate supervision and some treatment at a much lower cost than in hospitals.

2. Ambulatory Care Financing

For more than a decade, the U.S. government has supported research to develop an improved system to pay for ambulatory care, particularly to reduce the tendency to overpay for procedures and underpay for quality primary care. The first result of this research was the **resource-based relative value scale** (RBRVS), which sought to reimburse providers more equitably for outpatient care, based on their time spent on this care, their years of training, their level of skill, and their office equipment costs. At the same time, the government has been supporting research to determine how the general method used to develop DRGs could be applied to outpatient care. The result was the development of **ambulatory patient groups** (APGs) of conditions that require similar resources, based on the RBRVS. Thus, the two lines of research were combined with elements from the inpatient and outpatient care classification systems to produce the current **ambulatory payment classification** (APC) system. This federally mandated **outpatient** PPS is now being used by the federal government to reimburse for ambulatory care under Medicare.

3. Managed Care

Managed care is part of a complex balancing act created by society's struggles with two important questions.[20] First, how do we ensure that people receive needed health care without spending so much that we compromise other important social objectives? Second, how do we discourage unnecessary and inappropriate medical services without jeopardizing necessary high-quality care?

One answer to this dilemma was to develop standards of care to decide which patients can be admitted to the hospital, how long they may remain there, and what care must be done for them while they are hospitalized (**utilization management**). These determinations are variously referred to as **clinical pathways, medical protocols, best practices, practice guidelines,** or **clinical algorithms.** Another strategy to encourage high-quality care is to give providers financial incentives if they meet certain performance criteria

(**pay-for-performance** method). Administrative strategies aimed to discourage unnecessary services and keep costs low are described later. Techniques used by managed care companies to keep utilization down include **preadmission reviews and certification** (a reviewer, often a specially trained nurse, must approve a nonemergent hospital admission before it occurs), **concurrent review** (care is reviewed every day to determine if patient still needs to remain an inpatient), **second opinions** before expensive surgeries (second surgeon must agree service is indicated), and **gatekeeping** (referrals to specialists must be authorized by primary care provider).

4. Sharing Risk

In the first decade of the 21st century, policy makers have experimented with sharing the risk of medical care with providers. This trend takes various forms. Primary care providers can receive additional payments by providing expanded access and care. A **patient-centered medical home** (PCMH) is defined by the following principles[21]:

- *Personal physician.* Each patient has a personal physician who provides continuous and comprehensive care.
- *Physician-directed medical practice.* The personal physician leads a team that collectively takes responsibility for the ongoing care of the patient.
- *Whole-person orientation.* The practice addresses emotional, psychological, and medical needs of the patient.
- Care is *coordinated/integrated across systems* and facilitated by the use of registries.
- The practice engages in *continuous improvements* of quality and safety.
- *Enhanced access to care* is available through such systems as open scheduling, expanded hours, and new options for communication.
- *Payment appropriately recognizes* the added value.

Hospitals and providers can organize together to form **accountable care organizations** (ACOs). ACOs essentially function as traditional HMOs; hospitals, providers, and other institutions form a system to provide care and control costs. The difference is in the stress on patient engagement and that patients are free to choose their location and provider of care. The ACO is *accountable* to the patients and the third-party payer for the quality, appropriateness, and efficiency of the health care provided. The system provides and coordinates care, distributes payments, and shares in any cost savings.[22]

VII. ISSUES IN HEALTH POLICY

A. Complementary and Alternative Medicine

Trends in survey data indicate that the use of **complementary and alternative medicine** (CAM) is increasing in the United States, with more than a third of adults using some form of CAM.[23] Insurance plans and HMOs are rather timidly starting to cover certain CAM outpatient visits and procedures, and the survey data suggest that the total number of visits to CAM practitioners in the United States now exceeds the total number of primary care visits to allopathic (traditional medical) physicians.

A significant proportion of health care is now delivered by CAM practitioners and can no longer be ignored, even though everything about CAM is at least somewhat controversial. The boundaries of what constitutes CAM are not clearly defined. Some disciplines generally considered alternative, such as chiropractic and acupuncture, are increasingly embraced by allopathic medicine and may eventually become standard in the care of certain medical problems. Reimbursement for CAM by third-party payers is inconsistent, but increasingly some payment is being provided for chiropractic care and acupuncture for specified complaints. Other controversies relate to nomenclature and scientific evidence. Neither *alternative* nor *complementary* is thought to be an optimal designation for the field, and actually the terms are contradictory.

Efforts are ongoing to improve the evidence base for CAM.[24] Concerns persist that much of CAM lacks a rigorous evidence base, but most authorities agree that the effectiveness of nearly half of conventional medical practice is similarly unsubstantiated by the modern standards of evidence. Whether CAM use improves outcomes, reduces or increases the costs of care, or improves patient satisfaction is largely uncertain. The budget for the **National Center for Complementary and Alternative Medicine** (NCCAM) continues to grow, in testimony to the federal government's commitment to advancing this field and the evidence base underlying it. Currently, there are increasing efforts toward a creative and responsible synthesis of conventional medicine and CAM, which is often called **integrative medicine.**

B. The "Commons" and Moral Hazard

In 1968, Garrett Hardin[25] wrote about "the tragedy of the commons," perhaps the most famous contribution to the population-control debates of the 1960s. He noted that individuals and groups tend to maximize their own gains and use more than their fair share of any common good. This tendency is known in health policy as **moral hazard.** Because the shared resources of the earth (the "commons") are limited, Hardin argued that the attempt by one individual or group to maximize its own welfare would necessarily diminish the good that others can derive from the commons. This logic can be applied to the use of medical resources in the United States. Unless Americans are able and willing to organize, finance, and regulate medical care in light of the needs of the entire population, various individual groups (e.g., industries, hospitals, hospital chains, HMOs, insurance companies, nursing homes, home care programs) will continue to seek to maximize their benefits (their share of the commons) at the expense of others.

Apportioning resources from the medical commons is not simple, but a satisfactory resolution will not be achieved by piecemeal approaches. It is tempting to postulate that a single-payer system will improve the ability to achieve an ethical and rational allocation, but this method also has hazards. Health promotion and disease prevention will help, as would maximizing efficiency within the system, but these are not panaceas either. Any health care system has to find a balance among access to care, quality, and cost.[1] Independent of the Affordable Care Act, a national debate is needed on which health care services should be provided to all citizens and how limited resources should be distributed. With many large employers now pushing for solutions, the time for such a debate may finally be right.

VIII. SUMMARY

In the United States the medical care system has developed without strong direction from the local, state, or federal government. The result is a confusing mix of ways in which services are paid for and organized. The per-capita cost of medical care and the proportion of the GDP used for medical care are higher in the United States than anywhere in the world, yet approximately 17% of Americans still have no financial protection from the costs of medical care. The outcomes purchased for the enormous amount of money spent on health care are not consistently better than those of other countries. The inflation rate of U.S. medical care costs is one of the highest in the world.

Because of the high costs of U.S. medical care, cost-containment strategies are used extensively. In the prospective payment system, third-party payers reimburse hospitals for care at a predetermined rate, depending on the average duration and complexity of the medical care provided for each condition. Frequently used prospective payment systems include diagnosis-related groups and bundled payments for episodes of care. In managed care, hospitalizations are reimbursed by a third-party payer only if the payer has approved the admission (preadmission review and certification). If a patient is admitted through the emergency department, the admission is reviewed the next day and if not approved by the third-party payer, reimbursement may not be paid (emergency department admission review). Once a patient is in the hospital, the length of stay is closely monitored, and the patient may be denied coverage if the patient is deemed stable enough to be discharged from the hospital as soon as possible (concurrent review and discharge planning). Other aspects of managed care include second opinions before elective surgery, use of primary care physicians as gatekeepers, benefit design, and the provision of financial incentives for physicians to practice economically.

The main government funded health care financing mechanisms include social insurance (Medicare) and social welfare (Medicaid and State Children's Health Insurance Programs). The U.S. medical care system has many costly inefficiencies, and correcting these may require major changes. New care models aimed at improving these inefficiencies include the patient-centered medical home and the accountable care organization.

References

1. Kissick WL: *Medicine's dilemmas: infinite need versus finite resources*, New Haven, Conn, 1994, Yale University Press.
2. Keeler EB: Effects of cost sharing on use of medical services and health. *J Med Pract Manage* 8:317–321, 1992.
3. Commonwealth Report: Number of uninsured in United States.http://www.commonwealthfund.org/Blog/2011/Sep/Number-of-Uninsured-in-United-States-Grows.aspx
4. Kaiser Family Foundation. http://www.kff.org/insurance/snapshot/OECD042111.cfm
5. Total expenditure of health against life expectancy by country. http://www.theatlantic.com/business/archive/2011/04/oecd-us-outspends-average-developed-country-141-in-health-care/237171
6. Fineberg HV: A successful and sustainable health system—how to get there from here. *NEJM* 366:1020–1027, 2012.
7. Davies K, Schoen C, Stremikis K: Mirror, mirror on the wall: how the performance of the U.S. health care system compares internationally: 2010 update. http://www.commonwealthfund.org/~/

media/Files/Publications/Fund%20Report/2010/Jun/1400_Davis_Mirror_Mirror_on_the_wall_2010.pdf

8. Institute of Medicine: For the public's health: revitalizing law and policy to meet new challenges. http://www.iom.edu/Reports/2011/For-the-Publics-Health-Revitalizing-Law-and-Policy-to-Meet-New-Challenges.aspx

9. Environmental Data White Paper: http://tulane.edu/publichealth/caeph/epht/upload/Environmental-Data-White-Paper.pdf

10. http://www.kff.org/healthreform/upload/8061.pdf

11. Pande AH, Ross-Degnan D, Zaslavsky AM, et al: Effects of healthcare reforms on coverage, access, and disparities. *Am J Prev Med* 41:1–8, 2011.

12. Joyce TJ: Point/Counterpoint: What can Massachusetts teach us about national health insurance reform? *J Policy Analysis Manage* 30:177–195, 2011.

13. Musumeci MB: A guide to the Supreme Court's Affordable Care Decision. Policy Brief #8332. Available at http://www.kff.org/healthreform/upload/8332.pdf.

14. American College of Physicians: A shared statement of ethical principles for those who share and give healthcare: a working draft. http://www.acponline.org/clinical_information/journals_publications/ecp/mayjun99/tavistock.htm

15. Committee on the Costs of Medical Care: *Medical care for the American people*, Chicago, 1932, University of Chicago Press.

16. Povar GJ, Blumen H, Daniel J, et al: Ethics in practice: managed care and the changing health care environment. *Ann Intern Med* 141:131–136, 2004.

17. Fuchs VR, Emanuel EJ: Health care reform. Why? What? When? *Health Affairs* 24:1399–1414, 2005.

18. Enthoven AC: The history and principles of managed competition. *Health Affairs* Supplement 24–48, 1993.

19. Kruse M, Taillon H: *The clinical documentation improvement specialist's handbook*, ed 2, Danvers, Mass, 2011, HCPro. Available at http://www.hcmarketplace.com/supplemental/8876_browse.pdf

20. Gray BH, Field MJ, editors: *Controlling costs and changing patient care? The role of utilization management*, Washington, DC, 1989, National Academy Press.

21. http://www.pcpcc.net/content/joint-principles-patient-centered-medical-home

22. Health policy brief: Accountable care organizations. http://www.rwjf.org/files/research/66449.pdf

23. Barnes PM, Bloom B: Complementary and alternative medicine use among adults and children: United States, 2007. *National Health Statistics Reports*, 2008. http://nyscadistrict2.com/w/newspdf/ComplementaryAndAlternativeMedicineUseInUS2007.pdf

24. http://www.ncbi.nlm.nih.gov/pubmed/12868249

25. Hardin G: The tragedy of the commons. *Science* 162:1243–1248, 1968.

Select Readings

Fuchs VR, Emanuel EJ: Health care reform. Why? What? When? *Health Affairs* 24:1399–1414, 2005.

Gostin LO: *Public health law: power, duty, restraint*, ed 2, Los Angeles, 2008, University of California Press.

Kazmier JL: *Health care law*, Clifton Park, NY, 2008, Delmar Cengage Learning.

Kovner AR, Jonas S: *Health care delivery in the United States*, ed 10, New York, 2011, Springer.

Rognehaugh R: *The managed health care dictionary*, ed 2, Gaithersburg, Md, 1998, Aspen.

Stone D: *Policy paradox: the art of political decision making*, New York, 2002, WW Norton.

Websites

http://www.cms.hhs.gov [Center for Medicare and Medicaid Services]

http://www.dartmouthatlas.org/downloads/reports/supply_sensitive.pdf [Dartmouth Atlas Project: Supply-sensitive care]

http://www.epa.gov/lawsregs [Environmental Protection Agency: Laws and regulations]

http://www.hrsa.gov/ [Health Resources and Services Administration]

http://www.iom.edu [Institute of Medicine]

http://www.kff.org/ [The Henry J. Kaiser Family Foundation]

One Health: Interdependence of People, Other Species, and the Planet

Meredith A. Barrett and Steven A. Osofsky

I. UNPRECEDENTED CHALLENGES, HOLISTIC SOLUTIONS

Population growth and the globalization of economic networks have resulted in a rapidly changing, highly interconnected world. The global human population surpassed 7 billion inhabitants in 2011 and is expected to reach 9.3 billion by 2050 and 10 billion by 2100.[1] The resulting demands for living space, land, food, water, and energy have become an increasing challenge. Never before have global issues of environmental sustainability and the health of humans and animals been so closely interconnected. To broaden our thinking on the scope and magnitude of these

shifting global trends, we introduce a number of anthropological, environmental, and economic issues that ultimately relate to human health (Figure 30-1).

These health and sustainability consequences of global change are economically, socially, medically, and environmentally costly, and as such, their control can be considered a global public good.[2] The complexities and breadth of such threats demand interdisciplinary solutions that address the connections between human and animal health,[3] as well as the underlying environmental drivers that impact health. Traditionally, however, approaches to health have focused on interventions such as human-based clinical treatment, emergency response, or vaccines. Increasingly, there is a push in the global community to move from reductionist, reactionist approaches to more holistic, preventive approaches that rely on systems thinking.[4] One such approach, known as **One Health**, is a growing global strategy that is being adopted by a diversity of organizations and policy makers in response to the need for integrated approaches. This approach can be relevant to a wide range of global development goals, including the Millennium Development Goals themselves, which we explore in the Chapter 30 supplement on studentconsult.com.

In this chapter we define One Health; explore how it is relevant to public health, epidemiology, and medicine; follow its development; learn of its current supporters and applications; and consider implementation strategies for redefining health through transdisciplinary collaboration. Though this exploration of One Health, we hope to introduce a growing cadre of health professionals to a more holistic approach to health that will become increasingly important in the future.

II. WHAT IS ONE HEALTH?

One Health can be interpreted differently by various groups and tends to serve as a comprehensive framework that has been employed in different contexts.[5] This flexibility can strengthen its applicability rather than narrow its scope. Although different definitions and interpretations exist, a frequently used description follows:

> One Health is [characterized by] the collaborative efforts of multiple disciplines working locally, nationally and globally to attain optimal health for people, animals and our environment.[6]

The One Health approach calls for a paradigm shift in developing, implementing, and sustaining health policies that more proactively engage human medicine, veterinary

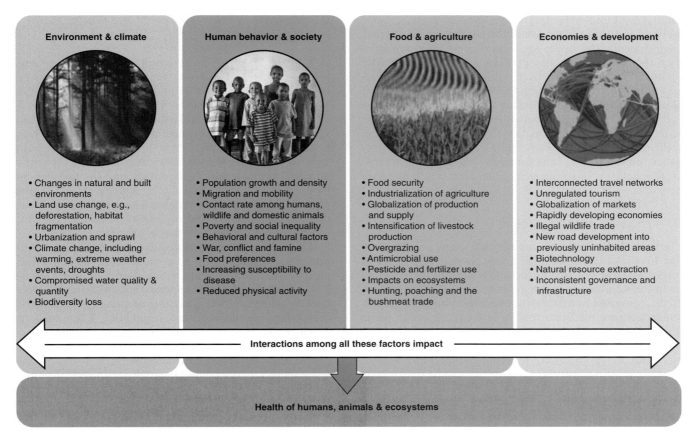

Figure 30-1 We are undergoing rapid shifts in our environment, in climate, in human behavior, in agriculture, and in economic development. All these factors interact to impact the health of humans, animals, and the environment. (Modified from World Bank: *People, pathogens and our planet: towards a One Health approach for controlling zoonotic diseases*, vol I, Washington, DC, 2010; and Institute of Medicine, National Research Council: *Sustaining global surveillance and response to emerging zoonotic diseases*, Washington, DC, 2009, National Academies Press.)

medicine, public health, environmental sciences, and a number of other disciplines that relate to health, land use, and the sustainability of human interactions with the natural world.[6-10] The use of this multifaceted perspective allows practitioners to work toward optimal health for people, domestic animals, wildlife, and the environment concurrently, over multiple spatial and temporal scales. Whereas some may view One Health as having a singular end goal of optimizing human health, we emphasize here that the maintenance and improvement of animal health and ecosystem functioning are also primary goals of One Health, with their own inherent value separate from their impact on human health.

Past global health interventions have generally tackled a single region or a single disease, but One Health offers an integrative, holistic health *systems* approach that also focuses on "upstream" prevention rather than reactive response. Just as the World Health Organization (WHO) maintains a multifaceted definition of health as "a state of complete physical, mental, and social well-being and not merely the absence of disease or infirmity," so too does One Health attempt to address the many different social, environmental, cultural, and physical determinants of human and animal health. Although different interpretations of One Health exist, certain unifying characteristics remain the same across all applications (Box 30-1).

Box 30-1	Shared Characteristics of One Health Applications

Goal of optimizing the health of people, animals, and the environment
Prevention-oriented
Collaborative
Transdisciplinary
Multiscale (local, national, global)
Systems-focused
Flexible
Innovative
Synergistic
Added value
Comprehensive
Holistic

A. Relevance to Epidemiology

One Health shares many of the same fundamental principles as the fields of epidemiology, biostatistics, public health, and preventive medicine and therefore is a relevant topic for these curricula. At its core, One Health calls for a shift from an individual, clinical-based treatment approach to a more holistic and preventive perspective that considers populations of multiple species and the context of their shared environments. The aim to apply this type of approach from local to global scales is also shared among these fields. The population/prevention focus of public health, epidemiology, and preventive medicine aligns perfectly with a One Health approach. However, One Health can move things a step further by enlarging the spatial, temporal, and organismal scope of these fields. Ultimately, One Health relies on the collaboration of multiple disciplines. Epidemiology, biostatistics, public health, and preventive medicine can serve as foundational disciplines in One Health collaborative networks.

B. Evolution of the Concept

The One Health concept is actually not a new one; its roots date back to ancient times. The Greek physician Hippocrates (ca. 460–370 BCE) wrote of the importance of the environment for maintaining health in his text, *On Airs, Waters and Places*.[11] Several centuries later, connections between human and veterinary medicine took shape in the 1800s when Rudolf Virchow (1821–1902), a German physician and pathologist known as the "Father of Comparative Pathology," laid the foundations for One Health thinking. He defined the term **zoonosis** (a disease that can be transmitted from animals to people) and stated, "Between animal and human medicine there are no dividing lines—nor should there be." A student of Virchow's, the Canadian physician Sir William Osler (1849–1919), once called the "Father of Modern Medicine," adopted similar ways of thinking about health across both human and veterinary medicine.[4] By the 1940s, this type of collaboration took a more distinct form. James Steele, veterinarian and the first U.S. Assistant Surgeon General for Veterinary Affairs, expanded the role of veterinarians by developing the first Veterinary Public Health program within the Centers for Disease Control and Prevention (CDC) and by incorporating veterinarians into the U.S. Public Health Service. Calvin Schwabe (1927–2006), a leading figure in veterinary epidemiology, re-emphasized the importance of veterinary medicine to human health and promoted the term **One Medicine** in his book, *Veterinary Medicine and Human Health*.[4,12,13]

The field of veterinary public health, which holds that the health of wildlife, domesticated animals, and humans is inherently intertwined, solidified as a result of collaborations among major international organizations such as the WHO and the United Nations Food and Agriculture Organization (FAO).[12,14] As the concept of sustainable development gained traction in the international arena during the late 1980s, a strengthened recognition of the role of the environment surfaced.[4,13] As a result of this trend, some new fields—notably conservation medicine and ecohealth—emerged with a particular emphasis on how the Earth's changing ecosystems affected the health of both animals and humans.[4,14-20] These approaches extended the One Medicine concept to include the whole ecosystem and brought in ideas of sustainable development and socio-ecological influences on health. This represented a move from a more clinical focus to a more holistic view that broadly incorporated the environment and social sciences. This type of perspective contributed greatly to the highly influential and informative **Millennium Ecosystem Assessment,**[21] which further delineated the reliance of human well-being on the environment.

C. Manhattan Principles on "One World, One Health"

In 2004 the **Wildlife Conservation Society** (WCS) brought together an array of partners to develop an unprecedented collaborative One Health framework to launch the **One World, One Health** initiative.[4,5,8] This launch resulted in the development of the **Manhattan Principles** (Box 30-2), which provide 12 recommendations for "establishing a more holistic approach to preventing epidemic/epizootic disease and for maintaining ecosystem integrity for the benefit of humans, their domesticated animals, and the foundational biodiversity that supports us all."[4,8,22] One World, One Health represented a proactive, collaborative effort among major international agencies and organizations and is seen as an important step in the evolution of One Health.

This type of interagency collaboration has led to several initiatives, including the subsequent 2006 Beijing Principles.[23] Notably, the World Organization for Animal Health (OIE), FAO, and the WHO released a joint strategic concept note to achieve a "world capable of preventing, detecting, containing, eliminating, and responding to animal and public health risks attributable to zoonoses and animal diseases with an impact on food security through multi-sectoral cooperation and strong partnerships."[22,23,24]

Other joint partnerships have emerged. In 2007, the American Veterinary Medical Association (AVMA) and the American Medical Association (AMA) both unanimously and explicitly supported One Health.[6] The AVMA-AMA collaboration called for the formation of a **One Health Commission** to work toward the "establishment of closer professional interactions, collaborations, and educational opportunities across the health sciences professions, together with their related disciplines, to improve the health of people, animals, and our environment" (see Websites list at end of chapter). In addition, the **One Health Initiative** has served as an important global clearinghouse for news and information related to One Health. It collaborates directly with the *One Health Newsletter,* an online quarterly for One Health articles sponsored by the Florida Department of Health. Through the newsletter and website, communication among One Health professionals all over the world has improved significantly.

Through the evolution of the One Health concept, different—yet complementary and related—approaches have emerged. All these approaches capture dimensions of One Health or have played an important role in the development of One Health. Relevant terms and fields complementary to One Health include One Medicine, comparative medicine, "One World, One Health," ecohealth, ecosystem approaches to health, veterinary public health, health in socio-ecological systems, conservation medicine, ecological medicine, environmental medicine, medical geology, and environmental health. Similarities also obviously exist between One Health and major fields such as global health, public health, and population health. As it continues to change and evolve, One Health will be strengthened and further defined, extending in scope and in its ability to address complex health and environmental challenges.[4]

D. Disciplines Engaged in One Health

Implementing One Health requires the cooperation of experts from numerous disciplines, including but not limited to the following: human medicine, veterinary medicine,

Box 30-2 Manhattan Principles on "One World, One Health"

Recent outbreaks of West Nile virus, Ebola hemorrhagic fever, SARS, monkeypox, mad cow disease, and avian influenza remind us that human and animal health are intimately connected. A broader understanding of health and disease demands a unity of approach achievable only through a consilience of human, domestic animal, and wildlife health—**One Health.** Phenomena such as species loss, habitat degradation, pollution, invasive alien species, and global climate change are fundamentally altering life on our planet, from terrestrial wilderness and ocean depths to the most densely populated cities. The rise of emerging and resurging infectious diseases threatens not only humans (and their food supplies and economies), but also the fauna and flora comprising the critically needed biodiversity that supports the living infrastructure of our world. The earnestness and effectiveness of humankind's environmental stewardship and our future health have never been more clearly linked. To win the disease battles of the 21st century while ensuring the biologic integrity of the Earth for future generations requires interdisciplinary and cross-sectoral approaches to disease prevention, surveillance, monitoring, control, and mitigation as well as to environmental conservation more broadly.

We urge the world's leaders, civil society, the global health community, and institutions of science to:

1. Recognize the essential link among human, domestic animal, and wildlife health and the threat that disease poses to people, their food supplies, and economies, as well as the biodiversity essential to maintaining the healthy environments and functioning ecosystems we all require.
2. Recognize that decisions regarding land and water use have real implications for health. Alterations in the resilience of ecosystems and shifts in patterns of disease emergence and spread manifest themselves when we fail to recognize this relationship.
3. Include wildlife health science as an essential component of global disease prevention, surveillance, monitoring, control, and mitigation.
4. Recognize that human health programs can greatly contribute to conservation efforts.
5. Devise adaptive, holistic, and forward-looking approaches to the prevention, surveillance, monitoring, control, and mitigation of emerging and resurging diseases that take the complex interconnections among species into full account.
6. Seek opportunities to fully integrate biodiversity conservation perspectives and human needs (including those related to domestic animal health) when developing solutions to infectious disease threats.
7. Reduce the demand for and better regulate the international live-wildlife and bushmeat trade not only to protect wildlife populations but to lessen the risks of disease movement, cross-species transmission, and the development of novel pathogen-host relationships. The costs of this worldwide trade in terms of impacts on public health, agriculture, and conservation are enormous, and the global community must address this trade as the real threat it is to global socioeconomic security.
8. Restrict the mass culling of free-ranging wildlife species for disease control to situations where there is a multidisciplinary, international scientific consensus that a wildlife population poses an urgent, significant threat to human health, food security, or wildlife health more broadly.
9. Increase investment in the global human and animal health infrastructure commensurate with the serious nature of emerging and resurging disease threats to people, domestic animals, and wildlife. Enhanced capacity for global human and animal health surveillance and for clear, timely information-sharing (that takes language barriers into account) can only help improve coordination of responses among governmental and nongovernmental agencies, public and animal health institutions, vaccine/pharmaceutical manufacturers, and other stakeholders.
10. Form collaborative relationships among governments, local people, and the private and public (i.e., nonprofit) sectors to meet the challenges of global health and biodiversity conservation.
11. Provide adequate resources and support for global wildlife health surveillance networks that exchange disease information with the public health and agricultural animal health communities as part of early-warning systems for the emergence and resurgence of disease threats.
12. Invest in educating and raising awareness among the world's people and in influencing the policy process to increase recognition that we must better understand the relationships between health and ecosystem integrity to succeed in improving prospects for a healthier planet.

It is clear that no one discipline or sector of society has enough knowledge and resources to prevent the emergence or resurgence of diseases in today's globalized world. No one nation can reverse the patterns of habitat loss and extinction that can and do undermine the health of people and animals. Only by breaking down the barriers among agencies, individuals, specialties, and sectors can we unleash the innovation and expertise needed to meet the many serious challenges to the health of people, domestic animals, and wildlife and to the integrity of ecosystems. Solving today's threats and tomorrow's problems cannot be accomplished with yesterday's approaches. We are in an era of "One World, One Health," and we must devise adaptive, forward-looking, and multidisciplinary solutions to the challenges that undoubtedly lie ahead.

From Cook RA, Karesh WB, Osofsky SA: *The Manhattan Principles on "One World, One Health": building interdisciplinary bridges to health in a globalized world,* New York, 2004, Wildlife Conservation Society. Available at http://www.oneworldonehealth.org/sept2004/owoh_sept04.html.

public health, environmental science, ecology, environmental health, conservation biology, dentistry, nursing, social sciences, the humanities, engineering, economics, education, and public policy. Although the foundations of the One Health concept originated within the veterinary and human medical professions, there is a strong push toward representation of a wider array of disciplines. One Health is not to be "owned" by certain disciplines. We illustrate the need for the participation of multiple disciplines when approaching health problems with a particularly relevant case study involving West Nile virus (WNV) (Fig. 30-2). When WNV emerged in New York City in 1999, discovery of the outbreak and development of a control strategy depended upon the involvement of multiple disciplines.[25]

III. BREADTH OF ONE HEALTH

A. Interdependence of Animal, Human, and Ecosystem Health

Fundamentally, the environment affects how organisms live, thrive, and interact and must be considered in order to achieve optimal health for people and animals.[21,26-28] By

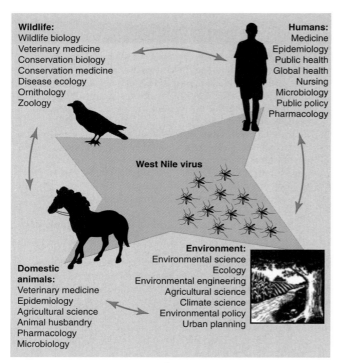

Figure 30-2 Emergence of West Nile virus (WNV) into the United States. The collaborative response to WNV in the U.S. provides a perfect case study for the One Health approach. In 1999, physicians noted a strange illness in elderly patients in New York City; simultaneously, veterinary pathologists and epidemiologists were exploring the mysterious deaths of large numbers of crows and exotic birds at the Bronx Zoo. Viral culture and polymerase chain reaction evidence concluded that the infections were related and later confirmed the outbreaks as the first emergence of WNV into the United States via the *Culex* mosquito vector. WNV can infect several wild bird species and a range of mammals, including: horses, squirrels, dogs, wolves, mountain goats, and humans. Combating WNV requires the collaboration of a multitude of disciplines. (From Barrett MA, Bouley TA, Stoertz AH, et al: Integrating a One Health approach in education to address global health and sustainability challenges. *Frontiers Ecol Environ* 9:239–245, 2010. Copyright Ecological Society of America.)

definition, the **environment** includes "all of the physical, chemical and biological factors and processes that determine the growth and survival of an organism or a community of organisms."[29] This definition encompasses many different contexts and scales, ranging from an individual's home environment, to social environments, to regional ecosystems, to the air that we breathe and the climate in which we exist. As such, the definition of environment can include both the *built* environment, such as urban systems, and more unmodified, *natural* ecosystems.

Human and animal well-being relies on the integrity of ecosystems. An **ecosystem** is "comprised of all of the organisms and their physical and chemical environment within a specific area."[29] Ecosystems underpin processes essential to our survival, known as **ecosystem services.**[21] The United Nations **Millennium Ecosystem Assessment,** a comprehensive global assessment of the world's ecosystems and what they mean to human well-being, deemed ecosystem services to be the "ultimate foundations of life and health."[21] These services include *supporting* services (nutrient cycling, soil formation, primary production); *regulating* services

(climate and flood regulation, disease buffering, water purification); *provisioning* services (food, water, fuel); and *cultural* services (aesthetic, spiritual, mental health) that make the persistence of human and animal life possible[21] (Figure 30-3). Many of these ecosystem services rely on the maintenance of **biodiversity** (including genes, species, and populations) and complex ecological relationships that make possible the growth of food, healthy diets, the development of new medicines, and the regulation of emerging infectious diseases.

Ecosystems can maintain healthy populations, but when mismanaged or rapidly altered due to human pressure, they can also be associated with disease emergence. Despite the importance of the environment to the preservation of human and animal well-being, we face increasing challenges to the maintenance of healthy ecosystems, including climate change, deforestation, intensification of agricultural systems, freshwater depletion, and resultant biodiversity loss[30,31] (Figure 30-4). In fact, human populations have altered ecosystems more rapidly and extensively over the last 60+ years than during any other period in history, causing some scientists to describe our current geologic time period as the **Anthropocene** ("age of man" or "age of human influence").[21,32] To enable assessment of this change, holistic indicators of ecosystem health (which incorporate environmental, social, and economic aspects of ecosystems) are being developed to assess ecological changes over space and time.[33] **Ecological indicators** can include measures such as water quality, tree canopy cover, soil organic matter, wildlife populations, land-use profiles, and vegetation characteristics.[34]

The growing global human population will continue to increase its need for land, food, and energy, yet already 60% of the essential ecosystem services of the planet are degraded or are under increasing threat. Addressing the environmental factors affecting health is essentially a public health–oriented prevention strategy, as it tackles the upstream drivers of disease. For example, an estimated 24% of the global burden of disease, and more than one third of the burden among children, originates from modifiable environmental causes.[35,36] Such issues are explored in One Health Case Study 1 on studentconsult.com, which examines a particularly salient case highlighting the emergence of Nipah virus in Malaysia caused by a combination of land-use, agricultural, and environmental factors.

B. Climate Change

Climate change is one of the most pressing human-driven environmental changes we face. The **Intergovernmental Panel on Climate Change** (IPCC) reported that three main components of climate change will continue to impact ecosystems and health in the future, including warming (1.1°-6.4° C increase in global mean surface temperature by 2100), shifting patterns of precipitation, and increased incidence of extreme climatic events.[37] The exact spatial occurrences of these shifts, as well as the resilience and responses of different ecosystems, are difficult to predict.

When examining the impact of climate change on disease, the picture grows more complex. Climate has affected spatial and temporal patterns of disease globally and has been identified as the greatest threat to global health for the 21st century,[38-40] yet there is still some debate about exactly how

Figure 30-3 Human health relies on essential ecosystem services derived from the environment. (From Corvalan C, Hales S, McMichael A, et al: Ecosystems and human well-being: health synthesis. Report of the Millennium Ecosystem Assessment, Geneva, 2005, World Health Organization. Figure from Rekacewicz P, Bournay E, United Nations Environment Programme/Grid-Arendal.)

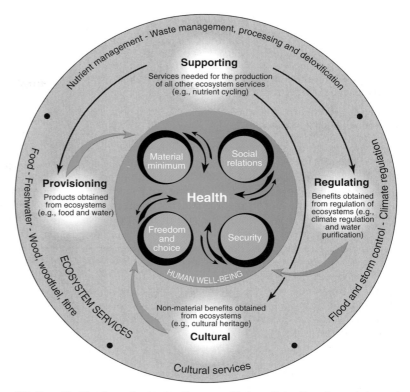

This figure identifies five main aspects of human well-being, with health as the central aspect. Human health is affected directly and indirectly by changes in ecosystems. The basic requirements for human well-being (i.e., material minimum, good social relations, security, freedom, and choice) are inherently connected to health.

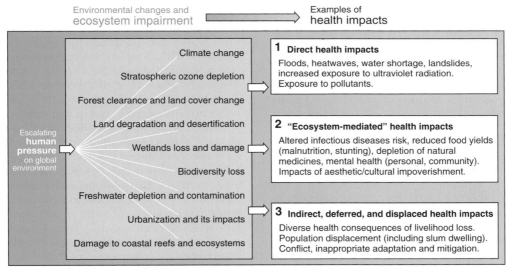

This figure describes the causal pathway from escalating human pressures on the environment to ecosystem changes resulting in diverse health consequences. Not all ecosystem changes are included, and some changes can have positive effects (e.g., food production).

Figure 30-4 Environmental change can degrade ecosystems and negatively affect health. (From Corvalan C, Hales S, McMichael A, et al: Ecosystems and human well-being: health synthesis. Report of the Millennium Ecosystem Assessment, Geneva, 2005, World Health Organization. Figure from Rekacewicz P, Bournay E, United Nations Environment Programme/Grid-Arendal.)

climate change will affect disease burden.[41] Changes in temperature, precipitation, and seasonality can influence infectious disease emergence, incidence, and spread (e.g., as seen with dengue, malaria, cholera).[42,43] These environmental changes can affect pathogen reproduction, abundance, environmental tolerance, virulence, and distributions.[44-47] For example, studies have documented that the chytrid fungus that decimated global amphibian populations partly emerged because of increasing temperatures,[48] and that the impacts of malaria, Ross River virus, plague, hantavirus, and cholera have been exacerbated by climate change.[39] In addition to disease, the potential health impacts of climate change will be broad and significant in terms of the following: heat and cold effects; wind, storms, and floods; drought, malnutrition, and food security; food safety; water quality; air quality; occupational health; and ultraviolet radiation.[37]

C. Biodiversity Loss

Land-use change such as deforestation leads to the loss of biodiversity and the increasing interactions of humans, wildlife, and domestic animals,[49-51] which can influence the spread of infectious diseases.[49,52,53] Strong evidence shows that in some vector-borne disease systems, more diverse species communities will reduce the risk of infection.[49,54,55] This pattern, termed the **dilution effect,** works because incompetent reservoir hosts "dilute" the likelihood of disease transmission among vectors and competent hosts.[54-58]

In the classic example of **Lyme disease,** higher levels of forest mammal biodiversity reduced infection risk because a greater proportion of species in more diverse systems were poor reservoirs for the *Borrelia* pathogen (see One Health Case Study 2 on studentconsult.com).

This pattern has also been seen in other vector-borne disease systems such as WNV, leishmaniasis, African trypanosomiasis, Chagas disease, and Rocky Mountain spotted fever.[59,60] In some cases, however, host diversity has also been linked to pathogen diversity. In a global study, zoonotic emerging infectious disease events were correlated with high wildlife biodiversity,[61] and another study found that the number of human pathogens was correlated with bird and mammal diversity in a region.[62]

Deforestation can also affect biodiversity by facilitating access for hunting opportunities. **Hunting** is important to consider for human health in a number of ways: as a source of nutrition, as a risk factor for disease emergence, as a driver of local biodiversity extinctions, and as a supplier for the global wildlife trade. Although hunting does provide valuable protein and micronutrient sources for populations relying on subsistence livelihoods,[63] the process of hunting, butchering, and cooking the animal creates opportunities for body fluid transfer and transmission of diseases from wildlife to humans. In fact, some of the world's most significant emerging diseases have been traced to zoonotic disease transmission via contact through hunting.[64,65] Regardless of whether wildlife is consumed or sold as clothing or ornamentals in wildlife markets, the wildlife trade contributes to the decimation of global biodiversity and the spread of pathogens.[66] A number of pathogens have been transmitted via wildlife trade, both into human populations and into novel wildlife hosts.[66] The global wildlife market is widespread and massive, generating more than an estimated $21 billion annually. The scale and risks associated with the wildlife trade demand an integrated approach to reduce and regulate it.

D. Food and Water Security

One Health offers new perspectives on addressing issues of food security for increasingly complex and connected global food networks. Factors such as specialization and intensification of livestock production; increasing spatial overlap of humans, wildlife, and domestic animals; deforestation for livestock grazing; globalization of livestock production; and climate change have led to escalating infectious disease occurrence in livestock animal populations,[22,38,57,67,68] raising serious conservation concerns and compromising food security and water quality.[50] Recent livestock diseases within the global food supply have been associated with subsequent occurrences of infectious disease in humans (e.g., bovine spongiform encephalopathy, Rift Valley fever, bovine tuberculosis, H1N1 influenza virus).[69,70] In 2005 alone, 1.8 million people died from food-borne bacterial infections with *Salmonella, Campylobacter,* or *Escherichia coli.*[2,71] One Health Case Study 3 on studentconsult.com explores Rift Valley fever and its intersection at the human-animal-environment interface.

Antimicrobial resistance presents another challenge for safe livestock production.[72] Resistant pathogens can cause morbidity and mortality in livestock, large economic consequences, and a danger to public health.[73] These pathogens can infect humans through direct contact with livestock or via unsafe food chains.[74] Other livestock-related diseases have not caused illness in humans, but have led to severe economic losses because of international trade regulations and the mass culling of livestock to prevent the spread of the infection. For example, foot-and-mouth disease in the United Kingdom resulted in the killing of 4 million livestock animals, a loss of £3.1 billion in revenue,[75] which was accompanied by a series of farmer suicides.

Global demand for animal-based protein is predicted to increase by nearly 50% by the year 2020,[76] a worrying forecast for the future of food, water, and ecosystem security worldwide. Agricultural production directly contributes to deforestation and associated land-use changes, further impacting hydrologic and climate systems. Livestock grazing is a main driver of deforestation in the Amazon basin, which boasts about 40% of the world's remaining tropical forests, yet has sustained the world's highest absolute rate of deforestation.[77] This deforestation has a global impact; a reduction in deforestation in the Amazon Basin could result in a 2% to 5% reduction in global carbon emissions.[78]

In light of ongoing agricultural intensification, issues of water quality, quantity, access, and impacts on biodiversity have become paramount worldwide. Widespread land cover change, urbanization, industrialization, and engineering have changed how we use and access water.[79] More than 1 billion people live in river basins vulnerable to the unpredictable effects of climate change, such as storms and droughts. Additionally, 80% of the world's population is under high levels of water insecurity, and an estimated 1 billion people lack access to clean water.[79,80] With water and food security problems growing, One Health can offer more effective solutions by bringing together relevant disciplines. By integrating expertise from agriculture, environmental science, regional planning, and public health, improvements in land-use planning and adaptive management can be achieved.

To highlight the relevance of the One Health approach to a medical and public health audience, we examine its applications to important health problems that a medical professional would confront regularly, in both domestic and international settings. We use the examples of *emerging diseases, neglected diseases, chronic diseases and mental health,* and *biomedical research frontiers* to illustrate the wide applicability of One Health approaches. Throughout these topics, environmental issues such as land use and climate change will be recurring themes.

E. Emerging Diseases

One of the most widely recognized target areas for One Health approaches is that of emerging and reemerging diseases, particularly those of animal origin. As defined by the WHO, an **emerging disease** is one that has appeared in a population for the first time, while a **reemerging disease** could have been present previously but may be increasing in occurrence and geographic scope.[81] Disease emergence rates have increased dramatically since the mid-20th century; 335 emerging infectious disease events have been identified in humans since 1940, and several rank as leading causes of mortality worldwide, with developing countries assuming a disproportionate burden.[8,61] Of these, more than 60% are zoonotic.[61,82,83] Of these emerging zoonoses, almost three quarters of them have originated in wildlife.[61] One of the most significant and devastating diseases of our time has been traced back to wildlife origins. The human immunodeficiency virus (HIV) evolved from a closely related simian immunodeficiency virus (SIV) found in chimpanzees.[84] HIV causes acquired immune deficiency syndrome (AIDS) and has grown into pandemic proportions within human populations since emergence (see One Health Case Study 4 on studentconsult.com).

Additional important zoonotic diseases and their common hosts are presented in Figure 30-5 on student consult.com. It is of the utmost importance to address the shifting ecological relationships among parasites, pathogens, vectors, and hosts that lead to the emergence of disease.[85,86] A One Health approach can help to accomplish this goal by:

- Integrating and coordinating disease prevention, surveillance, and response.
- Improving communication among human health, animal health, and environmental professionals.
- Addressing the upstream drivers of disease emergence, such as land-use change (e.g., deforestation, agriculture).
- Improving land-use planning to slow deforestation, enhance agricultural efficiency, and better manage livestock numbers and density.
- Adapting to and mitigating the predicted effects of climate change.
- Reducing contact among humans, livestock, and wildlife without compromising normal wildlife movements or wildlife access to critical habitat.
- Educating about safer practices for bushmeat hunting as well as providing alternative protein and income sources.

F. Neglected Diseases

Emerging diseases often receive global attention and high levels of funding, but many other diseases of equal distribution and consequence go comparatively unnoticed. These diseases, often referred to as **neglected diseases,** include some highly important diseases such as bovine tuberculosis, trypanosomiasis, anthrax, rabies, brucellosis, echinococcosis, cysticercosis, and leishmaniasis.[2,23,81,87] Their *neglected* status often stems from underreporting, poor diagnostics, and a lack of funding. These diseases have the largest effect on poorer communities in the developing world that rely on livestock for their livelihoods.[81] Neglected diseases could be addressed by incorporating One Health surveillance and treatment methods within both human and animal populations, but a lack of funding and communication often prevents this.[81,88] Additionally, improving agricultural practices with expertise from One Health disciplines could reduce infections. One Health Case Study 5 on studentconsult.com explores brucellosis for which mass vaccination of the animal reservoir is a cost-effective and successful public health intervention.

G. Chronic Diseases and Mental Health

Although most often applied in infectious disease settings, the One Health approach is also relevant for mental health and chronic diseases, such as cardiovascular diseases (CVD), cancer, chronic respiratory diseases, and diabetes. Once associated with high-income countries, chronic diseases now exert a heavier burden within low-income and middle-income countries and continue to increase in prevalence.[89] Global deaths from chronic diseases have more than doubled since 1990 and are expected to cause an estimated 7.63 million deaths in 2020 (66.7% of all deaths).[26,90,91] Because of this impending economic burden, many studies have examined the most effective interventions and recognized the important role of the built and natural environment in managing chronic disease.

One effective strategy for addressing CVD is through physical activity, which has been shown to increase within walkable communities with accessible open spaces for outdoor recreation. Evidence also shows that humans rely on the environment not only for physical activity, but also for psychological, emotional, and spiritual needs.[21,92-97] Contact with nature can reduce stress and improve work performance,[98] as well as enhance emotional and cognitive development in children.[99] As environments degrade, studies have shown that depression can result.[100] In an interesting example within hospitals, patients experienced reduced recovery times and improved outcomes when they could view trees from their hospital room.[101]

From this evidence, policy makers have begun to recognize the important role the environment plays, not just in regulating infectious disease, but also in maintaining healthy communities that can avoid and manage chronic disease. As an example, Australia's national health program has lauded the importance of access to healthy environments as a cornerstone of their general health promotion and prevention strategy.[26] They take an *upstream* approach in health promotion by encouraging citizens to spend time outside and access nature to improve physical activity and prevent disease. They see the benefits of natural environments as a "fundamental health resource" and have documented positive effects on blood pressure, cholesterol, stress reduction, and depression.[26] This type of activity and exposure to nature may have relevance for a range of health priorities, including cancer, injury prevention, mental health, asthma, arthritis, and musculoskeletal conditions, warranting further study.

A One Health perspective can additionally contribute to addressing chronic disease resulting from exposure to unhealthy environments. Chronic diseases such as asthma and cancer may result from prolonged exposure to particulates, chemicals, or toxins in the environment. Animals can play an important role as sentinels for such environmental

Table 30-1 **Different Types of Organisms Serving as Sentinels for Environmental Health Hazards**

Location	Organism	Sentinel for
Soil	Earthworms, soil insects, gophers, moles, mice, voles, ground-dwelling birds	Soil contamination
Air	Honeybees and other flying insects	Air pollution
Plants	Herbivorous animals	Plant contamination
Water	Fish, bivalves (e.g., mussels, oysters), gulls, ospreys, seals, some reptiles and amphibians	Toxic chemicals or pollutants in water can accumulate to higher concentrations in animal tissue
Homes	Domestic companion animals (e.g., cats, dogs)	Soil contamination, house dust, indoor air pollution, lead
Workplace	"Canary in a coal mine"	Chemical or air pollution

Modified from National Research Council: *Animals as sentinels of environmental health hazards*, Washington, DC, 1991, National Academy Press.

health toxins.[102] **Animal sentinel systems,** in which data on animals exposed to environmental contaminants are monitored and analyzed, have proved extremely helpful in identifying and addressing health hazards for many years.[103] These sentinel systems alert practitioners to hazards in homes, workplaces, agricultural settings, and aquatic and terrestrial ecosystems for risk characterization, hazard identification, dose-response assessment, and exposure assessment.[103] Animal sentinels may include domestic and companion animals, food animals, fish, wildlife, or even insects[103] (Table 30-1). It is important to note that sentinel systems not only benefit human health, but also the health of animals and the environment, because they can target interventions to reduce exposures and improve ecosystem quality. One program that aims to enhance the understanding and use of animal sentinels is the Canary Database of the Yale University Occupational and Environmental Medicine Department (http://canarydatabase.org/). This project accomplishes this goal by making scientific literature and studies of animal sentinels more accessible.

The **human-animal bond** is also an important component of One Health approaches to chronic disease. Evidence shows that the presence of companion animals in the home lowers systolic blood pressure, plasma cholesterol, and triglyceride values in owners.[104] Pet ownership has also been shown to improve survival after serious heart surgery.[105] One should take note, however, that pet ownership can increase the exposure to zoonotic disease due to close bodily contact.

H. Biomedical Research Frontiers

One Health can contribute to disease prevention, surveillance, and response and expand our research knowledge base. One Health–like approaches have been undertaken in the fields of biomedical research and comparative medicine for some time. These fields have long recognized the connections between humans and animals and have used animal models for developing vaccines, testing medications, and understanding diseases that are similar in humans and animals. The use of animal models has been extremely important when applied to a diverse variety of human health issues, including: mental disorders, infectious disease, stroke, tumor development, and osteoporosis. Studies of animal models of behavior can also elucidate human mental health disorders in terms of how stress, the environment, or social status can influence health. Additionally, the study of nonhuman genomes has facilitated important discoveries within the human genome. From a security standpoint, animal models can assist in preparing for possible bioterrorism.

Beyond animal models of disease, global biodiversity has contributed greatly to the development of novel medicines.[51] Many new species found in the soil, oceans, polar regions, and tropical rainforests have made a significant contribution to drug development. In fact, about half of the 100 most highly prescribed medications in the United States and about half the new drugs approved by the Food and Drug Administration (FDA) have been developed from nature.[106] New species continue to be discovered in nature every year. For example, despite 250 years of species classification and over 1.2 million species already catalogued, studies suggest that 86% of terrestrial species and 91% of marine species remain undiscovered.[107] Increasing ecosystem degradation and land-use change threaten to make these species discoveries impossible, which among other things would be a devastating loss to medical and pharmaceutical advancement. As such, it is important for the medical community to enhance public recognition of the importance of maintaining biodiversity and ecosystem quality.

IV. GOALS AND BENEFITS OF ONE HEALTH

Overarching benefits of the collaborative, integrative One Health approach are expected yet now need to be objectively evaluated through further research and economic analyses. Projected benefits include a synergy of systems, improved surveillance and preparedness, a shift toward prevention, and ultimately, economic savings. One Health is *synergistic,* as it aims to shift the focus from single diseases to strengthening public and animal health systems, while also recognizing the environmental and social drivers of health.[5] To achieve this synergy, there must be a delicate balance between improving collaboration and cooperation while also acknowledging the distinct objectives and management principles of each discipline involved. If One Health is successfully implemented, there should be improved reach and efficiency in logistics, the enhanced provisioning of services globally, and the strengthening of health systems.[108,109]

As a benefit of this integration, global health surveillance and preparedness should improve.[4,85] For example, an integrated One Health system could ultimately reduce the lag time for detecting emerging diseases, as well as improve response and, as importantly, prevention.[4] Recent outbreaks of emerging infectious diseases, including avian and swine influenza, WNV, and severe acute respiratory syndrome (SARS), have captured global attention with their significant effects on economies, biodiversity, and public health.[50,61,110,111] The World Bank estimates that infectious disease outbreaks over the last decade have cost more than $200 billion in direct and indirect costs, and a potential H5N1 or other pandemic could cost $3 trillion.[2,69,85,112]

The economic burden of emerging zoonoses underscores the urgent need for collaborative disease surveillance in both animals and humans, improved communication, integrated health systems, as well as a shift toward preventive actions against disease emergence.[113,114]

This type of integration would offer benefits in particular at the human-wildlife-livestock interface.[9] It would provide economic savings by adding value and allowing for cost-effective financing of programs that more efficiently address multiple objectives, as explored in the brucellosis case study[4,13] (see One Health Case Study 5 on student consult.com). As additional salient examples of the benefits of this type of integration, we briefly outline a few more programs that have addressed human and animal disease cooperatively. The HALI project in Tanzania simultaneously investigates the medical, ecological, socioeconomic, and policy issues that influence health outcomes caused by pathogens at the human-animal interface, such as *M. bovis*, *Brucella*, *Salmonella*, *Cryptosporidium*, *Giardia*, *E. coli*, and *Campylobacter*.[115] In Chad, joint human and cattle vaccination programs have proved successful[116] and have also been shown to be more cost-effective for addressing brucellosis than just human or animal control alone.[13,117] Several other studies demonstrate how control of an animal reservoir for disease can ultimately save money on human public health interventions, as seen with sleeping sickness in Uganda[118] and *Schistosoma japonicum* in China.[119-121] To further explore *S. japonicum* and the environmental, human, and animal health consequences of the construction of the Three Gorges Dam, see One Health Case Study 6 on studentconsult.com. Despite the potential cost savings of integrative approaches, this type of intervention is unfortunately not commonly implemented because of a lack of funding in resource-poor countries or the absence of a veterinary perspective in public health planning.[23]

V. INTERNATIONAL, INSTITUTIONAL, AND NATIONAL AGENCY SUPPORT

One Health has raised awareness of the increasing connections among the health of humans, animals, and the environment; increased scientific debate; fostered new research paradigms; and enhanced cooperation for disease surveillance and response.[4,23,116] Even before the current decade, the concepts behind what later became known as One Health began receiving attention from a diverse array of government agencies, nongovernmental organizations (NGOs), intergovernmental agencies, educational institutions, professional associations and others, and a number of different programs have evolved.[65,122] The strength of the movement has originated from consensus, shared interests, and common goals, and the weight and legitimacy of its supporters also lend it strength. The diverse stakeholders involved in the growth of One Health stem primarily from three groups at different scales[5]:

- International organizations that provide global leadership and buy-in
- Research networks and NGOs that provide analysis and expertise
- National agencies that provide political leadership and some funding

Intergovernmental organizations and agencies, including OIE, WHO, FAO, UN System Influenza Coordination Unit, World Bank, and U.S. agencies such as the United States Agency for International Development (USAID) and CDC, have come together in support of One Health around issues requiring cooperation, such as infectious disease monitoring and crisis management.[5]

Through partnerships built in part on these existing organizations' working relationships, integrative potential has been leveraged. Many research organizations, NGOs, professional associations, and national agencies have also taken the lead in building support for One Health through conferences, journal publications, and newsletters. Currently, these diverse agents are working together to determine how to operationalize One Health without duplication of effort. The Stone Mountain meeting focused on identifying clear steps toward One Health operationalization and implementation and has resulted in the creation of six ongoing working groups.[123] Several other key international meetings have been instrumental in moving toward this goal. Notably, the WHO, OIE, FAO, World Bank, and USAID came together with national partners through a series of international ministerial and interministerial meetings to focus on integrated preparedness for H5N1 influenza. These international meetings have represented a new, elevated level of cooperation among all these stakeholders.[2] Additionally, the International One Health Congress provided one of the first open conference opportunities to bring together professionals working across One Health–oriented disciplines. These meetings have provided a forum for scientific inquiry and a platform for discussion on how to operationalize One Health.

VI. ENVISIONING ONE HEALTH IN ACTION

A. Integrative Approaches to One Health

Now that we have explored contexts in which One Health is relevant, let's explore a few situations in which a One Health approach has been designed and implemented from the ground up. These programs are all explored in the Chapter 30 Supplement on studentconsult.com. One pioneering program of the Wildlife Conservation Society is Animal & Human Health for the Environment And Development (AHEAD), a landscape-level approach to addressing challenges at the interface of wildlife health, domestic animal health, human health and livelihoods, and environmental stewardship.[10] Another groundbreaking One Health program is PREDICT, part of USAID's Emerging Pandemic Threats Program that is building a global early-warning system. Also, the innovative HealthMap program uses technology to facilitate and visualize the integration of human and animal disease surveillance around the globe.[124] (See the Websites list.)

B. Implementation of One Health Framework

The One Health perspective offers a wealth of benefits for enhancing approaches to global health and sustainability challenges, but how will it be more consistently implemented? Although opinions and strategies differ, certain goals are shared across borders and disciplines. These goals include the enhancement of: research, communication, cooperation and priority setting across institutional lines, integrated surveillance, shared data systems, rapid-response mechanisms, preparedness and prevention, incentive frameworks, both horizontal and vertical health systems, institutional frameworks, methods for education, and joint funding.[2]

To accomplish these goals, a number of changes must occur to mainstream One Health.[125] We briefly discuss the communication, institutional, technical, and educational steps needed to operationalize the One Health approach on studentconsult.com.[5,85] In this online section, we provide recommendations for redesigning a more integrative and dynamic educational system, including the recognition of several "hot spot" areas of potential One Health collaboration across the United States.[126]

VII. SUMMARY

A. Growing Need for One Health Approaches

Issues of global environmental change, global health, emerging disease, and sustainability present some of the most complex and far-reaching challenges of the 21st century. Individual disciplines cannot address these issues in isolation, and the potential economic, health, and environmental consequences of inaction are enormous. One Health offers a logical path forward by recognizing the interconnected nature of human, animal, and ecosystem health in an attempt to inform health and environmental policy, expand scientific knowledge, improve health care training and delivery, improve conservation outcomes, identify *upstream* solutions, and address sustainability challenges.

One Health uniquely focuses on upstream approaches that tackle the root causes of global health and environmental challenges. By focusing on prevention, a One Health approach could, for example, not only reduce the response time to infectious disease outbreaks, but also predict and ideally prevent such disease emergence from occurring. It can also improve disease surveillance and response, strengthen health systems, enhance public health interventions, direct new avenues of research to enhance our understanding of health and the environment, improve vaccine development, augment medical care, strengthen conservation efforts, reinvigorate educational systems, and avoid large economic consequences of foreseeable and preventable disasters.[127,128] One Health can enhance strategies for sustainable development and conservation, especially surrounding protected areas, where health issues are relevant to threatened wildlife populations, people, and their domestic animals.[7,9]

We are at a turning point in which the sustainability of future human generations is increasingly reliant on proactive, earnest global stewardship.[67] Although challenges and barriers to realization of One Health certainly exist, this is an exciting and critical time in which to develop these collaborative, cross-sectoral approaches. Professionals from diverse disciplines are working together now to find collaborative solutions, at local, regional, and global scales.[38,129,130] We urge you to get involved.

B. Integrating One Health into Your Professional Career

One Health can add dynamism and broader relevance to health-related careers. As you enter your professional career, look for the following opportunities to become involved:

- Seek out local One Health research groups and seminar series.
- Attend One Health training workshops.
- Develop international, cross-sectoral professional networks.
- Develop collaborative, transdisciplinary research projects and grants.
- Publish transdisciplinary papers in traditional "unidisciplinary" journals (e.g., *JAMA*).
- Publish in transdisciplinary journals (e.g., *EcoHealth, Emerging Infectious Diseases, Environmental Health Perspectives, PLoS* journals).
- Attend transdisciplinary conferences (e.g., EcoHealth, AAAS, International One Health Congress).
- Participate in ongoing interdisciplinary education opportunities.
- Stay open to the importance of other perspectives on health and the environment.
- Keep updated on One Health progress through newsletters and online (see Websites).

References

1. United Nations, Department of Economic and Social Affairs, Population Division: World population prospects: the 2010 revision. Highlights and advance tables, Working Paper No ESA/P/WP.220, New York: 2011.
2. World Bank: *People, pathogens and our planet: towards a One Health approach for controlling zoonotic diseases*, vol 1, Washington, DC, 2010.
3. Institute of Medicine, National Research Council: *Sustaining global surveillance and response to emerging zoonotic diseases*, Washington, DC, 2009, National Academies Press.
4. Zinsstag J, Schelling E, Waltner-Toews D, et al: From "One Medicine" to "One Health" and systemic approaches to health and well-being. *Prev Vet Med* 101:148–156, 2011.
5. Leboeuf A: *Making sense of One Health: cooperating at the human-animal-ecosystem health interface, Health and Environment Reports No 7*, Paris, 2011, Institute Francais des Relations Internationales.
6. American Veterinary Medical Association: *One Health: a new professional imperative, One Health Initiative Task Force final report*, Washington, DC, 2008, AVMA.
7. Osofsky SA, Kock RA, Kock MD, et al: Building support for protected areas using a "One Health" perspective. In McNeely JA, editor: *Friends for life: new partners in support of protected areas*, Gland, Switzerland, 2005, International Union for the Conservation of Nature.
8. World Health Organization, Food and Agriculture Organization, United Nations Children Fund, World Bank, World Organization for Animal Health: *Contributing to "One World, One Health": a strategic framework for reducing risks of infectious diseases at the animal-human-ecosystems interface*, New York, 2008.
9. Osofsky SA, Cleaveland S, Karesh WB, et al, editors: *Conservation and development interventions at the wildlife/livestock interface: implications for wildlife, livestock and human health*, Gland, Switzerland, 2005, International Union for the Conservation of Nature.

10. Osofsky SA, Cumming DHM, Kock MD: Transboundary management of natural resources and the importance of a "One Health" approach: perspectives on southern Africa. In Fearn E, Redford KH, editors: *State of the wild 2008–2009: a global portrait of wildlife, wildlands, and oceans*, Washington, DC, 2008, Island Press.

11. Hippocrates: *Air, waters and places*, 400 BCE.

12. Schwabe CW: *Veterinary medicine and human health*, ed 3, Baltimore, 1984, Williams & Wilkins.

13. Zinsstag J, Schelling E, Wyss K, et al: Potential of cooperation between human and animal health to strengthen health systems. *Lancet* 366:2142–2145, 2005.

14. Aguirre AA: *Conservation medicine: ecological health in practice*, Oxford, 2002, Oxford University Press.

15. Rapport DJ, Costanza R, McMichael AJ: Assessing ecosystem health. *Trends Ecol Evol* 13:397–402, 1998.

16. Wilcox B: Ecosystem health in practice: Emerging areas of application in environment and human health. *Ecosystem Health* 7:317, 2001.

17. Van Leeuwen JA, Waltner-Toews D, Abernathy T, et al: Evolving models of human health toward an ecosystem context. *Ecosystem Health* 5:204–219, 1999.

18. Waltner-Toews D, Kay J: The evolution of an ecosystem approach: the diamond schematic and an adaptive methodology for ecosystem sustainability and health. *Ecol Soc* 10:38, 2005.

19. Rapport DJ, Mergler D: Expanding the practice of ecosystem health. *EcoHealth* 1:4–7, 2004.

20. Charron DF, editor: *Ecohealth research in practice: innovative applications of an ecosystem approach to health*, Ottawa, 2012, Springer and the International Development Research Center.

21. Millennium Ecosystem Assessment: Ecosystems and human well-being: current state and trends. In *Millennium ecosystem assessment*, vol. 1, Washington, DC, 2005, Island Press.

22. Cook RA, Karesh WB, Osofsky SA: *The Manhattan Principles on "One World, One Health": building interdisciplinary bridges to health in a globalized world*, New York, 2004, Wildlife Conservation Society. Available at http://www.oneworldonehealth.org/sept2004/owoh_sept04.html.

23. Welburn S: One Health: the 21st century challenge. *Vet Rec* 168:614–615, 2011.

24. Food and Agriculture Organization, World Organization for Animal Health, World Health Organization: *The FAO-OIE-WHO Collaboration: Sharing responsibilities and coordinating global activities to address health risks at the animal-human-ecosystems interfaces—a tripartite concept note*, Geneva, 2010.

25. Craven RB, Roehrig JT: West Nile virus. *JAMA* 286:651–653, 2001.

26. Maller C, Townsend M, St Leger L, et al: *Healthy parks, healthy people: the health benefits of contact with nature in a park context*, ed 2, Melbourne, Deakin University and Parks Victoria, 2008.

27. Wilkinson R, Marmot M: *Social determinants of health: the solid facts*, Geneva, 2003, World Health Organization.

28. Chu CM, Simpson R: *Ecological public health: from vision to practice*, Toronto, 1994, Centre for Health Promotion, University of Toronto.

29. Christensen N: *The environment and you*, Boston, 2012, Addison Wesley.

30. Myers S, Patz J: Emerging threats to human health from global environmental change. *Annu Rev Environ Resourc* 34:223–252, 2009.

31. Patz J, Daszak P, Tabor G, et al: Unhealthy landscapes: policy recommendations on land use change and infectious disease emergence. *Environ Health Perspect* 112:1092–1098, 2004.

32. McMichael AJ: Population health as the "bottom line" of sustainability: a contemporary challenge for public health researchers. *Eur J Public Health* 16:579–581, 2006.

33. Wiegand J, Raffaelli D, Smart JC, et al: Assessment of temporal trends in ecosystem health using an holistic indicator. *J Environ Manage* 91:1446–1455, 2010.

34. Muñoz-Erickson T, Aguilar-González B, Loeser M, et al: Framework to evaluate ecological and social outcomes of collaborative management: lessons from implementation with a northern Arizona collaborative group. *Environ Manage* 45:132–144, 2010.

35. Prüss-Üstün A, Corvalán C: *Preventing disease through healthy environments: towards an estimate of the environmental burden of disease*, Geneva, 2006, World Health Organization.

36. Prüss-Üstün A, Bonjour S, Corvalán C: The impact of the environment on health by country: a meta-synthesis. *Environ Health* 7(7), 2008.

37. Working Group I: Climate change 2007: the physical science basis. In Solomon S, Qin D, Manning M, et al, editors: *Fourth assessment report of the Intergovernmental Panel on Climate Change*, New York, 2007, Cambridge University Press.

38. Costello A, Abbas M, Allen A, et al: Managing the health effects of climate change. *Lancet* 373(9676):1693–1733, 2009.

39. Patz JA, Campbell-Lendrum D, Holloway T, et al: Impact of regional climate change on human health. *Nature* 438:310–317, 2005.

40. Patz JA, Gibbs HK, Foley JA, et al: Climate change and global health: quantifying a growing ethical crisis. *EcoHealth* 4:397–405, 2007.

41. Lafferty KD: The ecology of climate change and infectious diseases. *Ecology* 90:888–900, 2009.

42. Tanser FC, Sharp B, le Sueur D: Potential effect of climate change on malaria transmission in Africa. *Lancet* 362(9398):1792–1798, 2003.

43. McMichael AJ, Campbell-Lendrum DH, Corvalán CF, et al: *Climate change and human health: risks and responses*, Geneva, 2003, World Health Organization.

44. Brooks DR, Hoberg EP: How will global climate change affect parasite-host assemblages? *Trends Parasitol* 23:571–574, 2007.

45. Froeschke G, Harf R, Sommer S, et al: Effects of precipitation on parasite burden along a natural climatic gradient in southern Africa: implications for possible shifts in infestation patterns due to global changes. *Oikos* 119:1029–1039, 2010.

46. Kutz SJ, Hoberg EP, Polley L, et al: Global warming is changing the dynamics of Arctic host-parasite systems. *Proc R Soc Lond B Biol Sci* 272(1581):2571–2576, 2005.

47. Hoberg EP, Polley L, Jenkins EJ, et al: Pathogens of domestic and free-ranging ungulates: global climate change in temperate to boreal latitudes across North America. *Rev Sci Tech* 27:511–528, 2008.

48. Pounds JA, Bustamante MR, Coloma LA, et al: Widespread amphibian extinctions from epidemic disease driven by global warming. *Nature* 439(7073):161–167, 2006.

49. Keesing F, Belden LK, Daszak P, et al: Impacts of biodiversity on the emergence and transmission of infectious diseases. *Nature* 468(7324):647–652, 2010.

50. Daszak P, Cunningham AA, Hyatt AD: Emerging infectious diseases of wildlife: threats to biodiversity and human health. *Science* 287(5452):443–449, 2000.

51. Chivian E, Bernstein A, editors: *Sustaining life: how human health depends on biodiversity*, Oxford, 2008, Oxford University Press.

52. Ezenwa VO, Godsey MS, King RJ, et al: Avian diversity and West Nile virus: testing associations between biodiversity and infectious disease risk. *Proc R Soc Lond B Biol Sci* 273(1582):109–117, 2006.

53. Pongsiri MJ, Roman J, Ezenwa VO, et al: Biodiversity loss affects global disease ecology. *Bioscience* 59:945–954, 2009.

54. LoGiudice K, Ostfeld RS, Schmidt KA, et al: The ecology of infectious disease: effects of host diversity and community

composition on Lyme disease risk. *Proc Natl Acad Sci USA* 100:567–571, 2003.

55. Schmidt KA, Ostfeld RS: Biodiversity and the dilution effect in disease ecology. *Ecology* 82:609–619, 2001.

56. Johnson PTJ, Hartson RB, Larson DJ, et al: Diversity and disease: community structure drives parasite transmission and host fitness. *Ecol Lett* 11:1017–1026, 2008.

57. Keesing F, Holt RD, Ostfeld RS: Effects of species diversity on disease risk. *Ecol Lett* 9:485–498, 2006.

58. Begon M: Effects of host diversity in disease dynamics. In Ostfeld RS, Keesing F, Eviner VT, editors: *Infectious disease ecology: effects of ecosystems on disease and of disease on ecosystems*, Princeton, NJ, 2008, Princeton University Press.

59. Chivian E: *Biodiversity: its importance to human health. Interim executive summary*, Boston, 2002, Center for Health and the Global Environment, Harvard Medical School.

60. Chivian E, Bernstein AS: Embedded in nature: human health and biodiversity. *Environ Health Perspect* 112:A12, 2004.

61. Jones KE, Patel NG, Levy MA, et al: Global trends in emerging infectious diseases. *Nature* 451(7181):990–993, 2008.

62. Dunn RR, Davies TJ, Harris NC, et al: Global drivers of human pathogen richness and prevalence. *Proc R Soc Lond B Biol Sci* 277(1694):2587–2595, 2010.

63. Golden CD, Fernald LC, Brashares JS, et al: Benefits of wildlife consumption to child nutrition in a biodiversity hotspot. *Proc Natl Acad Sci USA* 2011.

64. Wolfe ND, Daszak P, Kilpatrick AM, et al: Bushmeat hunting, deforestation and prediction of zoonoses emergence. *Emerg Infect Dis* 11:1822–1827, 2005.

65. Wolfe ND, Switzer WM, Carr JK, et al: Naturally acquired simian retrovirus infections in central African hunters. *Lancet* 363(9413):932–937, 2004.

66. Travis D, Watson R, Tauer A: The spread of pathogens through trade in wildlife. *Rev Sci Tech* 1:219–239, 2011.

67. Osofsky SA, Karesh W, Deem SL: Conservation medicine: a veterinary perspective. *Conserv Biol* 14:336–337, 2000.

68. Dobson A, Cattadori I, Holt RD, et al: Sacred cows and sympathetic squirrels: the importance of biological diversity to human health. *PLoS Medicine* 3:714–718, 2006.

69. King DA, Peckham C, Waage JK, et al: Infectious diseases: preparing for the future. *Science* 313:1392–1393, 2006.

70. Cohen J: Out of Mexico? Scientists ponder swine flu's origins. *Science* 324:700–702, 2009.

71. World Health Organization: *Food Safety and Foodborne Illness*, vol 237, Geneva, 2007, WHO.

72. Call DR, Davis MA, Sawant AA: Antimicrobial resistance in beef and dairy cattle production. *Anim Health Res Rev* 9:159–167, 2008.

73. Mathew A, Cissell R, Liamthong S: Antibiotic resistance in bacteria associated with food animals: a United States perspective of livestock production. *Food-borne Pathogens Dis* 4:115–133, 2007.

74. Silbergeld E, Graham J, Price L: Industrial food animal production, antimicrobial resistance, and human health. *Annu Rev Public Health* 29:151–169, 2008.

75. Thompson D, Muriel P, Russell D, et al: Economic costs of the foot-mouth disease outbreak in the United Kingdom. *Rev Sci Tech* 21:675–687, 2002.

76. Delgado C, Rosegrant M, Steinfeld H, et al: *Livestock to 2020: the next food revolution. Food, Agriculture, and the Environment Discussion Paper 28*, Washington, DC, 1999, International Food Policy Research Institute.

77. Almeyda Zambrano A, Broadbent E, Schmink M, et al: Deforestation drivers in Southwest Amazonia: comparing smallholder farmers in Iñapari, Peru, and Assis Brasil, Brazil. *Conserv Soc* 8:157–170, 2010.

78. Nepstad D, Soares-Filho BS, Merry F, et al: The end of deforestation in the Brazilian Amazon. *Science* 326(5958):1350–1351, 2009.

79. Vorosmarty CJ, McIntyre PB, Gessner MO, et al: Global threats to human water security and river biodiversity. *Nature* 467(7315):555–561, 2010.

80. Naiman R, Dudgeon D: Global alteration of freshwaters: influences on human and environmental well-being. *Ecol Res* 26:865–873, 2011.

81. Maudlin I, Eisler MC, Welburn SC: Neglected and endemic zoonoses. *Philos Trans Proc R Soc Lond B Biol Sci* 364(1530):2777–2787, 2009.

82. Cleaveland S, Laurenson MK, Taylor LH: Diseases of humans and their domestic mammals: pathogen characteristics, host range and the risk of emergence. *Philos Trans R Soc Lond B Biol Sci* 356:991–999, 2001.

83. Taylor LH, Latham SM, Woolhouse MEJ: Risk factors for human disease emergence. *Philos Trans R Soc Lond B Biol Sci* 356:983–989, 2001.

84. Hahn BH, Shaw GM, De Cock KM, et al: AIDS as a zoonosis: Scientific and public health implications. *Science* 287(5453):607–614, 2000.

85. Chatham House: Shifting from emergency response to prevention of pandemic disease threats at source. Meeting report, London, 2010, Chatham House.

86. Clifford DL, Wolking DJ, Muse EA: *HALI Wildlife health handbook: recognizing, investigating, and reporting diseases of concern for wildlife conservation and human health*, Davis, 2011, University of California.

87. World Health Organization: *Integrated control of neglected zoonoses in Africa: applying the "One Health" concept. Report of a joint WHO/EU/ILRI/DBL/FAO/OIE/AU meeting*, Nairobi, 2009, WHO.

88. Okello AL, Gibbs EPJ, Vandersmissen A, et al: One Health and the neglected zoonoses: turning rhetoric into reality. *Vet Rec* 169:281–285, 2011.

89. Samb B, Desai N, Nishtar S, et al: Prevention and management of chronic disease: a litmus test for health-systems strengthening in low-income and middle-income countries. *Lancet* 376(9754):1785–1797, 2010.

90. World Health Organization: *Preventing chronic disease: a vital investment*. WHO Global Report, Geneva, 2005.

91. World Health Organization: *Global health risks: mortality and burden of disease attributable to selected major risks*, Geneva, 2009, WHO.

92. Gaffikin L: *Illustrative bibliography for exploring health as an ecosystem service*, New York, 2010, Wildlife Conservation Society.

93. Faber Taylor A, Kuo F, Sullivan W: Coping with ADD: the surprising connection to green play settings. *Environ Behav* 33:54–77, 2001.

94. Faber Taylor A, Kuo F, Sullivan W: Views of nature and self-discipline: evidence from inner city children. *J Environ Psychol* 22:49–64, 2002.

95. Frumkin H: Beyond toxicity: human health and the natural environment. *Am J Prev Med* 20:234–240, 2001.

96. Frumkin H: Healthy places: exploring the evidence. *Am J Public Health* 93:1451–1456, 2003.

97. Moore E: A prison environment's effect on health care service demands. *J Environ Syst* 11:17–34, 1981.

98. Kaplan R, Kaplan S: *The experience of nature: a psychological perspective*, New York, 1995, Cambridge University Press.

99. Kellert S: Experiencing nature: affective, cognitive, and evaluative development in children. In Kahn PH Jr, Kellert SR, editors: *Children and nature: psychological, sociocultural, and evolutionary investigations*, Cambridge, 2002, MIT Press.

100. Speldewinde PC, Cook A, Davies P, et al: A relationship between environmental degradation and mental health in rural Western Australia. *Health & Place* 15:880–887, 2009.

101. Ulrich RS: View through a window may influence recovery from surgery. *Science* 224:420–421, 1984.

102. Rabinowitz P, Odofin L, Dein F: From "us vs. them" to "shared risk": can animals help link environmental factors to human health? *EcoHealth* 5:224–229, 2008.

103. National Research Council: *Animals as sentinels of environmental health hazards*, Washington, DC, 1991, National Academy Press.

104. Anderson WP, Reid CM, Jennings GL: Pet ownership and risk factors for cardiovascular disease. *Med J Aust* 157:298–301, 1992.

105. Friedmann E, Thomas SA: Pet ownership, social support, and one-year survival after acute myocardial infarction in the Cardiac Arrhythmia Suppression Trial (CAST). *Am J Cardiol* 76:1213–1217, 1995.

106. Bernstein AS, Ludwig DS: The importance of biodiversity to medicine. *JAMA* 300:2297–2299, 2008.

107. Mora C, Tittensor DP, Adl S, et al: How many species are there on Earth and in the ocean? *PLoS Biol* 9:e1001127, 2011.

108. Alliance for Health Policy and Systems Research: *Strengthening health systems: the role and promise of policy and systems research*, Geneva, 2004, Global Forum for Health Research.

109. World Health Organization: *Adelaide Statement on health in all policies: moving towards a shared governance for health and well-being*, Adelaide, 2010, WHO and Government of South Australia.

110. Lloyd-Smith JO, George D, Pepin KM, et al: Epidemic dynamics at the human-animal interface. *Science* 326(5958):1362–1367, 2009.

111. Daszak P, Tabor GM, Kilpatrick AM, et al: Conservation medicine and a new agenda for emerging diseases. *Ann NY Acad Sci* 1026:1–11, 2004.

112. Gale J: Flu pandemic may cost world economy up to $3 trillion, Singapore. *Bloomberg News*, October 17, 2008.

113. Kahn LH: Confronting zoonoses, linking human and veterinary medicine. *Emerg Infect Dis* 12:556–561, 2006.

114. Kaplan B, Echols M: The case for a "One Health" paradigm shift. *ALN Europe*, September/October 2009.

115. Mazet JAK, Clifford DL, Coppolillo PB, et al: A "One Health" approach to address emerging zoonoses: the HALI Project in Tanzania. *PLoS Med* 6:1–6, 2009.

116. Zinsstag J, Schelling E, Bonfoh B, et al: Towards a "One Health" research and application tool box. *Vet Ital* 45:121–133, 2009.

117. Roth J, Zinsstag J, Orkhon D, et al: Human health benefits from livestock vaccination for brucellosis: case study. *Bull WHO* 81:867–876, 2003.

118. Picozzi K, Fevre EM, Odiit M, et al: Sleeping sickness in Uganda: a thin line between two fatal diseases. *British Medical Journal* 331:1238–1241, 2005.

119. Wang T, Zhang S, Wu W, et al: Treatment and reinfection of water buffaloes and cattle infected with *Schistosoma japonicum* in Yangtze River Valley, Anhui Province. *J Parasitol* 92:1088–1091, 2006.

120. Lin D, Zeng X, Chen H, et al: Cost-effectiveness and cost-benefit analysis on the integrated schistosomiasis control strategies with emphasis on infection source in Poyang Lake Region. *Chin J Parasitol Parasit Dis* 4:297–302, 2009.

121. McManus DP, Gray DJ, Li Y, et al: Schistosomiasis in the People's Republic of China: the era of the Three Gorges Dam. *Clin Microbiol Rev* 23:442–466, 2010.

122. Rockefeller Foundation: *Portfolio of One Health activities and case studies*, Bellagio, 2011, Rockefeller Foundation and Global Initiative for Food Systems Leadership, University of Minnesota.

123. Centers for Disease Control and Prevention: Operationalizing "One Health": a policy perspective—taking stock and shaping an implementation roadmap. Meeting Overview. Atlanta, GA, 2011. Available at http://www.cdc.gov/onehealth/archived-meetings/march2009-may2010.html#one.

124. Brownstein JS, Freifeld CC, Reis BY, et al: Surveillance Sans Frontières: Internet-based emerging infectious disease intelligence and the HealthMap Project. *PLoS Med* 5:e151, 2008.

125. Zinsstag J, Mackenzie JS, Jeggo M, et al: Mainstreaming One Health. *EcoHealth* 9:107–110. 2012.

126. Barrett MA, Bouley TA, Stoertz AH, et al: Integrating a One Health approach in education to address global health and sustainability challenges. *Frontiers Ecol Environ* 9:239–245, 2010.

127. Kaplan B, Kahn LH, Monath TP: One Health–One Medicine: linking human, animal and environmental health. *Vet Ital* 45:9–18, 2009.

128. Kaplan B, Kahn LH, Monath TP, et al: One Health and parasitology. *Parasites Vectors* 2:36, 2009.

129. Binder S, Levitt AM, Sacks JJ, et al: Emerging infectious diseases: public health issues for the 21st century. *Science* 284:1311–1313, 1999.

130. Parkes MW, Bienen L, Breilh J, et al: All hands on deck: transdisciplinary approaches to emerging infectious disease. *EcoHealth* 2:258–272, 2005.

Websites

www.wcs-ahead.org [Animal & Human Health for the Environment And Development]

www.healthmap.org [HealthMap program]

http://www.maweb.org/ [United Nations Millennium Ecosystem Assessment]

www.onehealthcommission.org/ [One Health Commission]

www.onehealthinitiative.com [One Health Initiative]

www.doh.state.fl.us/environment/medicine/One_Health/OneHealth.html [One Health Newsletter]

www.oneworldonehealth.org [One World, One Health]

www.vetmed.ucdavis.edu/ohi/predict [PREDICT, part of USAID's Emerging Pandemic Threats Program]

www.wcs.org [Wildlife Conservation Society]

Epidemiologic and Medical Glossary

Acceptability of medical care Measure of patients' satisfaction with available medical care. Acceptability is influenced by such factors as whether the health care professionals can communicate well with their patients, whether the care is seen as warm and humane and concerned with the whole person, and whether the patients believe in the confidentiality and privacy of information shared with their health care providers.

Accessibility of medical care Degree to which patients can receive care without undue geographic or financial obstacles.

Accountability of medical care Degree to which the health care system takes public responsibility for its actions. This involves public representation on the board of directors of the health care facility, regular review of financial records by certified public accountants, and appropriate public disclosure of financial records and of quality-of-care studies.

Accuracy Ability of a test to obtain the correct measure, on average.

Acquired immunodeficiency syndrome (AIDS) State of severe immunocompromise resulting from infection with human immunodeficiency virus (HIV) infection.

Active immunity Immunity conferred by exposure to an antigen that stimulates the host to produce antibody; far superior to passive immunity because active immunity lasts longer (a lifetime in some cases) and is rapidly stimulated to high levels by a reexposure to the same antigen or closely related antigens.

Active surveillance Occurs when public health officials initiate contact with physicians, laboratories, or hospitals to obtain information about diseases of interest.

Actuarial method Method of life table analysis in which proportionate survival is assessed at fixed intervals, such as months, that have been established before data accrual. *See also* **Life table analysis.**

Acute and convalescent sera *Acute sera* are the first serum samples collected soon after symptoms of an infectious disease occur. *Convalescent sera* are follow-up samples collected after a period of time that is sufficient to allow for antibody titers to rise. A significant increase in the titers is taken as proof of recent infection.

Acute tubular necrosis Sudden severe injury to renal tubule cells, often resulting from transient hypoperfusion.

Adequacy of medical care Sufficient volume of care to meet the needs of a community.

Adjusted rates *See* **Standardized rates.**

Advanced life support (ALS) Intervention protocols applied to resuscitate or stabilize the condition of critically ill or critically injured patients.

Air inversion Occurs when cooler air settles close to the surface of the Earth and warmer air rises above; thus the natural mixing of air does not occur, and pollution is concentrated.

Alcohol abuse *See* **Chemical substance abuse.**

Allostatic load Ongoing level of demand for adaptation in an individual. An elevated level may be an important contributor to many chronic diseases.

Alpha error *See* **Type I error.**

Alpha level Maximum probability of making a false-positive error that the investigator is willing to accept.

Alternative hypothesis The hypothesis that a real (true) difference exists between means or proportions of groups being compared, or that there is a real association between two variables. *Compare* **Null hypothesis.**

Ames test Quick, frequently used test to estimate the mutagenic potential of a chemical substance.

Analysis of covariance (ANCOVA) Method of significance testing based on the ratio of between-groups variance to within-groups variance. This method is used in multivariable analysis if the dependent variable is continuous, some of the independent variables are categorical (nominal, dichotomous, or ordinal), and some of the independent variables are continuous.

Analysis of variance (ANOVA) Method of significance testing based on the ratio of between-groups variance to within-groups variance. This method is used in statistical analysis if the dependent variable is continuous and the independent variable or variables are all categorical (nominal, dichotomous, or ordinal). If there is only one independent variable, the method is called **one-way** ANOVA. If there is more than one independent variable, the method is called **N-way** ANOVA, with *N* representing the number of independent variables.

Anergy panel Several prevalent antigens are injected to assess immunocompetence; at least one of the antigens should elicit a reaction if the immune system is not impaired.

Angina pectoris Chest pain resulting from periods of myocardial ischemia.

Antigenic drift Relatively minor change in the surface antigens of a viral influenza strain.

Antigenic shift Major change in the surface antigens of a viral influenza strain, with the potential to create worldwide epidemics (pandemics).

Appropriateness of medical care Procedures being performed are properly selected and carried out by trained personnel in the proper setting.

Asbestosis Pulmonary compromise resulting from an accumulation of asbestos fibers in the lungs and from the associated inflammatory response, ultimately leading to pulmonary fibrosis.

Assessability of medical care Data are available to evaluate the medical care regarding quality and medical errors.

Atherogenesis Development and accumulation of atherosclerotic plaque in arteries.

Attack rate Proportion of exposed persons who become ill; the customary measure used to establish the severity of a disease outbreak.

Attributable risk (AR) Of the total risk for a particular outcome, AR is the proportion attributable to a particular exposure. *See also* **Risk difference.**

Attributable risk percent in the exposed (AR%(exposed)) Answers the question, Among those with the risk factor, what percentage of the total risk for the disease is caused by the risk factor?

Availability of medical care Provision of care during the hours and days when people need it.

Avian influenza Caused by a strain of H5N1 influenza that ordinarily infects only birds, it has spread to many humans with close contact with birds, especially in Southeast Asia. It has a high case fatality ratio, and if it develops the ability to spread easily from one human being to another, it might cause a pandemic (a worldwide epidemic).

Bacille Calmette-Guérin (BCG) vaccine Live bacterial antigen vaccine that gives partial immunity against *Mycobacterium tuberculosis* infection.

Barthel index A validated, ordinal scale covering ten areas of self-care to measure an individual's capacity to attend to activities of daily living independently.

Bayes theorem Answers the two important questions that remain unanswered by sensitivity and specificity: (1) If the test results are positive, what is the probability that the patient has the disease? and (2) If the test results are negative, what is the probability that the patient does not have the disease? The theorem stipulates that the probability of a given condition in an individual is based on the presumed prevalence of that condition in the population of whom the individual is a member and on the characteristics of the test.

Berylliosis Poisoning by fumes or dust of the metal beryllium, usually resulting in pneumonitis.

Best estimate Estimate achieved with the statistical model that produces the smallest sum of the squared error terms.

Beta error *See* **Type II error.**

Between-groups mean square *See* **Between-groups variance.**

Between-groups variance Measurement of the variation between (or among) the means of more than one group, based on the independent variables under study.

Bias Introduction of error that produces deviations or distortions of data that are predominantly in one direction, as opposed to random error. *See also* **Differential error.**

Binary variables *See* **Dichotomous variables.**

Biochemical oxygen demand Quantity of oxygen that aerobic bacteria in sewage deplete from the water.

Bivariate analysis Analysis of the relationship between one independent variable and one dependent variable.

Black lung disease *See* **Coal worker's pneumoconiosis.**

Bonferroni adjustment to alpha Method for adjusting alpha when multiple hypotheses are being tested. To keep the risk of a false-positive finding in the entire study to no more than alpha (which is usually 0.05), the alpha level chosen for rejecting the null hypothesis is made more stringent by dividing alpha by the number of hypotheses being tested.

Botulism Poisoning by a neurotoxin produced by the bacterium *Clostridium botulinum;* usually results from ingestion of improperly canned or prepared food.

Break-even point The point at which costs and revenue are equal.

Bronchitis Inflammation of the bronchi, producing a clinical syndrome of cough, dyspnea, chest discomfort, and fever.

Byssinosis Asthmalike pulmonary syndrome resulting from inhalation of textile dust (e.g., cotton dust).

Capitation Basis for payment of primary care physicians on a "per head" basis. Although patients vary in their need for and use of medical services, the physician receives the same amount of money per patient per month or per year.

Case definition In the investigation of an acute disease outbreak, provides the inclusion and exclusion criteria that are used to determine which subjects are cases and which are not cases.

Case fatality ratio Proportion of clinically ill persons who die of the condition under study; a marker of virulence.

Case finding Process of searching for asymptomatic diseases or risk factors among people while they are in a clinical setting (i.e., under medical care). The distinction between **screening** and case finding is frequently ignored in the literature and in practice, but the distinction is important because many of the requirements for community screening do not need to be met during the process of case finding.

Case-control study Study groups are defined on the basis of disease (or outcome) status. The frequency of the risk factor (exposure) in the cases (diseased persons) is compared with the frequency of the risk factor (exposure) in the controls (nondiseased persons).

Case mix–adjusted mortality A method of comparing mortality rates that adjusts for differences in the types of patients, and the severity of their conditions, to allow for a more equitable analysis across sites. Without case-mix adjustment, tertiary care hospitals that take the sickest patients with the highest mortality rates will tend to have the worst performance assessments, which is a misrepresentation. Case-mix adjusted mortality rates correct for this.

Case-mix adjustment A method of adjusting analytical methods for variation in the type and severity of clinical cases. This is often applied when the performances of health care institutions are being compared.

Causality Some factor produces or contributes to the production of a specified outcome; *see also* **Direct causality** and **Indirect causality.**

Cause-specific rates Rates that provide numerators that are comparable with regard to diagnosis.

Cell-mediated immunity Tissue-based cellular response to foreign antigens that involves mobilization of killer T cells.

Central limit theorem For reasonably large samples, the distribution of the means of many samples is normal (gaussian), even though the data in individual samples may have skewness, kurtosis, or unevenness.

Chemical substance abuse Physical dependence (including tolerance) and psychological dependence on the use of chemicals (e.g., alcohol, tobacco, illegal or prescription drugs) to modify mood and performance and to escape from anxiety.

Chickenpox Illness that occurs most frequently during childhood, is caused by varicella-zoster virus (VZV) infection, and is characterized by fever and a papulovesicular rash; also called *varicella.*

Chi-square test of independence Statistical significance test used to analyze nominal or dichotomous data in a contingency table. The first step is to determine the chi-square value for each cell in the table, by calculating the square of the observed count (O) minus the expected count (E) in a cell and dividing the result by the expected count for that cell. The next step is to add the values for all cells in the table. The standard chi-square formula is $\Sigma[(O - E)^2/E]$.

Cholera Acute and sometimes fulminant diarrheal illness caused by an enterotoxin produced by the bacterium *Vibrio cholerae.*

Chronic renal failure Nonspecific term referring to a gradual decline in the functional capacity of the kidney, as measured by the creatinine clearance and glomerular filtration rate. The term is conventionally applied to renal insufficiency that is irreversible.

Coal worker's pneumoconiosis Disease caused by chronic inhalation of coal dust, characterized by pulmonary inflammation or fibrosis; also known as *black lung disease.*

Coefficient A weighting factor used in an equation, with the weight based on the relative importance of the factor in predicting the outcome.

Cohort Clearly defined group of persons studied over time.

Cohort study Study in which a clearly identified group is characterized by exposure and is followed for the outcome.

Completeness of medical care Adequate attention to all aspects of a medical problem, including prevention, early detection, diagnosis, treatment, follow-up measures, and rehabilitation.

Comprehensiveness of medical care Extent to which care is provided for all types of health problems, including dental and mental health problems.

Confounding Confusion of two supposedly causal variables, so that part or all of the purported effect of one variable is actually caused by the other.

Contingency table Table of counts used to determine whether the distribution of one variable is conditionally dependent (contingent) on the other variable.

Continuity of medical care Ideally, management of a patient's care over time is provided or coordinated by one provider.

Continuous variables Variables in which data are measured over the range of an uninterrupted numerical scale (e.g., height, weight, age); also called *dimensional variables.*

Convalescent sera *See* **Acute and convalescent sera.**

Copayment In copayments, patients pay a given percentage of medical expenses. In contrast to *deductibles,* copayments apply linearly to all costs.

Coronary artery disease (CAD) The accumulation of atherosclerotic plaque in the coronary arteries, which reduces perfusion of the myocardium and sometimes causes ischemia or infarction.

Cost-benefit analysis Measures and compares the costs and benefits of a proposed course of action in terms of the same units, usually monetary units such as dollars.

Cost-effectiveness analysis Summarizes the costs and benefits of various health interventions, usually with the help of a ratio, such as dollars/year of life saved.

Covariance Product of the deviation of an observation from the mean of the x variable, multiplied by the same observation's deviation from the mean of the y variable.

Cox method *See* **Proportional hazards method.**

Cox model *See* **Proportional hazards model.**

Crack cocaine Freebase cocaine, which is usually smoked and is the most potent and addictive form of cocaine.

Critical ratios Class of tests of statistical significance that depend on dividing some parameter (e.g., difference between means) by the standard error of that parameter.

Cross-sectional ecological study Study of the frequency with which some characteristic (e.g., smoking) and some outcome of interest (e.g., lung cancer) occur in the same geographically defined population at one particular time.

Cross-sectional survey Survey of a population at a single point in time.

Crude rates Rates that apply to an entire population, without reference to any characteristics of the individuals in it.

Cumulative incidence Total number of incident cases in a population over a specified period. Incident cases during the study period would be included in the cumulative incidence measure, but not in the point prevalence.

Data dredging Analysis of large data sets with modern computer techniques, permitting the assessment of hundreds of possible associations among the study variables. Unless alpha is adjusted, the testing of multiple hypotheses raises the risk of false-positive error.

Decision analysis Type of analysis intended to improve clinical decision making under conditions of uncertainty.

Deductible Out-of-pocket payments made by the patient, often at the beginning of the care process. Deductibles discourage the use of medical insurance for "unimportant" problems and reduce the amount of paperwork for the insurance companies.

Deductive reasoning Reasoning that proceeds from the general (assumptions, propositions, and formulas considered true) to the specific (specific members belonging to general category).

Degrees of freedom Number of observations in a data set free to vary when the parameters of the data set (e.g., mean) have been established.

Denominator data Data that define the population at risk.

Diabetes mellitus Impairment in glucose metabolism that results from a deficiency of insulin production (type 1) or from insulin resistance (type 2) or both. Hyperglycemia is the principal expression of the metabolic derangements associated with diabetes.

Diagnosis-related group (DRG) Part of a prospective payment system. A DRG may consist of a single diagnosis or procedure or several diagnoses or procedures that, on average, have similar hospital costs per admission. Hospitals are paid the same amount of money per DRG, independent of the actual costs incurred.

Dichotomous variables Variables with only two levels.

Diethylstilbestrol (DES) A synthetic estrogen once used to prevent preterm delivery. This use was discontinued in the 1970s when an association was recognized between use of DES in pregnant women, and increased risk of vaginal and cervical cancer in their female offspring.

Differential error Nonrandom, systematic, or consistent error in which the values tend to be inaccurate in a particular direction; *see also* **Bias.**

Dimensional variables *See* **Continuous variables.**

Diphtheria Acute and sometimes fatal infectious disease caused by *Corynebacterium diphtheriae* and acquired from a person who has the disease or is a disease carrier. Diphtheria usually involves the upper respiratory tract and is characterized by the formation of a pseudomembrane attached to the underlying tissue.

Direct causality Factor under consideration exerts its effect without intermediary factors.

Direct standardization Two populations to be compared are given the same age distribution. This distribution is applied to the observed age-specific death rates to determine the number of deaths that would have occurred in each of the two populations if they had been identical in age distribution.

Disability Social definition of limitation, based on the degree of impairment. The formal categories of disability

used in most states for reimbursement of workers who have job-related injuries or illnesses covered under a workers' compensation program are permanent total disability, permanent partial disability, temporary total disability, temporary partial disability, and death.

Disability-adjusted life years (DALYE) A measure of years of "healthy" life lost that combines years of life lost due to premature death with years of healthy life lost due to disability.

Disability limitation Medical and surgical measures aimed at controlling or correcting the anatomic and physiologic components of disease in symptomatic patients and preventing resultant limitations in functional ability.

Discounting Reduction in the present value of delayed benefits (or increase in present costs of benefits) to account for the time value of money.

Discrete variables Dichotomous variables and nominal variables are sometimes called discrete variables because the different categories are completely separate from each other.

Disease Medically definable process characterized by pathophysiology and pathology; *compare* **Illness.**

Dose-response relationship Exists when an increase in the intensity or duration of exposure increases the risk of an adverse outcome. The relationship is often shown in studies of chronic exposure (e.g., relationship between quantity of cigarette smoking and risk of lung cancer).

Double-blind study Study in which neither the subjects nor the investigators are aware of the treatment assignment (active agent or placebo) until the trial is terminated.

Drug abuse *See* **Chemical substance abuse.**

Dystress Harmful form of stress, the level of which must be low for an individual to have good health; opposite of *eustress.*

Early fetal death Delivery of a dead fetus during the first 20 weeks of gestation.

Ebola virus infection Virulent hemorrhagic disease with a high case fatality ratio.

Ecological fallacy Use of ecological data to draw inferences about causal relationships in individuals. If the frequency of an exposure and the frequency of an outcome are determined in the same population, but no information regarding the occurrence of exposure and outcome in the same individual is provided, the data cannot be construed to establish causality.

Effect modification Occurs when the strength (or even the direction) of the influence of a causal factor on outcome is altered by a third variable, the **effect modifier.**

Endemic disease Disease that is occurring regularly in a defined population.

Enzootic disease Disease that is occurring regularly in animal populations.

Eosinophilia-myalgia syndrome Syndrome of muscle pain and hypereosinophilia caused by a contaminant in one commercially prepared brand of the amino acid L-tryptophan.

Epidemic Occurrence of any disease at a frequency that is unusual (compared with baseline data) or unexpected.

Epidemic threshold Necessary degree of variation from usual patterns required for a disease to qualify as an outbreak.

Epidemiologic year Runs from the month of lowest incidence of a particular condition in one year to the same month in the next year.

Epidemiology Study of factors that influence the occurrence and distribution of disease in human populations.

Epizootic disease Disease outbreak in animals.

Error term Portion of variation in the dependent variable that is not explained by the statistical model; term needed to make an equation true if the prediction is not perfect.

Eustress Helpful form of stress that must be present for an individual to have good health, such as moderate exercise or early childhood stimulation; opposite of *dystress.*

Evidence-based medicine (EBM) The practice of clinical medicine informed by and consistent with the best available research evidence.

Evidence-based practice center (EPC) Centers funded by the Agency for Health Care Research and Quality (AHRQ) and devoted to the generation of reports and assessments to inform clinical practice and health care delivery.

External validity Present when the results of a study are true and meaningful for a larger population and not just for the study participants; same as *generalizability.*

***F*-test** Test of statistical significance used with ANOVA. The **F ratio** is the test statistic or *critical ratio,* the ratio of between-groups variance to within-groups variance.

Failure mode and effects analysis (FMEA) A systematic, proactive method for evaluating a process to identify where and how it might fail, and to assess the relative impact of different failures in order to identify the parts of the process that are most in need of change.

False-negative error *See* **Type II error.**

False-positive error *See* **Type I error.**

Fee-for-service Method of payment in which physicians are paid for each major item of service provided.

Fetal death Delivery of a dead fetus at any time during gestation.

Fisher exact probability test Statistical significance test that is used to analyze data in 2×2 contingency tables in which one or more of the expected counts are too small to satisfy conditions for the use of chi-square analysis.

Frequency distribution Plot of data displaying the value of each data point on one axis and the frequency with which that value occurs on the other axis.

General linear model General model depicting the linear (first-order) relationship between multiple independent variables and one dependent (outcome) variable. ANOVA, ANCOVA, multiple linear regression, and other multivariable techniques are variations of this basic model.

General well-being adjustment scale A validated survey instrument for measuring overall health status, useful in assessing side effects of pharmacotherapy in clinical trials.

German measles *See* **Rubella.**

Ghon complex Characteristic abnormality seen on chest x-ray after resolution of initial infection with *Mycobacterium tuberculosis.*

Gonorrhea Various clinical manifestations of infection with the sexually transmitted pathogen *Neisseria gonorrhoeae.*

Goodness-of-fit test General term used to describe the statistical comparison of actual data with the results predicted by a statistical model, such as the observed and expected counts generated by the use of chi-square analysis.

Granuloma Collection of inflammatory cells in a nodular formation that isolates the inflammatory agent (e.g., pathogen) within the complex.

Groundwater Water that is found in underground spaces called **aquifers.** When adequately protected from surface pollutants, aquifers represent an important source of potable water.

Group model HMO A health maintenance organization that does not directly hire medical staff as in a staff model HMO, but establishes contracts with clinicians in existing, multispecialty practices.

Haddon matrix A matrix of factors, and phases, developed by William Haddon in 1970, used to assess contributors to injury occurrence and severity in an effort to identify elements that can be modified for most effective injury prevention.

Hantavirus pulmonary syndrome Life-threatening syndrome characterized by respiratory distress and caused by infection with particular serotypes of hantavirus.

Health "A state of complete physical, mental, and social well-being and not merely the absence of disease or infirmity" (World Health Organization). Health is a difficult term to define, and some emphasize the importance of the ability to adapt to environmental stressors and the ability to function in society as important dimensions of health.

Health belief model Before seeking preventive measures, people generally must believe that the disease at issue is serious, if acquired; that they or their children are personally at risk for the disease; that the preventive measure is effective in warding off the disease; and that there are no serious risks or barriers involved in obtaining the preventive measure. Cues to action, consisting of information regarding how and when to obtain the preventive measure, are also needed, as well as encouragement and support of other people.

Health maintenance organization (HMO) Prepaid group practices that must include (1) a legal and fiscal entity that does the contracting and financial transactions and seeks to control the costs of medical care and either provides or arranges for (2) a group of physicians who provide the outpatient and inpatient medical care and (3) an associated hospital or hospitals.

Health risk assessments (HRAs) Use of questionnaires or computer programs to elicit and evaluate information concerning individuals in a clinical or industrial medical practice. Each assessed person receives information concerning estimates of life expectancy and the types of interventions likely to promote health or longevity.

Healthcare Effectiveness Data and Information Set (HEDIS) National data set of information about the performance of selected services by each managed care organization. HEDIS emphasizes data on preventive services.

Healthy worker effect Because people with jobs must be in reasonably good health to remain employed, their risk of death and illness is lower than that of the population as a whole. A carrier that insures a group of workers benefits from this effect.

Hepatitis Nonspecific term referring to inflammation of the liver. Common causes include viruses and toxins, especially excess alcohol consumption.

Herd immunity Immunity that results when a vaccine not only prevents the vaccinated person from contracting the disease, but also prevents the person from spreading the disease and protects even the unimmunized persons in the population.

Heritability Proportion of a disease's prevalence caused by genetic predisposition.

Herpes zoster Painful dermatomal rash that results from the reactivation of latent varicella-zoster virus, often many years after a case of chickenpox. Herpes zoster is also called *shingles.*

Homoscedasticity Homogeneity of variance across all independent-variable levels.

Hospice Skilled nursing facility that specializes in providing terminal care, especially for patients with cancer or AIDS.

Human immunodeficiency virus (HIV) Retrovirus that has a particular trophism for CD4 helper cells and is the infectious agent responsible for AIDS.

Hyperlipidemia Level of circulating lipoprotein particles or total cholesterol that exceeds the established reference range for a given population.

Hypersensitivity pneumonitis Pulmonary inflammation resulting from an allergic response to an inspired antigen.

Hypertension Usually defined as an average systolic blood pressure of 140 mm Hg or greater or an average diastolic blood pressure of 90 mm Hg or greater in an otherwise healthy person.

Iatrogenic Referring to diseases and injuries generated during the treatment process.

Iceberg phenomenon Earliest identified cases of a new disease are often fatal or severe (representing "tip of the iceberg"); however, as more becomes known about the disease, less severe cases and asymptomatic cases are usually discovered.

Illness What the patient experiences when he or she is sick; compare **Disease.**

Immunodeficiency Deficiency of the immune system, which may be long-term (as in AIDS) or may be transient (lasting for a short period after, e.g., infection or administration of chemotherapy).

Impairment Limitation of capacity or functional ability, usually as determined by a licensed physician.

Inactivated (Salk) polio vaccine (IVP) Injectable vaccine that provides individual humoral immunity to poliomyelitis, but is less effective at interrupting transmission than is the live attenuated vaccine.

Incidence Frequency (number) of new occurrences of disease, injury, or death in the study population during the period being examined.

Incidence density Frequency (density) of new events per person-time. Incidence density is especially useful in studying the frequency rates of diseases or events that occur more than once for an individual, such as otitis media, colds, or hospital admissions.

Incidence density measures Measures of the frequency of adverse health events that are used when the event of interest can occur more than once in the study period.

Incidence rate Number of incident cases over a defined study period, divided by the population at risk at the midpoint of that study period.

Independent practice association (IPA) Form of HMO. Patients enrolled in an IPA can choose a primary care physician from a list of physicians who have contracted to provide services for the IPA. The IPA pays an individual physician on a fee-for-service basis whenever a member uses that physician's services. The IPA physicians limit their fees to the rates specified in the contract and agree to certain quality review and practice controls often similar to those of managed care.

Index case The case (patient or other carrier) in whom the condition under investigation was first identified.

Indirect causality One factor influences one or more other factors that are directly causal.

Indirect standardization Used if age-specific death rates are unavailable in the study population, or if the study population is small and would yield age-specific death rates that would be statistically unstable. Death rates from the standard population are applied to the known age distribution of the study groups.

Individual practice association *See* **Independent practice association.**

Inductive reasoning Reasoning that proceeds from the specific (i.e., from data) to the general (i.e., to formulas or conclusions).

Infant death Death of a live-born child before that child's first birthday.

Infectiousness Measure of an organism's ability to infect, calculated as the proportion of exposed persons who become infected, although also influenced by the conditions of exposure and the immune status of the exposed person.

Influenza Infection of the upper respiratory tract by an influenza virus, resulting in an illness generally characterized by fever, sore throat, dry cough, and severe myalgia.

Interaction *See* **Effect modification.**

Intermediate care facility (ICF) Facility that is suitable if the patient's primary need is for help with the activities of daily living. An ICF is not required to have a registered (skilled) nurse on duty at all times.

Intermediate fetal death Delivery of a dead fetus between 20 and 28 weeks of gestation.

Intermediate hospital Medium to large community hospital that has a considerable amount of the latest technology, but less research and investigational activity than a tertiary medical center.

Internal validity Present when the results of a study are true and meaningful for the participants.

Interobserver variability Measure of disagreement between or among different observers.

Intervening variables Intermediary factors involved in indirect causality.

Interview survey Type of cross-sectional survey.

Intraobserver variability Measure of inconsistency in repeated assessments by a single observer.

Kaplan-Meier method Most frequently used approach to survival analysis in medicine. The Kaplan-Meier method of life table analysis is different from the actuarial method in that the occurrence of each death defines the end of one observation period and the beginning of the next. With this method, the duration of observation periods for which survival is determined varies throughout. *See also* **Life table analysis.**

Kappa test Measure of the extent to which agreement between two observers improves on chance agreement.

Kendall rank correlation test Nonparametric significance test of correlation used for ordinal data.

Kruskal-Wallis one-way ANOVA Nonparametric significance test used to compare three or more groups of ordinal data, analogous to the one-way ANOVA used for three or more groups of continuous data.

Kurtosis Vertical distortion of a frequency distribution.

Kwashiorkor Nutritional disease that tends to occur in children at weaning, when starchy foods replace breast milk, and there is protein deficiency despite nearly adequate calorie intake. The development of **ascites** (fluid in abdominal cavity) produces a distended abdomen, which suggests obesity, but is actually caused by severe undernutrition. Kwashiorkor also is called *visceral protein malnutrition.*

Late fetal death Death of a product of conception after 28 weeks of gestation but before birth; also called *stillbirth.*

Late-look bias Bias that occurs when mild, slowly progressive cases of a disease are preferentially detected in a survey because patients with this form of the disease live longer and can be interviewed, whereas more severe cases result in death and go undetected by the survey.

Lead-time bias Bias that occurs when screening detects disease earlier in its natural history than would otherwise have happened, so that the time from diagnosis to death is lengthened. Having additional lead time does not necessarily alter the natural history of the disease and may not indicate longer life.

Leavell's levels Three levels of preventive health care (primary, secondary, tertiary) based on the premise that all the activities of physicians and other health professionals have the goal of prevention, the focus of which depends on the stage of health or disease in the individual receiving preventive care.

Length bias Bias that occurs when milder, more indolent cases of disease are detected disproportionately in population screening programs, while more aggressive cases have already resulted in death or in symptoms requiring medical intervention; *see also* **Late-look bias.**

Life expectancy Traditionally defined as the average number of years of life remaining at a given age.

Life table analysis Statistical analysis of survival (or another dichotomous outcome) in which proportionate survival is assessed repeatedly over the intervals of observation. This shows the pattern of mortality over time and the rates of death and survival. *See also* **Actuarial method** and **Kaplan-Meier method,** the two methods of life table analysis in common use.

Likelihood ratio negative Ratio of the false-negative error rate of a test to the specificity of the test.

Likelihood ratio positive Ratio of the sensitivity of a test to the false-positive error rate of the test.

Linear regression analysis Statistical test of the strength of the linear relationship between one independent and one dependent variable, both of which must be continuous.

Live attenuated vaccines Created by altering infectious organisms so that they are no longer pathogenic but are still viable and antigenic.

Live birth Delivery of a product of conception that shows any sign of life after complete removal from the mother.

Local community hospital Hospital that provides services such as routine diagnosis, treatment, and surgery, but lacks the personnel and facilities for complex procedures.

Lockjaw *See* **Tetanus.**

Logrank test Test of statistical significance used to compare different rates of survival as determined by Kaplan-Meier life table analysis.

Longitudinal ecological studies Use of ongoing surveillance or frequent cross-sectional studies to measure trends in disease rates over years in a defined population.

Lyme disease Complex disease that affects multiple body systems and results from exposure to the tick-borne pathogen *Borrelia burgdorferi.*

Malaria Febrile illness caused by infection with a mosquito-borne protozoan of the genus *Plasmodium.* Plasmodia are obligate intracellular parasites.

Managed care System of administrative controls, the primary goal of which is to reduce the costs of medical care.

Mann-Whitney *U* test Nonparametric significance test used to compare two groups of ordinal data, analogous to Student's *t*-test for continuous data.

Marasmus Severe wasting syndrome in infants that results from malnutrition. It occurs when all nutrients in the diet are deficient, causing almost total growth retardation, and is usually caused by famine or failure of the mother's breast milk.

McNemar chi-square test Modification of the chi-square test for use with paired data; formula is $(|b - c| - 1)^2/(b + c)$.

Mean The average value, calculated as the sum of all the observed values divided by the total number of observations.

Mean deviation Average of the absolute values of the deviations of all observations from the mean.

Mean square Another name for variance, defined as a sum of squares divided by the appropriate number of degrees of freedom. Mean square in mainly used in analysis of variance (ANOVA).

Measles Highly contagious infection caused by a paramyxovirus and characterized by a maculopapular rash. Measles is effectively prevented by vaccination.

Measurement bias Bias resulting in distorted quantification of exposures or outcomes because of improper technique or subjectivity of the measurement scale.

Median Middle observation when data have been arranged in order from the lowest to the highest value.

Medicaid Program funded by general tax revenues of the federal and state governments. The benefits are considered to be social welfare, instead of social insurance.

Medical commons Shared medical resources. An attempt by one individual or group to maximize its own welfare by using more than its fair share would diminish the good that others can derive from the medical commons.

Medically indigent persons People whose incomes are too high to be eligible for Medicaid, who do not receive medical insurance in their jobs, and who are unable to pay for individual medical care insurance policies.

Medicare Federally administered program that pays for the health benefits of most persons 65 or older and those who receive Social Security disability benefits.

Meningitis Inflammation of the **meninges,** the sheaths of connective tissue surrounding the brain and spinal cord.

Meta-analysis Used increasingly in medicine to try to obtain a pooled quantitative or qualitative (methodologic) analysis of the research literature on a particular subject.

Metal fumes Gaseous metal oxides that come primarily from activities in occupational settings, such as welding without adequate ventilation.

Metal fume fever Acute syndrome that is usually characterized by flulike symptoms occurring a few hours after exposure to fumes from metalworking.

Miscarriage *See* **Early fetal death.**

Mode Most frequently observed value in a distribution (i.e., value with highest number of observations).

Moral hazard Patients who have health insurance are likely to use more medical care than uninsured patients.

Multidrug-resistant tuberculosis (MDRTB) Increasingly common type of tuberculosis that is resistant to more than one antimicrobial agent as a result of the failure of patients to complete the prescribed course of treatment with antituberculous drugs.

Multiple linear regression Method used in multivariable analysis if the dependent variable and all the independent variables are continuous.

Multivariable analysis Analysis of the relationship of more than one independent variable to a single dependent variable.

Multivariable models Statistical models that have one dependent (outcome) variable but include more than one independent variable.

Multivariate analysis Frequently used incorrectly; refers to methods for analyzing more than one dependent variable and more than one independent variable.

Mumps Infectious disease caused by a paramyxovirus. Mumps occurs most frequently during childhood, is characterized by **parotitis** (painful swelling of parotid glands), and is effectively prevented by vaccination.

Myocardial infarction Necrosis of the heart muscle as a result of protracted ischemia.

N-way ANOVA *See* **Analysis of variance.**

Natural booster phenomenon Augmentation of immunity that occurs with periodic exposure to an infectious agent. This effect may be lost when immunization prevents exposure.

Necessary cause Precedes a disease and has the following relationship with it: if the cause is absent, the disease cannot occur; if the cause is present, the disease may or may not occur.

Negative predictive value The proportion of subjects with negative test results who are truly free of the disease.

Network model HMO An expanded version of the Group Model HMO in which service is provided at multiple sites covering a larger geographical area.

Neyman bias *See* **Late-look bias.**

Nominal variables "Naming" or categorical variables that have no measurement scale.

Noncausal association The relationship between two variables is statistically significant, but no causal relationship exists, either because the temporal relationship is incorrect (presumed cause comes after, rather than before, presumed effect) or because another factor is responsible for the presumed cause and the presumed effect.

Nondifferential error Produces findings that are too high and too low in approximately equal amounts because of random factors.

Nonparametric data Data for which descriptive parameters such as the mean and standard deviation cannot be obtained because there is no measurement scale. No assumption is made about the underlying frequency distribution.

Nosocomial infections Hospital-acquired infections, which are more common than is often supposed.

Null hypothesis The hypothesis that no real (true) difference exists between means or proportions of the groups being compared, or that there is no real association between two continuous variables. *Compare* **Alternative hypothesis.**

Number needed to harm (NNH) The number of patients who would need to be treated, on average, for one of them to experience the adverse effects of a particular type of treatment. NNH is based on the absolute risk increase (ARI). If the risk of harm is 0.02 without the treatment and 0.05 with the treatment, the ARI = 0.03. The NNH is calculated as 1/ARI. In this example, it would be 1/0.03 = 33.3.

Number needed to treat (NNT) The number of patients who would need to be treated, on average, for one of them to experience the beneficial effects of a particular type of treatment. NNT is based on the absolute risk reduction (ARR). If the risk of benefit is 0.10 with the treatment and 0.04 without the treatment, the ARR = 0.06. The NNT is calculated as 1/ARR. In this example, it would be 1/0.06 = 16.7.

Numerator data Data that define the events or conditions of concern.

Nursing home *See* **Skilled nursing facility.**

Occupational asthma Bronchospastic disease with symptoms occurring during periods of exposure to respiratory tract irritants in the workplace and usually less pronounced during periods away from work, such as weekends.

Odds ratio (OR) The odds of exposure in the diseased group divided by the odds of exposure in the nondiseased group.

One-way ANOVA *See* **Analysis of variance.**

Oral polio vaccine (OPV) (Sabin) Vaccine that provides herd immunity to poliomyelitis and has resulted in the apparent eradication of wild virus from the Western Hemisphere. The oral vaccine is made from live virus and has produced clinical illness under certain circumstances.

Ordinal variables Medical data that can be characterized in terms of more than two values and have a clearly implied direction from better to worse, but are not measured on a continuous measurement scale.

Outbreak Often used to denote a local epidemic (may be considered interchangeable with the term *epidemic*).

Outliers Extreme values that are widely divergent from the mean (usually defined as at least three standard deviations from the mean).

Overall percent agreement Percentage of the total observations found in cells *a* and *d* of a 2×2 table.

***p* value** Probability that the observed difference could have been obtained by chance alone, given random variation and a single test of the null hypothesis.

Parametric data Data for which descriptive parameters (typically the mean and standard deviation) are known and define the underlying frequency distribution of the data. The underlying distribution is often assumed to be normal, as provided in the *central limit theorem*.

Particulate matter Small, solid particles dispersed in air, such as the matter that results from cigarette smoking or fuel combustion, which often contains carcinogenic substances.

Passive immunity Protection against an infectious disease provided by circulating antibodies made in another organism.

Passive surveillance Reporting of disease by physicians, laboratories, and hospitals on a voluntary basis.

Pathogenicity Ability of an organism to produce disease, calculated as the proportion of infected individuals who are clinically ill.

Pathognomonic test If positive, the results of this test are synonymous with having the disease.

Pathological gambling An inability to resist the impulse to gamble, despite potentially severe personal and/or social consequences.

Patient-centered medical home A health care delivery model in which the patient, family, and health care providers communicate by various means, including the Internet, so care is provided to the patient at home rather than only at encounters in health care settings. There is an emphasis on health maintenance, preventive care, cultural sensitivity, and patient-centeredness.

Pearson correlation coefficient Measure of strength of the linear relationship between two continuous variables.

Peptic ulcer disease Disease associated with hypersecretion of gastric acid and characterized by erosions of the stomach or duodenum; often caused by the bacterium *Helicobacter pylori*.

Period prevalence Number of persons who had the disease of interest at any time during the specified interval. It is the sum of the point prevalence at the beginning of the interval plus the incidence during the interval.

Person-time Unit of time used in studies during which persons are observed for unequal periods. For example, when one person is observed for 3 months, another for 14 months, and another for 7 months, the amount of time can be expressed as 24 person-months or 2 person-years.

Person-time methods of analysis Methods that control for the varying length of observation of persons in a study. These methods are used in calculating *incidence density*.

Pertussis Acute, highly contagious respiratory tract infection characterized by paroxysmal coughing and caused by the bacterium *Bordetella pertussis;* also called **whooping cough**.

Pneumococcal infection Infection caused by *Streptococcus pneumoniae;* this bacterium is a common cause of community-acquired pneumonia.

Pneumoconiosis Pulmonary injury caused by deposition of respirable particulate matter in the lungs and by the resulting inflammatory response.

Point prevalence Number of cases in the study population at one point in time.

Poliomyelitis Febrile viral disease that results in paralysis in severe cases. Polio is preventable by vaccination and is targeted for eradication by the World Health Organization.

Population attributable risk (PAR) The risk in the total population minus the risk in the unexposed group. PAR answers the question, Among the general population, how much of the total risk for the disease of interest is caused by the risk factor (exposure) of interest?

Population attributable risk percent (PAR%) Answers the question, Among the general population, what percentage of the total risk for the disease of interest is caused by the risk factor (exposure) of interest?

Positive predictive value The proportion of subjects with positive test results who actually have the disease.

Posterior probability Revised estimate of the probability of disease in a given patient after a diagnostic test or intervention.

Potable water Water that is safe to drink and to use for cooking.

Precision Ability of an instrument to provide the same or a very similar result with repeated measurements of the same factor.

Prediction model A statistical model, complete with coefficients, for use in predicting a particular outcome given the presence of a variety of independent variables.

Preferred provider organization (PPO) Formed when a third-party payer (e.g., insurance plan or company) establishes a network of contracts with independent practitioners. The patients in a PPO can see practitioners who are not members of the network, although they have to pay a surcharge for their services.

Prevalence Number of persons in a defined population who have a specified disease or condition at a point in time, usually the time a survey is done.

Prevalence rate Proportion of persons with a defined disease or condition at the time they are studied. This is not truly a "rate," although conventionally labeled as such.

Preventive medicine Medical specialty emphasizing practices that help individuals and populations promote and preserve health and avoid injury and illness.

Prior probability Probability of disease in a given patient that is estimated before the performance of laboratory or other tests and based on the estimated prevalence of a particular disease among patients with similar signs and symptoms.

Product-limit method *See* **Kaplan-Meier method.**

Prognostic stratification *See* **Stratified allocation.**

Propensity matching Typically used in observational cohort studies in which there are preexisting demographic and clinical differences between the people who received some treatment and those who did not, because the treatment was not randomized. A person who received treatment can be matched with a person who did not on the basis of a **propensity score**, which is based on multivariable analysis. This analysis seeks to make the treated and untreated groups comparable, as though they had been randomized.

Proportional hazards method Method used to test for differences between Kaplan-Meier survival curves while controlling for other variables. The method also is used to determine which variables are associated with better survival; also called *Cox method.*

Proportional hazards model Modification of multiple logistic regression to permit multivariable modeling of the data in a life table analysis; also called *Cox model.*

Prospective cohort study Investigator assembles the study groups in the present time on the basis of exposure, collects baseline data on them, and follows subjects over time for the outcomes of interest.

Prospective payment system (PPS) Based on diagnosis-related groups (DRGs). Each hospital admission is classified into one of the major diagnostic categories based on organ systems, which are subdivided further into DRGs. A DRG may consist of a single diagnosis or procedure or several diagnoses or procedures that, on average, have similar hospital costs per admission.

Public health (1) The health status of the public (i.e., of a defined population). (2) The organized social efforts made to preserve and improve the health of a defined population.

Publication bias Reluctance to publish papers reporting negative results; introducing potential distortion into the literature due to preferential publication of positive findings.

Qualitative characteristic Characteristic that must be described in detail, but cannot be quantified.

Quantitative characteristic Characteristic that can be described by a rigid, dimensional measurement scale.

Quality-adjusted life years (QALY) Health status index that incorporates life expectancy and the perceived impact of illness and disability on the quality of life.

Rabies Highly virulent viral infection of the central nervous system, spread to humans from infected animals and usually preventable by postexposure prophylaxis.

Random error Produces findings that are too high and too low in approximately equal amounts, because of random factors.

Random sampling Entails *selecting* a small group for study from a much larger group of potential study subjects by the use of one of several possible random methods.

Randomization Entails *allocating* the available subjects to one or another study group using a random method; generally used in clinical studies of treatment or prevention methods.

Randomized controlled clinical trials (RCCTs, RCTs) Studies designed to test a therapeutic measure. Subjects are randomly assigned to one of the following groups: (1) the intervention group, which receives the experimental treatment, or (2) the control group, which receives the nonexperimental treatment, consisting of either a placebo (inert substance) or a standard method of treatment.

Randomized controlled field trials (RCFTs) Studies that are similar to RCCTs, but are designed to test a preventive measure, such as a vaccine. Susceptible persons in the population are randomized into two groups and are given the vaccine or a placebo, usually at the beginning of the high-risk season of the year. Testing the efficacy of vaccines by RCFTs is costly, but it may be required the first time a new vaccine is introduced.

Ranked variables *See* **Ordinal variables.**

Rank-order test Statistical analysis based on the ordinal distribution of observations rather than their absolute values.

Rapid sand filtration Technique for purifying water by adding a flocculent (usually aluminum sulfate, called alum) to the water before filtration. The flocculent coagulates and traps suspended materials, preventing them from passing through the sand with the filtered water. The flocculent is removed periodically by backflushing, and new flocculent is added to the next batch of water.

Rate Frequency (number) of events that occur in a defined time, divided by the average population at risk.

Rate difference Similar to *risk difference,* but applied to rates.

Ratio variables Variables derived from a continuous scale that has a true 0 point.

Recall bias Bias resulting from differential recall of exposure to causal factors among those who have a disease compared with those who do not.

Regression toward mean Patients chosen to participate in a study precisely because they had an extreme measurement on some variable are likely to have a measurement that is closer to average at a later time for reasons unrelated to the type or efficacy of the treatment they are given. Regression toward the mean also is known as the *statistical regression effect.*

Rehabilitation Attempt to mitigate the effects of disease by preventing or limiting social and functional disability.

Relative risk (RR) Ratio of the risk in the exposed group to the risk in the unexposed group; expressed as $RR = Risk_{(exposed)} / Risk_{(unexposed)} = [a/(a + b)] / [c/(c + d)]$.

Resource-based relative value scale (RBRVS) Method of rating the relative value of outpatient diagnosis and treatment, based on the average time that the caregiver (physician or other practitioner) spends with the patient, the years of training and skill required by the caregiver, and the cost of the equipment needed. The RBRVS was created to reimburse primary care practitioners more fairly in a reimbursement system that tended to pay more for procedures than for clinical time and judgment.

Retrospective cohort study Cohorts are identified on the basis of *past* exposure and followed forward to the present for the occurrence of the outcome of interest.

Rheumatic fever Immune-mediated inflammatory condition that occurs after streptococcal infection and can result in permanent damage to the kidneys and heart valves.

Risk Calculated as the proportion of persons who are unaffected at the beginning of a study period, but who undergo the risk event during the study period.

Risk difference Risk in the exposed group minus the risk in the unexposed group.

Risk event Occurrence of a death, an injury, or a new case of disease.

Risk factor Characteristic that, if present and active, increases the probability of a particular disease in a group of persons who have the factor compared with an otherwise similar group of persons who do not. A risk factor is neither a necessary cause nor a sufficient cause of the disease.

Risk ratio *See* **Relative risk.**

Root cause analysis (RCA) A structured error analysis method, widely used in health care, designed to identify active and latent errors that can cause adverse outcomes.

Rubella Acute respiratory tract infection caused by a togavirus. Although usually benign and self-limited, the infection can cause death or severe injury to an embryo if maternal infection occurs during the first trimester. Rubella is prevented by vaccination; also known as *German measles.*

Screening Process of identifying a subgroup of people with a high probability of having asymptomatic disease or who have a risk factor that puts them at high risk for developing a disease or becoming injured. Screening occurs in a community setting and is applied to a community population, such as students in a school or workers in an industry. Compare **Case finding.**

Selection bias Bias resulting when the allocation of individuals to a study or to a particular study group is influenced by individual characteristics that also influence the probability of the outcome.

Sensitivity Ability of a test to detect a disease when it is present.

Sentinel health event Adverse health event (death, disease, or impairment) that serves to identify a potential threat to the public health.

Severe acute respiratory syndrome (SARS) Often fatal respiratory syndrome caused by a coronavirus, SARS resulted in a worldwide outbreak; apparently initially acquired by humans in close contact with certain animals in Southeast Asia.

Shingles *See* **Herpes zoster.**

Sick building syndrome Group of workers may have a constellation of symptoms (e.g., headache, watery eyes, wheezing) ascribed to their work environment. The syndrome often, but not always, occurs in buildings that are tightly sealed for energy conservation or are not well ventilated. The specific cause of the symptoms seems to vary from one building to the next, but usually is unknown.

Sign of life A breath, a cry, a pulse, a pulsation of the umbilical cord, or any spontaneous movement at the time of birth.

Sign test Nonparametric significance test for use with continuous, ordinal, or dichotomous data. The sign test is used to determine whether or not, on average, one group experienced a better outcome on significantly more variables than a comparison group.

Silicosis Type of pneumoconiosis that results from inhalation of the dust of stones or sand containing silicon dioxide. *See* **Pneumoconiosis.**

Skewness Horizontal distortion of a frequency distribution, so that one tail of the plot is longer and contains more observations than the other.

Skilled nursing facility (SNF) Usually provides specialized care, such as intravenous fluids and medicines. A registered (skilled) nurse must be on duty at all times.

Sleeping sickness Form of trypanosomiasis endemic in parts of Africa, spread by the bite of the tsetse fly.

Slow sand filtration Technique for purifying water by filtering it through a large bed of packed sand, on which an organic layer (the *Schmutzdecke,* German for "dirt cover") forms and assists in the filtration process.

Smallpox Acute infectious disease characterized by distinctive skin eruptions. Smallpox has now been eradicated worldwide as a result of successful vaccination.

Spearman rank correlation test Analogous to **Pearson correlation coefficient** but used for ranked data.

Specific rates Rates that pertain to some homogeneous subgroup of the population, such as an age group, gender group, or ethnic group.

Specificity Ability of a test to indicate nondisease when no disease is present.

Staff model health maintenance organization Most physicians in a staff model HMO are salaried, full-time employees who work exclusively for the HMO or belong to a physician group that contracts to provide all of the medical services to the HMO. Some specialists may be retained on part-time contracts. The HMO may have its own hospitals or may hospitalize its patients in one or more local hospitals, in which case the local hospitals are not usually a formal part of the HMO. Other types are network model and group model HMOs.

Standard deviation (SD) Square root of the variance.

Standard error (SE) Standard deviation (SD) of a population of sample means, rather than of individual observations. The SE is calculated as the observed SD divided by the square root of N.

Standard error of difference between means (SED) Square root of the sum of the respective population variances, each divided by its own sample size.

Standardized mortality ratio (SMR) Observed total events in the study group, divided by the expected number of events based on the standard population rates applied to the study group. The constant multiplier for this measure is 100.

Standardized rates Crude rates that have been modified to allow for valid comparisons of rates. Standardization is usually necessary to correct for differing age distributions in different populations. *See* **Direct standardization** and **Indirect standardization.**

Statistical regression effect *See* **Regression toward mean.**

Statistical significance Result is statistically significant whenever a significance test produces a p value less than the preset value of alpha, which is conventionally 0.05. The implication of statistical significance at an alpha of 0.05 is that chance would produce such a difference between comparison groups no more often than 5 times in 100. This is taken to mean that chance is not responsible for the outcome.

Stillbirth *See* **Late fetal death.**

Stratified allocation Assignment of patients to different risk groups on the basis of variables such as the severity of disease (e.g., stage of cancer) and age.

Strength of association Degree to which variation in one variable explains variation in another. The greater the strength of association between variables, the more completely variation in one predicts variation in the other.

Strep throat Infection of the oropharynx by group A beta-hemolytic streptococci *(Streptococcus pyogenes).*

Sufficient cause Precedes a disease and has the following relationship with it: if the cause is present, the disease always occurs.

Surface water Surface sources of potable water, including protected surface reservoirs, lakes, and rivers.

Surveillance *See* **Active surveillance** and **Passive surveillance.**

Synergy Present when the combined impact of two or more factors on an individual or population is greater than the sum of the separate effects of each factor.

Syphilis Sexually transmitted infectious disease caused by the spirochete *Treponema pallidum.* The disease is most communicable in its early stages. Early treatment with penicillin prevents disease progression to late stages, but consequently permits reinfection. Reinfection may lead to greater rates of transmission if the highly infectious early stages of the disease occur repeatedly in the same individual.

t-**test** Test that compares differences between two means.

Tertiary medical center Hospital that has most or all of the latest technology and usually participates actively in medical education and even in clinical research.

Tetanus Acute infection with the bacterium *Clostridium tetani.* The bacterium produces a neurotoxin that can cause severe muscle spasm and paralysis. Tetanus is also known as *lockjaw.*

Threshold level Level below which the body can adapt to an adverse exposure successfully with little or no harm resulting. Such a threshold level exists for most chemical and physical agents and even for most microbes. Usually, *nonthreshold* exposures are limited to those that alter genetic material, producing genetic mutations and potentially causing cancer. Ionizing radiation is currently considered a nonthreshold exposure.

Total variation Equal to the sum of the squared deviations from the mean; usually called the total sum of squares (TSS) but also simply the sum of squares (SS).

Toxoids Inactivated or altered bacterial exotoxins, such as diphtheria vaccine and tetanus vaccine.

Trypanosomiasis Infection with protozoa of the genus *Trypanosoma.*

Tuberculosis Diverse clinical manifestations resulting from infection with *Mycobacterium tuberculosis.*

Type I error Error that occurs when data lead one to conclude that something is true when it is not true. Type I error also is called *alpha error* and *false-positive error.*

Type II error Error that occurs when data lead one to conclude that something is false when it is true. Type II error also is called *beta error* and *false-negative error.*

Typhoid Acute febrile illness caused by ingestion of food contaminated with *Salmonella typhi.* Typhoid is also known as *typhoid fever.*

Unit of observation Source of data in a medical study. The *unit* is usually a study participant.

Utilization management Component of managed care.

Validity *See* **External validity** and **Internal validity.**

Variable Measure of a single characteristic.

Variance For a sample, this is the sum of the squared deviations from the mean, divided by the number of observations minus 1.

Varicella *See* **Chickenpox.**

Vector Factor in disease transmission, often an insect that carries the agent to the host.

Visceral protein malnutrition *See* **Kwashiorkor.**

Whooping cough *See* **Pertussis.**

Wilcoxon matched-pairs signed-ranks test Nonparametric significance test used to compare paired, ordinal data, analogous to the paired *t*-test for continuous data.

Within-groups mean square *See* **Within-groups variance.**

Within-groups variance Measurement based on the variation within each group (i.e., variation around a single group mean).

Workers' compensation Based on laws stipulating that people with a job-related injury or illness have their medical and rehabilitation expenses paid and receive a certain amount of cash payments as wages while they are recuperating. The expenses are paid by the company, which usually is freed from further liability, unless the injury or illness was caused by the company breaking some federal or state occupational or environmental law.

Yates correction for continuity Adjustment to the chi-square value sometimes recommended when counts in the contingency table are small, because the binomial distribution is discontinuous.

Yellow fever Acute, often fatal, mosquito-borne infectious disease caused by a flavivirus. The clinical manifestations vary.

z-test Significance test based on the normal distribution and used to compare differences between proportions.

Index

Page numbers followed by f refer to figures; t, tables; and b, boxes.